Marcus Ang • Tien Y. Wong
Editors

Updates on Myopia

A Clinical Perspective

Editors
Marcus Ang
Singapore National Eye Center
Duke-NUS Medical School
National University of Singapore
Singapore

Tien Y. Wong
Singapore National Eye Center
Duke-NUS Medical School
National University of Singapore
Singapore

https://doi.org/10.1007/978-981-13-8491-2

Preface

Myopia is now being recognized as a significant global public health problem that will affect billions of people in the next decades, especially in Asia. Currently, pathologic myopia is already a major cause of visual impairment in both Asian and Western populations. As the prevalence of myopia and pathological myopia increases around the world, there is increasing need for active prevention of myopia progression and management of its potential complications.

The purpose of this book is to provide updates on current understanding of myopia, new methods of evaluation of the myopic eye, and a focus on clinical management of myopia and its complications. This book will provide a unique perspective from the current world experts on the subject, with a focus on clinical aspects of understanding, evaluation, and management of myopia.

Chapter 1 provides a concise summary of all the key points from the book for busy readers who want a quick overview on clinical myopia. The rest of the book is comprehensive and provides updates on almost all aspects with regard to myopia. Chapters 2 and 3 describe epidemiology and economic burden; Chaps. 4 and 5 discuss genetic and pathogenetic mechanisms; Chaps. 6 to 8 describe risk factors and ways to prevent myopia development or progression. Next, Chaps. 9 and 10 discuss pathological myopia and advances (and challenges) in imaging myopic eyes. Finally, Chaps. 11 to 14 provide clinical pearls of managing myopia complications, i.e., glaucoma, retina, and choroidal neovascularization in adults.

As new data is constantly emerging, this book was generated with the inputs of all authors within 6 months to ensure that the evidence shared is as current as possible. Thus, it is important to keep updated with online material and literature review. Nonetheless, we hope you will find this book as a useful reference for optometry students, ophthalmology residents, and eye care professionals to have a comprehensive update on myopia with a clinical perspective.

Singapore, Singapore — Marcus Ang
Singapore, Singapore — Tien Y. Wong

Acknowledgments

Singapore National Eye Centre, Singapore

Singapore Eye Research Institute, Singapore

Duke National University of Singapore (DUKE NUS), Singapore

Singapore National Eye Centre Myopia Centre, Singapore

Contents

About the Editors

Marcus Ang is consultant ophthalmologist at the Corneal and External Eye Disease Department of the Singapore National Eye Center (SNEC) and Duke-NUS Medical School, National University of Singapore, as well as Clinical Director of the SNEC Myopia Centre. His clinical and research areas of expertise include the treatment, and prevention of visual impairment in adult myopia. He also has special research interests in corneal transplantation, such as Descemet membrane endothelial keratoplasty (DMEK) and anterior segment imaging including novel optical coherence tomography systems for the cornea. Dr. Ang has published over 120 peer-reviewed articles journals, coauthored several book chapters on corneal transplantation, and received numerous international awards.

Tien Y. Wong is Arthur Lim Professor in Ophthalmology and Medical Director at the Singapore National Eye Center (SNEC). He is concurrently Academic Chair of Ophthalmology and Vice-Dean of Duke-NUS Medical School, National University of Singapore. Prior to his current appointments, Prof. Wong was Executive Director of the Singapore Eye Research Institute; Chairman of the Department of Ophthalmology, National University of Singapore; Chairman of the Department of Ophthalmology at the University of Melbourne; and Managing Director of the Centre for Eye Research Australia, Australia. Professor Wong is a retinal specialist, whose clinical practice focuses on major retinal diseases. His research covers epidemiological, clinical, and translational studies of eye diseases, including epidemiology and risk factors of myopia, imaging in myopic macular degeneration, and clinical trials on treatment of myopic choroidal neovascularization. He has published more than 1000 papers in peer-reviewed journals, including the *New England Journal of Medicine* and the *Lancet*. Prof. Wong has received a number of national and international awards.

Introduction and Overview on Myopia: A Clinical Perspective

1

Chee Wai Wong, Noel Brennan, and Marcus Ang

Key Points

- Myopia is a significant global public health and socioeconomic problem.
- Pathologic myopia has become a major cause of blindness or visual impairment in both Asian and Western populations.
- Myopia may be a highly heritable trait, with environmental influences such as outdoor activity playing important roles in its development and progression.
- Control of myopia in children is important, and various strategies including pharmacologic and lens-related interventions have proven efficacy.
- Imaging is important to detect complications of pathologic myopia, and both medical and surgical interventions may be useful for their management.

C. W. Wong · M. Ang (✉)
Singapore National Eye Centre, Singapore Eye Research Institute, Singapore, Singapore

Duke-NUS Medical School, Singapore, Singapore
e-mail: marcus.ang@snec.com.sg

N. Brennan
R&D, Johnson & Johnson Vision Care, Inc, Jacksonville, FL, USA

M. Ang, T. Y. Wong (eds.), *Updates on Myopia*,
https://doi.org/10.1007/978-981-13-8491-2_1

1.1 Global Epidemiology

Myopia has become a significant global public health and socioeconomic problem [1–4]. East Asia, and other parts of the world to a lesser extent, has been faced with an increasing prevalence of myopia [5, 6]. The prevalence of myopia and high myopia (HM) (the definition of myopia and HM is spherical equivalence (SE) of −0.50 diopters (D) or less and SE −5.00 D or −6.00 D, respectively) in young adults in urban areas of East Asian countries has risen to 80–90% and around 20%, respectively [7, 8]. According to a summary of 145 studies regarding the global prevalence of myopia and HM, there are approximately 1950 million with myopia (28.3% of the global population) and 277 million with HM (4.0% of the global population), and these numbers are predicted to increase to 4758 million (49.8% of the global population) for myopia, and 938 million (9.8% of the global population) for HM by 2050 [9].

The prevalence of childhood myopia is substantially higher in urban East Asian countries (49.7–62.0% among 12-year-old children) [7, 10] compared with other countries (6.0–20.0% among 12-year-old children) [9]. Similarly, in teenagers and young adults, the prevalence of myopia is higher in East Asian countries (65.5–96.5%) [8] compared with other countries (12.8–35.0%) [9]. However, the geographic difference of myopia prevalence in older populations is less than that in younger populations. The prevalence rates of myopia in adults in urban East Asian countries are only slightly higher than in Western countries.

The prevalence of myopia has remained consistently high among Chinese children in urban settings, but the evidence does not support the idea that it is caused by purely genetic difference [10]. The association of an urbanized setting with high myopia rates is likely to be influenced by possible modifiable risk factors such as near work and outdoor time.

Despite the relatively low prevalence in the general population, pathologic myopia (PM) is a major cause of blindness or visual impairment in both Asian and Western populations. One study has shown that the prevalence of PM was 28.7% among high myopes and 65% of those with HM and were over 70 years old had PM [11]. Based on the global prediction of HM on 2050, PM may increase to over 200 million in future [9]. Treatment strategies against PM have not been effective [12].

Generational differences in prevalence are seen with the highest rates in young adults (myopia 65.5–96.5% and HM 6.8–21.6%) and the lowest rates in older adults (myopia 25.0–40.0% and HM 2.4–8.2%). The disease progression pattern of HM and subsequent development of PM may be different between young adults and older adults due to generational differences, or changes in the lifestyle factors such as the education system, near work, and outdoor time exposure in rapidly developing urban Asian countries.

1.2 Pathogenesis of Myopia

Ocular Biometric Changes in Human Myopia The axial length of the eye or, more precisely, the vitreous chamber depth is the primary individual biometric contributor to refractive error in children, young adults, and the elderly [13–15], with the vitreous chamber depth accounting for over 50% of the observed variation in spherical equivalent refractive error (SER), followed by the cornea (~15%) and crystalline lens (~1%) [15]. However, the dimensions, curvature, and refractive index of each individual ocular structure contribute to the final refractive state. The choroid is typically thinner in myopic compared to non-myopic eyes (most pronounced at the fovea [16, 17]) and thins with increasing myopia and axial length in both adults [18–25] and children [26–28]. Significant choroidal thinning is also observed in eyes with posterior staphyloma [29], and has been associated with the presence of lacquer cracks [30], choroidal neovascularization [31], and reduced visual acuity [32]. The choroid also appears to be a biomarker of ocular processes regulating eye growth given that the central macular choroid thins during the initial development and progression of myopia [33–35] and thickens in response to imposed peripheral myopic retinal image defocus [36, 37], topical anti-muscarinic agents [38, 39], and increased light exposure [40]; clinical interventions associated with a slowing of eye growth in children.

Visual Environment, Emmetropization, and Myopia Much of the knowledge on vision-dependent changes in ocular growth has emanated from animal experiments in which either the quality of image formed on the retina is degraded (known as form deprivation [FD]), or the focal point of the image is altered with respect to the retinal plane (known as lens defocus). Both FD and lens defocus result in abnormal eye growth and development of refractive errors.

Monochromatic Higher-Order Aberrations as a Myopigenic Stimulus Myopia may develop due to the eye's emmetropization response to inherent ocular aberrations that degrade retinal image quality and trigger axial elongation [41]. Evidence concerning the relationship between higher order abberation (HOAs) during distance viewing and refractive error from cross-sectional studies is conflicting [41, 42]. However, during or following near-work tasks, adult myopic eyes tend to display a transient increase in corneal and total ocular HOAs, suggesting a potential role for near-work-induced retinal image degradation in myopia development [43, 44]. Longitudinal studies of myopic children also indicate that eyes with greater positive spherical aberration demonstrate slower eye growth [45, 46].

Accommodation Given the association between near work and the development and progression of childhood myopia [47], numerous studies have compared various characteristics of accommodation between refractive error groups. Typically, this involves the accuracy of the accommodation response, since lag of accommodation (hyperopic retinal defocus) may stimulate axial elongation as observed in some animal models. The slowing of myopia progression during childhood with progressive addition or bifocal lenses, designed to improve accommodation accuracy and minimize lag of accommodation, adds some weight to the role of accommodation in myopia development and progression [48, 49]. However, the exact underlying mechanism of myopia control with such lenses may be related to imposed peripheral retinal defocus or a reduction in the near vergence demand [50]. Certainly, elevations in measured lag observed in myopes arise after rather than before onset [51].

1.3 Key Environmental Factors on Myopia

Near work and education: Many studies have established a strong link between myopia and education [52–57]. Moreover, Mountjoy et al. have shown that exposure to longer duration of education was a causal risk factor for myopia [53]. The exact mechanism linking increased education with myopia is unclear. Although it is possible that optical [43, 58] or biomechanical [59, 60] ocular changes associated with near work could potentially promote myopic eye growth in those with higher levels of education (and hence near-work demands), population studies examining the link between near-work activities and myopia have been conflicting, with some studies suggesting an association between near work and myopia [47, 61], and others indicating no significant effects [62]. The relatively inconsistent findings linking near work with myopia development suggests a potential role for other factors in the association between education and myopia.

Outdoor Activity A number of recent studies report that the time children spend engaged in outdoor activities is negatively associated with their risk of myopia [62–68]. Both cross-sectional and longitudinal studies indicate that greater time spent outdoors is associated with a significantly lower myopia prevalence and reduced risk of myopia onset in childhood. Although some studies report significant associations between myopia progression and outdoor activity [66, 68], this is not a consistent finding across all longitudinal studies [69]. A recent meta-analysis of studies examining the relationship between outdoor time and myopia indicated that there was a 2% reduction in the odds of having myopia for each additional hour per week spent outdoors [70].

Duration of Outdoor Activity and Myopia In a large longitudinal study, Jones and colleagues [62] reported that children who engaged in outdoor activities for 14 h per week or more exhibited the lowest odds of developing myopia. A number of recent randomized controlled trials have reported that interventions that increase children's outdoor time (by 40–80 min a day) significantly reduce the onset of myopia in childhood [71–73]. In the "Role of outdoor activity in myopia study" [74], children who were habitually exposed to low ambient light levels (on average less than 60 min exposure to outdoor light per day) had significantly faster axial eye growth compared to children habitually exposed to moderate and high light. These findings from human studies suggest that children who are exposed to less than 60 min a day of bright outdoor light are at an increased risk of more rapid eye growth and myopia development, and that approximately 2 h or more of outdoor exposure each day is required to provide protection against myopia development in the human eye.

1.4 Genetics of Myopia

Myopia is highly heritable; genes explain up to 80% of the variance in refractive error in twin studies. For the last decade, genome-wide association study (GWAS) approaches have revealed that myopia is a complex trait, with many genetic variants of small effect influencing retinal signaling, eye growth, and the normal process of emmetropization. Particularly notable are genes encoding extracellular matrix-related proteins (COL1A1, COL2A1 [75, 76], and MMP1, MMP2, MMP3, MMP9, MMP10 [77, 78]). For candidates such as PAX6 and TGFB1, the results were replicated in multiple independent extreme/high myopia studies and validated in a large GWAS meta-analysis in 2018, respectively [79, 80]. However, the genetic architecture and its molecular mechanisms are still to be clarified, and while genetic risk score prediction models are improving, this knowledge must be expanded to have impact on clinical practice.

Gene–environment (GxE) interaction analysis has focused primarily on education. An early study in North American samples examined GxE for myopia and the matrix metalloproteinases genes (MMP1–MMP10): a subset of single nucleotide polymorphism (SNPs) was only associated with refraction in the lower education level [78, 81]. A subsequent study in five Singapore cohorts found variants in DNAH9, GJD2, and ZMAT4, which had a larger effect on myopia in a high education subset [82]. Subsequent efforts to examine GxE considered the aggregate effects of many SNPs together. A study in Europeans found that a genetic risk score comprising 26 genetic variants was most strongly associated with myopia in individuals with a university level education [83]. A study examining GxE in children considered near work and time outdoors in association with 39 SNPs and found weak evidence for an interaction with near work [83, 84]. Finally, a Consortium for Refractive Error and Myopia (CREAM) study was able to identify additional myopia risk loci by allowing for a GxE approach [85].

Mendelian randomization (MR) offers a better assessment of causality than that available from observational studies [86, 87]. Two MR studies found a causal effect of education on the development of myopia [53, 80]. Both found a larger effect through MR than that estimated from observational studies suggesting that confounding in observational studies may have been obscuring the true relationship [55, 79]. As expected, there was little evidence of myopia affecting education (−0.008 years/diopter, $P = 0.6$). Another study focused on the causality of low vitamin D on myopia found only a small estimated effect on refractive error [88] suggesting that previous observational findings were likely confounded by the effects of time spent outdoors.

Due to the high polygenicity of myopia and low explained phenotypic variance by genetic factors (7.8%), clinical applications derived from genetic analyses of myopia are currently limited. Risk predictions for myopia in children are based on family history, education level of the parents, the amount of outdoor exposure, and the easily measurable refractive error and axial length. Currently, we are able to make a distinction between high myopes and high hyperopes based on the polygenic risk scores derived from CREAM studies: persons in the highest decile for the polygenic risk score had a 40-fold greater risk of myopia relative to those in the lowest decile. A prediction model, including age, sex, and polygenic risk score, achieved an area under curve (AUC) of 0.77 (95% CI = 0.75–0.79) for myopia versus hyperopia in adults (Rotterdam Study I–III) [80]. To date, one study has assessed both environmental and genetic factors together and showed that modeling both genes and environment improved prediction accuracy [89].

1.5 Prevention of the Onset of Myopia

The vast majority of literature suggests that most cases of myopia develop during the school-going age in children. After the age of 6 years, the prevalence of myopia starts to rise [90–94]. The highest annual incidence of myopia is reported among school children from urban mainland China [92] and Taiwan [95], ranging from 20% to 30% through ages 7–14 years, with earlier onset of myopia also being identified [94]. A study in Japan showed that while the prevalence of myopia has been increasing from 1984 to 1996, the prevalence among children aged 6 or younger has remained unchanged. This suggests that the majority of increased myopia onset is secondary to increased educational intensity [94].

Rates of progression increase dramatically with the year of onset and this has been suggested by spherical equivalent refraction and axial length [96]. Myopic refractions tend to stabilize in late adolescent but can remain progressive until adulthood. The mean age at myopia stabilization is 15.6 years but this can vary among children of different ethnicities [97].

Several factors have been found to be associated with the development of incident myopia in school. Asian ethnicity [93, 98], parental history of myopia [62, 99], reduced time outdoors [62], and level of near-work activity [47, 100] are risk factors for incident myopia, although the evidence can be seen as controversial in some instances.

Evidence of time spent outdoors as a risk factor for myopia progression was first presented in a 3-year follow-up study of myopia in school children, showing that those who spent more time outdoors were less likely to progress [64]. Consistent results were reported in various studies, such as the Sydney Myopia Study, Orinda Study, as well as the Singapore Cohort Study of Risk Factors for Myopia [63, 65, 101]. This led to the commencement of several clinical trials which confirmed the protective effect and indicated a dose-dependent effect, among them, the randomized clinical trial in Guangzhou which reported that an additional 40 min of outdoor activity can reduce the incidence of myopia by 23% [63]. Additionally, the trial in Taiwan suggested that an extra 80 min may further reduce incidence by 50% [72, 73].

Near-work activity as a risk factor for myopia has not been entirely consistent. A meta-analysis reported a modest, but statistically significant, association between time spent performing near work and myopia (odds ratio, 1.14) [47]. Core techniques to implementing interventions of near-work activities include effective measures of near-work-related parameters, real-time data analyses, and alert systems. Wearable devices that possess these techniques have emerged in the last decade.

It has been estimated that without any effective controls or interventions the proportion of myopes in the population will reach up to 50% and 10% for high myopes by 2050 [9]. Approaches that have produced a reduction of at least 50% in incidence, such as time outdoors, lead to delayed onset and have the potential to make a significant difference on the impending myopia epidemic.

Another critical issue is the need to balance educational achievement and interventions to prevent myopia progression in East Asia. This balance can be seen in Australia [102], with not only some of the highest educational ranks in the world but also high levels of outdoor activity and light intensity. Preventing the onset of myopia is certainly challenging in the East Asian population and requires a collaborative effort among clinics, schools, parents, and the entire society.

1.6 Understanding Pathologic Myopia

Pathologic myopia (PM) is a major cause of blindness in the world, especially in East Asian countries [103–107]. The cause of blindness in patients with PM includes myopic maculopathy with or without posterior staphyloma, myopic macular retinoschisis, and glaucoma or glaucoma-like optic neuropathy. The term "pathologic myopia" describes the situation of pathologic consequences of a myopic axial elongation. According to a recent consensus article by Ohno-Matsui et al. [108], pathologic myopia was defined by a myopic chorioretinal atrophy equal to or more serious than diffuse atrophy (by Meta-analysis for pathologic myopia (META-PM) study group classification [109]) and/or the presence of posterior staphylomas.

A posterior staphyloma is an outpouching of a circumscribed area of the posterior fundus, where the radius of curvature is less than the curvature radius of the surrounding eye wall [110], and can be associated with, or lead to, vision-threatening complications such as myopic maculopathy [109, 111–114] and myopic optic neuropathy/glaucoma [115, 116]. Based upon and modifying Curtin's [117] classical categorization of posterior staphylomas, with types I–V as primary staphylomas and types VI–X as compound staphylomas, Ohno-Matsui [118] used 3D-magnetic resonance imaging (3D-MRI) and wide-field fundus imaging to re-classify staphylomas into six types: wide macular, narrow macular, peripapillary, nasal, inferior, and others.

In the META-PM classification [109], myopic maculopathy lesions have been categorized into five categories from "no myopic retinal lesions" (category 0), "tessellated fundus only" (category 1), "diffuse chorioretinal atrophy" (category 2), "patchy chorioretinal atrophy" (category 3), to "macular atrophy" (category 4). These categories were defined based on long-term clinical observations that showed the progression patterns and associated factors of the development of myopic choroidal neovascularization (CNV) for each stage. Three additional features were added to these categories and were included as "plus signs": (1) lacquer cracks, (2) fuch spot and (3) myopic CNV.

Myopic CNV is a major sight-threatening complication of pathologic myopia. It is the most common cause of CNV in individuals younger than 50 years, and it is the second most common cause of CNV overall [119, 120]. Anti-vascular endothelial growth factor (anti-VEGF) therapy is the first-line treatment for myopic CNV, as shown by the RADIANCE study [121] and the MYRROR study [122].

Panozzo and Mercanti proposed the term "myopic traction maculopathy (MTM)" to encompass various findings characterized by a traction as visualized by optical coherence tomography (OCT) in highly myopic eyes [123]. A dome-shaped macula (DSM) is an inward protrusion of the macula as visualized by OCT [124–126]. Imamura, Spaide, and coworkers reported that a DSM was associated with, and caused by, a local thickening of the subfoveal sclera [127]. It was postulated that the local thickening of the subfoveal sclera was an adaptive or compensatory response to the defocus of the image on the fovea in highly myopic eyes.

1.7 Imaging in Myopia

Imaging the myopic eye can be challenging due to various structural changes (abnormal eye elongation, scleral and corneal curvature irregularities, cataracts leading to poor clarity; or retinal thinning causing abnormal projections of the final image [128, 129]).

Optic disc imaging can also be used to predict the development of glaucoma, where visualization of myopic tilting of the optic disc with peripapillary atrophy (PPA) and pitting of the optic disc [130] is a possible predisposing factor [131, 132]. Serial imaging investigative measures can therefore be utilized for monitoring the development of open-angle, normal-tension glaucoma [133]. Features such as optic disc tilt, PPA, and abnormally large or small optic discs are the earliest known structural alterations that potentially predict the development of pathological myopia and can be observed even in young highly myopic adults. Unfortunately, these features (some also with associations to glaucoma) also interfere with the visualization of optic disc margins [134, 135] and are also not easy to discern in highly myopic eyes [136]. There is also added difficulty in eyes with myopic maculopathy, where visual field defects result in further interference [137]. As such, the answer to these challenges may lie in imaging deep optic nerve head structures (such as parapapillary sclera, scleral wall, and lamina cribosa) [138] in highly myopic eyes for more precise diagnoses of glaucoma.

The ability to view distinct retinal layers with OCT has enhanced visualization of myopic traction maculopathy (MTM). Examples of features that can be seen include inner or outer retinal schisis, foveal detachment, lamellar or full-thickness macular hole, and/or macular detachment [139, 140]. Non-stereoscopic fundus photographs are inadequate for detailed studies of posterior staphylomas as the change in contour at the staphyloma edge is not always discernible. The OCT overcomes this limitation because of its excellent depth resolution [141, 142].

The OCT itself has its shortcomings; the sclera cannot be visualized using the OCT. These limitations also extend to the use of OCT angiography (OCTA). There is currently no standard protocol for segmentation; the outcome parameters for OCTA have not been clearly defined either. Although some authors have tried to use analysis of flow voids or signal voids in the choriocapillaris to quantify the area taken up by the microvasculature [143, 144], the data pertaining to myopic patients are but insufficient [145]. Looking into the future, there is, however, incipient research suggesting that the comprehension of blood supply and changes in vasculature from the anterior to the posterior segment of the myopic eye is crucial to the understanding of the disease [146–149].

Photoacoustic imaging has shown promise recently to fill the gaps between OCT and ultrasound in terms of penetration depth [150]. This modality has been used before to image the posterior pole of the eye in vitro and in animal models *in vivo*. This can also be used in concurrence with angiography, measuring oxygen saturation and pigment imaging [151]. However, there are some limitations pertaining to this modality notwithstanding moderate depth resolution, pure optical absorption sensing, need for contact detection with ultrasound sensor, and a relatively long acquisition time. In view of these limitations, we are yet to receive tangible results from photoacoustic imaging for posterior pole imaging in humans.

1.8 Glaucoma in Myopia

Axial myopization leads to marked changes of the optic nerve head: (1) an enlargement of all three layers of the optic disc (i.e., optic disc Bruch's membrane opening, optic disc choroidal opening, optic disc scleral opening) with the development of a secondary macrodisc, (2) an enlargement and shallowing of the cup, (3) an elongation and thinning of the lamina cribrosa with a secondary reduction in the distance between the intraocular space with the intraocular pressure (IOP) and the retro-lamina compartment with the orbital cerebrospinal fluid pressure, (4) a direct exposure of the peripheral posterior lamina cribrosa surface to the orbital cerebrospinal fluid space, (5) an elongation and thinning of the peripapillary scleral flange with development and enlargement of the parapapillary gamma zone and delta zone, (6) an elongation and thinning of the peripapillary border tissue of the choroid, and (7) a rotation of the optic disc around the vertical axis, and less often and to a minor degree around the horizontal axis und the sagittal axis. These changes make it more difficult to differentiate between myopic changes and (additional) glaucoma-associated changes such as a loss of neuroretinal rim and thinning of the retinal nerve fiber layer, and these changes may make the optic nerve head more vulnerable, potentially explaining the increased prevalence of glaucomatous optic neuropathy in highly myopic eyes.

Population-based investigations and hospital-based studies have shown that the prevalence of glaucomatous optic neuropathy (GON) was higher in highly myopic eyes than in emmetropic eyes [152–166]. A previous study revealed that at a given IOP in patients with chronic open-angle glaucoma, the amount of optic nerve damage was more marked in highly myopic eyes with large optic discs than in non-highly myopic eyes [165].

Highly myopic glaucomatous eyes as compared with non-highly myopic glaucomatous eyes may have a markedly lower IOP threshold to develop optic nerve damage. It could indicate that an IOP of perhaps lower than 10 mmHg might be necessary to prevent the development of GON in these highly myopic eyes, and that in highly myopic eyes with axial elongation-associated enlargement and stretching of the optic disc and parapapillary region as the main risk factors for GON in high myopia a normal IOP may be sufficient to lead to GON [136].

Although it has not yet been firmly proven that GON in high myopia is dependent on IOP, most researchers recommend lowering IOP in highly myopic patients with glaucoma. Based on the morphological findings described above, the target pressure in highly myopic glaucoma may be lower than in non-highly myopic glaucoma. Due to the peculiar anatomy of the optic nerve head in highly myopic eyes, most diagnostic procedures fail in precisely assessing the status of the optic nerve in highly myopic eyes with glaucoma. It includes factors such as a decreased spatial and color contrast between the neuroretinal rim and the optic cup making a delineation of both structures more difficult; a peripapillary retinoschisis leading to an incorrect segmentation of the retinal nerve fiber layer upon optical coherence tomography; a large gamma zone (and delta zone) which makes using the end of Bruch's membrane as reference point for the measurement of the neuroretinal rim useless; and macular Bruch's membrane defects and other reasons for non-glaucomatous visual field defects which reduces the diagnostic precision of perimetry for the detection of presence and progression of GON.

1.9 Management of Myopic Choroidal Neovascularization

Myopic choroidal neovascularization (myopic CNV) is the second most common cause of CNV after age-related macular degeneration (AMD) [167, 168]. It is one of the most sight-threatening complications of pathological myopia [119, 169] and is the most common cause of CNV in those 50 years or younger [167], with significant social and economic burden. The prevalence of myopic CNV is between 5.2% and 11.3% in individuals with pathological myopia [12], with female preponderance seen in most studies [167–170]. The long-term outcome of CNV is poor if left untreated. In a 10-year follow-up study of 25 patients with myopic CNV, visual acuity deteriorated to 20/200 or worse in 89% and 96% of eyes in 5 years and 10 years, respectively [168].

On slit-lamp biomicroscopy, myopic CNV manifests as a small, flat, grayish subretinal lesion adjacent to or beneath the fovea [109, 168, 169, 171]. On SD-OCT, myopic CNV presents as a hyper-reflective material above the retinal pigment epithelium band (type 2 CNV), with variable amount of subretinal fluid. Clinical diagnosis is confirmed by fundus fluorescein angiography (FFA). Most myopic CNVs are type 2 neovascularization and present with a "classic" pattern on FA. OCT angiography (OCTA) was able to detect flow within myopic CNV vascular complexes and hence delineate vascular networks in these myopic neovascular membranes that lie above the retinal pigment epithelium (RPE) where flow signals are spared from attenuation [172].

Prior to the advent of anti-VEGF therapy, the main treatment options for myopic CNV were limited to thermal laser photocoagulation [173], photodynamic therapy with verteporfin (vPDT) [174, 175]. These treatments had limited efficacy in improving vision significantly and have now largely been relegated to the annals of history by anti-vascular endothelial growth factor (anti-VEGF) therapy [176]. Once active myopic CNV is diagnosed, prompt treatment with intravitreal anti-VEGF therapy should be administered as soon as possible [121, 177]. Current evidence suggests a pro-re-nata (PRN) regimen without a loading phase can be considered in most patients. Patients should be monitored monthly with OCT and treatment administered until cessation of disease activity on OCT or visual stabilization.

1.10 Management of Myopia-Related Retinal Complications

Myopic traction maculopathy (MTM) [123] is estimated to occur in approximately 8–34% in individuals with high myopia [178–180] and encompasses retinal thickening, macular retinoschisis, foveal detachment, lamellar macular hole with or without epiretinal membrane and/or vitreomacular traction [123], and/or full-thickness macular hole (HM) with or without retinal detachment. Central to the pathogenesis of MTM is traction, which was postulated to arise from one or more of the following mechanisms [181]: vitreomacular traction associated with perifoveal posterior vitreous detachment (PVD) [182–184]; relative incompliance of the internal limiting membrane (ILM) [185–189], epiretinal membrane (ERM) [180, 182, 190–192], and cortical vitreous remnant after PVD [193] to the outer retina which conforms to the shape of the posterior staphyloma; and traction exerted by retinal arterioles [188, 194, 195]. Not all patients with MTM require interventions [184, 196, 197]. There are numerous reported interventions for MTM. The principles of the treatment are: (1) to relieve traction, mainly achieved through pars plana vitrectomy (PPV) with or without ILM peeling; (2) to minimize surgical damage to the weakened macula through technique modifications in order to prevent the formation of postoperative MH; and (3) in the presence of full-thickness MH, to maximize the chance of hole closure through the use of various surgical adjuncts.

1.10.1 Proposed Adjuncts to Improve Outcome of Macular Hole Surgery

Inverted Internal Limiting Membrane Flap This technique involves leaving a hinge of ILM flap at the edge of MH during ILM peeling. This ILM flap is then inverted upside-down to cover or fill the MH [198].

Autologous Internal Limiting Membrane Transplantation In eyes where ILM around the macula hole has already been removed, an appropriately sized ILM can be peeled off from a distant site and placed as a free flap onto the persistent MH [199, 200].

Autologous Blood In order to prevent subretinal migration of dye and the resultant retinal toxicity associated with vital stains, it was proposed to use autologous blood to cover the MH before injection of brilliant blue dye. It has been demonstrated that compared to conventional method, the use of pre-staining autologous blood led to better visual acuity outcomes and continuity of ellipsoid zone at all post-operative time points [201].

Lens Capsular Flap Transplantation Chen et al. demonstrated a 100% MH closure rate with anterior capsular transplantation among patients with refractory MH,

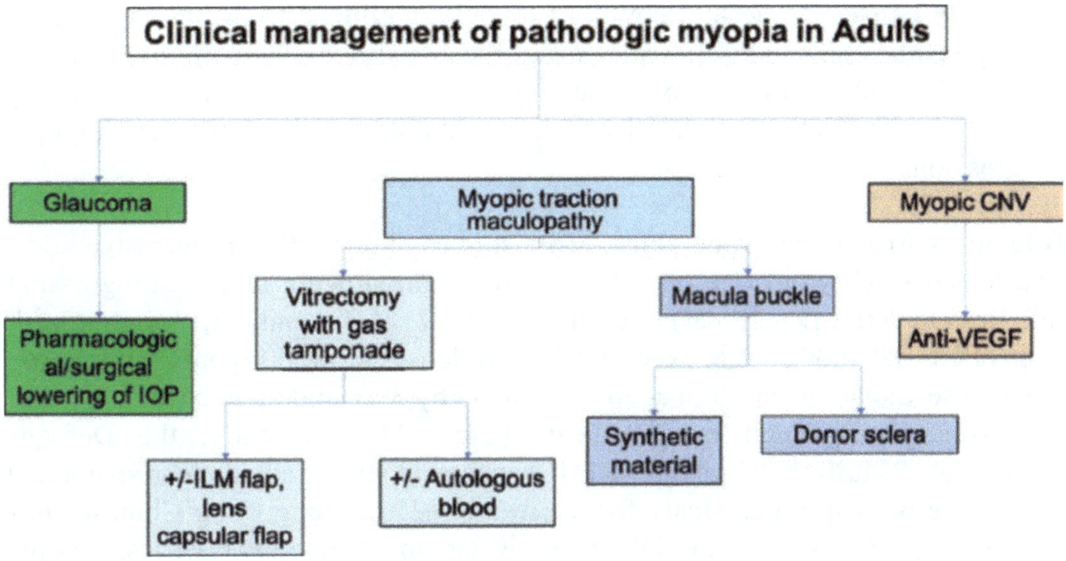

Fig. 1.1 Summary of the clinical management of pathologic myopia in adults

whereas the complete closure rate of MH after posterior capsular transplantation was only 50% and with another 30% enjoyed partial MH closure [202].

Macular Buckle Macular buckles have been used to shorten the axial length of myopic eyeballs in conditions such as macular hole retinal detachment (MHRD), myopic foveoschisis with or without foveal detachment, and MH with foveoschisis. There are many types of macular buckle, including scleral sponge, T-shaped or L-shaped buckle, Ando Plombe, wire-strengthened sponge exoplant, and even donor sclera and suprachoroidal injectable long-acting hyaluronic acid [203].

Autologous Neurosensory Retinal Transplantation The technique involves bimanually harvesting a free flap of neurosensory retina superior to the superotemporal arcade, with the harvest site first secured by endolaser barricade and endodiathermy. The free flap was translocated in its correct orientation over the macular hole and perfluoro-*n*-octane heavy liquid (PFC) was instilled over it, followed by direct PFC–silicone oil exchange [204].

Figure 1.1 presents an overview of the management of myopia-related complications in adults.

1.11 Management and Control of Myopia in Children

Currently, there are many types of interventions to slow myopia progression in children, including spectacle lenses, contact lenses, pharmaceuticals, and environmental or behavioral modification. However, none of these myopia control methods have been proven to stop the development or progression of myopia completely and each method has their own limitations.

Spectacle Lenses Under-correction of myopia in clinical trials has shown conflicting results and small, clinically insignificant effect on slowing myopia progression [205–207]. In view of these conflicting results, there is no convincing evidence to indicate that under-correction should be used to slow myopia progression.

Bifocal or Multifocal Spectacles Most studies showed that progressive addition lenses (PALs) have an insignificant effect on slowing myopia progression rate (less than 0.2 D per year) overall [48, 208–214]. In contrast, a randomized, controlled trial showed that executive bifocal lenses slowed myopia progression in Chinese-Canadian children aged 8–13 years by 39% and up to 51% with base-in prisms incorporated over 3 years [215]. More recently, the Defocus Incorporated Multiple Segments (DIMS) spectacle lens enabled clear vision and myopic defocus simultaneously for the wearer [216]. Hong Kong Chinese children aged 8–13 years wearing DIMS lenses had approximately 60% less myopia progression and axial elongation when compared with children wearing single vision spectacle lenses over 2 years. Moreover, about 20% of the DIMS lens wearers had no myopia progression during the study period.

Peripheral Myopic Defocus Glasses In 2010, Sankaridurg et al. published their results of three novel peripheral defocus spectacle lens. Unfortunately, there was no significant effect on myopic progression with all three designs [217]. In a recent randomized controlled trial (RCT) conducted in Japanese children with peripheral defocus lenses, no difference in myopia reduction was found [218].

Rigid Gas Permeable Contact Lenses Two randomized clinical trials [219, 220] showed that rigid gas permeable (RGP) contact lenses did not retard axial eye growth. However, Walline et al. [219] reported significant slower myopia progression in the group of RGP lenses compared with soft contact lenses, despite that no differences were found in axial elongation between the groups. The proposed reason for a treatment effect on refraction may be due to the changes in corneal curvature.

Orthokeratology Orthokeratology (Ortho-K) lenses are specially designed RGP contact lenses that are worn overnight to reshape the cornea and thereby temporarily correct low-to-moderate myopia. Various clinical studies have demonstrated the effectiveness of inhibiting myopic progression with Ortho-K. Individual studies and meta-analyses have shown a 32–63% reduction in the rate of axial elongation in East Asian children initially aged from 7 to 16 years and followed for up to 5 years [221–227]. Efficacy may decrease over time [224, 228], with a potential "rebound" after discontinuation, especially in children under 14 years [229]. There is also a potential non-response rate of 7–12% [223]. Interestingly, a recent study in Japan [230] showed that the combination of Ortho-K and low-concentration atropine (0.01%) eyedrops was more effective in slowing axial elongation over 12 months than Ortho-K treatment alone in myopic children. The risk of infective keratitis remains [231].

Soft Bifocal and Multifocal Contact Lenses These lenses are worn during the daytime. Compared to spectacles, contact lenses are more cosmetically acceptable, more easily handled, and are more convenient for daily activities of some children, especially during sports [232, 233]. For most of eye-care practitioners, the fitting procedures of soft bifocal contact lenses are relatively simpler than Ortho-K. Overall, soft bifocal and multifocal contact lenses slow the progression of myopia in children by an amount comparable to that of Ortho-K lenses. Studies exploring the effect of these bifocal soft contact lenses indicate slowing of myopia progression by 25–50% and axial length by 27–32% in children aged 8–16 of various ethnicities over a period of 24 months [234, 235].

Atropine The initial high doses of atropine (i.e., 0.5% or 1.0%) slowed myopia progression by more than 70% in Asian children aged 6–13 years over 1–2 years [229, 236–238]. However, lower doses (0.1% or less) can also slow refractive progression by 30–60% with less side effects (pupil dilation, glare, or blur) [238]. The Atropine Treatment of Myopia (ATOM) studies showed that there was a myopic rebound if atropine was stopped suddenly, especially at higher doses and in younger children [239, 240].

Time Spent Outdoors In the Sydney Myopia Study, exposure to more than 2 h of outdoor activity per day decreased the odds of myopia and countered the effects of near work [65]. Interventions involving increasing time outdoors appeared to reduce the onset of myopia and also its progression in myopic children [71]. A meta-analysis has suggested a 2% reduced odds of myopia per additional hour of time spent outdoors per week [70].

Environmental Interventions Based on new evidence, the advice has shifted from spending at least 2 h per day outdoors in addition to avoiding excessive near work. This has changed health and school messaging in many East Asian countries [71].

Higher Light Intensities and Dopamine Potential reasons why time outdoors may be protective include higher light intensities [241], differences in chromatic composition [242], the reduction in dioptric accommodative focus and psychometric influences encountered outdoors [243]. The role of chromaticity (red and blue) and ultraviolet (UV) light is still uncertain [244], while that of higher vitamin D levels has been debunked [88].

Figure 1.2 presents an overview of the management and prevention of myopia in children.

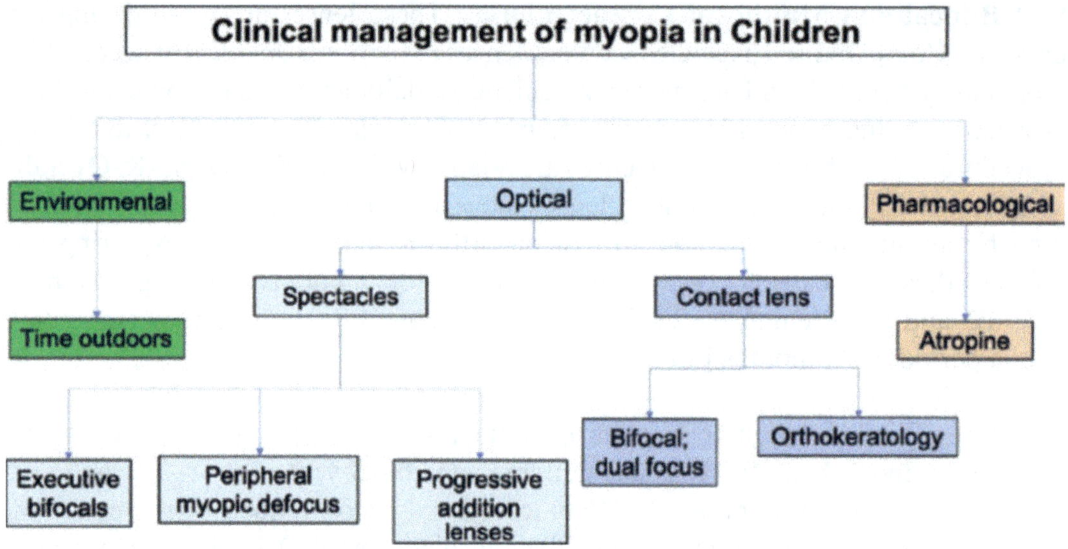

Fig. 1.2 Summary of the clinical management of myopia in children

References

1. Dolgin E. The myopia boom. Nature. 2015;519(7543):276–8.
2. Vitale S, Cotch MF, Sperduto RD. Prevalence of visual impairment in the United States. JAMA. 2006;295(18):2158–63.
3. Zheng YF, Pan CW, Chay J, Wong TY, Finkelstein E, Saw SM. The economic cost of myopia in adults aged over 40 years in Singapore. Invest Ophthalmol Vis Sci. 2013;54(12):7532–7.
4. Liang YB, Wong TY, Sun LP, et al. Refractive errors in a rural Chinese adult population the Handan eye study. Ophthalmology. 2009;116(11):2119–27.
5. Morgan IG, Ohno-Matsui K, Saw S-M. Myopia. Lancet. 2012;379(9827):1739–48.
6. Morgan IG. What public policies should be developed to deal with the epidemic of myopia? Optom Vis Sci. 2016;93(9):1058–60.
7. Lin LL, Shih YF, Hsiao CK, Chen CJ. Prevalence of myopia in Taiwanese school children: 1983 to 2000. Ann Acad Med Singap. 2004;33(1):27–33.
8. Jung SK, Lee JH, Kakizaki H, Jee D. Prevalence of myopia and its association with body stature and educational level in 19-year-old male conscripts in Seoul, South Korea. Invest Ophthalmol Vis Sci. 2012;53(9):5579–83.
9. Holden BA, Fricke TR, Wilson DA, et al. Global prevalence of myopia and high myopia and temporal trends from 2000 through 2050. Ophthalmology. 2016;123(5):1036–42.
10. Ding BY, Shih YF, Lin LLK, Hsiao CK, Wang IJ. Myopia among school children in East Asia and Singapore. Surv Ophthalmol. 2017;62(5):677–97.
11. Wong YL, Sabanayagam C, Ding Y, et al. Prevalence, risk factors, and impact of myopic macular degeneration on visual impairment and functioning among adults in Singapore. Invest Ophthalmol Vis Sci. 2018;59(11):4603–13.

12. Wong TY, Ferreira A, Hughes R, Carter G, Mitchell P. Epidemiology and disease burden of pathologic myopia and myopic choroidal neovascularization: an evidence-based systematic review. Am J Ophthalmol. 2014;157(1):9–25 e12.
13. Xie R, Zhou XT, Lu F, et al. Correlation between myopia and major biometric parameters of the eye: a retrospective clinical study. Optom Vis Sci. 2009;86(5):E503–8.
14. Li SM, Li SY, Kang MT, et al. Distribution of ocular biometry in 7- and 14-year-old Chinese children. Optom Vis Sci. 2015;92(5):566–72.
15. Richter GM, Wang M, Jiang X, et al. Ocular determinants of refractive error and its age- and sex-related variations in the Chinese American eye study. JAMA Ophthalmol. 2017;135(7):724–32.
16. Read SA, Collins MJ, Vincent SJ, Alonso-Caneiro D. Choroidal thickness in myopic and non-myopic children assessed with enhanced depth imaging optical coherence tomography. Invest Ophthalmol Vis Sci. 2013;54(12):7578–86.
17. Xiong S, He X, Deng J, et al. Choroidal thickness in 3001 Chinese children aged 6 to 19 years using swept-source OCT. Sci Rep. 2017;7:45059.
18. Chen FK, Yeoh J, Rahman W, Patel PJ, Tufail A, Da Cruz L. Topographic variation and interocular symmetry of macular choroidal thickness using enhanced depth imaging optical coherence tomography. Invest Ophthalmol Vis Sci. 2012;53(2):975–85.
19. Esmaeelpour M, Povazay B, Hermann B, et al. Three-dimensional 1060-nm OCT: choroidal thickness maps in normal subjects and improved posterior segment visualization in cataract patients. Invest Ophthalmol Vis Sci. 2010;51(10):5260–6.
20. Gupta P, Jing T, Marziliano P, et al. Distribution and determinants of choroidal thickness and volume using automated segmentation software in a population-based study. Am J Ophthalmol. 2015;159(2):293–301.e293.
21. Li XQ, Munkholm A, Larsen M, Munch IC. Choroidal thickness in relation to birth parameters in 11- to 12-year-old children: the Copenhagen child cohort 2000 eye study. Invest Ophthalmol Vis Sci. 2014;56(1):617–24.
22. Ouyang Y, Heussen FM, Mokwa N, et al. Spatial distribution of posterior pole choroidal thickness by spectral domain optical coherence tomography. Invest Ophthalmol Vis Sci. 2011;52(9):7019–26.
23. Tan CS, Cheong KX. Macular choroidal thicknesses in healthy adults--relationship with ocular and demographic factors. Invest Ophthalmol Vis Sci. 2014;55(10):6452–8.
24. Wei WB, Xu L, Jonas JB, et al. Subfoveal choroidal thickness: the Beijing eye study. Ophthalmology. 2013;120(1):175–80.
25. Sanchez-Cano A, Orduna E, Segura F, et al. Choroidal thickness and volume in healthy young white adults and the relationships between them and axial length, ammetropy and sex. Am J Ophthalmol. 2014;158(3):574–583.e571.
26. He X, Jin P, Zou H, et al. Choroidal thickness in healthy Chinese children aged 6 to 12: the Shanghai children eye study. Retina. 2017;37(2):368–75.
27. Jin P, Zou H, Zhu J, et al. Choroidal and retinal thickness in children with different refractive status measured by swept-source optical coherence tomography. Am J Ophthalmol. 2016;168:164–76.
28. Zhang JM, Wu JF, Chen JH, et al. Macular choroidal thickness in children: the Shandong children eye study. Invest Ophthalmol Vis Sci. 2015;56(13):7646–52.
29. Zhou LX, Shao L, Xu L, Wei WB, Wang YX, You QS. The relationship between scleral staphyloma and choroidal thinning in highly myopic eyes: the Beijing eye study. Sci Rep. 2017;7(1):9825.
30. Wang NK, Lai CC, Chou CL, et al. Choroidal thickness and biometric markers for the screening of lacquer cracks in patients with high myopia. PLoS One. 2013;8(1):e53660.
31. Ikuno Y, Jo Y, Hamasaki T, Tano Y. Ocular risk factors for choroidal neovascularization in pathologic myopia. Invest Ophthalmol Vis Sci. 2010;51(7):3721–5.
32. Nishida Y, Fujiwara T, Imamura Y, Lima LH, Kurosaka D, Spaide RF. Choroidal thickness and visual acuity in highly myopic eyes. Retina. 2012;32(7):1229–36.

33. Read SA, Alonso-Caneiro D, Vincent SJ, Collins MJ. Longitudinal changes in choroidal thickness and eye growth in childhood. Invest Ophthalmol Vis Sci. 2015;56(5):3103–12.
34. Fontaine M, Gaucher D, Sauer A, Speeg-Schatz C. Choroidal thickness and ametropia in children: a longitudinal study. Eur J Ophthalmol. 2017;27:730–4.
35. Jin P, Zou H, Xu X, et al. Longitudinal changes in choroidal and retinal thicknesses in children with myopic shift. Retina. 2018. https://doi.org/10.1097/IAE.0000000000002090.
36. Chen Z, Xue F, Zhou J, Qu X, Zhou X. Effects of orthokeratology on choroidal thickness and axial length. Optom Vis Sci. 2016;93(9):1064–71.
37. Li Z, Cui D, Hu Y, Ao S, Zeng J, Yang X. Choroidal thickness and axial length changes in myopic children treated with orthokeratology. Cont Lens Anterior Eye. 2017;40(6):417–23.
38. Sander BP, Collins MJ, Read SA. The effect of topical adrenergic and anticholinergic agents on the choroidal thickness of young healthy adults. Exp Eye Res. 2014;128:181–9.
39. Zhang Z, Zhou Y, Xie Z, et al. The effect of topical atropine on the choroidal thickness of healthy children. Sci Rep. 2016;6:34936.
40. Read SA. Ocular and environmental factors associated with eye growth in childhood. Optom Vis Sci. 2016;93(9):1031–41.
41. Charman WN. Aberrations and myopia. Ophthalmic Physiol Opt. 2005;25(4):285–301.
42. Little JA, McCullough SJ, Breslin KM, Saunders KJ. Higher order ocular aberrations and their relation to refractive error and ocular biometry in children. Invest Ophthalmol Vis Sci. 2014;55(8):4791–800.
43. Buehren T, Collins MJ, Carney LG. Near work induced wavefront aberrations in myopia. Vis Res. 2005;45(10):1297–312.
44. Vincent SJ, Collins MJ, Read SA, Carney LG, Yap MK. Corneal changes following near work in myopic anisometropia. Ophthalmic Physiol Opt. 2013;33(1):15–25.
45. Lau JK, Vincent SJ, Collins MJ, Cheung SW, Cho P. Ocular higher-order aberrations and axial eye growth in young Hong Kong children. Sci Rep. 2018;8(1):6726.
46. Hiraoka T, Kotsuka J, Kakita T, Okamoto F, Oshika T. Relationship between higher-order wavefront aberrations and natural progression of myopia in schoolchildren. Sci Rep. 2017;7(1):7876.
47. Huang HM, Chang DS, Wu PC. The association between near work activities and myopia in children-a systematic review and meta-analysis. PLoS One. 2015;10(10):e0140419.
48. Gwiazda J, Hyman L, Hussein M, et al. A randomized clinical trial of progressive addition lenses versus single vision lenses on the progression of myopia in children. Invest Ophthalmol Vis Sci. 2003;44(4):1492–500.
49. Cheng D, Schmid KL, Woo GC, Drobe B. Randomized trial of effect of bifocal and prismatic bifocal spectacles on myopic progression: two-year results. Arch Ophthalmol. 2010;128(1):12–9.
50. Berntsen DA, Barr CD, Mutti DO, Zadnik K. Peripheral defocus and myopia progression in myopic children randomly assigned to wear single vision and progressive addition lenses. Invest Ophthalmol Vis Sci. 2013;54(8):5761–70.
51. Mutti DO, Mitchell GL, Hayes JR, et al. Accommodative lag before and after the onset of myopia. Invest Ophthalmol Vis Sci. 2006;47(3):837–46.
52. Nickels S, Hopf S, Pfeiffer N, Schuster AK. Myopia is associated with education: results from NHANES 1999-2008. PLoS One. 2019;14(1):e0211196.
53. Mountjoy E, Davies NM, Plotnikov D, et al. Education and myopia: assessing the direction of causality by mendelian randomisation. BMJ. 2018;361:k2022.
54. Morgan IG, French AN, Ashby RS, et al. The epidemics of myopia: aetiology and prevention. Prog Retin Eye Res. 2018;62:134–49.
55. Cuellar-Partida G, Lu Y, Kho PF, et al. Assessing the genetic predisposition of education on myopia: a mendelian randomization study. Genet Epidemiol. 2016;40(1):66–72.
56. Williams KM, Bertelsen G, Cumberland P, et al. Increasing prevalence of myopia in Europe and the impact of education. Ophthalmology. 2015;122(7):1489–97.

57. Han SB, Jang J, Yang HK, Hwang JM, Park SK. Prevalence and risk factors of myopia in adult Korean population: Korea national health and nutrition examination survey 2013-2014 (KNHANES VI). PLoS One. 2019;14(1):e0211204.
58. Gwiazda J, Thorn F, Bauer J, Held R. Myopic children show insufficient accommodative response to blur. Invest Ophthalmol Vis Sci. 1993;34(3):690–4.
59. Read SA, Collins MJ, Woodman EC, Cheong SH. Axial length changes during accommodation in myopes and emmetropes. Optom Vis Sci. 2010;87(9):656–62.
60. Woodman-Pieterse EC, Read SA, Collins MJ, Alonso-Caneiro D. Regional changes in choroidal thickness associated with accommodation. Invest Ophthalmol Vis Sci. 2015;56(11):6414–22.
61. Hepsen IF, Evereklioglu C, Bayramlar H. The effect of reading and near-work on the development of myopia in emmetropic boys: a prospective, controlled, three-year follow-up study. Vis Res. 2001;41(19):2511–20.
62. Jones LA, Sinnott LT, Mutti DO, Mitchell GL, Moeschberger ML, Zadnik K. Parental history of myopia, sports and outdoor activities, and future myopia. Invest Ophthalmol Vis Sci. 2007;48(8):3524–32.
63. Mutti DO, Mitchell GL, Moeschberger ML, Jones LA, Zadnik K. Parental myopia, near work, school achievement, and children's refractive error. Invest Ophthalmol Vis Sci. 2002;43(12):3633–40.
64. Parssinen O, Lyyra AL. Myopia and myopic progression among school children: a three-year follow-up study. Invest Ophthalmol Vis Sci. 1993;34(9):2794–802.
65. Rose KA, Morgan IG, Ip J, et al. Outdoor activity reduces the prevalence of myopia in children. Ophthalmology. 2008;115(8):1279–85.
66. Guo Y, Liu LJ, Tang P, et al. Outdoor activity and myopia progression in 4-year follow-up of Chinese primary school children: The Beijing Children Eye Study. PLoS One. 2017;12(4):e0175921.
67. Guggenheim JA, Northstone K, McMahon G, et al. Time outdoors and physical activity as predictors of incident myopia in childhood: a prospective cohort study. Invest Ophthalmol Vis Sci. 2012;53(6):2856–65.
68. Parssinen O, Kauppinen M, Viljanen A. The progression of myopia from its onset at age 8-12 to adulthood and the influence of heredity and external factors on myopic progression. A 23-year follow-up study. Acta Ophthalmol. 2014;92(8):730–9.
69. Jones-Jordan LA, Sinnott LT, Cotter SA, et al. Time outdoors, visual activity, and myopia progression in juvenile-onset myopes. Invest Ophthalmol Vis Sci. 2012;53(11):7169–75.
70. Sherwin JC, Reacher MH, Keogh RH, Khawaja AP, Mackey DA, Foster PJ. The association between time spent outdoors and myopia in children and adolescents: a systematic review and meta-analysis. Ophthalmology. 2012;119(10):2141–51.
71. Wu PC, Chen CT, Lin KK, et al. Myopia prevention and outdoor light intensity in a school-based cluster randomized trial. Ophthalmology. 2018;125:1239–50.
72. He M, Xiang F, Zeng Y, et al. Effect of time spent outdoors at school on the development of myopia among children in China: a randomized clinical trial. JAMA. 2015;314(11):1142–8.
73. Wu PC, Tsai CL, Wu HL, Yang YH, Kuo HK. Outdoor activity during class recess reduces myopia onset and progression in school children. Ophthalmology. 2013;120(5):1080–5.
74. Read SA, Collins MJ, Vincent SJ. Light exposure and eye growth in childhood. Invest Ophthalmol Vis Sci. 2015;56(11):6779–87.
75. Metlapally R, Li YJ, Tran-Viet KN, et al. COL1A1 and COL2A1 genes and myopia susceptibility: evidence of association and suggestive linkage to the COL2A1 locus. Invest Ophthalmol Vis Sci. 2009;50(9):4080–6.
76. Mutti DO, Cooper ME, O'Brien S, et al. Candidate gene and locus analysis of myopia. Mol Vis. 2007;13:1012–9.
77. Hall NF, Gale CR, Ye S, Martyn CN. Myopia and polymorphisms in genes for matrix metalloproteinases. Invest Ophthalmol Vis Sci. 2009;50(6):2632–6.
78. Wojciechowski R, Yee SS, Simpson CL, Bailey-Wilson JE, Stambolian D. Matrix metalloproteinases and educational attainment in refractive error: evidence of gene-environment interactions in the age-related eye disease study. Ophthalmology. 2013;120(2):298–305.

79. Tang SM, Rong SS, Young AL, Tam PO, Pang CP, Chen LJ. PAX6 gene associated with high myopia: a meta-analysis. Optom Vis Sci. 2014;91(4):419–29.
80. Tedja MS, Wojciechowski R, Hysi PG, et al. Genome-wide association meta-analysis highlights light-induced signaling as a driver for refractive error. Nat Genet. 2018;50(6):834–48.
81. Wojciechowski R, Bailey-Wilson JE, Stambolian D. Association of matrix metalloproteinase gene polymorphisms with refractive error in Amish and Ashkenazi families. Invest Ophthalmol Vis Sci. 2010;51(10):4989–95.
82. Fan Q, Wojciechowski R, Kamran Ikram M, et al. Education influences the association between genetic variants and refractive error: a meta-analysis of five Singapore studies. Hum Mol Genet. 2014;23(2):546–54.
83. Verhoeven VJ, Buitendijk GH, Consortium for Refractive E, et al. Education influences the role of genetics in myopia. Eur J Epidemiol. 2013;28(12):973–80.
84. Fan Q, Guo X, Tideman JW, et al. Childhood gene-environment interactions and age-dependent effects of genetic variants associated with refractive error and myopia: The CREAM Consortium. Sci Rep. 2016;6:25853.
85. Fan Q, Verhoeven VJ, Wojciechowski R, et al. Meta-analysis of gene-environment-wide association scans accounting for education level identifies additional loci for refractive error. Nat Commun. 2016;7:11008.
86. Ebrahim S, Davey Smith G. Mendelian randomization: can genetic epidemiology help redress the failures of observational epidemiology? Hum Genet. 2008;123(1):15–33.
87. Smith GD, Ebrahim S. Mendelian randomization: prospects, potentials, and limitations. Int J Epidemiol. 2004;33(1):30–42.
88. Cuellar-Partida G, Williams KM, Yazar S, et al. Genetically low vitamin D concentrations and myopic refractive error: a Mendelian randomization study. Int J Epidemiol. 2017;46(6):1882–90.
89. Ghorbani Mojarrad N, Williams C, Guggenheim JA. A genetic risk score and number of myopic parents independently predict myopia. Ophthalmic Physiol Opt. 2018;38(5):492–502.
90. Zhao J, Mao J, Luo R, Li F, Munoz SR, Ellwein LB. The progression of refractive error in school-age children: Shunyi district, China. Am J Ophthalmol. 2002;134(5):735–43.
91. Xiang F, He M, Zeng Y, Mai J, Rose KA, Morgan IG. Increases in the prevalence of reduced visual acuity and myopia in Chinese children in Guangzhou over the past 20 years. Eye. 2013;27(12):1353–8.
92. Wang SK, Guo Y, Liao C, et al. Incidence of and factors associated with myopia and high myopia in Chinese children, based on refraction without cycloplegia. JAMA Ophthalmol. 2018;136(9):1017–24.
93. Saw SM, Tong L, Chua WH, et al. Incidence and progression of myopia in Singaporean school children. Invest Ophthalmol Vis Sci. 2005;46(1):51–7.
94. Matsumura H, Hirai H. Prevalence of myopia and refractive changes in students from 3 to 17 years of age. Surv Ophthalmol. 1999;44(Suppl 1):S109–15.
95. Tsai DC, Fang SY, Huang N, et al. Myopia development among young school children: the myopia investigation study in Taipei. Invest Ophthalmol Vis Sci. 2016;57(15):6852–60.
96. Xiang F, He M, Morgan IG. Annual changes in refractive errors and ocular components before and after the onset of myopia in Chinese children. Ophthalmology. 2012;119(7):1478–84.
97. COMET Group. Myopia stabilization and associated factors among participants in the Correction of Myopia Evaluation Trial (COMET). Invest Ophthalmol Vis Sci. 2013;54(13):7871–84.
98. French AN, Morgan IG, Burlutsky G, Mitchell P, Rose KA. Prevalence and 5- to 6-year incidence and progression of myopia and hyperopia in Australian schoolchildren. Ophthalmology. 2013;120(7):1482–91.
99. Jones-Jordan LA, Sinnott LT, Manny RE, et al. Early childhood refractive error and parental history of myopia as predictors of myopia. Invest Ophthalmol Vis Sci. 2010;51(1):115–21.
100. Williams C, Miller LL, Gazzard G, Saw SM. A comparison of measures of reading and intelligence as risk factors for the development of myopia in a UK cohort of children. Br J Ophthalmol. 2008;92(8):1117–21.

101. Dirani M, Tong L, Gazzard G, et al. Outdoor activity and myopia in Singapore teenage children. Br J Ophthalmol. 2009;93(8):997.
102. Morgan IG. New perspectives on the prevention of myopia. Eye Sci. 2011;26(1):3.
103. Iwase A, Araie M, Tomidokoro A, et al. Prevalence and causes of low vision and blindness in a Japanese adult population: the Tajimi Study. Ophthalmology. 2006;113(8):1354–62.
104. Xu L, Wang Y, Li Y, Cui T, Li J, Jonas JB. Causes of blindness and visual impairment in urban and rural areas in Beijing: the Beijing Eye Study. Ophthalmology. 2006;113(7):1134 e1131–11.
105. You QS, Xu L, Yang H, Wang YX, Jonas JB. Five-year incidence of visual impairment and blindness in adult Chinese the Beijing Eye Study. Ophthalmology. 2011;118(6):1069–75.
106. Yamada M, Hiratsuka Y, Roberts CB, et al. Prevalence of visual impairment in the adult Japanese population by cause and severity and future projections. Ophthalmic Epidemiol. 2010;17(1):50–7.
107. Hsu WM, Cheng CY, Liu JH, Tsai SY, Chou P. Prevalence and causes of visual impairment in an elderly Chinese population in Taiwan: the Shihpai Eye Study. Ophthalmology. 2004;111(1):62–9.
108. Ohno-Matsui K, Lai TYY, Cheung CMG, Lai CC. Updates of pathologic myopia. Prog Retin Eye Res. 2016;52(5):156–87.
109. Ohno-Matsui K, Kawasaki R, Jonas JB, et al. International photographic classification and grading system for myopic maculopathy. Am J Ophthalmol. 2015;159(5):877–883 e877.
110. Spaide RF. Staphyloma: part 1. New York: Springer; 2014.
111. Fang Y, Yokoi T, Nagaoka N, et al. Progression of myopic maculopathy during 18-year follow-up. Ophthalmology. 2018;125:863–77.
112. Hayashi K, Ohno-Matsui K, Shimada N, et al. Long-term pattern of progression of myopic maculopathy: a natural history study. Ophthalmology. 2010;117(8):1595–611.
113. Yan YN, Wang YX, Yang Y, et al. Ten-year progression of myopic maculopathy: The Beijing Eye Study 2001-2011. Ophthalmology. 2018;125:1253–63.
114. Vongphanit J, Mitchell P, Wang JJ. Prevalence and progression of myopic retinopathy in an older population. Ophthalmology. 2002;109(4):704–11.
115. Xu L, Wang Y, Wang S, Jonas JB. High myopia and glaucoma susceptibility the Beijing Eye Study. Ophthalmology. 2007;114(2):216–20.
116. Nagaoka N, Jonas JB, Morohoshi K, et al. Glaucomatous-type optic discs in high myopia. PLoS One. 2015;10(10):e0138825.
117. Curtin BJ. The posterior staphyloma of pathologic myopia. Trans Am Ophthalmol Soc. 1977;75:67–86.
118. Ohno-Matsui K. Proposed classification of posterior staphylomas based on analyses of eye shape by three-dimensional magnetic resonance imaging. Ophthalmology. 2014;121(9):1798–809.
119. Neelam K, Cheung CM, Ohno-Matsui K, Lai TY, Wong TY. Choroidal neovascularization in pathological myopia. Prog Retin Eye Res. 2012;31(5):495–525.
120. Ohno-Matsui K, Yoshida T, Futagami S, et al. Patchy atrophy and lacquer cracks predispose to the development of choroidal neovascularisation in pathological myopia. Br J Ophthalmol. 2003;87(5):570–3.
121. Wolf S, Balciuniene VJ, Laganovska G, et al. RADIANCE: a randomized controlled study of ranibizumab in patients with choroidal neovascularization secondary to pathologic myopia. Ophthalmology. 2014;121(3):682–92.
122. Ikuno Y, Ohno-Matsui K, Wong TY, et al. Intravitreal aflibercept injection in patients with myopic choroidal neovascularization: The MYRROR Study. Ophthalmology. 2015;122(6):1220–7.
123. Panozzo G, Mercanti A. Optical coherence tomography findings in myopic traction maculopathy. Arch Ophthalmol. 2004;122(10):1455–60.
124. Gaucher D, Erginay A, Lecleire-Collet A, et al. Dome-shaped macula in eyes with myopic posterior staphyloma. Am J Ophthalmol. 2008;145(5):909–14.

125. Caillaux V, Gaucher D, Gualino V, Massin P, Tadayoni R, Gaudric A. Morphologic characterization of dome-shaped macula in myopic eyes with serous macular detachment. Am J Ophthalmol. 2013;156(5):958–67.
126. Ellabban AA, Tsujikawa A, Matsumoto A, et al. Three-dimensional tomographic features of dome-shaped macula by swept-source optical coherence tomography. Am J Ophthalmol. 2012;3(12):578.
127. Imamura Y, Iida T, Maruko I, Zweifel SA, Spaide RF. Enhanced depth imaging optical coherence tomography of the sclera in dome-shaped macula. Am J Ophthalmol. 2011;151(2):297–302.
128. Pope JM, Verkicharla PK, Sepehrband F, Suheimat M, Schmid KL, Atchison DA. Three-dimensional MRI study of the relationship between eye dimensions, retinal shape and myopia. Biomed Opt Express. 2017;8(5):2386–95.
129. Kuo AN, Verkicharla PK, McNabb RP, et al. Posterior eye shape measurement with retinal OCT compared to MRI. Invest Ophthalmol Vis Sci. 2016;57(9):196–203.
130. Samarawickrama C, Mitchell P, Tong L, et al. Myopia-related optic disc and retinal changes in adolescent children from singapore. Ophthalmology. 2011;118(10):2050–7.
131. Jonas JB, Jonas SB, Jonas RA, Holbach L, Panda-Jonas S. Histology of the parapapillary region in high myopia. Am J Ophthalmol. 2011;152(6):1021–9.
132. Park HY, Lee K, Park CK. Optic disc torsion direction predicts the location of glaucomatous damage in normal-tension glaucoma patients with myopia. Ophthalmology. 2012;119(9):1844–51.
133. Marcus MW, de Vries MM, Junoy Montolio FG, Jansonius NM. Myopia as a risk factor for open-angle glaucoma: a systematic review and meta-analysis. Ophthalmology. 2011;118(10):1989–1994.e1982.
134. Chang RT, Singh K. Myopia and glaucoma: diagnostic and therapeutic challenges. Curr Opin Ophthalmol. 2013;24(2):96–101.
135. Jonas JB, Gusek GC, Naumann GO. Optic disk morphometry in high myopia. Graefes Arch Clin Exp Ophthalmol. 1988;226(6):587–90.
136. Jonas JB, Nagaoka N, Fang YX, Weber P, Ohno-Matsui K. Intraocular pressure and glaucomatous optic neuropathy in high myopia. Invest Ophthalmol Vis Sci. 2017;58(13):5897–906.
137. Ohno-Matsui K, Shimada N, Yasuzumi K, et al. Long-term development of significant visual field defects in highly myopic eyes. Am J Ophthalmol. 2011;152(2):256–265 e251.
138. Han JC, Lee EJ, Kim SB, Kee C. The Characteristics of deep optic nerve head morphology in myopic normal tension glaucoma. Invest Ophthalmol Vis Sci. 2017;58(5):2695–704.
139. Johnson MW. Myopic traction maculopathy: pathogenic mechanisms and surgical treatment. Retina. 2012;32(Suppl 2):S205–10.
140. Wong CW, Phua V, Lee SY, Wong TY, Cheung CM. Is Choroidal or scleral thickness related to myopic macular degeneration? Invest Ophthalmol Vis Sci. 2017;58(2):907–13.
141. Ohno-Matsui K, Akiba M, Modegi T, et al. Association between shape of sclera and myopic retinochoroidal lesions in patients with pathologic myopia. Invest Ophthalmol Vis Sci. 2012;53(10):6046–61.
142. Shinohara K, Moriyama M, Shimada N, Yoshida T, Ohno-Matsui K. Characteristics of peripapillary staphylomas associated with high myopia determined by swept-source optical coherence tomography. Am J Ophthalmol. 2016;169:138–44.
143. Spaide RF. Choriocapillaris flow features follow a power law distribution: implications for characterization and mechanisms of disease progression. Am J Ophthalmol. 2016;170:58–67.
144. Zhang Q, Zheng F, Motulsky EH, et al. A novel strategy for quantifying choriocapillaris flow voids using swept-source OCT angiography. Invest Ophthalmol Vis Sci. 2018;59(1):203–11.
145. Al-Sheikh M, Phasukkijwatana N, Dolz-Marco R, et al. Quantitative OCT angiography of the retinal microvasculature and the choriocapillaris in myopic eyes. Invest Ophthalmol Vis Sci. 2017;58(4):2063–9.
146. Ang M, Devarajan K, Das S, et al. Comparison of anterior segment optical coherence tomography angiography systems for corneal vascularisation. Br J Ophthalmol. 2018;102(7):873–7.

147. Cai Y, Alio Del Barrio JL, Wilkins MR, Ang M. Serial optical coherence tomography angiography for corneal vascularization. Graefes Arch Clin Exp Ophthalmol. 2017;255(1):135–9.
148. Ang M, Cai Y, Shahipasand S, et al. En face optical coherence tomography angiography for corneal neovascularisation. Br J Ophthalmol. 2016;100(5):616–21.
149. Grudzinska E, Modrzejewska M. Modern diagnostic techniques for the assessment of ocular blood flow in myopia: current state of knowledge. J Ophthalmol. 2018;2018:8.
150. Silverman RH, Cannata J, Shung KK, et al. 75 MHz ultrasound biomicroscopy of anterior segment of eye. Ultrason Imaging. 2006;28(3):179–88.
151. Xie D, Li Q, Gao Q, Song W, Zhang HF, Yuan X. In vivo blind-deconvolution photoacoustic ophthalmoscopy with total variation regularization. J Biophotonics. 2018;11(9):e201700360.
152. Xu L, Wang Y, Wang S, Wang Y, Jonas JB. High myopia and glaucoma susceptibility the Beijing Eye Study. Ophthalmology. 2007;114(2):216–20.
153. Podos SM, Becker B, Morton WR. High myopia and primary open-angle glaucoma. Am J Ophthalmol. 1966;62(6):1038–43.
154. Greve EL, Furuno F. Myopia and glaucoma. Albrecht Von Graefes Arch Klin Exp Ophthalmol. 1980;213(1):33–41.
155. Daubs JG, Crick RP. Effect of refractive error on the risk of ocular hypertension and open angle glaucoma. Trans Ophthalmol Soc Aust. 1981;101(1):121–6.
156. Phelps CD. Effect of myopia on prognosis in treated primary open-angle glaucoma. Am J Ophthalmol. 1982;93(5):622–8.
157. Perkins ES, Phelps CD. Open angle glaucoma, ocular hypertension, low-tension glaucoma, and refraction. Arch Ophthalmol. 1982;100(9):1464–7.
158. Leske MC, Connell AM, Wu SY, Hyman LG, Schachat AP. Risk factors for open-angle glaucoma. The Barbados Eye Study. Arch Ophthalmol. 1995;113(7):918–24.
159. Chihara E, Liu X, Dong J, et al. Severe myopia as a risk factor for progressive visual field loss in primary open-angle glaucoma. Ophthalmologica. 1997;211(2):66–71.
160. Mitchell P, Hourihan F, Sandbach J, Wang JJ. The relationship between glaucoma and myopia: the Blue Mountains Eye Study. Ophthalmology. 1999;106(10):2010–5.
161. Grodum K, Heijl A, Bengtsson B. Refractive error and glaucoma. Acta Ophthalmol Scand. 2001;79(6):560–6.
162. Jonas JB, Martus P, Budde WM. Anisometropia and degree of optic nerve damage in chronic open-angle glaucoma. Am J Ophthalmol. 2002;134(4):547–51.
163. Wong TY, Klein BE, Klein R, Knudtson M, Lee KE. Refractive errors, intraocular pressure, and glaucoma in a white population. Ophthalmology. 2003;110(1):211–7.
164. Leske MC, Heijl A, Hussein M, et al. Factors for glaucoma progression and the effect of treatment: the early manifest glaucoma trial. Arch Ophthalmol. 2003;121(1):48–56.
165. Jonas JB, Budde WM. Optic nerve damage in highly myopic eyes with chronic open-angle glaucoma. Eur J Ophthalmol. 2005;15(1):41–7.
166. Kuzin AA, Varma R, Reddy HS, Torres M, Azen SP, Los Angeles Latino Eye Study G. Ocular biometry and open-angle glaucoma: the Los Angeles Latino Eye Study. Ophthalmology. 2010;117(9):1713–9.
167. Cohen SY, Laroche A, Leguen Y, Soubrane G, Coscas GJ. Etiology of choroidal neovascularization in young patients. Ophthalmology. 1996;103(8):1241–4.
168. Yoshida T, Ohno-Matsui K, Yasuzumi K, et al. Myopic choroidal neovascularization: a 10-year follow-up. Ophthalmology. 2003;110(7):1297–305.
169. Avila MP, Weiter JJ, Jalkh AE, Trempe CL, Pruett RC, Schepens CL. Natural history of choroidal neovascularization in degenerative myopia. Ophthalmology. 1984;91(12):1573–81.
170. Curtin BJ, Karlin DB. Axial length measurements and fundus changes of the myopic eye. I. The posterior fundus. Trans Am Ophthalmol Soc. 1970;68:312–34.
171. Lai TY, Cheung CM. Myopic choroidal neovascularization: diagnosis and treatment. Retina. 2016;36(9):1614–21.
172. Jia Y, Bailey ST, Wilson DJ, et al. Quantitative optical coherence tomography angiography of choroidal neovascularization in age-related macular degeneration. Ophthalmology. 2014;121(7):1435–44.

173. Virgili G, Menchini F. Laser photocoagulation for choroidal neovascularisation in pathologic myopia. Cochrane Database Syst Rev. 2005;4:CD004765.
174. Blinder KJ, Blumenkranz MS, Bressler NM, et al. Verteporfin therapy of subfoveal choroidal neovascularization in pathologic myopia: 2-year results of a randomized clinical trial--VIP report no. 3. Ophthalmology. 2003;110(4):667–73.
175. Verteporfin in Photodynamic Therapy Study G. Photodynamic therapy of subfoveal choroidal neovascularization in pathologic myopia with verteporfin. 1-year results of a randomized clinical trial--VIP report no. 1. Ophthalmology. 2001;108(5):841–52.
176. Chen Y, Sharma T, Li X, et al. Ranibizumab versus verteporfin photodynamic therapy in Asian patients with myopic choroidal neovascularization: brilliance, a 12-month, randomized, double-masked study. Retina. 2018. https://doi.org/10.1097/IAE.0000000000002292.
177. Tufail A, Narendran N, Patel PJ, et al. Ranibizumab in myopic choroidal neovascularization: the 12-month results from the REPAIR study. Ophthalmology. 2013;120(9):1944–1945.e1941.
178. Wu PC, Chen YJ, Chen YH, et al. Factors associated with foveoschisis and foveal detachment without macular hole in high myopia. Eye. 2009;23(2):356–61.
179. Baba T, Ohno-Matsui K, Futagami S, et al. Prevalence and characteristics of foveal retinal detachment without macular hole in high myopia. Am J Ophthalmol. 2003;135(3):338–42.
180. Fang X, Weng Y, Xu S, et al. Optical coherence tomographic characteristics and surgical outcome of eyes with myopic foveoschisis. Eye. 2009;23(6):1336–42.
181. VanderBeek BL, Johnson MW. The diversity of traction mechanisms in myopic traction maculopathy. Am J Ophthalmol. 2012;153(1):93–102.
182. Yeh SI, Chang WC, Chen LJ. Vitrectomy without internal limiting membrane peeling for macular retinoschisis and foveal detachment in highly myopic eyes. Acta Ophthalmol. 2008;86(2):219–24.
183. Smiddy WE, Kim SS, Lujan BJ, Gregori G. Myopic traction maculopathy: spectral domain optical coherence tomographic imaging and a hypothesized mechanism. Ophthalmic Surg Lasers Imaging. 2009;40(2):169–73.
184. Gaucher D, Haouchine B, Tadayoni R, et al. Long-term follow-up of high myopic foveoschisis: natural course and surgical outcome. Am J Ophthalmol. 2007;143(3):455–62.
185. Ikuno Y, Sayanagi K, Soga K, Oshima Y, Ohji M, Tano Y. Foveal anatomical status and surgical results in vitrectomy for myopic foveoschisis. Jpn J Ophthalmol. 2008;52(4):269–76.
186. Ikuno Y, Sayanagi K, Ohji M, et al. Vitrectomy and internal limiting membrane peeling for myopic foveoschisis. Am J Ophthalmol. 2004;137(4):719–24.
187. Kuhn F. Internal limiting membrane removal for macular detachment in highly myopic eyes. Am J Ophthalmol. 2003;135(4):547–9.
188. Panozzo G, Mercanti A. Vitrectomy for myopic traction maculopathy. Arch Ophthalmol. 2007;125(6):767–72.
189. Kumagai K, Furukawa M, Ogino N, Larson E. Factors correlated with postoperative visual acuity after vitrectomy and internal limiting membrane peeling for myopic foveoschisis. Retina. 2010;30(6):874–80.
190. Kwok AK, Lai TY, Yip WW. Vitrectomy and gas tamponade without internal limiting membrane peeling for myopic foveoschisis. Br J Ophthalmol. 2005;89(9):1180–3.
191. Tang J, Rivers MB, Moshfeghi AA, Flynn HW, Chan CC. Pathology of macular foveoschisis associated with degenerative myopia. J Ophthalmol. 2010;2010:175613.
192. Sayanagi K, Morimoto Y, Ikuno Y, Tano Y. Spectral-domain optical coherence tomographic findings in myopic foveoschisis. Retina. 2010;30(4):623–8.
193. Spaide RF, Fisher Y. Removal of adherent cortical vitreous plaques without removing the internal limiting membrane in the repair of macular detachments in highly myopic eyes. Retina. 2005;25(3):290–5.
194. Ikuno Y, Gomi F, Tano Y. Potent retinal arteriolar traction as a possible cause of myopic foveoschisis. Am J Ophthalmol. 2005;139(3):462–7.
195. Sayanagi K, Ikuno Y, Gomi F, Tano Y. Retinal vascular microfolds in highly myopic eyes. Am J Ophthalmol. 2005;139(4):658–63.

196. Benhamou N, Massin P, Haouchine B, Erginay A, Gaudric A. Macular retinoschisis in highly myopic eyes. Am J Ophthalmol. 2002;133(6):794–800.
197. Ripandelli G, Rossi T, Scarinci F, Scassa C, Parisi V, Stirpe M. Macular vitreoretinal interface abnormalities in highly myopic eyes with posterior staphyloma: 5-year follow-up. Retina. 2012;32(8):1531–8.
198. Michalewska Z, Michalewski J, Adelman RA, Nawrocki J. Inverted internal limiting membrane flap technique for large macular holes. Ophthalmology. 2010;117(10):2018–25.
199. Morizane Y, Shiraga F, Kimura S, et al. Autologous transplantation of the internal limiting membrane for refractory macular holes. Am J Ophthalmol. 2014;157(4):861–869 e861.
200. Leisser C, Hirnschall N, Doller B, et al. Internal limiting membrane flap transposition for surgical repair of macular holes in primary surgery and in persistent macular holes. Eur J Ophthalmol. 2018;28(2):225–8.
201. Ghosh B, Arora S, Goel N, et al. Comparative evaluation of sequential intraoperative use of whole blood followed by brilliant blue versus conventional brilliant blue staining of internal limiting membrane in macular hole surgery. Retina. 2016;36(8):1463–8.
202. Chen SN, Yang CM. Lens capsular flap transplantation in the management of refractory macular hole from multiple etiologies. Retina. 2016;36(1):163–70.
203. Alkabes M, Mateo C. Macular buckle technique in myopic traction maculopathy: a 16-year review of the literature and a comparison with vitreous surgery. Graefes Arch Clin Exp Ophthalmol. 2018;256(5):863–77.
204. Grewal DS, Mahmoud TH. Autologous neurosensory retinal free flap for closure of refractory myopic macular holes. JAMA Ophthalmol. 2016;134(2):229–30.
205. Chung K, Mohidin N, O'Leary DJ. Undercorrection of myopia enhances rather than inhibits myopia progression. Vis Res. 2002;42(22):2555–9.
206. Adler D, Millodot M. The possible effect of undercorrection on myopic progression in children. Clin Exp Optom. 2006;89(5):315–21.
207. Sun YY, Li SM, Li SY, et al. Effect of uncorrection versus full correction on myopia progression in 12-year-old children. Graefes Arch Clin Exp Ophthalmol. 2017;255(1):189–95.
208. Edwards MH, Li RW, Lam CS, Lew JK, Yu BS. The Hong Kong progressive lens myopia control study: study design and main findings. Invest Ophthalmol Vis Sci. 2002;43(9):2852–8.
209. Yang Z, Lan W, Ge J, et al. The effectiveness of progressive addition lenses on the progression of myopia in Chinese children. Ophthalmic Physiol Opt. 2009;29(1):41–8.
210. Correction of Myopia Evaluation Trial 2 Study Group for the Pediatric Eye Disease Investigator Group. Progressive-addition lenses versus single-vision lenses for slowing progression of myopia in children with high accommodative lag and near esophoria. Invest Ophthalmol Vis Sci. 2011;52(5):2749–57.
211. Berntsen DA, Sinnott LT, Mutti DO, Zadnik K. A randomized trial using progressive addition lenses to evaluate theories of myopia progression in children with a high lag of accommodation. Invest Ophthalmol Vis Sci. 2012;53(2):640–9.
212. Hasebe S, Jun J, Varnas SR. Myopia control with positively aspherized progressive addition lenses: a 2-year, multicenter, randomized, controlled trial. Invest Ophthalmol Vis Sci. 2014;55(11):7177–88.
213. Walline JJ, Lindsley K, Vedula SS, Cotter SA, Mutti DO, Twelker JD. Interventions to slow progression of myopia in children. Cochrane Database Syst Rev. 2011;12:CD004916.
214. Hasebe S, Ohtsuki H, Nonaka T, et al. Effect of progressive addition lenses on myopia progression in Japanese children: a prospective, randomized, double-masked, crossover trial. Invest Ophthalmol Vis Sci. 2008;49(7):2781–9.
215. Cheng D, Woo GC, Drobe B, Schmid KL. Effect of bifocal and prismatic bifocal spectacles on myopia progression in children: three-year results of a randomized clinical trial. JAMA Ophthalmol. 2014;132(3):258–64.
216. Lam CSY, Lee PK, Lam CSY, Tang WC, Lee PK, et al. Myopic control with multi-segment of myopic defocus (MSMD) spectacle lens: a randomized clinical trial. Birmingham, UK. 2017.
217. Sankaridurg P, Donovan L, Varnas S, et al. Spectacle lenses designed to reduce progression of myopia: 12-month results. Optom Vis Sci. 2010;87(9):631–41.

218. Kanda H, Oshika T, Hiraoka T, et al. Effect of spectacle lenses designed to reduce relative peripheral hyperopia on myopia progression in Japanese children: a 2-year multicenter randomized controlled trial. Jpn J Ophthalmol. 2018;62(5):537–43.
219. Walline JJ, Jones LA, Mutti DO, Zadnik K. A randomized trial of the effects of rigid contact lenses on myopia progression. Arch Ophthalmol. 2004;122(12):1760–6.
220. Katz J, Schein OD, Levy B, et al. A randomized trial of rigid gas permeable contact lenses to reduce progression of children's myopia. Am J Ophthalmol. 2003;136(1):82–90.
221. Cho P, Cheung SW, Edwards M. The longitudinal orthokeratology research in children (LORIC) in Hong Kong: a pilot study on refractive changes and myopic control. Curr Eye Res. 2005;30(1):71–80.
222. Kakita T, Hiraoka T, Oshika T. Influence of overnight orthokeratology on axial elongation in childhood myopia. Invest Ophthalmol Vis Sci. 2011;52(5):2170–4.
223. Cho P, Cheung SW. Retardation of myopia in Orthokeratology (ROMIO) study: a 2-year randomized clinical trial. Invest Ophthalmol Vis Sci. 2012;53(11):7077–85.
224. Hiraoka T, Kakita T, Okamoto F, Takahashi H, Oshika T. Long-term effect of overnight orthokeratology on axial length elongation in childhood myopia: a 5-year follow-up study. Invest Ophthalmol Vis Sci. 2012;53(7):3913–9.
225. Charm J, Cho P. High myopia-partial reduction ortho-k: a 2-year randomized study. Optom Vis Sci. 2013;90(6):530–9.
226. Wen D, Huang J, Chen H, et al. Efficacy and acceptability of orthokeratology for slowing myopic progression in children: a systematic review and meta-analysis. J Ophthalmol. 2015;2015:360806.
227. Sun Y, Xu F, Zhang T, et al. Orthokeratology to control myopia progression: a meta-analysis. PLoS One. 2015;10(4):e0124535.
228. Lee YC, Wang JH, Chiu CJ. Effect of orthokeratology on myopia progression: twelve-year results of a retrospective cohort study. BMC Ophthalmol. 2017;17(1):243.
229. Yen MY, Liu JH, Kao SC, Shiao CH. Comparison of the effect of atropine and cyclopentolate on myopia. Ann Ophthalmol. 1989;21(5):180–182, 187.
230. Kinoshita N, Konno Y, Hamada N, Kanda Y, Shimmura-Tomita M, Kakehashi A. Additive effects of orthokeratology and atropine 0.01% ophthalmic solution in slowing axial elongation in children with myopia: first year results. Jpn J Ophthalmol. 2018;62(5):544–53.
231. Young AL, Leung AT, Cheng LL, Law RW, Wong AK, Lam DS. Orthokeratology lens-related corneal ulcers in children: a case series. Ophthalmology. 2004;111(3):590–5.
232. Rah MJ, Walline JJ, Jones-Jordan LA, et al. Vision specific quality of life of pediatric contact lens wearers. Optom Vis Sci. 2010;87(8):560–6.
233. Walline JJ, Gaume A, Jones LA, et al. Benefits of contact lens wear for children and teens. Eye Contact Lens. 2007;33(6 Pt 1):317–21.
234. Benavente-Perez A, Nour A, Troilo D. Axial eye growth and refractive error development can be modified by exposing the peripheral retina to relative myopic or hyperopic defocus. Invest Ophthalmol Vis Sci. 2014;55(10):6765–73.
235. Li SM, Kang MT, Wu SS, et al. Studies using concentric ring bifocal and peripheral add multifocal contact lenses to slow myopia progression in school-aged children: a meta-analysis. Ophthalmic Physiol Opt. 2017;37(1):51–9.
236. Shih YF, Chen CH, Chou AC, Ho TC, Lin LL, Hung PT. Effects of different concentrations of atropine on controlling myopia in myopic children. J Ocul Pharmacol Ther. 1999;15(1):85–90.
237. Chua WH, Balakrishnan V, Chan YH, et al. Atropine for the treatment of childhood myopia. Ophthalmology. 2006;113(12):2285–91.
238. Chia A, Chua WH, Cheung YB, et al. Atropine for the treatment of childhood myopia: safety and efficacy of 0.5%, 0.1%, and 0.01% doses (Atropine for the Treatment of Myopia 2). Ophthalmology. 2012;119(2):347–54.
239. Tong L, Huang XL, Koh AL, Zhang X, Tan DT, Chua WH. Atropine for the treatment of childhood myopia: effect on myopia progression after cessation of atropine. Ophthalmology. 2009;116(3):572–9.

240. Chia A, Chua WH, Wen L, Fong A, Goon YY, Tan D. Atropine for the treatment of childhood myopia: changes after stopping atropine 0.01%, 0.1% and 0.5%. Am J Ophthalmol. 2014;157(2):451–457 e451.
241. Ashby R, Ohlendorf A, Schaeffel F. The effect of ambient illuminance on the development of deprivation myopia in chicks. Invest Ophthalmol Vis Sci. 2009;50(11):5348–54.
242. Seidemann A, Schaeffel F. Effects of longitudinal chromatic aberration on accommodation and emmetropization. Vis Res. 2002;42(21):2409–17.
243. Flitcroft DI. The complex interactions of retinal, optical and environmental factors in myopia aetiology. Prog Retin Eye Res. 2012;31(6):622–60.
244. Hung LF, Arumugam B, She Z, Ostrin L, Smith EL. Narrow-band, long-wavelength lighting promotes hyperopia and retards vision-induced myopia in infant rhesus monkeys. Exp Eye Res. 2018;176:147–60.

Global Epidemiology of Myopia

2

Saiko Matsumura, Cheng Ching-Yu, and Seang-Mei Saw

Key Points

- The prevalence of myopia in children is high in urban East Asian countries.
- The myopia and HM prevalence among young adults is much higher in East Asia than in Western countries.
- The burden of HM is huge because HM can cause PM changes and visual impairment.
- The prevalence of PM among adults has been relatively low, but it is likely to increase in future.
- It is important to develop public policies and preventive measures to retard the epidemic myopia.

S. Matsumura
Singapore Eye Research Institute, Singapore, Singapore
e-mail: matsumura.saiko@seri.com.sg

C. Ching-Yu
Singapore National Eye Centre, Singapore, Singapore

National University of Singapore, Singapore, Singapore

Duke-NUS Medical School, Singapore, Singapore
e-mail: chingyu.cheng@duke-nus.edu.sg

S.-M. Saw (✉)
Singapore Eye Research Institute, Singapore, Singapore

National University of Singapore, Singapore, Singapore

Saw Swee Hock School of Public Health, National University of Singapore, Singapore, Singapore
e-mail: ephssm@nus.edu.sg, saw.seang.mei@seri.com.sg

M. Ang, T. Y. Wong (eds.), *Updates on Myopia*,
https://doi.org/10.1007/978-981-13-8491-2_2

2.1 Introduction

Myopia has become a significant global public health and socioeconomic problem [1–4]. Developed countries, especially among East Asia, have been faced with high prevalence of myopia and high myopia (HM) and the same trend has been shown in other parts of the world with less extent [5, 6]. (The definition of myopia and HM is spherical equivalence (SE) of −0.50 diopters (D) or less and SE −5.00 D or −6.00 D, respectively.) The prevalence of myopia and HM in young adults in urban area of East Asian countries has risen to 80–90% and around 20%, respectively [7, 8]. According to a summary of 145 studies regarding the global prevalence of myopia and HM, there are approximately 1950 million (28.3% of the global population) and 277 million (4.0% of the global population) cases, and they are predicted to increase to 4758 million (49.8% of the global population) for myopia, and 938 million (9.8% of the global population) for HM by 2050 [9].

Most cases of myopia are considered as a benign condition because vision is corrected with spectacles, contact lenses, or refractive surgery. However, severe cases of myopia are associated with the risk of irreversible vision impairment and blindness due to pathological changes in retina, choroid, and sclera. One study has shown that 25% of HM will develop pathologic myopia (PM) and 50% of those with PM will have low vision as older adults. Thus, HM and PM are likely to increase drastically in the older generation. Based on the global prediction of HM on 2050, PM may increase to over 200 million in future [9]. Treatment strategies against PM have not been effective and costly [10]. Considering the burden of PM in the future, it is important to develop public policies and preventive and early interventional measures to retard the epidemic myopia. In this chapter, we summarize data on the prevalence of myopia and HM in different generations and the prevalence of PM from recent epidemiological studies.

2.2 Prevalence of Myopia in Children

In children, cycloplegic refraction is a common procedure to measure refractive error because children have a possibility to have an overestimation of myopic refraction, due to increased tone of the ciliary muscle and a constant accommodative effort during the examination, and makes the refraction overestimated approximately over −1 to −2 D [11, 12]. Many population-based studies on children have proved that the prevalence of myopia is higher in urbanized East Asian countries. In surveys of 12-year-old children, the prevalence of myopia is higher in Singapore (62.0%) [13], Hong Kong (53.1%) [14], and Guangzhou, China (49.7%) [15] than in the United States (20.0%) [16], Northern Ireland (17.7%) [17], Australia (11.9%) [18], urban India (9.7%) [19], Nepal (16.5%) [20], and Cambodia (6.0%) [21]. We summarized the prevalence of myopia among children in population studies using cycloplegic refraction between Asian countries (Table 2.1) and non-Asian countries (Table 2.2).

Table 2.1 Summary of prevalence of myopia and high myopia in children in population-based studies using cycloplegic refraction in Asian countries

Study (authors, year)	Location	Number	Race	Age (year)	Response rate (%)	Description of source	Prevalence (%)	95%CI
East Asian countries								
Hsu et al. (2016) [22]	Taipei, Taiwan	$N = 11{,}590$	Taiwanese	8	59.8	Citywide cohort study	M: 36.4% HM: –	NA
Lai et al. (2009) [23]	Kaohsiung, Taiwan	$N = 618$	Taiwanese	3–6	97.7	The screening nationwide programs for schools	M: 5.5% HM: –	(3.6–7.4%)
Lin et al. (2004) [7]	Taiwan	$N = 10{,}889$	Taiwanese	7–18	91.0	Cross-sectional surveys	M: 20.0% (7 years) M: 61.0% (12 years) M: 81.0% (15 years)	NA
Li (2017) [24]	Beijing, China	$N = 3676$	Chinese	15.25 ± 0.46	NA	School-based longitudinal study	M: 65.5% HM: 6.7% (≤ −6.0 D)	NA
Ma et al. (2016) [25]	Shanghai, China	$N = 8398$	Chinese	3–10	70.0	Random selection of 7 kindergartens and 7 primary schools	M: 20.1% HM: 0.33%	NA
Li et al. (2013) [26]	Rural area, China	$N = 1675$	Chinese	5–18	90.8	Random selection of geographically defined clusters	M: 5.0% HM: –	(4.8–5.4%)
Pi et al. (2012) [27]	Yongchuan, Suburban area, China	$N = 3070$	Chinese	6–15	NA	Random cluster sampling door-to-door surveys	M: 13.7% HM: –	NA
He (2007) [28]	Rural area, Guangdong, China	$N = 2454$	Chinese	13–17	NA	Stratified cluster sampling in 17 county schools	M: 42.4% HM: –	(35.8–49.0%)

(continued)

Table 2.1 (continued)

Study (authors, year)	Location	Number	Race	Age (year)	Response rate (%)	Description of source	Prevalence (%)	95%CI
He et al. (2004) [15]	Urban area, Guangzhou, China	$N = 4364$	Chinese	5–15	86.4	Random selection of geographically defined clusters	M: 38.1% HM: –	(36.3–39.8%)
Zhao et al. (2000) [29]	Shunyi, North east of Beijing, China	$N = 5884$	Chinese	5–15	95.9	Random selection of village-based clusters	M: 14.9% HM: –	NA
Fan et al. (2011) [30]	Hong Kong	$N = 601$ $N = 823$	Chinese	3–6	96.5 99.3	Random selection of kindergartens	M: 2.3% M: 6.3%	NA
Dirani et al. (2010) [31]	Singapore	$N = 2369$	Chinese	6M–6	72.3	Stratified random sampling, door-to-door surveys	M: 11.0% HM: 0.2%	(10.9–11.2%) (0.08–0.50%)
Saw et al. (2005) [13]	Singapore	$N = 1453$	Chinese	7–9	67.6	School-based cross-sectional study	M: 36.7% HM:	(34.2–39.2%)
Rest of Asian countries								
Murthy et al. (2002) [19]	New Delhi, India	$N = 6447$	Indian	5–15	92.0	Random selection of geographically defined clusters	M: 7.4%	(5.0%–9.7%)
Dandona et al. (2002) [32]	1 urban 3 rural areas, India	$N = 11786$	Indian	<15 >15	NA	Stratified random cluster sampling	M: 3.19% (<15) M: 19.45% (>15) HM: –	(2.24–4.13%) (17.88–21.02%)
Yekta et al. (2010) [33]	Shiraz, Iran	$N = 1854$	Iranian	7–15	87.9	Random cluster sampling	M: 4.4% HM:	(2.89–5.82%)
Jamali et al. (2009) [34]	Shahrood, Iran	$N = 815$	Iranian	6	NA	Random selection of primary schools	M: 1.7% HM: –	NA

Fotouhi et al. (2007) [35]	Rural area Dezful, Iran	$N = 5544$	Iranian	7–15	96.8	Random cluster sampling, selection of 460 schools	M: 3.4% HM: –	(2.5–4.4%)
Hashemi et al. (2004) [36]	Tehran, Iran	$N = 809$	Iranian	5–15	70.3	Stratified random cluster sampling, door-to-door surveys	M: 7.2% HM: –	(5.3–9.2%)
Sapkota et al. (2008) [20]	Rural area Kathmandu, Nepal	$N = 4282$	Aryan Mongol Tibetan	10–15	95.1	Stratified random selection of classes from secondary private schools	M: 19.0% HM: –	(17.8–20.2%)
Yingyong et al. (2010) [37]	Thailand	$N = 2360$	Thai	6–12	NA	Random selection of geographically defined clusters	M: 11.1% HM: –	NA

NA not applicable, ***M*** myopia, ***HM*** high myopia

Table 2.2 Summary of prevalence of myopia and high myopia in children in population-based studies using cycloplegic refraction in non-Asian countries

Study (authors, year)	Location	Number	Race	Age (year)	Response rate (%)	Description of source	Prevalence (%)	95%CI
Wen et al. (2013) [38]	LA, USA	$N = 1501$ $N = 1507$	NHW Asian	6M–6	NA	Population-based cohort study, door-to-door surveys	M: 1.2% (NHM) M: 3.98% (Asian) HM: –	(0.76–1.89%) (3.11–5.09%)
Giordano et al. (2009) [39]	Baltimore, USA	$N = 2298$	White A-A	6M–6	62	Population-based cohort study, door-to-door surveys	M: 0.7% (White) M: 5.5% (A-A) (Myopia <−1.0 D) HM: –	NA
Tideman (2018) [40]	The Netherlands	$N = 5711$	Euro non-Euro	6	68.4	Population-based birth cohort study	M: 2.4% HM: –	(2.13–5.10%)
Logan et al. (2011) [41]	England	$N = 327$ $N = 269$	Mix ethnicity	6–7 12–13	NA	Random selection of geographically defined clusters	M: 9.4% (6–7 years) M: 29.4% (12–13 years) HM: –	NA
O'Donoghue et al. (2010) [42]	Northern Ireland	$N = 661$ $N = 392$	Euro non-Euro	6–7 12–13	65.0	Random cluster sampling	M: 2.8% (6–7 years) M: 17.7% (12–13 years) HM: –	(1.3–4.3%) (13.2–22.2%)
Czepita et al. (2007) [43]	Poland	$N = 4422$	Euro	6–18	95.8	Random selection of elementary and secondary schools	M: 13.3% HM: –	NA
French et al. (2013) [44]	Sydney, Australia	$N = 2760$	Mix ethnicity	12	50.5	Random stratified cluster-sample of 55 schools	M: 18.9% (12 years) HM: 0.1% (12 years)	(7.5–30.4%)

Ip et al. (2008) [18]	Australia	$N = 2353$	Mix ethnicity	11–15	75.3	Random cluster-sample of 21 secondary schools	M: 11.9% HM: –	(6.6–17.2%)
Ojaimi et al. (2005) [45]	Australia	$N = 1765$	Mix ethnicity	5–8	79.0	Random stratified cluster-sample of schools	M: 1.43% HM: –	(0.94–2.18%)
Kumah et al. (2013) [46]	Ghana	$N = 2435$	African	12–15	99.2	Random selection of geographically defined clusters	M: 3.4% HM: –	(2.7–4.2%)
Naidoo et al. (2003) [47]	South Africa	$N = 4890$	African	5–15	87.3	Random selection of geographically defined clusters	M: 4.0% HM: –	(3.3–4.8%)

NA not applicable, *NHW* non-Hispanic White, *A-A* African-American, *Euro* European, *M* myopia, *HM* high myopia

2.2.1 Asian Countries

2.2.1.1 East Asian Countries and Singapore

Taiwanese school children have the highest prevalence of myopia among all school children worldwide. The prevalence of myopia among 8-year-old children is 36.4% in Taiwan [22], followed by 34.7% in Singapore [13], 30.8% in Shanghai [25] and 14.0% in Malaysia [48]. Lai et al. reported that the prevalence of myopia among 618 preschool Taiwanese children were also as high as 3.0%, 4.2%, 4.7%, and 12.2% in the age groups of 3, 4, 5, and 6 years, respectively [23]. A nationwide myopia survey in Taiwan showed that the prevalence of myopia among 7-year-olds increased from 5.8% in 1983 to 21% in 2000. At the age of 12, the prevalence of myopia was 36.7% in 1983 increasing to 61% in 2000, corresponding figures for 15-year-olds being 64.2% and 81%, respectively [7]. In China, Ma et al. reported that the prevalence of myopia in Shanghai was 20.1% among 3-year-old to 10-year-old children. They also showed that the prevalence increased dramatically from 5.2% in 6-year-old children and 14.3% in 7-year-old children to 52.2% in 10-year-old children [25]. In the urban city of Guangzhou, the prevalence of myopia was 7.7% in 7-year-old, 30.1% in 10-year-old, and 78.4% in 15-year-old children, with an overall prevalence of 38.1% among 4364 children aged 5–15 years [15]. In a rural area of Beijing, Zhao et al. reported that the prevalence of myopia among school children aged 5–7 and 14–15 years were 1.2% and 38.8%, respectively, with an overall prevalence of 14.9% among 5884 children aged 5–15 years [29]. In a suburban area, the prevalence of myopia among 3070 school children aged 6, 7, 10, and 14 years was 0.42%, 1.92%, 9.4%, and 28.8%, respectively [27]. In another rural area of northern China, the prevalence of myopia among 1675 school children aged 5–9, 10–14, and 15–18 years was 0.9%, 4.5%, and 8.2%, respectively, with an overall prevalence rate of 5.0% [49]. In Hong-Kong, 2 population-based surveys were conducted in children aged 3–6 years during 1996–1997 and 2006–2007, which revealed that prevalence of myopia increased 2.3–6.3% in a decade [30]. In Singapore, the school-based population study of the Singapore Cohort Study of Risk factors for Myopia (SCORM) showed that the prevalence of myopia was 29.0% in 7-year-olds, 34.7% in 8-year-olds, and 53.1% in 9-year-olds [50]. In younger ages from 6 months to 6 years, the Strabismus, Amblyopia, and Refractive Error in Singapore (STARS) Study reported that the prevalence of myopia was 11.0% in Chinese children [31].

2.2.1.2 Rest of Asian Countries

On the other hand, the prevalence of myopia is generally lower in other countries in Asia. In India, 6447 school children aged 5–15 years had 7.4% of the myopia prevalence in an urban population in New Delhi [19]. A population-based cross-sectional study was conducted among children in 1 urban and 3 rural areas. It reported that the prevalence of myopia among children ≤15 years of age and >15 years of age was 3.2% and 20.0%, respectively [32]. In Iran, the prevalence of myopia among 1854 school children aged 7, 10, and 14 years were 1.7%, 2.4%, and 7.6%, respectively, with an overall prevalence rate of 4.4% among 7-year-old to 15-year-old children in Shiraz [33]. In 4282 Nepalese secondary school children aged 10–15 years, the myopia prevalence was ranged from 10.9% in 10-year-olds to 27.3% in 15-year-olds [20]. In Thailand, the prevalence of myopia was 11.1% in 2360 children aged 6–12 years [37].

2.2.2 Non-Asian Countries

Nowadays, a rise of the myopia prevalence has also been shown in non-East-Asian countries that previously were only mildly or moderately affected, such as the UK, Australia, and the United States, although the prevalence is still lower than that in Asian countries. In the United States, the prevalence of myopia among 6–month-old to 6-year-old children was 1.20% and 3.98% in 1501 non-Hispanic White and 1507 Asian ethnicity children, respectively, as per the Multi-Ethnic Pediatric Eye Disease Study [38]. In the Baltimore Eye Study, the prevalence of myopia (SE <−1.00 D) was 1.2% in Whites, 6.6% in African-Americans among children aged 6 years, and an overall prevalence among 6-month-old to 71-month-old children was 0.7% and 5.5% in 1030 Whites and 1268 African-Americans, respectively [39]. Although few reports have been published on the prevalence of myopia in children in Europe, regional differences from country to country were shown even within the same geographical area. In England, the Aston Eye Study (AES) reported that the prevalence was 9.4% among children aged 6–7 years, and 29.4% among children aged 12–13 years, whereas the prevalence was 2.8% and 17.7% among children in the same age groups in Northern Ireland [17, 41]. In the Netherlands, the myopia prevalence rate was as low as 2.4% in 5711 children aged 6 years [40]. In Poland, the myopia prevalence was lower: 2.0% in 6-year-old, 8.4% in 8-year-old, and 14.7% in 12-year-old children [43]. In Australia, the Sydney Myopia Study (SMS) reported that myopia was present in 1.43% in 1765 children aged 7 years, with 0.79% in European children and 2.73% in other ethnicity children [45]. The Sydney Adolescent Vascular and Eye Study (SAVES) reported the myopia prevalence to be 18.9% among 12-year-old children, with 52.5% in East Asian, 8.6% in European Caucasian, and 12.0% in other ethnicity groups [44]. However, these ethnic differences may not be based solely on genetic differences. Studies on migrant populations suggest that the prevalence of myopia among Asian children living in non-Asian countries such as Australia is not as high as those living in East Asian countries [51]. Finally, in population-based studies, the lowest prevalence appears to be in Africa. The prevalence of myopia was 3.4% in 12-year-old to 15-year-old children in Ghana and 4.0% in 5-year-old to 15-year-old children in South Africa [46].

2.2.3 Urban and Rural Areas

Collectively, there are significant differences in the prevalence of myopia between urban areas and rural areas. In China, the prevalence of myopia was 38.1% in children aged 5–15 years in urban area, Guangzhou, whereas the prevalence of myopia was 5.0% in children aged 5–18 years in rural area. In an urban area,

Tehran, the prevalence of myopia was 7.2% in 809 children aged 5–15 years in the Tehran Eye Study, while a rural area, Dezful, had a lower prevalence of myopia which was 3.4% in children aged 7–15 years [35, 36]. A recent meta-analysis found a 2.6 times higher risk of developing myopia in children of urban residence compared with those who lived in rural areas [52]. These differences in the myopia prevalence among children may be caused by a rigorous education system which children especially living in urbanized are exposed to. Especially in Eastern Asian countries, academic success is important, and most children are enrolled in competitive, academically oriented schooling at a very early age [51]. It is influenced by enduring patterns of behavior and cultural attitudes that may result in the myopic environmental factors, such as higher levels of more intense near-work and lower levels of outdoor activity.

In summary, the prevalence of myopia in children is higher in East Asian countries (49.7–62.0% among 12-year-old children) compared with non-Asian countries and other Asian countries (6.0–20.0%). The prevalence of myopia has remained consistently high among Chinese children in urban settings, but the evidence does not support the idea that it is caused by purely genetic difference [53]. The association of an urbanized setting with high myopia rates is likely to be influenced by possible modifiable risk factors such as near-work and outdoor time.

2.3 Prevalence of Myopia and HM in Teenagers and Young Adults

2.3.1 East Asian Countries

The prevalence of myopia in young adults is more than 80% in urbanized East Asian countries (Table 2.3). A remarkable increase in the myopia and HM prevalence was seen in the past decades. In China, Chen et al. conducted a 15-year population-based survey using noncycloplegic autorefraction to investigate trends in the prevalence of myopia among 43,858 high school students in Fenghua city, eastern China, from 2001 to 2015. The overall prevalence of myopia and HM increased from 79.5% to 87.7% and 7.9% to 16.6%, respectively, during the 15-year period [54]. In Shandong, another city in eastern China, the prevalence of myopia and HM using cycloplegic autorefraction in school children aged 17 years was 84.6% and 13.9%, respectively [55]. A cross-sectional study among 5083 university students in Shanghai showed that 95.5% were myopic and 19.5% were high myopic (SE <−6.0 D) [56]. In Korea, the prevalence of myopia and HM (SE <−6.0 D) using cycloplegic autorefraction was higher in an urban population (96.5% and 21.6%) [8], compared to a rural population (83.3% and 6.8%) [26], among 19-year-old males in military conscripts. In Taiwan, the prevalence of myopia and HM (SE <−6.0 D) was 86.1% and 21.2%, respectively, in males aged 18–24 years in military conscripts [57]. In Singapore, the overall myopia and HM prevalence in 28,906 young males aged 16–25 years increased from 79.2% and 13.1% in 1996–1997 to 81.6% and 14.7% in 2009–2010, respectively [58].

Table 2.3 Summary of prevalence of myopia and high myopia in teenager and adolescent in East Asian countries

Study (authors, year)	Location	Number	Race gender	Age (year)	Refraction method	Response rate (%)	Description of source	Prevalence (%)	95% CI
Chen et al. (2018) [54]	Fenghua suburban, China	$N = 2932$	Chinese male/female	18.31 ± 0.60	Noncycloplegic autorefraction	NA	Population-based national college entrance examination	M: 87.7% HM: 16.6% (≤−6.0 D)	NA
Wu et al. (2013) [55]	Shandong, China	$N = 6026$	Chinese male/female	17	Cycloplegic autorefraction	94.7	Random cluster sampling in a cross-sectional school-based study design	M: 84.6% HM: 13.9%	(78.0–91.0%) (7.8–19.9%)
Sun et al. (2012) [56]	Shanghai, China	$N = 5083$	Chinese male/female	20.2 ± 2.8	Noncycloplegic autorefraction	92.8	Specific population of Chinese University students	M: 95.5% HM: 19.5% (≤−6.0 D)	(94.9–96.1%) (18.4–20.6%)
Lee et al. (2013) [26]	Rural area, South Korea	$N = 02805$	Korean male	19	Cycloplegic autorefraction	100	Population-based male compulsory conscripts	M: 83.3% HM: 6.8% (≤−6.0 D)	(81.8–84.7%)
Jung et al. (2012) [8]	South Korea	$N = 23{,}616$	Korean male	19	Cycloplegic autorefraction	100	Population-based male compulsory conscripts	M: 96.5% HM: 21.6% (≤−6.0 D)	(96.3–96.8%) (20.5–22.8%)
Lee et al. (2013) [57]	Taiwan	$N = 5048$	Chinese male	18–24	Noncycloplegic autorefraction	98.1	Population-based Male compulsory conscripts	M: 86.1% HM: 21.2% (≤−6.0 D)	NA
Koh et al. (2014) [58]	Singapore	$N = 28{,}908$	Chinese Malay Indian male	19.8 ± 1.2	Noncycloplegic autorefraction	99.9	Population-based male compulsory conscripts	M: 81.6% HM: 14.7%	(81.1–82.0%) (14.3–15.1%)

NA not applicable, *M* myopia, *HM* high myopia

2.3.2 Rest of East Asian Countries

In contrast to the uniformly high prevalence in Eastern Asian countries, the prevalence of myopia and HM in young adult populations in other countries varies among different ethnicity and geography (Table 2.4). In Israel, a 13-year series of population-based prevalence survey was conducted on young adults aged 16–22 years during the years 1990–2002. The overall prevalence of myopia and HM (SE <−6.0 D) using noncycloplegic autorefraction increased from 20.3% and 1.7% in 1990 to 28.3% and 2.05% in 2002, respectively [59]. In the Tehran Eye Study, the prevalence of myopia using cycloplegic autorefraction was 29.3% among young adults aged 16–25 years [36]. In Australia, the prevalence of myopia was 20.4% in a population-based cohort using cycloplegic autorefraction in mostly White subjects aged 19–22 years [60]. In the Sydney Adolescent Vascular and Eye Study (SAVES), myopia was present in 30.8%, with 59.1% in East Asian, 17.7% in European Caucasian, and 34.9% in other ethnicity group; and HM (SE <−6.00 D) was present in 1.9% among 17-year-old young adults [44]. In Europe, the prevalence of myopia and HM (SE <−6.50 D) among 4681 Danish conscripts was 12.8% and 0.3%, respectively [61]. A population-based study in Norway reported that 35.0% were myopic among 1248 young adults aged 20–25 years [62]. In the United States, the myopic prevalence rate was 27.7% in young adults aged 18–24 years [63].

As shown above, the myopia prevalence among young adults in East Asia is much higher than in Western countries. This is most likely reflecting the higher myopia prevalence among school children in Eastern Asia and can be further accelerated by their education system. This age population usually spend much time in study and are expected to achieve high scores for competitive college entrance examination, especially in Asia. In one study conducted in China, the prevalence of myopia in postgraduates was higher than in undergraduates [56], suggesting that associated factors, such as higher school achievement and prolonged near-work and less outdoor time, might contribute to the increasing prevalence of myopia [51]. We summarized the myopia prevalence in East Asian countries (Table 2.3) and rest of East Asian countries (Table 2.4). When comparing the results, we must be cautious because some conscript-based studies investigated only men, and conducted eye examination without cycloplegic refraction, which may make the refraction overestimated approximately over −0.50 D in younger adults [64].

2.4 Prevalence of Myopia and HM in Adults

In adults, the prevalence rates of myopia vary widely with age reflecting the hyperopic shift by aging in older generations. According to the results from the Beaver Dam Eye Study, the prevalence of myopia was likely to decrease with age among individuals aged above 43 years [65]. Wong et al. showed that the highest prevalence of myopia was in the age group of 40 years and above 70 years among Chinese-Singaporean adults aged 40–81 years old [66]. It suggested that the prevalence in elderly adults older 70 years could be overestimated due to lens nuclear sclerosis

Table 2.4 Summary of prevalence of myopia and high myopia in teenager and adolescent in rest of East Asian countries

Study (authors, year)	Location	Number	Race gender	Age (year)	Refraction method	Response rate (%)	Description of source	Prevalence (%)	95%CI
Bar Dayan et al. (2005) [59]	Israel	$N = 919{,}929$	Male/ female	16–22	Noncycloplegic autorefraction		Retrospective study, based on 13 repeated prevalence surveys	M: 28.3% HM: 2.0% (M) HM: 2.3% (F) (≤−6.0 D)	NA
Hashemi (2004) [36]	Tehran, Iran	$N = 974$	Iranian male/ female	16–25	Cycloplegic autorefraction	70.3	Stratified random cluster sampling, door-to-door surveys	M: 29.3%	(26.0–32.7%)
McKnight et al. (2014) [60]	Australia	$N = 1315$	Mix ethnicity male/ female	19–22	Cycloplegic autorefraction	97.8	Population-based cross-sectional study	M: 20.4% HM: –	(21.4–25.9%)
French (2013) [44]	Australia	$N = 1157$	Mix ethnicity male/ female	17	Cycloplegic autorefraction	51.5	Random stratified cluster-sample of 55 schools	M: 30.8% HM: 1.9%	(22.5–39.0%)
Jacobsen et al. (2007) [61]	Denmark	$N = 4681$	Danish male	19.3 ± 1.6	Noncycloplegic autorefraction	NA	Population-based male compulsory conscripts	M: 12.8% HM: 0.3% (≤−6.5 D)	(11.8–13.8%) (0.2–0.5%)
Midelfart et al. (2002) [62]	Norway	$N = 1248$	Euro male/ female	20–25	Noncycloplegic autorefraction	NA	Population-based sample in a health study (HUNT)	M: 35.0% HM: –	NA
Sperduto et al. (1983) [63]	USA	$N = 9882$	Mix male/ female	18–24	Noncycloplegic autorefraction	69.9	Population-based sample in a National Health Nutrition Examination Survey	M: 27.7%	NA

NA not applicable, *Euro* European, *M* myopia, *HM* high myopia

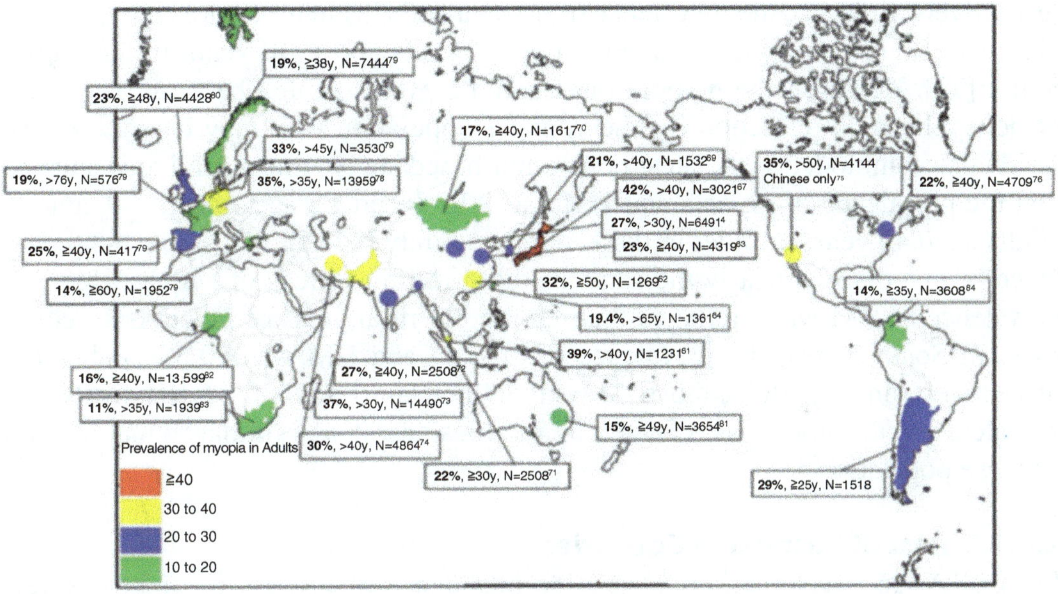

Fig. 2.1 Reported prevalence of myopia in adult population based on population studies

inducing refractive myopia. Population-based data indicate that Asian adult population is more susceptible to myopia compared with similarly aged western population. However, compared to the prevalence of myopia in children, the regional difference is not obvious in adults. We summarized the prevalence of myopia in adult population-based studies in the world (Fig. 2.1). It must be noted that there is lack of consensus in definitions of myopia and HM, and the definition varies among studies and that there is a difference of age population affecting by nuclear cataract, thus not directly comparable among different studies.

2.4.1 Asian Countries

2.4.1.1 East Asian Countries

In China, the prevalence of myopia and HM (SE <−6.0 D) was 32.3% and 5.0%, respectively, in 1269 adults aged 50 or more years in the Liwan Eye Study [67] conducted in an urban city of Guangzhou. In rural areas, 26.7% were myopic and 1.8% were high myopic in 6491 adults aged 30 or more years in the Handan Eye Study [4]. The Beijing Eye Study reported that the myopia and HM (SE <−6.0 D) prevalence was 22.9% and 2.6%, respectively, in 4319 adults aged 40 or more years in urban and rural Chinese populations [68]. However, these data may lead to substantial underestimation of the myopia prevalence because refraction data were obtained only from those with visual impairment. In Taiwan, the Shinpai Eye Study in adults aged over 65 years reported that the prevalence of myopia and HM (SD <−6.0 D) was 19.4% and 2.4%, respectively [69]. In Singapore, the prevalence of myopia in Singaporean-Chinese, Malay, and Indians was 38.7% [66], 26.2% [70], and 28.0% [71], and corresponding figures for HM being 9.1%, 3.9%, and 4.1%, respectively. In Japan, the prevalence of myopia and HM in urban areas is relatively high, 41.8% and 8.2%, respectively, in 3021 adults above 40 years in the Tajimi Study [72]. However, the myopia rates may be overestimated because of the use of noncycloplegic refraction for the younger population who may have excessive residual accommodation. A latest population-based study from a rural area showed that the prevalence of myopia and HM was 29.5% and 1.9%, respectively, among adults aged 40 years or older in the Kumejima Study [73]. In this study, the prevalence of myopia was nearly the same as those in urban areas of China, while the prevalence of HM was similar to that reported in rural areas of other Asian countries. In South Korea, the prevalence of myopia and HM was 20.5% and 1.0%, respectively, among adults above 40 years in the Namil Study [74]. Relatively low prevalence in the study was reflected by rural lesions, it was similar to that of rural Chinese population.

2.4.1.2 Rest of East Asian Countries

In other Asian developing countries, the prevalence of myopia is slightly lower: 17.2% among adults aged 40 or more years in Mongolia, and 22.1% among adults aged 30 or more years in Bangladesh [75, 76]. Further, the myopia rate in the Bangladesh study may be overestimated because of the use of noncycloplegic refraction for the younger group aged 30–39 years who may have excessive residual accommodation. In a rural area in India, the prevalence of myopia and HM was 27.0% and 3.7%, respectively, in 2508 Indian adults aged above 39 years [77]. Relatively high prevalence in rural Indian population may be caused by higher rates of nuclear cataract. The prevalence of myopia is slightly higher at 36.5% among adults aged 30 or more years in Pakistan, and at 30.2% among adults aged 40 or more years in Iran [78, 79]. The myopia rate in the Pakistan study may be overestimated because of the cohort effect of younger group aged 30–39 years.

2.4.2 Non-Asian Countries

In the USA, the latest report in the Chinese American study showed the relatively high prevalence of myopia and HM, 35.1% and 7.4%, respectively, in 4144 Chinese adults aged 50 years or older [80]. This result is similar to or slightly higher than same Chinese populations from other studies in urban Asian countries (38.7% in the Tanjong Pagar Study, Singapore and 32.3% in the Liwan Eye Study). The Barbados Eye Study reported the prevalence of myopia was 21.9% in 4709 African-Americans aged 40–84 years [81]. Another population-based study in Latino showed that the overall prevalence of myopia (SE <-1.00 D) and HM in the worse eye was 16.8% and 2.4%, respectively, among 5927 adults aged 40 years or older [82]. In Europe, although the myopia rate varies across the countries, two latest population-based studies proved that it was nearly the same as those in urban Asian countries. The Gutenburg Health Study in Germany reported that the prevalence of myopia and HM was 35.1% and 5.6%, respectively, in 13,959 adults aged 35–74 years. The high prevalence of myopia in the study can be explained by the fact that this cohort had younger participants than most other studies [83]. In the Netherlands, the prevalence of myopia was 32.5% in a total of 3530 adults aged above 46 years in the Rotterdam study [84]. This study may have overestimated the prevalence of myopia because the refraction method was subjective refraction. In UK, a population-based study showed that 23.0% were myopic among a total of 7444 adults aged above 48 years [85]. In other European countries, the prevalence of myopia is slightly lower: 19.4% among adults aged 38 or more years in Norway, 19.1% among adults aged 76 or more years in France, and 14.2% among adults aged 60 or more years in Greece [84]. In Australia, the prevalence of myopia was relatively lower, 15.0% in 3654 adults aged over 49 years in the Blue Mountain Eye Study in 1999 [86]. In the two population-based studies, the lowest prevalence appears to be in Africa. In Nigeria, the prevalence of myopia and HM was 16.1% and 2.1%, respectively, among 13,599 adults aged over 40 years as per the Nigeria National Blindness and Visual Impairment Study [87]. In South Africa, the prevalence of myopia was 11.4% in 1939 adults aged over 35 years [88]. In the same vein, the prevalence of myopia was relatively low 14.4% among adults aged 35–55 years in MIROR Study in Colombia [89].

2.4.3 Generational Gap

There is a difference in myopia and HM prevalence among age groups. In general, the generational differences of prevalence of myopia and HM are seen with the highest rates in young adults and the lowest rates in older adults. We have shown the higher prevalence rates of myopia (65.5–96.5%) and HM (14.7–21.6%) in East Asian young adults in the previous section [8, 57, 58]. By contrast, the lower prevalence rates of myopia (approximately 25–40%) and HM (2.4–8.2%) were reported among East Asian middle-aged and elderly adults [69, 72, 90]. Particularly, the burden of HM is important because HM is more likely to develop PM changes that tend to be visually disabling. Some studies supported the idea of two types of HM, one is related to educational parameters such as near-work and frequent among young adults, and the other is more likely related to the earlier onset of myopia by genetic factors in contrast to environmental factors and occurs in older adults [91, 92]. Jonas et al. compared highly myopic young individuals and highly myopic adult individuals and assessed the association of the prevalence of HM with parameters of education. It revealed that education-related parameters did not show a clear association with HM in older generation, while in contrast, HM in school children showed a strong association with education [91]. Thus, it has been assumed that the development of pathologic myopia (PM) in later life may be different depending on two forms of HM with different etiologies. One form of HM is caused by mutations of genes responsible to scleral modeling and leading to abnormal deformity and thin sclera [93], while the other form caused by insufficient outdoor time in younger adults may be driven by reduced release of retinal dopamine [1].

In summary, the higher prevalence rates of myopia were also seen in urban East Asian countries (approximately 25–40%) and in Western Europe or the United States (approximately 20–35%), compared to other developing Asian countries and some countries in Western populations such as Australia (approximately 15–20%). Similarly, urban Asian countries have higher prevalence rates of HM (5–9%), compared with other Asian countries (2–5%) or non-Asian countries (2–7%). However, the geographic difference of myopia prevalence in older populations is not pronounced compared to that in younger populations. From a viewpoint of ethnicity difference, Chinese have a substantially higher prevalence of myopia compared with other racial groups, and a similar pattern of even greater magnitude was seen in HM prevalence. The prevalence of myopia and HM in Chinese ethnicity in western countries is similar to other studies of Chinese in urban Asian countries [80].

2.5 The Prevalence of PM

Pathologic myopia (PM) has been reported as one of the most common causes of blindness worldwide. Studies reported that PM is the major cause of blindness or visual impairment (VI) in 7% in Western populations and in 12–27% in Asian populations [94–99]. According to a review to estimate blindness and VI with myopic macular degeneration (MMD), 10.0 million people had VI from MMD (0.13%), 3.3 million of whom were blind (0.04%) in 2015, and furthermore 55.7 million people will have VI from MMD (0.33%), 18.5 million of whom will be blind (0.19%) in 2050 [100].

Before we discuss the prevalence of PM in detail, it must be noted that the definition of PM has been inconsistent in previous studies. Avila et al. proposed a definition of myopic maculopathy that included posterior staphyloma, and it has been used most frequently in earlier studies [101]. However, this classification was not based on the actual progression pattern. In 2015, the META-analysis for Pathologic Myopia (META-PM) study group proposed a new classification system for PM for use in future studies [102]. In this classification, myopic macular degeneration (MMD) is categorized into 5 categories according to severity: no myopic retinal lesions (category 0); tessellated fundus only (category 1); diffuse chorioretinal atrophy (category 2); patchy chorioretinal atrophy (category 3); and macula atrophy (category 4). And three additional lesions of MMD that cause central vision loss were included as plus sign: lacquer cracks, myopic choroidal neovascularization (CNV), Fuchs spot. PM is defined if an eye has category 2 or above, or presence of plus sign, or the presence of posterior staphyloma. We summarized population-based studies on PM prevalence in adult populations (Fig. 2.2).

In China, the Beijing Eye Study showed a high PM prevalence, 3.1%, among 4319 Chinese subjects aged 40 years or older [103]. PM was defined with myopic chorioretinal atrophy or staphyloma or lacquer cracks or Fuch's spot. In the same definition, the Handan Eye Study showed that the prevalence of PM and HM was 0.9% and 2.1%, respectively, among 6603 Chinese subjects aged 30 years or older

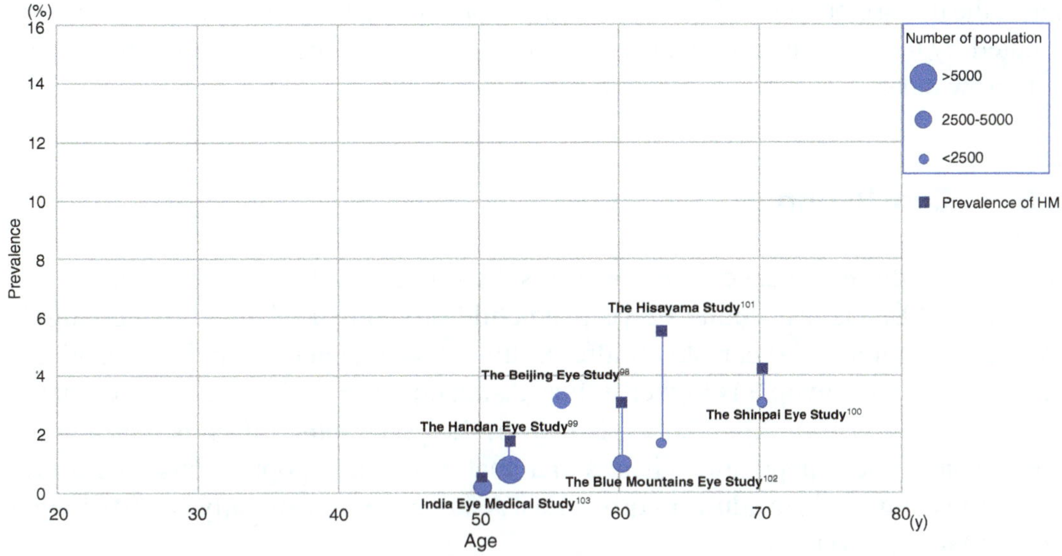

Fig. 2.2 Prevalence of pathologic myopia (PM) among adults in population-based studies

[104]. The much lower prevalence in this study than Beijing might be due to urban and rural differences. Among 1058 Taiwanese subjects aged 65 years or older in the Shinpai Eye study, the prevalence of PM and HM was 3% and 4.2%, respectively, with the definition by Avila et al. [105]. The high prevalence was influenced by its older population than other population-based studies. The Hisayama study reported the prevalence of PM and HM was 1.7% and 5.7%, respectively, among 1892 Japanese aged 40 years or older with the definition of PM as myopic chorioretinal atrophy, lacquer cracks, or Fuch's spot [106]. However, this study cannot exclude the possibility of sampling bias because the response rate was only 44.4%. In Western countries, the Blue Mountain Eye Study was performed in 3583 adults aged 49 years or older, who were mainly White urban population of Australia, using the same PM definition with two studies in China [107]. The prevalence of PM and HM was 1.2% and 2.7%, respectively. Using the new META-PM classification, the prevalence of PM and HM was 0.2% and 0.5%, respectively, among 4561 Indian subjects aged 30 years or older in rural central India [108]. However, the population in this study may not be adequately representative of the whole population of India because this study was conducted in rural tribal regions.

As shown above, the prevalence of PM among adult populations was relatively low in the world. Furthermore, the prevalence of PM among middle-aged and elderly adults is higher in urban East Asian populations (1.7–3.1%) than rural Asian populations (0.2–0.9%) and non-Asian populations (1.2%) [109]. It is consistent with the results of higher prevalence of HM in East Asian countries because the risk of PM increases with HM [109]. Both the prevalence and severity of PM become higher in adult population aged 40 years and with severe high myopia. Compared to the PM prevalence in adult populations, adolescents and children have significantly lower prevalence [27, 110]. It supports the idea that myopic macular changes are time-dependent changes as a result of mechanical stretching of the retina from axial elongation. However, a recent report revealed that myopia-related changes of the optic disc and macula were commonly found in highly myopic eyes in young adults [111].

Thus, the disease burden of PM due to high myopia is likely to increase in future, contributed by the aging effect where young adults who have high rates of high myopia will grow older.

2.6 Conclusion

In children, the prevalence of myopia is substantially higher in urban East Asian countries (49.7–62.0% among 12-year-old children) compared with other countries (6.0–20.0% among 12-year-old children). Similarly, in teenagers and young adults, the prevalence of myopia is higher in East Asian countries (65.5–96.5%) compared with other countries (12.8–35.0%). However, the geographic difference of myopia prevalence in older populations is less than that of younger populations. The prevalence rates of myopia in adults in urban East Asian countries are only slightly higher than in Western countries.

A relationship between myopia prevalence and community development is apparent, and most data have shown urban areas have a higher prevalence of myopia than rural areas. The association of an urbanized environment with myopia development in Asia could be mediated by factors such as intensive education and greater levels of near-work and less outdoor time. Overall, the prevalence of myopia in child population seems to be strongly related to the region where they grow up and the environmental factors such as urbanization, economy, and education.

Generational differences are seen with the highest rates in young adults (myopia 65.5–96.5% and HM 6.8–21.6%) and the lowest rates in older adults (myopia 25.0–40.0% and HM 2.4–8.2%). The disease progression pattern of HM and subsequent development of PM may be different between young adults and older adults due to generational differences, or changes in the lifestyle factors such as the education system and near-work and outdoor time exposure in rapidly developing urban Asian countries.

Current data show a relatively low prevalence of PM among middle-aged and elderly adults so far, and PM increases with age over 40 years and severity of myopia. Despite the relatively low prevalence in general population, PM is the major cause of blindness or visual impairment in both Asian populations and Western populations. According to a previous study, early grades of PM lesions are observed in young highly myopic adults in urban Asian population, and these structure changes are likely to worsen with age [111]. Considering the increasing prevalence of HM among young generations, we must be prepared for the expected increase of disease burden of PM in the near future.

References

1. Dolgin E. The myopia boom. Nature. 2015;519(7543):276–8.
2. Vitale S, Cotch MF, Sperduto RD. Prevalence of visual impairment in the United States. JAMA. 2006;295(18):2158–63.
3. Zheng YF, Pan CW, Chay J, Wong TY, Finkelstein E, Saw SM. The economic cost of myopia in adults aged over 40 years in Singapore. Invest Ophthalmol Vis Sci. 2013;54(12):7532–7.

4. Liang YB, Wong TY, Sun LP, Tao QS, Wang JJ, Yang XH, et al. Refractive errors in a rural Chinese adult population the Handan eye study. Ophthalmology. 2009;116(11):2119–27.
5. Morgan IG, Ohno-Matsui K, Saw S-M. Myopia. Lancet. 2012;379(9827):1739–48.
6. Morgan IG. What public policies should be developed to deal with the epidemic of myopia? Optom Vis Sci. 2016;93(9):1058–60.
7. Lin LL, Shih YF, Hsiao CK, Chen CJ. Prevalence of myopia in Taiwanese school children: 1983 to 2000. Ann Acad Med. 2004;33(1):27–33.
8. Jung SK, Lee JH, Kakizaki H, Jee D. Prevalence of myopia and its association with body stature and educational level in 19-year-old male conscripts in Seoul, South Korea. Invest Ophthalmol Vis Sci. 2012;53(9):5579–83.
9. Holden BA, Fricke TR, Wilson DA, Jong M, Naidoo KS, Sankaridurg P, et al. Global prevalence of myopia and high myopia and temporal trends from 2000 through 2050. Ophthalmology. 2016;123(5):1036–42.
10. Wong TY, Ferreira A, Hughes R, Carter G, Mitchell P. Epidemiology and disease burden of pathologic myopia and myopic choroidal neovascularization: an evidence-based systematic review. Am J Ophthalmol. 2014;157(1):9–25.e12.
11. Zhao J, Mao J, Luo R, Li F, Pokharel GP, Ellwein LB. Accuracy of noncycloplegic autorefraction in school-age children in China. Optom Vis Sci. 2004;81(1):49–55.
12. Fotedar R, Rochtchina E, Morgan I, Wang JJ, Mitchell P, Rose KA. Necessity of cycloplegia for assessing refractive error in 12-year-old children: a population-based study. Am J Ophthalmol. 2007;144(2):307–9.
13. Saw SM, Tong L, Chua WH, Chia KS, Koh D, Tan DT, et al. Incidence and progression of myopia in Singaporean school children. Invest Ophthalmol Vis Sci. 2005;46(1):51–7.
14. Fan DS, Lam DS, Lam RF, Lau JT, Chong KS, Cheung EY, et al. Prevalence, incidence, and progression of myopia of school children in Hong Kong. Invest Ophthalmol Vis Sci. 2004;45(4):1071–5.
15. He M, Zeng J, Liu Y, Xu J, Pokharel GP, Ellwein LB. Refractive error and visual impairment in urban children in Southern China. Invest Ophthalmol Vis Sci. 2004;45(3):793–9.
16. Zadnik K. The Glenn A. Fry Award Lecture (1995). Myopia development in childhood. Optom Vis Sci. 1997;74(8):603–8.
17. O'Donoghue L, Kapetanankis VV, McClelland JF, Logan NS, Owen CG, Saunders KJ, et al. Risk factors for childhood myopia: findings from the NICER study. Invest Ophthalmol Vis Sci. 2015;56(3):1524–30.
18. Ip JM, Huynh SC, Robaei D, Kifley A, Rose KA, Morgan IG, et al. Ethnic differences in refraction and ocular biometry in a population-based sample of 11-15-year-old Australian children. Eye. 2008;22(5):649–56.
19. Murthy GV, Gupta SK, Ellwein LB, Munoz SR, Pokharel GP, Sanga L, et al. Refractive error in children in an urban population in New Delhi. Invest Ophthalmol Vis Sci. 2002;43(3):623–31.
20. Sapkota YD, Adhikari BN, Pokharel GP, Poudyal BK, Ellwein LB. The prevalence of visual impairment in school children of upper-middle socioeconomic status in Kathmandu. Ophthalmic Epidemiol. 2008;15(1):17–23.
21. Gao Z, Meng N, Muecke J, Chan WO, Piseth H, Kong A, et al. Refractive error in school children in an urban and rural setting in Cambodia. Ophthalmic Epidemiol. 2012;19(1):16–22.
22. Hsu CC, Huang N, Lin PY, Tsai DC, Tsai CY, Woung LC, et al. Prevalence and risk factors for myopia in second-grade primary school children in Taipei: a population-based study. J Chin Med Assoc. 2016;79(11):625–32.
23. Lai YH, Hsu HT, Wang HZ, Chang SJ, Wu WC. The visual status of children ages 3 to 6 years in the vision screening program in Taiwan. J AAPOS. 2009;13(1):58–62.
24. Li Y, Liu J, Qi P. The increasing prevalence of myopia in junior high school students in the haidian district of beijing, china: A 10-year population-based survey. BMC Ophthalmol. 2017;17:88.
25. Ma Y, Qu X, Zhu X, Xu X, Zhu J, Sankaridurg P, et al. Age-specific prevalence of visual impairment and refractive error in children aged 3-10 years in Shanghai, China. Invest Ophthalmol Vis Sci. 2016;57(14):6188–96.

26. Lee JH, Jee D, Kwon JW, Lee WK. Prevalence and risk factors for myopia in a rural Korean population. Invest Ophthalmol Vis Sci. 2013;54(8):5466–71.
27. Pi LH, Chen L, Liu Q, Ke N, Fang J, Zhang S, et al. Prevalence of eye diseases and causes of visual impairment in school-aged children in Western China. J Epidemiol. 2012;22(1):37–44.
28. He M, Huang W, Zheng Y, Huang L, Ellwein LB. Refractive error and visual impairment in school children in rural southern china. Ophthalmology. 2007;114:374–82.
29. Zhao J, Pan X, Sui R, Munoz SR, Sperduto RD, Ellwein LB. Refractive error study in children: results from Shunyi District, China. Am J Ophthalmol. 2000;129(4):427–35.
30. Fan DS, Lai C, Lau HH, Cheung EY, Lam DS. Change in vision disorders among Hong Kong preschoolers in 10 years. Clin Exp Ophthalmol. 2011;39(5):398–403.
31. Dirani M, Chan YH, Gazzard G, Hornbeak DM, Leo SW, Selvaraj P, et al. Prevalence of refractive error in Singaporean Chinese children: the strabismus, amblyopia, and refractive error in young Singaporean Children (STARS) study. Invest Ophthalmol Vis Sci. 2010;51(3):1348–55.
32. Dandona R, Dandona L, Srinivas M, Giridhar P, McCarty CA, Rao GN. Population-based assessment of refractive error in India: the Andhra Pradesh eye disease study. Clin Exp Ophthalmol. 2002;30(2):84–93.
33. Yekta A, Fotouhi A, Hashemi H, Dehghani C, Ostadimoghaddam H, Heravian J, et al. Prevalence of refractive errors among schoolchildren in Shiraz, Iran. Clin Exp Ophthalmol. 2010;38(3):242–8.
34. Jamali P, Fotouhi A, Hashemi H, Younesian M, Jafari A. Refractive errors and amblyopia in children entering school: Shahrood, iran. Optom Vis Sci. 2009;86:364–9.
35. Fotouhi A, Hashemi H, Khabazkhoob M, Mohammad K. The prevalence of refractive errors among schoolchildren in Dezful, Iran. Br J Ophthalmol. 2007;91(3):287–92.
36. Hashemi H, Fotouhi A, Mohammad K. The age- and gender-specific prevalences of refractive errors in Tehran: the Tehran Eye Study. Ophthalmic Epidemiol. 2004;11(3):213–25.
37. Yingyong P. Refractive errors survey in primary school children (6-12 year old) in 2 provinces: Bangkok and Nakhonpathom (one year result). J Med Assoc Thail. 2010;93(10):1205–10.
38. Wen G, Tarczy-Hornoch K, McKean-Cowdin R, Cotter SA, Borchert M, Lin J, et al. Prevalence of myopia, hyperopia, and astigmatism in non-Hispanic white and Asian children: multi-ethnic pediatric eye disease study. Ophthalmology. 2013;120(10):2109–16.
39. Giordano L, Friedman DS, Repka MX, Katz J, Ibironke J, Hawes P, et al. Prevalence of refractive error among preschool children in an urban population: the Baltimore Pediatric Eye Disease Study. Ophthalmology. 2009;116(4):739–46.
40. Tideman JWL, Polling JR, Hofman A, Jaddoe VW, Mackenbach JP, Klaver CC. Environmental factors explain socioeconomic prevalence differences in myopia in 6-year-old children. Br J Ophthalmol. 2018;102(2):243–7.
41. Logan NS, Shah P, Rudnicka AR, Gilmartin B, Owen CG. Childhood ethnic differences in ametropia and ocular biometry: the Aston Eye Study. Ophthalmic Physiol Opt. 2011;31(5):550–8.
42. O'Donoghue L, McClelland JF, Logan NS, Rudnicka AR, Owen CG, Saunders KJ. Refractive error and visual impairment in school children in northern ireland. Br J Ophthalmol. 2010;94:1155–9.
43. Czepita D, Zejmo M, Mojsa A. Prevalence of myopia and hyperopia in a population of polish school children. Ophthalmic Physiol Opt. 2007;27(1):60–5.
44. French AN, Morgan IG, Burlutsky G, Mitchell P, Rose KA. Prevalence and 5- to 6-year incidence and progression of myopia and hyperopia in Australian school children. Ophthalmology. 2013;120(7):1482–91.
45. Ojaimi E, Rose KA, Morgan IG, Smith W, Martin FJ, Kifley A, et al. Distribution of ocular biometric parameters and refraction in a population-based study of Australian children. Invest Ophthalmol Vis Sci. 2005;46(8):2748–54.
46. Kumah BD, Ebri A, Abdul-Kabir M, Ahmed AS, Koomson NY, Aikins S, et al. Refractive error and visual impairment in private school children in Ghana. Optom Vis Sci. 2013;90(12):1456–61.
47. Naidoo KS, Raghunandan A, Mashige KP, Govender P, Holden BA, Pokharel GP, Ellwein LB. Refractive error and visual impairment in african children in south africa. Invest Ophthalmol Vis Sci. 2003;44:3764–70.

48. Goh PP, Abqariyah Y, Pokharel GP, Ellwein LB. Refractive error and visual impairment in school-age children in Gombak District, Malaysia. Ophthalmology. 2005;112(4):678–85.
49. Li Z, Xu K, Wu S, Lv J, Jin D, Song Z, et al. Population-based survey of refractive error among school-aged children in rural northern China: the Heilongjiang eye study. Clin Exp Ophthalmol. 2014;42(4):379–84.
50. Saw SM, Carkeet A, Chia KS, Stone RA, Tan DT. Component dependent risk factors for ocular parameters in Singapore Chinese children. Ophthalmology. 2002;109(11):2065–71.
51. Rose KA, Morgan IG, Smith W, Burlutsky G, Mitchell P, Saw SM. Myopia, lifestyle, and schooling in students of Chinese ethnicity in Singapore and Sydney. Arch Ophthalmol. 2008;126(4):527–30.
52. Rudnicka AR, Kapetanakis VV, Wathern AK, Logan NS, Gilmartin B, Whincup PH, et al. Global variations and time trends in the prevalence of childhood myopia, a systematic review and quantitative meta-analysis: implications for aetiology and early prevention. Br J Ophthalmol. 2016;100(7):882–90.
53. Ding BY, Shih YF, Lin LLK, Hsiao CK, Wang IJ. Myopia among schoolchildren in East Asia and Singapore. Surv Ophthalmol. 2017;62(5):677–97.
54. Chen M, Wu A, Zhang L, Wang W, Chen X, Yu X, et al. The increasing prevalence of myopia and high myopia among high school students in Fenghua city, eastern China: a 15-year population-based survey. BMC Ophthalmol. 2018;18(1):159.
55. Wu JF, Bi HS, Wang SM, Hu YY, Wu H, Sun W, et al. Refractive error, visual acuity and causes of vision loss in children in Shandong, China. The Shandong Children Eye Study. PLoS One. 2013;8(12):e82763.
56. Sun J, Zhou J, Zhao P, Lian J, Zhu H, Zhou Y, et al. High prevalence of myopia and high myopia in 5060 Chinese university students in Shanghai. Invest Ophthalmol Vis Sci. 2012;53(12):7504–9.
57. Lee YY, Lo CT, Sheu SJ, Lin JL. What factors are associated with myopia in young adults? A survey study in Taiwan Military Conscripts. Invest Ophthalmol Vis Sci. 2013;54(2):1026–33.
58. Koh V, Yang A, Saw SM, Chan YH, Lin ST, Tan MM, et al. Differences in prevalence of refractive errors in young Asian males in Singapore between 1996-1997 and 2009-2010. Ophthalmic Epidemiol. 2014;21(4):247–55.
59. Bar Dayan Y, Levin A, Morad Y, Grotto I, Ben-David R, Goldberg A, et al. The changing prevalence of myopia in young adults: a 13-year series of population-based prevalence surveys. Invest Ophthalmol Vis Sci. 2005;46(8):2760–5.
60. McKnight CM, Sherwin JC, Yazar S, Forward H, Tan AX, Hewitt AW, et al. Myopia in young adults is inversely related to an objective marker of ocular sun exposure: the Western Australian Raine cohort study. Am J Ophthalmol. 2014;158(5):1079–85.
61. Jacobsen N, Jensen H, Goldschmidt E. Prevalence of myopia in Danish conscripts. Acta Ophthalmol Scand. 2007;85(2):165–70.
62. Midelfart A, Kinge B, Midelfart S, Lydersen S. Prevalence of refractive errors in young and middle-aged adults in Norway. Acta Ophthalmol Scand. 2002;80(5):501–5.
63. Sperduto RD, Seigel D, Roberts J, Rowland M. Prevalence of myopia in the United States. Arch Ophthalmol. 1983;101(3):405–7.
64. Mimouni M, Zoller L, Horowitz J, Wygnanski-Jaffe T, Morad Y, Mezer E. Cycloplegic autorefraction in young adults: is it mandatory? Graefes Arch Clin Exp Ophthalmol. 2016;254(2):395–8.
65. Wang Q, Klein BE, Klein R, Moss SE. Refractive status in the Beaver Dam Eye Study. Invest Ophthalmol Vis Sci. 1994;35(13):4344–7.
66. Wong TY, Foster PJ, Hee J, Ng TP, Tielsch JM, Chew SJ, et al. Prevalence and risk factors for refractive errors in adult Chinese in Singapore. Invest Ophthalmol Vis Sci. 2000;41(9):2486–94.
67. He M, Huang W, Li Y, Zheng Y, Yin Q, Foster PJ. Refractive error and biometry in older Chinese adults: the Liwan eye study. Invest Ophthalmol Vis Sci. 2009;50(11):5130–6.
68. Xu L, Li J, Cui T, Hu A, Fan G, Zhang R, et al. Refractive error in urban and rural adult Chinese in Beijing. Ophthalmology. 2005;112(10):1676–83.
69. Cheng CY, Hsu WM, Liu JH, Tsai SY, Chou P. Refractive errors in an elderly Chinese population in Taiwan: the Shihpai Eye Study. Invest Ophthalmol Vis Sci. 2003;44(11):4630–8.

70. Saw SM, Chan YH, Wong WL, Shankar A, Sandar M, Aung T, et al. Prevalence and risk factors for refractive errors in the Singapore Malay Eye Survey. Ophthalmology. 2008;115(10):1713–9.
71. Pan CW, Wong TY, Lavanya R, Wu RY, Zheng YF, Lin XY, et al. Prevalence and risk factors for refractive errors in Indians: the Singapore Indian Eye Study (SINDI). Invest Ophthalmol Vis Sci. 2011;52(6):3166–73.
72. Sawada A, Tomidokoro A, Araie M, Iwase A, Yamamoto T. Refractive errors in an elderly Japanese population: the Tajimi study. Ophthalmology. 2008;115(2):363–70.e3.
73. Nakamura Y, Nakamura Y, Higa A, Sawaguchi S, Tomidokoro A, Iwase A, et al. Refractive errors in an elderly rural Japanese population: the Kumejima study. PLoS One. 2018;13(11):e0207180.
74. Yoo YC, Kim JM, Park KH, Kim CY, Kim TW. Refractive errors in a rural Korean adult population: the Namil Study. Eye. 2013;27(12):1368–75.
75. Wickremasinghe S, Foster PJ, Uranchimeg D, Lee PS, Devereux JG, Alsbirk PH, et al. Ocular biometry and refraction in Mongolian adults. Invest Ophthalmol Vis Sci. 2004;45(3):776–83.
76. Bourne RR, Dineen BP, Ali SM, Noorul Huq DM, Johnson GJ. Prevalence of refractive error in Bangladeshi adults: results of the national blindness and low vision survey of Bangladesh. Ophthalmology. 2004;111(6):1150–60.
77. Raju P, Ramesh SV, Arvind H, George R, Baskaran M, Paul PG, et al. Prevalence of refractive errors in a rural South Indian population. Invest Ophthalmol Vis Sci. 2004;45(12):4268–72.
78. Shah SP, Jadoon MZ, Dineen B, Bourne RR, Johnson GJ, Gilbert CE, et al. Refractive errors in the adult pakistani population: the national blindness and visual impairment survey. Ophthalmic Epidemiol. 2008;15(3):183–90.
79. Hashemi H, Khabazkhoob M, Jafarzadehpur E, Yekta AA, Emamian MH, Shariati M, et al. High prevalence of myopia in an adult population, Shahroud, Iran. Optom Vis Sci. 2012;89(7):993–9.
80. Varma R, Torres M, McKean-Cowdin R, Rong F, Hsu C, Jiang X. Prevalence and risk factors for refractive error in adult Chinese Americans: The Chinese American Eye Study. Am J Ophthalmol. 2017;175:201–12.
81. Wu SY, Nemesure B, Leske MC. Refractive errors in a black adult population: the Barbados Eye Study. Invest Ophthalmol Vis Sci. 1999;40(10):2179–84.
82. Tarczy-Hornoch K, Ying-Lai M, Varma R. Myopic refractive error in adult Latinos: the Los Angeles Latino Eye Study. Invest Ophthalmol Vis Sci. 2006;47(5):1845–52.
83. Wolfram C, Hohn R, Kottler U, Wild P, Blettner M, Buhren J, et al. Prevalence of refractive errors in the European adult population: the Gutenberg Health Study (GHS). Br J Ophthalmol. 2014;98(7):857–61.
84. Williams KM, Verhoeven VJ, Cumberland P, Bertelsen G, Wolfram C, Buitendijk GH, et al. Prevalence of refractive error in Europe: the European Eye Epidemiology (E(3)) Consortium. Eur J Epidemiol. 2015;30(4):305–15.
85. Sherwin JC, Khawaja AP, Broadway D, Luben R, Hayat S, Dalzell N, et al. Uncorrected refractive error in older British adults: the EPIC-Norfolk Eye Study. Br J Ophthalmol. 2012;96(7):991–6.
86. Attebo K, Ivers RQ, Mitchell P. Refractive errors in an older population: the Blue Mountains Eye Study. Ophthalmology. 1999;106(6):1066–72.
87. Ezelum C, Razavi H, Sivasubramaniam S, Gilbert CE, Murthy GV, Entekume G, et al. Refractive error in Nigerian adults: prevalence, type, and spectacle coverage. Invest Ophthalmol Vis Sci. 2011;52(8):5449–56.
88. Mashige KP, Jaggernath J, Ramson P, Martin C, Chinanayi FS, Naidoo KS. Prevalence of refractive errors in the INK Area, Durban, South Africa. Optom Vis Sci. 2016;93(3):243–50.
89. Galvis V, Tello A, Otero J, Serrano AA, Gomez LM, Camacho PA, et al. Prevalence of refractive errors in Colombia: MIOPUR study. Br J Ophthalmol. 2018;102(10):1320–3.
90. Pan CW, Zheng YF, Anuar AR, Chew M, Gazzard G, Aung T, et al. Prevalence of refractive errors in a multiethnic Asian population: the Singapore epidemiology of eye disease study. Invest Ophthalmol Vis Sci. 2013;54(4):2590–8.

91. Jonas JB, Xu L, Wang YX, Bi HS, Wu JF, Jiang WJ, et al. Education-related parameters in high myopia: adults versus school children. PLoS One. 2016;11(5):e0154554.
92. Morgan I, Rose K. How genetic is school myopia? Prog Retin Eye Res. 2005;24(1):1–38.
93. Li YT, Xie MK, Wu J. Association between ocular axial length-related genes and high myopia in a Han Chinese Population. Ophthalmologica. 2016;235(1):57–60.
94. Ohno-Matsui K, Lai TY, Lai CC, Cheung CM. Updates of pathologic myopia. Prog Retin Eye Res. 2016;52:156–87.
95. Cedrone C, Culasso F, Cesareo M, Nucci C, Palma S, Mancino R, et al. Incidence of blindness and low vision in a sample population: the Priverno Eye Study, Italy. Ophthalmology. 2003;110(3):584–8.
96. Klaver CC, Wolfs RC, Vingerling JR, Hofman A, de Jong PT. Age-specific prevalence and causes of blindness and visual impairment in an older population: the Rotterdam Study. Arch Ophthalmol. 1998;116(5):653–8.
97. Iwase A, Araie M, Tomidokoro A, Yamamoto T, Shimizu H, Kitazawa Y. Prevalence and causes of low vision and blindness in a Japanese adult population: the Tajimi Study. Ophthalmology. 2006;113(8):1354–62.
98. Xu L, Wang Y, Li Y, Wang Y, Cui T, Li J, et al. Causes of blindness and visual impairment in urban and rural areas in Beijing: the Beijing Eye Study. Ophthalmology. 2006;113(7):1134.e1–11.
99. Yamada M, Hiratsuka Y, Roberts CB, Pezzullo ML, Yates K, Takano S, et al. Prevalence of visual impairment in the adult Japanese population by cause and severity and future projections. Ophthalmic Epidemiol. 2010;17(1):50–7.
100. Fricke TR, Jong M, Naidoo KS, Sankaridurg P, Naduvilath TJ, Ho SM, et al. Global prevalence of visual impairment associated with myopic macular degeneration and temporal trends from 2000 through 2050: systematic review, meta-analysis and modelling. Br J Ophthalmol. 2018;102(7):855–62.
101. Avila MP, Weiter JJ, Jalkh AE, Trempe CL, Pruett RC, Schepens CL. Natural history of choroidal neovascularization in degenerative myopia. Ophthalmology. 1984;91(12):1573–81.
102. Ohno-Matsui K, Kawasaki R, Jonas JB, Cheung CM, Saw SM, Verhoeven VJ, et al. International photographic classification and grading system for myopic maculopathy. Am J Ophthalmol. 2015;159(5):877–83.e7.
103. Liu HH, Xu L, Wang YX, Wang S, You QS, Jonas JB. Prevalence and progression of myopic retinopathy in Chinese adults: the Beijing Eye Study. Ophthalmology. 2010;117(9):1763–8.
104. Gao LQ, Liu W, Liang YB, Zhang F, Wang JJ, Peng Y, et al. Prevalence and characteristics of myopic retinopathy in a rural Chinese adult population: the Handan Eye Study. Arch Ophthalmol. 2011;129(9):1199–204.
105. Chen SJ, Cheng CY, Li AF, Peng KL, Chou P, Chiou SH, et al. Prevalence and associated risk factors of myopic maculopathy in elderly Chinese: the Shihpai eye study. Invest Ophthalmol Vis Sci. 2012;53(8):4868–73.
106. Asakuma T, Yasuda M, Ninomiya T, Noda Y, Arakawa S, Hashimoto S, et al. Prevalence and risk factors for myopic retinopathy in a Japanese population: the Hisayama Study. Ophthalmology. 2012;119(9):1760–5.
107. Vongphanit J, Mitchell P, Wang JJ. Prevalence and progression of myopic retinopathy in an older population. Ophthalmology. 2002;109(4):704–11.
108. Jonas JB, Nangia V, Gupta R, Bhojwani K, Nangia P, Panda-Jonas S. Prevalence of myopic retinopathy in rural Central India. Acta Ophthalmol. 2017;95(5):e399–404.
109. Wong YL, Saw SM. Epidemiology of pathologic myopia in Asia and worldwide. Asia-Pac J Ophthalmol. 2016;5(6):394–402.
110. Samarawickrama C, Mitchell P, Tong L, Gazzard G, Lim L, Wong TY, et al. Myopia-related optic disc and retinal changes in adolescent children from singapore. Ophthalmology. 2011;118(10):2050–7.
111. Koh V, Tan C, Tan PT, Tan M, Balla V, Nah G, et al. Myopic maculopathy and optic disc changes in highly myopic young asian eyes and impact on visual acuity. Am J Ophthalmol. 2016;164:69–79.

The Economic and Societal Impact of Myopia and High Myopia

3

Sharon Yu Lin Chua and Paul J. Foster

Key Points

- The prevalence of myopia has increased rapidly throughout Asia. In urban areas, 80–90% of young adults are myopic and 10–20% have high myopia. By 2050, it is estimated that five billion people will be myopic. Of these, one billion people will be highly myopic. World Health Organization lists uncorrected or under-corrected myopia as a major cause of visual impairment.
- Myopia may impair many aspects of life including educational and occupational activities. The annual direct cost of myopia correction for Asian adults has been estimated at US $328 billion/annum. The cost of care is also likely to increase significantly and will be exacerbated by an even greater increase in the prevalence of high myopia.
- High myopes have greater risk of developing several vision-threatening conditions including myopic macular degeneration, retinal detachment, glaucoma, and cataract. Those affected individuals incur costs for specialist eye care, or specialist optical aids for patients with visual impairment. These costs are in the region of US $250 billion/annum.

S. Y. L. Chua · P. J. Foster (✉)
Integrative Epidemiology Cluster, NIHR Biomedical Research Centre, UCL Institute of Ophthalmology and Moorfields Eye Hospital NHS Foundation Trust, London, UK
e-mail: p.foster@ucl.ac.uk

M. Ang, T. Y. Wong (eds.), *Updates on Myopia*,
https://doi.org/10.1007/978-981-13-8491-2_3

- Myopes, especially high myopes, tend to have reduced quality of life due to adverse influences from psychological, cosmetic, practical and financial factors. Hence, affecting productivity, mobility, and activities of daily living.
- Treatments such as under-correction of myopia, gas permeable contact lenses, and bifocal or multifocal spectacles have all been proven to be ineffective for myopia control. The most effective methods are the use of orthokeratology contact lenses, soft bifocal contact lenses, and topical pharmaceutical agents, such as low-dose atropine or pirenzepine. These will have differing implications for personal finances and quality of life. Hence, the best modality should be selected by the eye care practitioner, parent or individual, based on the lifestyle of the individual.

3.1 Introduction

The prevalence of myopia is most pronounced in the industrialized nations of East Asia, where rates of 95% among young adults have been recorded [1]. In this context, the impact of myopia is profound and far reaching, and recent study by Naidoo et al. [2] suggests that myopia has a global economic impact, with the greatest burden throughout Asia. Its economic impact is very significant. This chapter seeks to examine the impact of myopia on individuals and the wider society, both from the monetary perspective and also in terms of emotional well-being and quality of life. Peer-reviewed data on this subject are comparatively sparse, and in some areas, it is necessary to make inferences on the basis of indirect evidence.

The impact of myopia illustrates an interesting dichotomy. The condition appears to be an exaggerated adaptive response which has a predilection for the most affluent and educated in society. Low myopia [up to around −3 D (diopters)] is arguably an ideal state for the older urban professional, in that the frustration of presbyopia is avoided, and hence maximum efficiency in an office-based career is maintained, and the ability to pursue leisure activities, such as reading, creative arts, and many household tasks, is enhanced. Myopes are among the best educated and thus highest earning members of any society. Furthermore, they confer on their children a range of advantages—they are typically well educated, and in turn benefit from higher career prospects and incomes. The offspring are also more likely to be myopes [3].

3.2 Economic Impact of Myopia

Myopia is the most common distance refractive error. The global prevalence of myopia is expected to increase from 27% of the world's population in 2010 to 52% by 2050 [4]—a 2.6-fold increase. A recent meta-analysis estimated a significant increase in the global prevalence of myopia and high myopia, affecting nearly five billion people and one billion people, respectively, by 2050 [4]. The projected increases in myopia and high myopia may be due to environmental factors, such as a combination of decreased time outdoors and increased near work activities, among other factors [5]. Uncorrected distance refractive error was estimated in 2013 to affect 108 million people globally, and myopia is the most common refractive error [6]. It is the leading cause of moderate and severe vision impairment (VI; 42%) and a major cause of blindness (3%) [2]. Uncorrected myopia as low as −1.50 D will result in moderate VI, and uncorrected myopia of −4.00 D is sufficient refractive error to be classified as blindness [7]. Depending on national legislation, people with moderate VI may not be allowed to drive. Moderate VI may also require the use of aids and/or accommodations/adaptions for some tasks in the learning environment.

If the increasing prevalence of myopia is not addressed, a similar increase in uncorrected refractive error can be expected. These projections are based on conservative assumptions and, given the published relationship between level of education and myopia, increased provision of education could markedly increase these trends. Furthermore, uncorrected distance refractive error has been estimated to result in a global loss of productivity of international dollar (I$) 269 billion [8] (US $202 billion) annually [9], which will also increase if there is a significant increase in uncorrected myopia. International dollar allows comparison of prices and currency values between countries after adjustment of currency exchange rate. An international dollar has the same purchasing power as the U.S. dollar has in the United States [10]. A recent meta-analysis estimated the global potential loss associated with VI in 2015 was US $244 billion/annum [95% confidence interval (CI) US $49 billion—US $697 billion] from uncorrected myopia and US $6 billion/annum (95% CI US $2 billion–US $17 billion) from myopic macular degeneration [2]. The cost of care is also likely to increase significantly, and will be exacerbated by an even greater increase in the prevalence of high myopia, from 2.8% (190 million people) to 9.7% (924 million people) by 2050 [4], representing a 4.9-fold increase in high myopia. In some populations of young adults in Asia, the prevalence of high myopia has already reached 38% [11]. The annual direct cost of optical correction of myopia for Singaporean adults has been estimated at US $755 million. Refractive correction comprising of optometry visits, spectacles, and/or contact lenses is the most significant cost domain and it accounts for 65.2% of the total costs [12]. In Singapore, the estimates in an adult (SG $587 or US $455 per patient per year) is significantly higher than a child aged 7–9 years (SG $222 or US $175 per patient per year) [13]. The higher cost could be because of the greater likelihood that adults may undergo laser-assisted in situ keratomileusis (LASIK), wear contact lens, or develop ocular complications due to high myopia. Furthermore, adults tend to have higher spending power compared to a child. It has been estimated that if such prevalence rates were extrapolated to all cities in Asia in which the prevalence of myopia is approximately equal to the rates in Singapore, the estimated direct cost would be US $328 billion/annum. It is estimated that US $8.1 billion/annum was spent on vision products including eyeglass frames, lenses, and contact lenses in the USA in 1990 [14]. In United States, a cross-sectional study demonstrated that 110 million Americans could achieve normal vision with refractive correction and the estimated cost was US $3.8 billion/annum [15]. Of this amount, the annual cost of providing distance vision correction for adults older than 65 years old was US $780 million. The types of refractive error included correction for myopia, hyperopia, and presbyopia. This represents approximately US $35 per person or US $13 per capita annually, based on the cost of a pair of spectacles and refractive examination. Possible reasons for the difference in direct costs of refractive correction are the treatment costs may be borne by the individual, who may be willing to pay for other factors such as aesthetics. Whereas in some countries (e.g., the United Kingdom), some segments of the population are entitled to free eye glasses subsidized by the government. As the prevalence of myopia increase in East Asia, the total cost of treating myopia will be high. There is likely to be an increase in the demand for optical services as the number of older people increases and if, as suggested, the number of younger people with myopia increases. It is estimated that partial sight and blindness in adults costs the UK economy around £22 billion per year [16].

The cost of spectacles varies, but there may some individuals who may not be able to afford a basic pair of spectacles, and hence refractive error may not be fully corrected. Health economic analyses in the United States and Australia have reported the economic burden of refractive correction associated with medical care expenditure, informal care days, and healthy utility is greater than age-related macular degeneration, primary open-angle glaucoma, and diabetic retinopathy, while it was secondary to the medical cost of age-related cataract [17, 18]. As the economic costs of myopia are high, more efforts and resources could be directed toward having new strategies to prevent and slow down myopia progression to high myopia and its associated visually disabling ocular complications.

3.3 Secondary Impact of Myopia from Other Eye Diseases and Sight Loss

High myopia increases the risk of other eye diseases such as cataract, glaucoma, retinal detachment, and myopic macular degeneration (MMD), which may lead to irreversible vision loss. MMD has been reported to cause 12.1% of VI (approximately 200,000 people) in Japan [19]. Visual impairment and blindness impact the individuals, their families, caregivers, and the community, which lead to a significant cost burden. In Australia, visual disorders were ranked seventh among diseases in terms of economic burden on the health system, which is ahead of coronary heart disease, diabetes, depression, and stroke [20]. Naidoo et al. estimated the potential global economic productivity loss resulting from VI and blindness as a result of uncorrected myopia and MMD in 2015 [2]. Their study suggests that the greatest burden of VI resulting from uncorrected refractive error is older people in rural areas of the least developed countries. The regional productivity loss owing to VI resulting from myopia may be reflected in Southeast Asia, South Asia, and East Asia as having a percentage gross domestic product (GDP) of 1.35%, 1.3%, and 1.27%, respectively. Differences in productivity loss arises from the interplay between country-specific variables, such as myopia and high myopia prevalence, demographics, Health Development Index (HDI), health expenditure, urbanization, labor force participation, employment, GDP, and population. There are other components that contribute to the overall burden of myopia, such as cost of eye examinations, refractive corrections, managing pathologic consequences of myopia such as MMD, and related opportunity costs. The value of any investment to prevent myopia, slow progression of myopia, improve spectacle correction rates, and improve outcomes in MMD depends on a comparison of lost productivity owing to VI resulting from myopia with the cost of prevention and management interventions. Fricke et al. estimated the global cost of facilities and personnel for establishing refractive care services US $20 billion over 5 years [9]. Direct medical costs occur mostly due to hospitalization, the use of direct medical services, and medical products. Hospitalization and use of medical services around diagnosis and treatment at the onset of VI and blindness were the two largest components related to direct medical costs. The mean annual expenses per patient to be US$ purchasing power parities (PPPs) 12,175–14,029 for moderate VI, US$ PPPs 13,154–16,321 for severe VI, and US$ PPPs 14,882–24,180 for blindness [21]. PPPs account for differences in price levels between countries, and convert local currencies into international dollars by taking into account the purchasing power of different national currencies and eliminates the difference in price levels between countries [22]. Direct nonmedical costs include assistive devices and aids, home modifications, and costs for healthcare services such as home-based nursing or nursing home placements. The cost for support services and assistive devices increased from US$ PPP 54 for a person with visual acuity (VA) 20/20 or better up to US$ PPP 609 for a person with VA 20/80 or worse. Indirect costs include productivity losses, changes in employment (employer and/or area of work), loss of income, premature mortality, and dead-weight losses [21]. Dead-weight losses, also known as excess burden, describe the costs to society created by market inefficiency. In the study by Köberlein et al., it is referred to as an excess financial burden on society caused by VI and blindness [21]. The annual estimates of productivity losses and absenteeism range from US$ PPP 4974 to 5724 million and a decrease in workforce participation range was estimated to be US$ PPP 7.4 billion [21].

Value of the Commercial Optical Good Sector

In the UK in 2017, the optical goods and services industry had total consumer spending estimated at £3.1 billion (2.0 billion US$ = @ 0.66 £:$). Growth was estimated at 2% for 2017, and forecasts projected further 3.2% growth in 2018. Market research suggests this was primarily driven by an aging population. In the UK, 70% of consumers are reported to wear some form of prescription eyewear. Just 11% of those with vision correction need wear contact lenses, with this sector characterized by a high rate of premium and daily wear lenses. Contact lenses account for 20% of the total spending on optical products, with the sale of contact lens solutions made up an additional 3% of the market, compared to 60% market share for spectacle frames and lenses. Only one in six (18%) people have purchased optical products online. Reports suggest that consumers perceive buying prescriptions eyewear online as harder—49% of people buying prescription eyewear saying it is more difficult than buying in-store, although 45% of consumers who said they have not bought optical products online before, would consider doing so in the future [23].

3.4 Quality of Life

Quality of life is a multidimensional construct with different domains. The identified domains related to ophthalmic quality of life include activity limitation, mobility, convenience, health concerns, visual symptoms, ocular-comfort symptoms, general symptoms, emotional well-being, and social and economic issues [24]. Impaired vision will lead to significant reduction in activities associated with participation in society and religion, mobility, daily living, and visually intensive tasks. This may impact education, employment, child development, mental health, and functional capacity in older people, increasing the risk of hip fractures and the need for community or family support or nursing home placement [25–27]. A cross-sectional study in Germany reported that mild VI affected emotional well-being [28]. Depression was considered to cause further functional decline in visually impaired patients by reducing motivation, initiative, and resiliency [29–31]. Visual impairment and blindness associated with myopic macular degeneration will increase significantly, hence affecting the quality of life and causing socioeconomic impact [32]. A cross-sectional study reported the functional status in daily life and quality of life of pathologic myopia patients were reduced compared with control subjects [33]. The influence of pathologic myopia on a patient's daily life was primarily the result of three major factors: handicap, disability, and support. Wong et al. reported that those with VI, measured in terms of presenting vision (i.e., wearing their habitual correction), had statistically significantly lower scores for total quality of life (−3.8; 95% CI −7.1 to −0.5; $P = 0.03$), psychosocial functioning (−4.2; 95% CI −8.1 to −0.3; $P = 0.03$), and school functioning (−5.5; 95% CI −10.2 to −0.9; $P = 0.02$) [34]. Another study indicates that correction of refractive errors by the provision of spectacles in low socioeconomic areas in China would markedly improve educational outcomes since the major medium of instruction is the blackboard [35].

Patients with cataract may experience vision-related problems, such as decreased visual acuity, loss of contrast sensitivity, problems under glare conditions, and altered color recognition [36]. Studies in Japan and Canada reported a loss of well-being as disability adjusted life years (DALYs) and an associated cost of US$ PPP 51.8 billion/annum and US$ PPP 15.11 billion/annum, respectively [37, 38]. The global burden of diseases study 2010 estimated the burden of disease related to vision disorders has increased by 47% from 12,858,000 disability adjusted life years (DALYs) in 1990 to 18,837,000 DALYs in 2010 [39]. The Melbourne Visual Impairment Project (VIP) cohort showed the association between VI and mortality to increase linearly from 4.5% in people with a VA of 20/20 or better to 22.2% in blind people with VA of 20/200 or worse [40].

3.5 Impact of Myopia Treatments on Quality of Life

Current treatment options for control of myopia progression include optical correction such as bifocal spectacle lenses, progressive addition spectacle lenses, under-correction, orthokeratology, multifocal contact lenses, increased exposure to outdoor activities, and the use of atropine eye drops. Surgical techniques, such as LASIK, have become increasingly popular and over a million surgical procedures are performed annually in the United States [41]. Choice of refractive correction leads to various quality-of-life implications. Often, the type of refractive correction depends on prescription, lifestyle including occupational and recreational needs, economic issues, and personality. If refractive error may be corrected through the provision of corrective spectacles, visual acuity, and therefore functional vision could be improved. Patient reported outcomes (PROs) have been used to assess the outcomes of interventions on people's lives. A PRO is described as a report that comes directly from a patient regarding the impact of the condition and outcome of an intervention [42]. The Quality of Life Impact of Refractive Correction (QIRC) is useful to detect differences in quality of life impact from various refractive corrections (spectacles, contact lenses, and refractive surgery). Pesudovs et al. reported that QIRC score was highest in refractive surgery patients (mean QIRC score of 50.2 ± 6.3), followed by contact lens wearers (mean QIRC score 46.7 ± 5.5), and spectacle wears (mean QIRC score 44.1 ± 5.9) [43]. Orthokeratology (OrthoK) contact lenses (CL) are worn while sleeping to reshape the cornea and are used to correct refractive error and slow the progression of myopia [44]. Quality of life using the National Eye Institute Refractive Error Quality of Life (NEI RQL)-42 questionnaire was evaluated in a group of subjects with low to moderate myopia who had undergone four types of refractive correction, namely, LASIK, OrthoK, soft contact lens (SCL), and spectacles [45]. Results showed decrease in quality of life for most of the subscales in the treatment groups compared to emmetropic subjects. The average decrease in quality of life compared with emmetropes were −7.1% ($P = 0.021$) for LASIK, −13.0% ($P = 0.001$) for OrthoK, −15.8% ($P = 0.001$) for spectacles, and −17.3% ($P = 0.001$) for SCL. The subscales which were affected in LASIK and OrthoK patients compared to emmetropes were as follows: clarity of vision, expectations, glare, and worry. This suggests that both types of treatment affected the quality of life due to high-order aberrations [46]. LASIK and OrthoK are commonly associated with experiencing haloes and glare because of the dramatic changes in the corneal shape [47]. Spectacle wearers had the worse scores in expectations, dependence on correction, worry, and appearance as compared to the other three treatment modalities [45]. The primary motivation for undergoing LASIK was a desire to improve uncorrected visual acuity, without a need to wear glasses and improved ease to pursue sports or recreational activities [48]. Although LASIK patients may have excellent vision during day time, they may experience disturbances in night vision such as halo and glare disability [49]. An estimated 12–57% of patients experience night vision symptoms and 30% have difficulty with night driving after undergoing photorefractive keratectomy (PRK) and LASIK [50, 51]. In addition, these patients may experience poor vision in low light setting due to contrast sensitivity decreasing initially after LASIK [52].

OrthoK allows patients to enjoy good vision without needing to wear vision correction during their waking hours. This benefits patients who have an active lifestyle as they are more mobile without the need for refractive correction. OrthoK provides excellent vision and improves vision related quality of life [45, 53]. Side effects of OrthoK include halos secondary to spherical aberration, which may reduce visual acuity and contrast sensitivity or discomfort from the lenses [54]. Although the most serious complication with CL wear is infection, these occurrences are relatively rare [55, 56]. Most common complaints are related to intolerance or limited wearing time due to fluctuations of vision, dryness and discomfort [57]. Atropine has been used to control myopia progression [58]. As atropine causes pupil dilation and temporary paralysis of accommodation, patients may experience glare, discomfort, blurred vision, or allergic/hypersensitivity reactions. Complications of LASIK include corneal ectasia [59], dry eyes [60], and night vision disturbances [49].

Cataract surgery is a highly effective, cost-effective health-care intervention [61], and results in almost immediate visual rehabilitation. In addition to visual rehabilitation from media opacities, it offers once in a lifetime opportunity for refractive manipulation that benefits the majority of people with a refractive error. Previous studies have utilized Visual Functioning Index-14 (VF-14) or similar vision-functioning tools and reported the impact of cataract surgery can be translated beyond visual acuity. Evidence has shown several fold improvements in other critical daily tasks such as read critical daily living tasks such as reading newspapers or books; driving; watching TV; cooking; negotiating steps; sewing, knitting, crocheting, or doing handicrafts; noticing traffic, information or shop signs; and recognizing people [62]. In addition, there are improvements in several psychosocial aspects such as social interaction; mental and emotional well-being; psychological distress; adaptation; and coping.

3.6 Summary

Myopia is a major global public health concern due to its high and increasing prevalence in Asian countries, where it is a common cause of vision dysfunction. Uncorrected myopia is a leading cause of visual impairment. People with high myopia have increased risk of developing myopic pathologies which may lead to blindness. The economic burden of uncorrected distance refractive error, largely caused by myopia, is estimated to be US $202 billion annually. Direct cost of refractive correction comprises of cost from spectacles, contact lenses, and refractive surgeries. Other medical costs include those associated with treatment of ocular complications from high myopia, such as retinal detachment, myopic macular degeneration, glaucoma and cataract, and its associated visual impairment and blindness. This global cost will continue to increase as the number of people with myopia rises. Patients with higher myopic refractive error tend to have adverse effect on the quality of life and lead to lower health, economic, and social outcomes. Effective methods to control or correct myopia include the use of optical devices, pharmacological drops, surgical, or outdoor exposure. Each treatment method will have various quality of life implications; thus, it is important to ensure prescription, lifestyle including occupational and recreational needs, and economic issues are discussed. Although a broader societal perspective is useful for informing policy, the patient's perspective is essential for designing service models to improve the social interaction and mental and emotional well-being of these individuals. In conclusion, the impact that myopia and its associated visual impairment have on individuals is substantial. Myopia preferentially affects the more highly educated and potentially most productive sectors of the population, the individual and societal costs involved. Developing appropriate public health policies to prevent and reduce myopia progression will benefit the individual and the wider society.

References

1. Lin LL, Shih YF, Hsiao CK, Chen CJ. Prevalence of myopia in Taiwanese schoolchildren: 1983 to 2000. Ann Acad Med Singap. 2004;33(1):27–33.
2. Naidoo KS, Fricke TR, Frick KD, et al. Potential lost productivity resulting from the global burden of myopia: systematic review, meta-analysis, and modeling. Ophthalmology. 2018;126(3):338–46.
3. Mutti DO, Mitchell GL, Moeschberger ML, et al. Parental myopia, near work, school achievement, and children's refractive error. Invest Ophthalmol Vis Sci. 2002;43(12):3633–40.
4. Holden BA, Fricke TR, Wilson DA, et al. Global prevalence of myopia and high myopia and temporal trends from 2000 through 2050. Ophthalmology. 2016;123(5):1036–42.
5. Morgan IG, Ohno-Matsui K, Saw S-M. Myopia. Lancet. 2012;379(9827):1739–48.
6. Bourne RRA, Stevens GA, White RA, et al. Causes of vision loss worldwide, 1990–2010: a systematic analysis. Lancet Glob Health. 2013;1(6):e339–e49.
7. Rabbetts RB. Bennett & Rabbetts' clinical visual optics. New York: Elsevier/Butterworth Heinemann; 2007.
8. Smith TS, Frick KD, Holden BA, et al. Potential lost productivity resulting from the global burden of uncorrected refractive error. Bull World Health Organ. 2009;87(6):431–7.
9. Fricke T, Holden B, Wilson D. Global cost of correcting vision impairment from uncorrected refractive error. Bull World Health Organ. 2012;90:728–38.
10. World Health Organization. Purchasing power parity. 2005. https://www.who.int/choice/costs/ppp/en/. Accessed 20 June 2019.
11. Wang TJ, Chiang TH, Wang TH, et al. Changes of the ocular refraction among freshmen in National Taiwan University between 1988 and 2005. Eye. 2009;23(5):1168–9.
12. Zheng YF, Pan CW, Chay J, et al. The economic cost of myopia in adults aged over 40 years in Singapore. Invest Ophthalmol Vis Sci. 2013;54(12):7532–7.
13. Lim MC, Gazzard G, Sim EL, et al. Direct costs of myopia in Singapore. Eye. 2009;23(5):1086–9.
14. Letsch SW, Lazenby HC, Levit KR, Cowan CA. National health expenditures, 1991. Health Care Financ Rev. 1992;14(2):1–30.
15. Vitale S, Cotch MF, Sperduto R, Ellwein L. Costs of refractive correction of distance vision impairment in the United States, 1999-2002. Ophthalmology. 2006;113(12):2163–70.
16. England N. Improving eye health and reducing sight loss: a call to action. 2014. https://www.england.nhs.uk/2014/06/eye-cta/. Accessed 6 Feb 2019.
17. Frick KD, Gower EW, Kempen JH, Wolff JL. Economic impact of visual impairment and blindness in the United States. Arch Ophthalmol. 2007;125(4):544–50.
18. Keeffe JE, Chou SL, Lamoureux EL. The cost of care for people with impaired vision in Australia. Arch Ophthalmol. 2009;127(10):1377–81.
19. Yamada M, Hiratsuka Y, Roberts CB, et al. Prevalence of visual impairment in the adult Japanese population by cause and severity and future projections. Ophthalmic Epidemiol. 2010;17(1):50–7.
20. Taylor HR, Pezzullo ML, Keeffe JE. The economic impact and cost of visual impairment in Australia. Br J Ophthalmol. 2006;90(3):272–5.
21. Koberlein J, Beifus K, Schaffert C, Finger RP. The economic burden of visual impairment and blindness: a systematic review. BMJ Open. 2013;3(11):e003471.

22. Organisation for Economic Co-operation and Development. OECD health statistics. 2018. http://www.oecd.org/els/health-systems/health-data.htm. Accessed 6 Feb 2019.
23. Mintel. Optical goods retailing: UK. 2018. http://reports.mintel.com/display/858753/. Accessed 6 Feb 2019.
24. Khadka J, Fenwick E, Lamoureux E, Pesudovs K. Methods to develop the eye-tem bank to measure ophthalmic quality of life. Optom Vis Sci. 2016;93(12):1485–94.
25. Cieza A, Kocur I, Mariotti S, McCoy M. The future of eye care in a changing world. Bull World Health Organ. 2017;95:667.
26. Klein BE, Klein R, Lee KE, Cruickshanks KJ. Performance-based and self-assessed measures of visual function as related to history of falls, hip fractures, and measured gait time. The Beaver Dam Eye Study. Ophthalmology. 1998;105(1):160–4.
27. Mitchell P, Hayes P, Wang JJ. Visual impairment in nursing home residents: the Blue Mountains Eye Study. Med J Aust. 1997;166(2):73–6.
28. Finger RP, Fenwick E, Marella M, et al. The impact of vision impairment on vision-specific quality of life in Germany. Invest Ophthalmol Vis Sci. 2011;52(6):3613–9.
29. Rovner BW, Casten RJ, Tasman WS. Effect of depression on vision function in age-related macular degeneration. Arch Ophthalmol. 2002;120(8):1041–4.
30. Horowitz A, Reinhardt JP, Boerner K, Travis LA. The influence of health, social support quality and rehabilitation on depression among disabled elders. Aging Ment Health. 2003;7(5):342–50.
31. Tolman J, Hill RD, Kleinschmidt JJ, Gregg CH. Psychosocial adaptation to visual impairment and its relationship to depressive affect in older adults with age-related macular degeneration. Gerontologist. 2005;45(6):747–53.
32. Fricke TR, Jong M, Naidoo KS, et al. Global prevalence of visual impairment associated with myopic macular degeneration and temporal trends from 2000 through 2050: systematic review, meta-analysis and modelling. Br J Ophthalmol. 2018;102(7):855–62.
33. Takashima T, Yokoyama T, Futagami S, et al. The quality of life in patients with pathologic myopia. Jpn J Ophthalmol. 2001;45(1):84–92.
34. Wong HB, Machin D, Tan SB, et al. Visual impairment and its impact on health-related quality of life in adolescents. Am J Ophthalmol. 2009;147(3):505–11.e1.
35. Ma X, Zhou Z, Yi H, et al. Effect of providing free glasses on children's educational outcomes in China: cluster randomized controlled trial. BMJ. 2014;349:g5740.
36. Crabtree HL, Hildreth AJ, O'Connell JE, et al. Measuring visual symptoms in British cataract patients: the cataract symptom scale. Br J Ophthalmol. 1999;83(5):519–23.
37. Cruess AF, Gordon KD, Bellan L, et al. The cost of vision loss in Canada. 2. Results. Can J Ophthalmol. 2011;46(4):315–8.
38. Roberts CB, Hiratsuka Y, Yamada M, et al. Economic cost of visual impairment in Japan. Arch Ophthalmol. 2010;128(6):766–71.
39. Murray CJ, Vos T, Lozano R, et al. Disability-adjusted life years (DALYs) for 291 diseases and injuries in 21 regions, 1990-2010: a systematic analysis for the Global Burden of Disease Study 2010. Lancet. 2012;380(9859):2197–223.
40. McCarty CA, Nanjan MB, Taylor HR. Vision impairment predicts 5 year mortality. Br J Ophthalmol. 2001;85(3):322–6.
41. Hammond MD, Madigan WP, Bower KS. Refractive surgery in the United States Army, 2000-2003. Ophthalmology. 2005;112(2):184–90.
42. Denniston AK, Kyte D, Calvert M, Burr JM. An introduction to patient-reported outcome measures in ophthalmic research. Eye. 2014;28(6):637–45.
43. Pesudovs K, Garamendi E. Elliott DB. A quality of life comparison of people wearing spectacles or contact lenses or having undergone refractive surgery. J Refract Surg. 2006;22(1):19–27.
44. Lipson MJ, Brooks MM, Koffler BH. The role of orthokeratology in myopia control: a review. Eye Contact Lens. 2018;44(4):224–30.
45. Queiros A, Villa-Collar C, Gutierrez AR, et al. Quality of life of myopic subjects with different methods of visual correction using the NEI RQL-42 questionnaire. Eye Contact Lens. 2012;38(2):116–21.

46. Queiros A, Villa-Collar C, Gonzalez-Meijome JM, et al. Effect of pupil size on corneal aberrations before and after standard laser in situ keratomileusis, custom laser in situ keratomileusis, and corneal refractive therapy. Am J Ophthalmol. 2010;150(1):97–109.e1.
47. al-Kaff AS. Patient satisfaction after photorefractive keratectomy. J Refract Surg. 1997;13(5 Suppl):S459–60.
48. McGhee CN, Craig JP, Sachdev N, et al. Functional, psychological, and satisfaction outcomes of laser in situ keratomileusis for high myopia. J Cataract Refract Surg. 2000;26(4):497–509.
49. Villa C, Gutierrez R, Jimenez JR, Gonzalez-Meijome JM. Night vision disturbances after successful LASIK surgery. Br J Ophthalmol. 2007;91(8):1031–7.
50. Bailey MD, Mitchell GL, Dhaliwal DK, et al. Patient satisfaction and visual symptoms after laser in situ keratomileusis. Ophthalmology. 2003;110(7):1371–8.
51. Schein OD, Vitale S, Cassard SD, Steinberg EP. Patient outcomes of refractive surgery. The refractive status and vision profile. J Cataract Refract Surg. 2001;27(5):665–73.
52. Chan JWW, Edwards MH, Woo GC, Woo VCP. Contrast sensitivity after laser in situ keratomileusis: one-year follow-up. J Cataract Refract Surg. 2002;28(10):1774–9.
53. Hiraoka T, Okamoto C, Ishii Y, et al. Patient satisfaction and clinical outcomes after overnight orthokeratology. Optom Vis Sci. 2009;86(7):875–82.
54. Johnson KL, Carney LG, Mountford JA, et al. Visual performance after overnight orthokeratology. Cont Lens Anterior Eye. 2007;30(1):29–36.
55. Morgan PB, Efron N, Hill EA, et al. Incidence of keratitis of varying severity among contact lens wearers. Br J Ophthalmol. 2005;89(4):430.
56. Schein OD. Microbial keratitis associated with overnight orthokeratology: what we need to know. Cornea. 2005;24(7):767–9.
57. Pritchard N, Fonn D. Dehydration, lens movement and dryness ratings of hydrogel contact lenses. Ophthalmic Physiol Opt. 1995;15(4):281–6.
58. Pineles SL, Kraker RT, VanderVeen DK, et al. Atropine for the prevention of myopia progression in children: a report by the American Academy of Ophthalmology. Ophthalmology. 2017;124(12):1857–66.
59. Randleman JB, Russell B, Ward MA, et al. Risk factors and prognosis for corneal ectasia after LASIK. Ophthalmology. 2003;110(2):267–75.
60. De Paiva CS, Chen Z, Koch DD, et al. The incidence and risk factors for developing dry eye after myopic LASIK. Am J Ophthalmol. 2006;141(3):438–45.
61. Lansingh VC, Carter MJ, Martens M. Global cost-effectiveness of cataract surgery. Ophthalmology. 2007;114(9):1670–8.
62. Lamoureux EL, Fenwick E, Pesudovs K, Tan D. The impact of cataract surgery on quality of life. Curr Opin Ophthalmol. 2011;22(1):19–27.

Understanding Myopia: Pathogenesis and Mechanisms

4

Ranjay Chakraborty, Scott A. Read, and Stephen J. Vincent

Key Points

- Visual environment (or the quality of the retinal image) modulates the refractive development of the eye.
- Ocular response to form-deprivation and lens induced defocus is evident across a wide range of animal species, including humans.
- The visual system appears to be more sensitive to myopic than hyperopic defocus.
- Evidence suggests that greater time spent outdoors is protective against development and progression of myopia in children.

4.1 Emmetropization and Normal Ocular Growth in Human Eyes

When incident parallel rays of light from distant objects are brought to a focus upon the retina without accommodation, it is known as emmetropia. During postnatal eye growth, the precise matching of the axial length (the distance from the anterior corneal surface to the retina along the visual axis) and the optical power of the eye brings the eye to emmetropia [1, 2]. This active regulatory process that harmonizes the expansion of the eye with the optical power of the cornea and the crystalline lens

R. Chakraborty (✉)
Flinders University, Adelaide, SA, Australia
e-mail: ranjay.chakraborty@flinders.edu.au

S. A. Read · S. J. Vincent
Queensland University of Technology, Brisbane, QLD, Australia

M. Ang, T. Y. Wong (eds.), *Updates on Myopia*,
https://doi.org/10.1007/978-981-13-8491-2_4

is known as emmetropization [1]. Any disruption to these highly coordinated ocular changes results in the development of refractive errors, wherein distant images are focused either behind (hyperopia) or in front (myopia) of the retina [1].

Human eyes exhibit a distinctive pattern of eye growth during the early period of visual development. The distribution of refractive errors at birth appears to be normally distributed [3, 4]. Apart from some exceptions [5], the majority of newborn infants are moderately hyperopic (~+2.00 to +4.00 D) and this refractive error reduces significantly during the first 18 months of life [3, 6–8] (Fig. 4.1). By about 2–5 years of age, the distribution becomes leptokurtic with a peak around emmetropia to low hyperopia of about +0.50 to +1.00 D [5, 6, 8, 11, 12]. Although studies have reported small reductions in hyperopic refraction until the middle to late teen years [13, 14], emmetropization is believed to be largely completed by 5–6 years of age [5, 6, 8, 14].

Based on the visually guided ocular growth observed in a variety of animal models [15–17] (see Sect. 4.3), the growth of the human eye is also believed to be modulated by an active visual feedback from the hyperopic refractive error in neonatal eyes [18]. Studies have found a strong correlation between the rapid reduction in hyperopia and the changes in axial length during early ocular development [18, 19]. Human eyes are ~17 mm long after birth and grow to about 20 mm after the first year [11, 18–20]. This rapid expansion of the eye is largely attributed to the

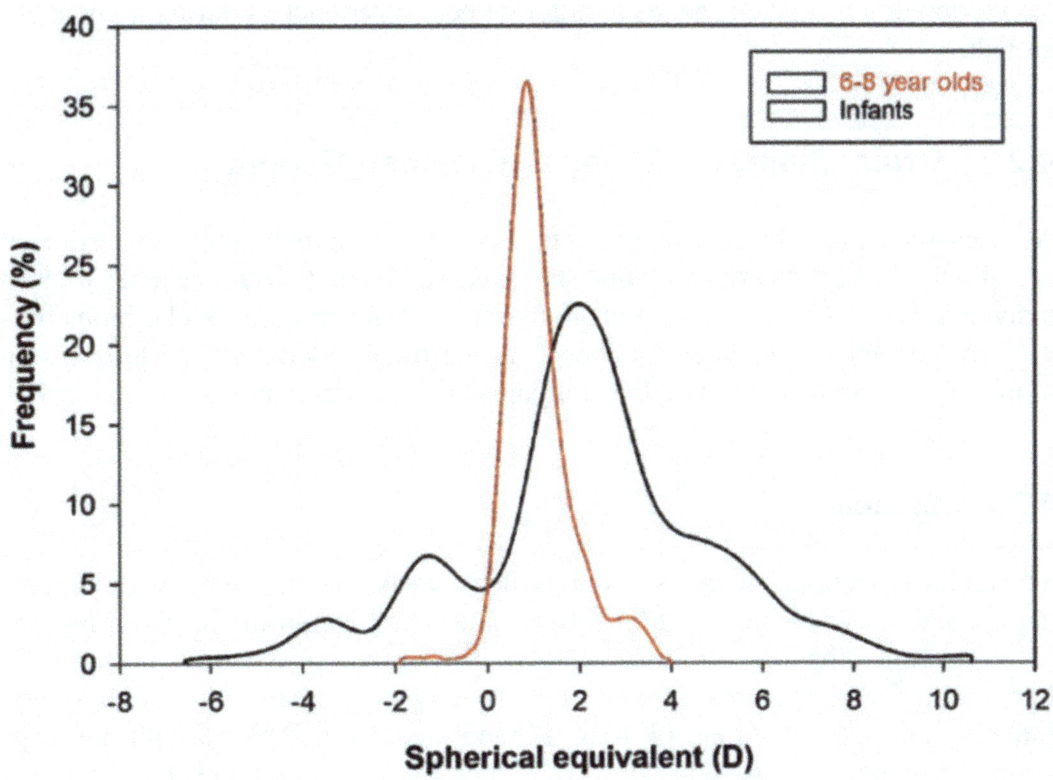

Fig. 4.1 Comparison of refractive error distribution among newborns [3] and 6–8-year-old children [9]. The distribution of refractive errors narrows between infancy to early childhood during the process of emmetropization. Adapted from FitzGerald and Duckman [10]

expansion of the vitreous chamber [18, 21]. From 2–3 years of age, axial elongation slows to approximately 0.4 mm/year until preschool age [11]. Consistent with changes in ocular refraction, the growth of the eye stabilizes further at 5–6 years, and only increases by 1–1.5 mm through the teenage years [11, 20, 21]. Together, these studies suggest that axial length is the most influential factor for emmetropization in human eyes.

In addition to changes in axial length, there is also a significant reduction in the refractive power of the cornea and the crystalline lens that contributes to the overall reduction in hyperopia in the first year of life [11, 18, 22]. Mutti et al. [18] reported a reduction of 1.07 and 3.62 D in corneal and crystalline lens powers, respectively, associated with flattening of the corneal and lens radii in newborn infants, between the ages of 3 and 9 months. Studies have also found higher degrees of corneal astigmatism in newborn infants [23–28], which reduces during the first 4 years of life and is associated with corneal flattening [24, 27, 29, 30]. Overall, these studies suggest that emmetropization in human eyes is largely attributed to the changes in axial length with minor contributions from corneal and crystalline lens powers.

Refractive errors occur as a result of either variations in (a) axial length with respect to the total refractive power of the eye (termed axial myopia or hyperopia) or (b) refractive power of the cornea and the crystalline lens with respect to the axial length of the eye (termed refractive myopia or hyperopia). This chapter focuses on the pathogenesis and potential underlying mechanisms of myopia, and the following section discusses the changes in different ocular parameters during myopic eye growth.

4.2 Ocular Biometric Changes in Human Myopia

As discussed earlier, the axial length of the eye is the primary biometric determinant of refractive error; however, the dimensions, curvature, and refractive index of each individual ocular structure contribute to the final refractive state. Ocular biometrics vary considerably throughout childhood, during the development and progression of myopia, and in response to clinical myopia control interventions.

4.2.1 Cornea

Several cross-sectional analyses have revealed a weak association between increasing corneal power (a steeper radius of curvature) and increasing levels of myopia [31–33], while others report no association [34], or the opposite relationship [35]. Longitudinal studies indicate that changes in corneal curvature during childhood [36–38] and early adulthood [39] are minimal and not associated with the magnitude of myopia progression. However, since the correlation between spherical equivalent refraction (SER) and the axial length to corneal radius ratio is typically stronger than that of axial length alone (by 15–20%) [40–43], corneal curvature does appear to make a modest contribution to the magnitude of myopia. Although corneal thickness does not vary systematically with refractive error [44–47], a reduction in corneal hysteresis (an estimate of corneal biomechanical strength or viscoelasticity) has been observed with increasing levels of myopia in children [48, 49] and adults [50–52]. However, the causal nature of this relationship remains unclear, or if such corneal metrics correlate with posterior scleral biomechanics.

4.2.2 Crystalline Lens and Anterior Chamber Depth

While the cornea flattens substantially during infancy and then remains relatively stable throughout childhood, the crystalline lens continues to thin, flatten, and reduce in optical power until approximately 10 years (a 0.25–0.50 D reduction per year), concurrent with lens fiber compaction [53–55]. These changes may be part of an emmetropization mechanism to compensate for continued axial elongation or a mechanical consequence of equatorial eye growth. Across a range of ethnicities, Mutti et al. [56] observed that within 1 year of myopia onset, compensatory crystalline lens thinning and flattening abruptly halted compared to children who remained emmetropic (Fig. 4.2), suggesting that childhood myopia is not purely axial in nature, but involves a decoupling of highly correlated anterior and posterior segment eye growth. In Singaporean children, Iribarren et al. [57] reported a transient acceleration in the reduction of lens power during myopia onset when the rate

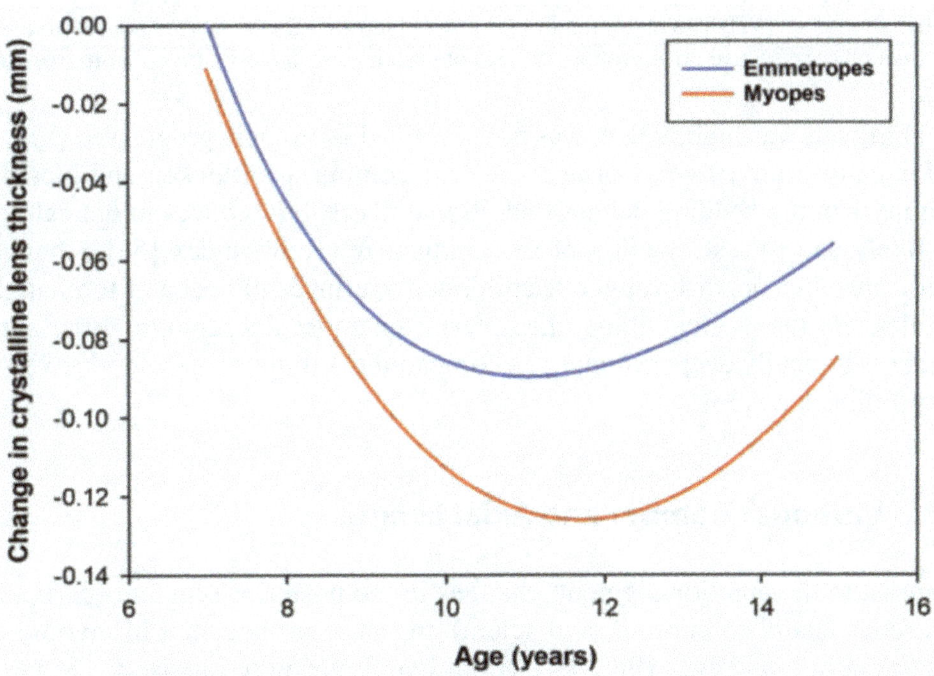

Fig. 4.2 The change in crystalline lens thickness as a function of age in myopes and emmetropes during childhood (after Mutti et al. [56]). Shortly after myopia onset (10–12 years), compensatory crystalline lens thinning abruptly halted compared to children who remained emmetropic suggesting that myopia development involves a decoupling of anterior and posterior segment eye growth

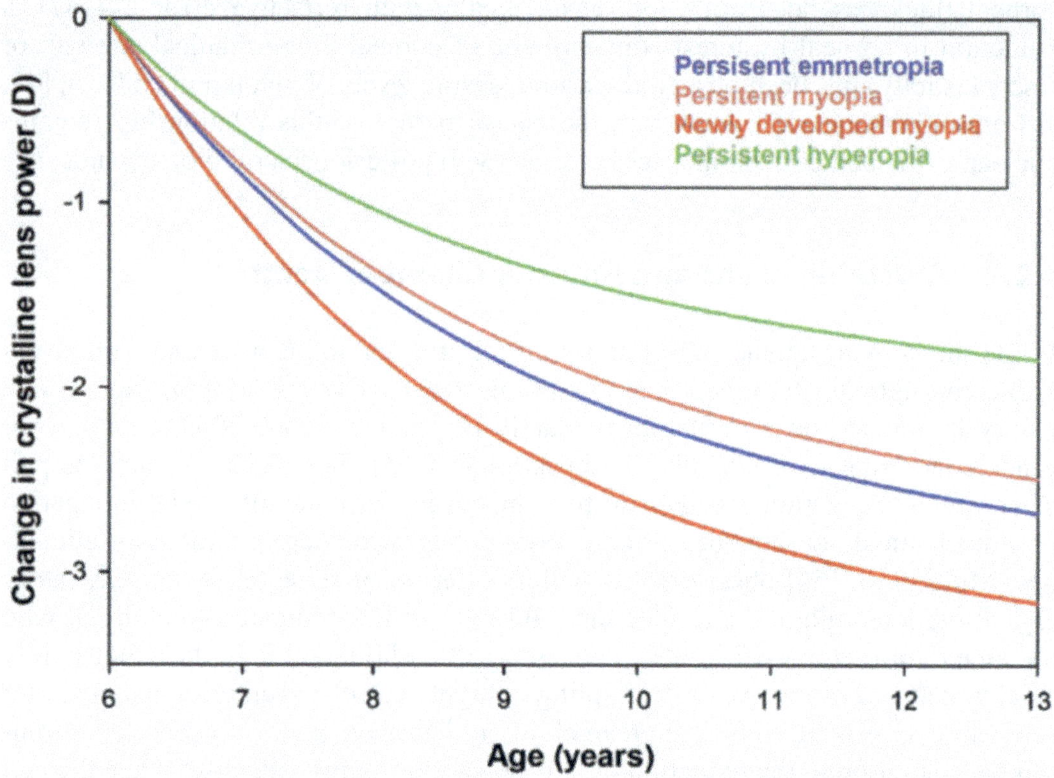

Fig. 4.3 The change in crystalline lens power during childhood (calculated from refraction and biometric measurements) in young Singaporean children for a range of refractive error groups (after Iribarren et al. [57]) The reduction in lens power increases during myopia onset (to a greater extent than other refractive error groups), but is not sustained throughout myopia progression

of axial growth was high, which was not sustained as myopia progressed (Fig. 4.3). Paradoxically, after 10 years of age, the lens continues to thicken and increase in curvature with the bedding down of additional fibers, but reduces in optical power, most likely due to a steepening of the gradient refractive index [58]. Changes in anterior chamber depth throughout childhood are inversely related to changes in lens thickness (as the lens thins, the anterior chamber deepens), and the anterior chamber is typically deeper in myopes compared to emmetropes and vice versa for the crystalline lens [53].

4.2.3 Vitreous Chamber and Axial Length

In contrast to the anterior segment, changes in the posterior segment (particularly, the vitreous chamber, choroid, and sclera) are more pronounced in myopic compared to non-myopic eyes (Fig. 4.4). Axial length, or more precisely, the vitreous chamber depth is the primary individual biometric contributor to refractive error in children, young adults, and the elderly [34, 59, 60], with the vitreous chamber depth accounting for over 50% of the observed variation in SER, followed by the cornea (~15%) and crystalline lens (~1%) [60]. Modeling of cross-sectional and

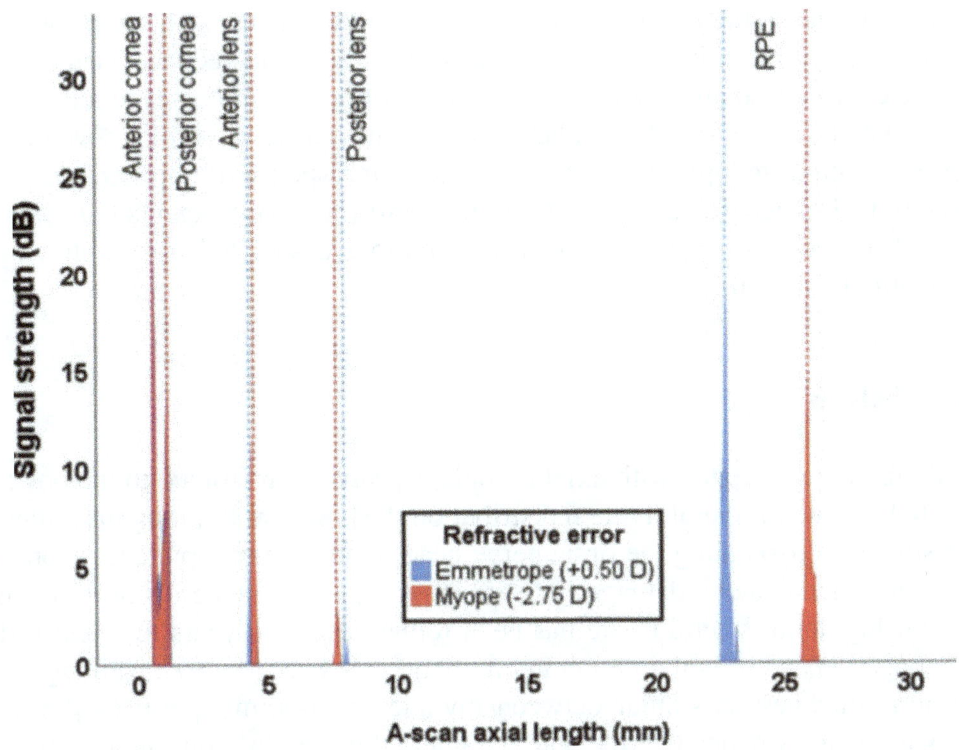

Fig. 4.4 Optical low coherence reflectometry A-Scan output from two 11-year-old males (one myope and one emmetrope). The predominant biometric differences are the deeper vitreous chamber (19.05 mm compared to 15.47 mm) and the longer axial length (25.87 mm compared to 22.69 mm) in the myopic eye. The anterior chamber depth is slightly shallower in the emmetropic eye (by 0.13 mm) while the crystalline lens is thicker (by 0.49 mm) in comparison to the myopic eye. The corneal thickness varies by only 0.04 mm

longitudinal data from emmetropic children indicates that axial length and vitreous chamber depth increase by approximately 0.16 mm per year from age 6–10 years, slowing to 0.05 mm per year from 11 to 14 years [61]. In myopic children aged between 6 and 11 years (corrected with single vision spectacles or contact lenses) average growth rates of approximately 0.30 mm per year have been reported [37, 62, 63], with greater vitreous chamber and axial elongation observed in younger females with myopic parents [37]. A range of myopia control interventions significantly slow the rate of eye growth and myopia progression during childhood, in some cases by up to 50% [64], and this reduction in axial elongation appears to be initially modulated by changes in the choroid underlying the retina.

4.2.4 Choroid

The choroid supplies the outer retina with oxygen and nutrients and regulates intraocular pressure and ocular temperature. The choroid is typically thinner in myopic compared to non-myopic eyes (most pronounced at the fovea [65, 66]) and thins with increasing myopia and axial length in both adults [67–74] and children [75–77]. Significant choroidal thinning is also observed in high myopia (<−6.00 D) or eyes with posterior staphyloma [78], and has been associated with the presence of lacquer cracks [79], choroidal neovascularization [80], and reduced visual acuity [81]. The choroid also appears to be a biomarker of ocular processes regulating eye growth given that the central macular choroid thins during the initial development and progression of myopia [82–84] and thickens in response to imposed peripheral myopic retinal image defocus [85, 86], topical anti-muscarinic agents [87, 88], and increased light exposure [89] (clinical interventions associated with a slowing of eye growth in children).

4.2.5 Sclera

Scleral thinning associated with axial myopia is primarily restricted to the posterior pole [90–92], due to scleral tissue redistribution [93]. Scleral thinning may alter the tissue strength surrounding the optic nerve head, rendering myopic eyes more susceptible to glaucomatous damage [94, 95]. Consequently, posterior reinforcement surgery using donor scleral tissue has been refined over the years to arrest further axial elongation and scleral thinning in highly myopic eyes [96, 97]. Although anterior scleral thickness is similar between myopic and non-myopic eyes [98–100], there is growing evidence that the anterior sclera thins slightly during accommodation, particularly in myopic eyes [101, 102], most likely due to biomechanical forces of the ciliary muscle. A greater thinning observed in myopic eyes may be a result of a thicker posterior ciliary muscle [103–105] or changes in biomechanical properties of the sclera reported in animal models of form-deprivation myopia [106, 107].

4.3 Visual Environment, Emmetropization, and Myopia: Evidence from Animal Models

Over the last four decades, numerous animal models have provided valuable insight into the mechanisms underlying emmetropization and refractive error development. Much of the knowledge on vision-dependent changes in ocular growth has emanated from animal experiments in which either the quality of image formed on the retina is degraded (known as form-deprivation [FD]), or the focal point of the image is altered with respect to the retinal plane (known as lens induced defocus). Both FD and lens induced defocus result in abnormal eye growth and development of refractive errors. This section summarizes the attributes of experimental ametropias derived from these two visual manipulations, their differences, and significance for understanding refractive error development in humans.

4.3.1 Form-Deprivation Myopia

FD is the most commonly used experimental paradigm to model axial myopia in animals. Depriving the retina of form or patterned vision through eyelid suture

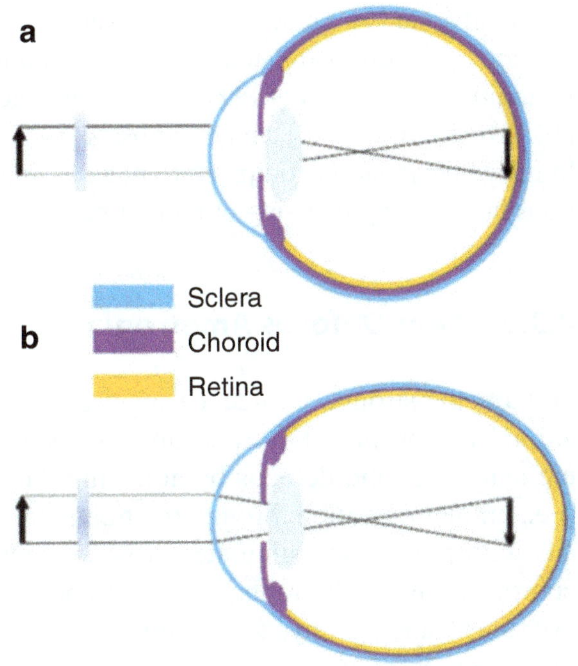

Fig. 4.5 Ocular compensation for form-deprivation (FD). (**a**) A diffuser causes nondirectional blur and a reduction in contrast of the retinal image. (**b**) The absence of visual feedback related to the effective refractive state of the eye causes a thinning of the posterior choroid and an increase in ocular growth, resulting in myopia

[108–110], or translucent diffusers [2, 15, 111–114] consistently produces axial myopia (Fig. 4.5). The use of noncontact translucent diffusers offers a more reliable representation of ocular changes with FD since they do not induce corneal changes (unlike eyelid fusion techniques). The ocular changes observed in response to FD clearly illustrate that degrading retinal image quality can produce robust myopic changes. Schaeffel et al. [115] proposed that FD is an open-loop condition, in which myopia develops as a result of uncoordinated ocular growth due to reduced retinal image contrast (or mid-range spatial frequency vision) [116] and the absence of visual feedback related to the effective refractive state of the eye [117].

The myopic response to FD varies among different animals. It is generally greatest in chickens (−9 D after 5 days of FD) [118], followed by tree shrews (−8 D after 12 days in young animals) [119] and guinea pigs (−6.6 D after 11 days) [113], and is less pronounced and much more variable in marmosets (−8 D after 4.5 weeks) [120] and rhesus monkeys (~−5 to −6 D after 17 weeks) [121, 122]. Variations observed between individual studies and animal models may be due to differences in experimental paradigms, the duration and extent of FD, inherent ocular anatomical variations, and/or differences in susceptibility to environmental myopia. Nevertheless, the myopic response to FD is conserved across a wide range of animal species (including fish, rabbit, mouse, and kestrel) [123]. In all species, axial myopia is predominantly caused by a significant elongation of the vitreous chamber, along with thinning of the choroid and the sclera [16, 17, 113, 124–132]. Few studies have also reported changes in corneal curvature and lens thickness with FD [131, 133–135]. Interestingly, ocular conditions that cause varying degrees of visual deprivation in humans such as ptosis [136], congenital cataract [137], corneal opacity [138], and vitreous hemorrhage [139] are associated with myopia, which may result from mechanisms similar to FD myopia observed in animals.

FD myopia is a graded phenomenon, where increasing degrees of image degradation are positively correlated with the magnitude of induced axial myopia [129, 140]. In addition, the effects of FD declines with age. Younger chicks [141, 142], macaques [143], tree shrews [119], and marmosets [144] show greater ocular changes in response to image degradation compared to older animals, potentially due to age-related reductions in sensory processing of blur stimuli or changes in scleral growth [144].

4.3.2 Lens Defocus Ametropias

Perhaps the strongest evidence of visual regulation of ocular growth comes from animal studies that show eyes can actively compensate for artificially induced myopic and hyperopic defocus by adjusting the axial length to the altered focal plane (i.e., emmetropization through the treatment lenses) (Fig. 4.6) [145]. Myopic defocus with plus lenses simulates artificial myopia that leads to a thickening of the choroid (moving the retina forward) and a reduction in the overall growth of the eye, thus, causing a hyperopic refractive error. Conversely, hyperopic defocus with minus lenses induces artificial hyperopia that leads to a thinning of the choroid

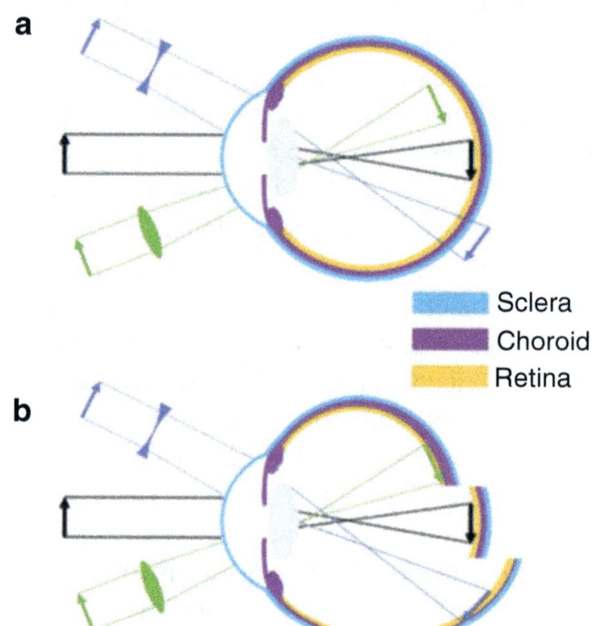

Fig. 4.6 (**a**) Schematic of imposed lens defocus. With no lens (black arrow), incident parallel rays of light from distant objects are focused on the retina. A plus lens (green, convex) causes the retinal image to focus in front of the retina known as myopic defocus, whereas a minus lens (blue, concave) focuses the image behind the retina known as hyperopic defocus. (**b**) A normal eye with no imposed lens defocus (black) exhibits normal ocular growth and choroidal thickness. Myopic defocus with plus lenses (green) causes a thickening of the choroid (moving the retina forward) and a reduction in the overall growth of the eye, causing a hyperopic refractive error. Hyperopic defocus with minus lenses (blue) leads to a thinning of the choroid (moving the retina backward) and an increase in ocular growth, resulting in myopia. Adapted from Wallman J and Winawer J, 2004 [1]

(moving the retina backward) and an increase in ocular growth, resulting in myopia to re-establish the optimal refractive state. This phenomenon was first documented in chicks [145], and has been extensively studied in chicks [16, 17, 146–148], tree shrews [149], rhesus monkeys [15, 150], marmosets [151], guinea pigs [152, 153], and mice [154] thereafter, indicating that the mechanisms regulating ocular growth can distinguish the sign of the imposed defocus in a wide range of animal species.

Chick eyes can compensate for a remarkable range of +15 to −10 D of imposed defocus [16, 147]. However, the operating range of defocus is much smaller for other animal species (monkey: −2 to +8 D [15], marmosets: −8 to <+4 D [151], tree shrew: −10 to +4 D [155], guinea pig: −7 to +4 D) [152, 156]. Compared to birds, the inability of primates to compensate for greater magnitudes of defocus may be due to bigger eye size [15, 150], the process of emmetropization [150], differences in the accommodative response to defocus stimuli, and/or the degree of independent accommodation between fellow eyes [15, 150, 157]. In all animals, the axial response to lens induced defocus is dependent upon the power of the treatment lens [147, 149–152, 158], and is predominantly attributed to the changes in vitreous chamber depth [16, 147, 159]. Similar to FD, the ocular response to lens induced defocus decreases with age [16]. Recent evidence suggests that the human visual system may also be able to detect the sign and magnitude of imposed defocus and make compensatory changes in axial length, similar to other animals. A number of studies have reported small bidirectional changes in axial length and choroidal thickness in response to 1–2 h of myopic and hyperopic defocus in children and young adults [160–165].

Studies have shown that the biological mechanisms underlying alterations in ocular growth to myopic and hyperopic defocus may be completely different (and not merely opposite to each other), and that the visual system is perhaps more sensitive to myopic defocus [166, 167]. In fact, the ocular response to lens induced defocus depends on the frequency and duration of lens wear, and not simply the "total duration" per day [166–169]. These findings argue for a nonlinear processing of myopic and hyperopic defocus signals across the retina [166, 167].

4.3.3 Comparing Form-Deprivation and Lens Defocus

Although FD and lens induced defocus use different visual stimuli to induce compensatory changes in ocular growth, there are features that are common to both visual manipulations. Removal of the visual manipulation triggers "recovery" from both FD and lens induced defocus [16, 17, 170]. During this recovery phase, the eyes quickly return to emmetropia by reversing the changes in choroidal thickness and axial eye growth (mainly by changing the vitreous chamber depth) [16, 17, 119, 150, 151, 170–173].

Further evidence from animal work suggests that the elimination of accommodation by cycloplegia, ciliary nerve section or damage to the Edinger-Westphal nucleus does not prevent the response to imposed FD [145, 174] or lens induced defocus [148, 175]. These results suggest that intact accommodation is not essential for visually guided growth [176] or there might be another accommodative pathway (not through ciliary and iris sphincter muscles) underlying optical defocus induced alterations in ocular growth [175].

Other studies argue that mechanisms underlying the response to FD and lens induced defocus may not be the same [177]. Some studies show different light paradigms selectively disrupt the response to FD or lens induced defocus [178–180]. For instance, high luminance levels inhibit myopia caused by FD in monkeys and chicks, but only slow the response to negative lenses [181, 182]. Furthermore, dopamine (a strong ocular growth inhibitor, see Sect. 4.4.1) may not signal eye growth in a similar manner for these two forms of experimental myopia [183]. While most studies indicate that dopamine agonists block increased axial elongation [177], one study reported that dopamine agonists inhibit FD, but not lens-induced myopia in guinea pigs [184]. More studies are needed to determine if these contradictory results are due to different regulatory mechanisms of eye growth or other parameters of the experimental paradigm.

4.4 Other Visual Cues for Emmetropization

Whilst the clarity of the retinal image dominates the nature of ocular growth, other visual cues may also influence the process of emmetropization. This section examines some of the important cues that could significantly affect retinal image quality, and hence ocular growth in human eyes.

4.4.1 Retinal Physiology

Work from animal models suggests that retinal defocus (or visual blur) initiates a signaling cascade that leads to a number of cellular and biochemical changes in the retina and the retinal pigment epithelium (RPE), which signal changes to the choroid, and eventually the sclera, leading to alterations in the overall growth and refractive state of the eye (Fig. 4.7) [16, 17, 185]. The retina is an integral part of this visual signaling as it is the first layer of photosensory neurons that detect

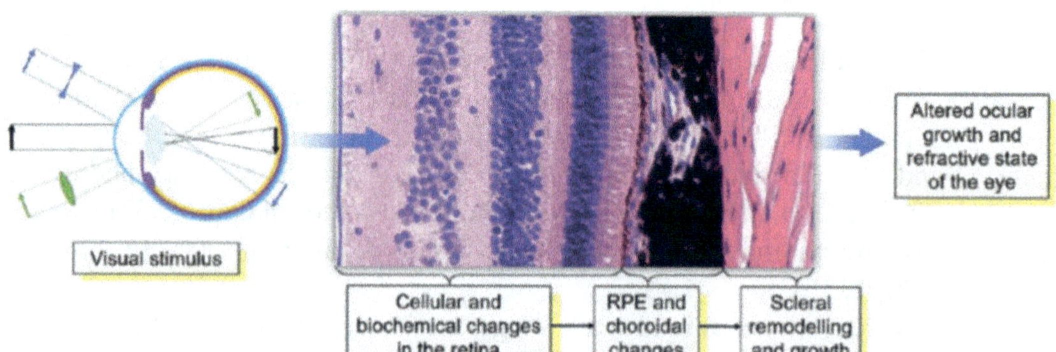

Fig. 4.7 A biochemical signal cascade beginning at the retina and ending at the sclera regulating ocular growth and the refractive state. Retinal defocus may initiate a signaling cascade that leads to a number of cellular and biochemical changes in the retina and the retinal pigment epithelium (RPE), the choroid, and eventually the sclera, leading to alterations in the overall growth and the refractive state of the eye

defocus [186]. Furthermore, ocular compensation for both FD and lens induced defocus are largely regulated at the retinal level. Severing the optic nerve in young chicks does not prevent the development of refractive errors in response to spectacle lenses [16, 187] or diffusers [130]. In both chicks [17, 188, 189] and primates [190], partial diffusers and hemifield spectacle lenses restricted to only half of the visual field cause corresponding myopic changes only in the visually deprived part of the globe. These studies demonstrate that the visual regulation of ocular growth in response to diffusers and lenses primarily occurs within the retina, with minimal input from the brain.

Retinal neurons also secrete a number of growth regulatory neurotransmitters (such as dopamine [191, 192], retinoic acid [153], nitric oxide [193, 194] and glucagon [195]) that can directly alter ocular growth in mammalian eyes. Dopamine, one of the most widely studied neurotransmitters with regard to myopia in animal models, has been implicated as a potent stop signal for myopic eye growth [183, 196]. In both chickens [191, 197] and primates [198], FD myopia is associated with lower levels of 3,4-dihydroxyphenylacetate (DOPAC, the primary metabolite of dopamine) and dopamine in the retina. Although the protective effects of outdoor light exposure on myopia development in children has been hypothesized to be mediated by greater dopamine synthesis in the eye (see Sect. 4.5), the exact mechanisms underlying the protective effects of dopamine on myopia are not fully known. Together, these studies suggest that alterations in normal retinal physiology and/or changes in retinal neurotransmitters may lead to the development of refractive errors, as shown in chickens [186, 199, 200] and mice [201–206]. Some features of retinal abnormalities and refractive errors are evident in humans as well; for instance, NYX [207] and GRM6 [208] retinal ON pathway mutations and retinal degenerations such as cone-rod dystrophy [209] and retinitis pigmentosa [210] are associated with myopia.

4.4.2 Aberrations

A long held belief is that myopia may develop due to the eye's emmetropization response to inherent ocular aberrations that degrade retinal image quality and trigger axial elongation [211]. Since there is minimal variation in longitudinal chromatic aberration between individuals or refractive error groups in humans [212], most investigations have focused on monochromatic higher order aberrations (HOAs) as a potential myopigenic stimulus. Evidence concerning the relationship between HOAs during distance viewing and refractive error from cross-sectional studies is conflicting [211, 213]. However, during or following near work tasks, adult myopic eyes tend to display a transient increase in corneal and total ocular HOAs (Figs. 4.8 and 4.9), suggesting a potential role for near work induced retinal image degradation in myopia development [214, 215]. Longitudinal studies of myopic children also indicate that eyes with greater positive spherical aberration demonstrate slower eye growth [63, 216].

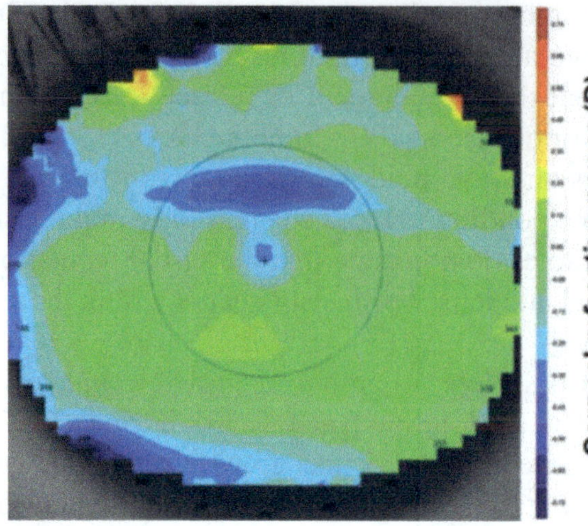

Fig. 4.8 Corneal refractive power difference map following a 10 min reading task at 25° downward gaze. The black circle denotes the pupil outline detected by the video keratoscope. A horizontal band of corneal flattening is observed in the superior aspect of the pupil corresponding to the position of the upper eyelid during downward gaze. This refractive change is equivalent to a 0.20 D hyperopic shift over the central 4 mm

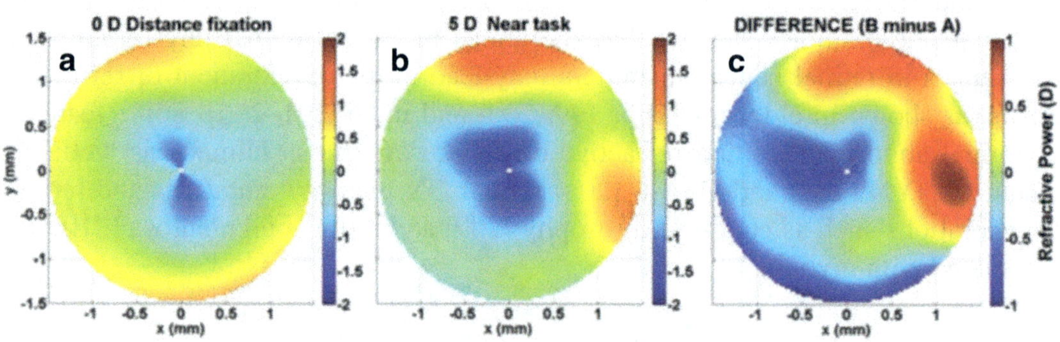

Fig. 4.9 Refractive power maps, a graphical representation of total ocular higher order aberrations, during (**a**) distance fixation (0 D accommodation demand), (**b**) a 5 D accommodation task, and (**c**) the difference (B minus A) over a 3 mm pupil diameter. A significant increase in negative spherical aberration of −0.10 μm is displayed

A number of myopia control interventions also alter the HOA and peripheral refraction profile. While relative peripheral refraction was initially thought to modulate central eye growth, recent longitudinal studies have found no association between peripheral refraction and myopia progression in children [217, 218]. Multifocal soft contact lenses and orthokeratology significantly increase the magnitude of positive spherical aberration [219, 220]. The anticholinergic agent atropine may also provide visual feedback that influences eye growth due to an increase in positive spherical aberration or horizontal coma associated with cycloplegia and pupil mydriasis, respectively [221]. Collectively, these findings suggest that changes in HOAs may influence eye growth and refractive development during childhood.

4.4.3 Accommodation

Given the association between near work and the development and progression of childhood myopia [222], numerous studies have compared various characteristics of accommodation between refractive error groups, typically the accuracy of the accommodation response, since a lag of accommodation (hyperopic retinal defocus) may stimulate axial elongation as observed in animal models. Using a range of experimental approaches, the accommodative response to a 3 D accommodative stimulus is ~0.25 to 1.00 D less in myopic adults compared to emmetropes [223–227]. The slowing of myopia progression during childhood with progressive addition or bifocal lenses, designed to improve accommodation accuracy and minimize a lag of accommodation, adds some weight to the role of accommodation in myopia development and progression [62, 228]. However, the exact underlying mechanism of myopia control with such lenses may be related to imposed peripheral retinal defocus or a reduction in the near vergence demand [229]. In a longitudinal study of young infants [230], a significant relationship was observed between the accommodative response and the reduction in neonatal refractive error in the first 2 years of life, supporting a potential role for accommodation-guided eye growth.

4.4.4 Circadian Rhythms

Like many of the human body's physiological processes, numerous ocular structures and functions exhibit cyclic variations over the course of the day. Visual inputs such as daily patterns of light exposure are considered critical factors in entraining the timing of these circadian rhythms. Findings from animal studies demonstrate that normal eye growth exhibits significant circadian variations, with the eye generally being longest during the day and shorter at night [231]. Choroidal thickness also exhibits a circadian rhythm in normal eyes, which is generally in antiphase to the rhythms in axial length [172]. Similar patterns of diurnal variation in axial length and choroidal thickness have also been documented in normal human eyes [232–234].

It has also been suggested that ocular circadian rhythms may play a role in eye growth regulation and the development of myopia, since altering the visual inputs that drive circadian rhythms (e.g., rearing animals in constant light [235] or constant darkness [236], or exposing the eye to bright light at night time [237]) can result in alterations in normal eye growth in animal models. Furthermore, when refractive errors (both hyperopic and myopic) are induced experimentally in animals, changes in the magnitude and phase of the normal circadian rhythms of axial length and choroidal thickness also occur, which also supports a potential role of circadian rhythms in the development of refractive errors [172, 238]. These findings from animal research were paralleled by studies in young adult humans, where changes in the normal diurnal rhythms of axial length and choroidal thickness occurred in response to short-term (12-h) exposure to monocular myopic [165], and hyperopic blur [163]. Although the exact role played by circadian rhythms in the regulation of human eye growth is not fully understood, human studies also indicate that myopes exhibit alterations in their systemic melatonin levels [239], and also exhibit altered sleep patterns [240] compared to non-myopic individuals.

4.5 Effects of Key Environmental Factors on Myopia

As discussed in Chaps. 1 and 2, myopia represents a "complex" disorder with both environmental and genetic origins [241, 242]. This section discusses some of the important environmental factors, and their influence on myopia.

4.5.1 Near Work and Education

Since the age when myopia normally develops and progresses coincides with the school years, myopia has long been suggested to be connected with increased levels of education. Indeed, numerous studies conducted across a range of different populations have consistently found that higher levels of education are associated with a higher prevalence of myopia [243–245]. The exact mechanism linking increased education with myopia, however, is less clear. Although it is possible that optical [214, 224] or biomechanical [246, 247] ocular changes associated with near work could potentially promote myopic eye growth in those with higher levels of education (and hence near work demands), population studies examining the link between near work activities and myopia have been conflicting, with some studies suggesting an association between near work and myopia [222, 248], and others indicating no significant effects [249]. The relatively inconsistent findings linking near work with myopia development suggests a potential role for other factors in the association between education and myopia, such as a lack of outdoor light exposure, discussed further below.

4.5.2 Urbanization

Aspects of the living environment may also be involved in the development and progression of myopia, since population-based studies consistently report a higher prevalence of myopia in children living in urban regions, compared to children living in rural regions [250, 251]. These associations between the urban environment and myopia could at least partially be explained by socioeconomic and educational differences between urban and rural regions, which could in turn result in differences in near work and outdoor activities. However, a number of recent studies indicate that a higher population density is significantly associated with increased myopia prevalence in children, independent of near work and outdoor activities [252, 253]. This suggests other aspects of the urban environment may potentially impact upon eye growth. Studies have also reported associations between housing type and myopia, with children living in smaller homes reported to have a significantly higher prevalence of myopia [253, 254]. Although further research is required to establish the causative nature and mechanisms underlying these associations, it has been hypothesized that a constricted living space may result in an increased exposure to hyperopic blur, thus promoting myopia.

4.5.3 Light Exposure

A number of recent studies report that the time children spend engaged in outdoor activities is negatively associated with their risk of myopia [241, 249, 255–259]. Both cross-sectional and longitudinal studies indicate that greater time spent outdoors is associated with a significantly lower myopia prevalence and reduced risk of myopia onset in childhood. Although some studies report significant associations between myopia progression and outdoor activity [257, 259], this is not a consistent finding across all longitudinal studies [260]. A recent meta-analysis of studies examining the relationship between outdoor time and myopia indicated that there was a 2% reduction in the odds of having myopia for each additional hour per week spent outdoors [261].

These associations [241, 255, 256] have prompted recent interest in the potential influence of light exposure in the regulation of eye growth and myopia. Since outdoor activity typically involves exposure to high intensity light, it has been hypothesized that increased exposure to bright light may be the important factor underlying these protective effects of outdoor activity [256]. Other factors, such as the typical pattern of retinal focus experienced in outdoor environments (which is likely to involve less near focusing and potentially less exposure to hyperopic blur), may also play a role [262].

Light Intensity and Myopia Animal studies indicate that the intensity of daily light exposure can influence refractive development. In normal growing young chickens, rearing animals under a normal daily light-dark cycle, but with daily bright ambient lighting (~10,000 lux) resulted in significantly less myopic refractive errors than when animals were reared under dim ambient lighting during the day (50 lux) [263]. Bright light exposure also inhibits the development of FD myopia in a range of different animal species [114, 181, 264], with the strength of inhibitory effects correlating significantly with the log of the intensity of ambient light exposure [264]. The effects of increased light intensity upon lens induced myopia (through imposing hyperopic defocus) in animals however are less consistent, with either a slowing of lens compensation (with no change in refractive endpoint) [182], or no significant effects on lens compensation reported [265].

Recent observational longitudinal studies in humans utilizing wearable light sensors to assess ambient light exposure have enabled the relationship between light exposure and axial eye growth in childhood to be examined [266, 267]. Similar to findings in animals, both of these recent studies have reported that slower axial eye growth is associated with greater daily ambient light exposure (with a 1-log unit increase in light exposure being associated with ~0.1 mm/year slower axial eye growth), with this relationship reaching statistical significance in the study with the larger sample size ($n = 102$) [266], and bordering on significance ($p = 0.07$, $n = 60$) in the other study [267]. A recent randomized, controlled trial in Taiwan examined the effect of increasing outdoor time during the school day (an extra 40 min of outdoor time during school recess) upon myopia development and axial eye growth over 12 months [268]. In this study, light exposure was also monitored using wearable light sensors, and a significant association between greater light exposure and slower myopia progression was also documented. Collectively, these studies suggest that increased light exposure is associated with slower axial eye growth in the human eye.

Increased light exposure may also underlie some of the differences in myopia prevalence found in different geographic locations. A recent study compared the habitual ambient light exposure (captured with wearable light sensors) of children living in Singapore (a country with some of the highest reported levels of childhood myopia prevalence [269]) with children living in Australia (where myopia prevalence is generally reported to be relatively low [270]) and found substantially lower levels of outdoor light exposure in the children living in Singapore (Fig. 4.10) [271].

Duration of Light Exposure and Myopia Animal studies examining the effects of increased light exposure upon myopia development have generally used experimental paradigms where elevated light levels were applied continuously for the full day. Lan et al. [272] examined the influence of different daily durations of bright light exposure upon inhibition of myopia in chickens. They found bright light applied for

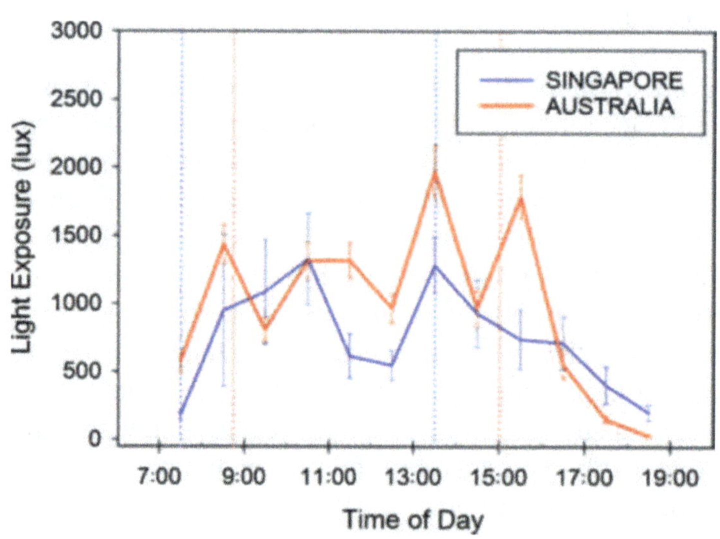

Fig. 4.10 Average hourly light exposure of Australian (red lines) and Singaporean (blue lines) children assessed during school weekdays using wearable light sensors. Note the substantially greater light exposure for the Australian children at a number of periods throughout the day [271]. This lower daily exposure to bright outdoor light may be one factor underlying the higher myopia prevalence typically observed in Singaporean children. Dashed lines indicate the average school start and finish times in Australia (red) and Singapore (blue). Error bars represent the standard error of the mean

only 1 or 2 h per day did not inhibit myopia, but 5 h of exposure did significantly protect against the development of FD myopia. Extending exposure duration further to 10 h per day did not appear to offer further protective benefit.

In a large longitudinal study, Jones et al. [249] reported that children who engaged in outdoor activities for 14 h per week or more, exhibited the lowest odds of developing myopia. A number of recent randomized controlled trials have reported that interventions that increase children's outdoor time (by 40–80 min a day) significantly reduce the onset of myopia in childhood [268, 273, 274]. In the "Role of outdoor activity in myopia study" [266], children who were habitually exposed to low ambient light levels (on average less than 60 min exposure to outdoor light per day) had significantly faster axial eye growth compared to children habitually exposed to moderate and high light levels. These findings from human studies suggest that children who are exposed to less than 60 min a day of bright outdoor light are at an increased risk of more rapid eye growth and myopia development, and that approximately 2 h or more of outdoor exposure each day is required to provide protection against myopia development in the human eye.

Spectral Composition of Light and Myopia Since the spectral characteristics of outdoor light are significantly different to typical indoor light, it has been suggested that the spectral composition of outdoor light may be an additional factor that underlies the protective effects of outdoor activity upon myopia development. Although some studies in humans suggest exposure to short-wavelength light may protect against myopia [275], there has only been limited work in humans examining the possible impact of the spectral composition of light on myopia.

Animal studies do suggest that the spectral content of light can influence the growth of the eye, since altered eye growth is observed in animals reared under narrow band spectral lighting conditions. However, the effects of the spectral content of light shows substantial interspecies differences [276–279]. In chickens and guineas pigs, raising animals in short-wavelength light appears to slow eye growth and reduce myopia development, whereas long-wavelength light appears to increase eye growth and lead to myopia development [276, 279]. Conversely long-wavelength light appears to slow eye growth and reduce myopia development in tree shrews and rhesus monkeys [277, 278]. Further research is required to understand the mechanisms underlying these effects (and interspecies differences) and to establish the impact of the spectral composition of light upon human myopia.

4.6 Conclusion

In conclusion, over the last 40 years, remarkable progress has been made in understanding the possible mechanisms and pathogenesis of myopia, with a large contribution to this knowledge coming from an extensive body of work in animal models. Importantly, laboratory research in animals have shown that the visual environment (i.e., quality and/or focus of the retinal image) influences ocular growth and refractive development, which has been a key to our current understanding of the process of emmetropization in humans. Similarities in features of defocus induced ocular changes in humans and experimental models of myopia, such as the eye's ability to detect the sign of retinal defocus and make compensatory changes in axial length, suggest that mechanisms of visually guided eye growth and refractive error development in animal models may be present in human eyes as well. Alongside animal research, a large body of clinical and epidemiological research has identified a number of other visual cues (e.g., aberrations, accommodation, and circadian rhythms) and environmental factors (e.g., light exposure, near work, and education) that could affect normal ocular growth and lead to the development of refractive errors. Experimental models continue to provide valuable information on cellular and biochemical mechanisms of eye growth, enabling the identification of potential new therapeutic targets for early diagnosis and treatment of myopia.

References

1. Wallman J, Winawer J. Homeostasis of eye growth and the question of myopia. Neuron. 2004;43:447–68.
2. Smith EL. Spectacle lenses and emmetropization: the role of optical defocus in regulating ocular development. Optom Vis Sci. 1998;75:388–98.
3. Cook RC, Glasscock R. Refractive and ocular findings in the newborn. Am J Ophthalmol. 1951;34:1407–13.
4. Banks MS. Infant refraction and accommodation. Int Ophthalmol Clin. 1980;20:205–32.
5. Mohindra I, Held R. Refraction in humans from birth to five years. In: Third International Conference on Myopia Copenhagen, August 24–27, 1980. New York: Springer; 1981. p. 19–27.
6. Ingram R, Barr A. Changes in refraction between the ages of 1 and 3 1/2 years. Br J Ophthalmol. 1979;63:339–42.
7. Wood I, Hodi S, Morgan L. Longitudinal change of refractive error in infants during the first year of life. Eye. 1995;9:551–7.
8. Gwiazda J, Thorn F, Bauer J, Held R. Emmetropization and the progression of manifest refraction in children followed from infancy to puberty. Clin Vis Sci. 1993;8:337–44.
9. Kempf GA, Collins SD, Jarman BL. Refractive errors in the eyes of children as determined by retinoscopie examination with a cycloplegic. Results of eye examinations of 1,860 white school children in Washington, DC. Public Health Bulletin. 1928;182:56.
10. Fitzgerald DE, Duckman R. Refractive error. In: Visual development, diagnosis, and treatment of the pediatric patient. Philadelphia: Lippincott Williams & Wilkins; 2006. p. 69–88.
11. Gordon RA, Donzis PB. Refractive development of the human eye. Arch Ophthalmol. 1985;103:785–9.
12. Saunders KJ. Early refractive development in humans. Surv Ophthalmol. 1995;40:207–16.
13. Hirsch MJ. Predictability of refraction at age 14 on the basis of testing at age 6—interim report from the Ojai Longitudinal Study of Refraction. Optom Vis Sci. 1964;41:567–73.
14. Zadnik K, Mutti DO, Friedman NE, Adams AJ. Initial cross-sectional results from the Orinda Longitudinal Study of Myopia. Optom Vis Sci. 1993;70:750–8.
15. Smith EL, Hung LF. The role of optical defocus in regulating refractive development in infant monkeys. Vis Res. 1999;39:1415–35.
16. Wildsoet C, Wallman J. Choroidal and scleral mechanisms of compensation for spectacle lenses in chicks. Vis Res. 1995;35:1175–94.

17. Wallman J, Wildsoet C, Xu A, et al. Moving the retina: choroidal modulation of refractive state. Vis Res. 1995;35:37–50.
18. Mutti DO, Mitchell GL, Jones LA, et al. Axial growth and changes in lenticular and corneal power during emmetropization in infants. Invest Ophthalmol Vis Sci. 2005;46:3074–80.
19. Pennie FC, Wood IC, Olsen C, White S, Charman WN. A longitudinal study of the biometric and refractive changes in full-term infants during the first year of life. Vis Res. 2001;41:2799–810.
20. Larsen JS. The sagittal growth of the eye: IV. Ultrasonic measurement of the axial length of the eye from birth to puberty. Acta Ophthalmol. 1971;49:873–86.
21. Larsen JS. The sagittal growth of the eye. 3. Ultrasonic measurement of the posterior segment (axial length of the vitreous) from birth to puberty. Acta Ophthalmol. 1971;49:441–53.
22. Sorsby A, Leary G, Richards MJ. Correlation ametropia and component ametropia. Vis Res. 1962;2:309–13.
23. Isenberg SJ, Del Signore M, Chen A, Wei J, Christenson PD. Corneal topography of neonates and infants. Arch Ophthalmol. 2004;122:1767–71.
24. Ehrlich DL, Braddick OJ, Atkinson J, et al. Infant emmetropization: longitudinal changes in refraction components from nine to twenty months of age. Optom Vis Sci. 1997;74:822–43.
25. Varughese S, Varghese RM, Gupta N, Ojha R, Sreenivas V, Puliyel JM. Refractive error at birth and its relation to gestational age. Curr Eye Res. 2005;30:423–8.
26. Friling R, Weinberger D, Kremer I, Avisar R, Sirota L, Snir M. Keratometry measurements in preterm and full term newborn infants. Br J Ophthalmol. 2004;88:8–10.
27. Rowland HC, Sayles N. Photokeratometric and photorefractive measurements of astigmatism in infants and young children. Vis Res. 1985;25:73–81.
28. Gwiazda J, Scheiman M, Mohindra I, Held R. Astigmatism in children: changes in axis and amount from birth to six years. Invest Ophthalmol Vis Sci. 1984;25:88–92.
29. Atkinson J, Braddick O, French J. Infant astigmatism: its disappearance with age. Vis Res. 1980;20:891–3.
30. Dobson V, Fulton A, Sebris SL. Cycloplegic refractions of infants and young children: the axis of astigmatism. Invest Ophthalmol Vis Sci. 1984;25:83–7.
31. Li SM, Iribarren R, Kang MT, et al. Corneal power, anterior segment length and lens power in 14-year-old Chinese children: the Anyang Childhood Eye Study. Sci Rep. 2016;6:20243.
32. Carney LG, Mainstone JC, Henderson BA. Corneal topography and myopia. A cross-sectional study. Invest Ophthalmol Vis Sci. 1997;38:311–20.
33. AlMahmoud T, Priest D, Munger R, Jackson WB. Correlation between refractive error, corneal power, and thickness in a large population with a wide range of ametropia. Invest Ophthalmol Vis Sci. 2011;52:1235–42.
34. Xie R, Zhou XT, Lu F, et al. Correlation between myopia and major biometric parameters of the eye: a retrospective clinical study. Optom Vis Sci. 2009;86:E503–8.
35. Zhang YY, Jiang WJ, Teng ZE, et al. Corneal curvature radius and associated factors in Chinese children: the Shandong Children Eye Study. PLoS One. 2015;10:e0117481.
36. Breslin KM, O'Donoghue L, Saunders KJ. A prospective study of spherical refractive error and ocular components among Northern Irish schoolchildren (the NICER study). Invest Ophthalmol Vis Sci. 2013;54:4843–50.
37. Saw SM, Chua WH, Gazzard G, Koh D, Tan DT, Stone RA. Eye growth changes in myopic children in Singapore. Br J Ophthalmol. 2005;89:1489–94.
38. Scheiman M, Gwiazda J, Zhang Q, et al. Longitudinal changes in corneal curvature and its relationship to axial length in the Correction of Myopia Evaluation Trial (COMET) cohort. J Opt. 2016;9:13–21.
39. Lin LL, Shih YF, Lee YC, Hung PT, Hou PK. Changes in ocular refraction and its components among medical studentsDOUBLEHYPHENa 5-year longitudinal study. Optom Vis Sci. 1996;73:495–8.
40. Ojaimi E, Rose KA, Morgan IG, et al. Distribution of ocular biometric parameters and refraction in a population-based study of Australian children. Invest Ophthalmol Vis Sci. 2005;46:2748–54.

41. He X, Zou H, Lu L, et al. Axial length/corneal radius ratio: association with refractive state and role on myopia detection combined with visual acuity in Chinese schoolchildren. PLoS One. 2015;10:e0111766.
42. Gonzalez Blanco F, Sanz Fernandez JC, Munoz Sanz MA. Axial length, corneal radius, and age of myopia onset. Optom Vis Sci. 2008;85:89–96.
43. Foo VH, Verkicharla PK, Ikram MK, et al. Axial length/corneal radius of curvature ratio and myopia in 3-year-old children. Transl Vis Sci Technol. 2016;5:5.
44. Ortiz S, Mena L, Rio-San Cristobal A, Martin R. Relationships between central and peripheral corneal thickness in different degrees of myopia. J Opt. 2014;7:44–50.
45. Pedersen L, Hjortdal J, Ehlers N. Central corneal thickness in high myopia. Acta Ophthalmol Scand. 2005;83:539–42.
46. Tong L, Saw SM, Siak JK, Gazzard G, Tan D. Corneal thickness determination and correlates in Singaporean schoolchildren. Invest Ophthalmol Vis Sci. 2004;45:4004–9.
47. Fam HB, How AC, Baskaran M, Lim KL, Chan YH, Aung T. Central corneal thickness and its relationship to myopia in Chinese adults. Br J Ophthalmol. 2006;90:1451–3.
48. Huang Y, Huang C, Li L, et al. Corneal biomechanics, refractive error, and axial length in Chinese primary school children. Invest Ophthalmol Vis Sci. 2011;52:4923–8.
49. Chang PY, Chang SW, Wang JY. Assessment of corneal biomechanical properties and intraocular pressure with the Ocular Response Analyzer in childhood myopia. Br J Ophthalmol. 2010;94:877–81.
50. Jiang Z, Shen M, Mao G, et al. Association between corneal biomechanical properties and myopia in Chinese subjects. Eye. 2011;25:1083–9.
51. Wang W, He M, He H, Zhang C, Jin H, Zhong X. Corneal biomechanical metrics of healthy Chinese adults using Corvis ST. Cont Lens Anterior Eye. 2017;40:97–103.
52. Shen M, Fan F, Xue A, Wang J, Zhou X, Lu F. Biomechanical properties of the cornea in high myopia. Vis Res. 2008;48:2167–71.
53. Shih YF, Chiang TH, Lin LL. Lens thickness changes among school children in Taiwan. Invest Ophthalmol Vis Sci. 2009;50:2637–44.
54. Wong HB, Machin D, Tan SB, Wong TY, Saw SM. Ocular component growth curves among Singaporean children with different refractive error status. Invest Ophthalmol Vis Sci. 2010;51:1341–7.
55. Jones LA, Mitchell GL, Mutti DO, Hayes JR, Moeschberger ML, Zadnik K. Comparison of ocular component growth curves among refractive error groups in children. Invest Ophthalmol Vis Sci. 2005;46:2317–27.
56. Mutti DO, Mitchell GL, Sinnott LT, et al. Corneal and crystalline lens dimensions before and after myopia onset. Optom Vis Sci. 2012;89:251–62.
57. Iribarren R, Morgan IG, Chan YH, Lin X, Saw SM. Changes in lens power in Singapore Chinese children during refractive development. Invest Ophthalmol Vis Sci. 2012;53:5124–30.
58. Dubbelman M, Van der Heijde GL. The shape of the aging human lens: curvature, equivalent refractive index and the lens paradox. Vis Res. 2001;41:1867–77.
59. Li SM, Li SY, Kang MT, et al. Distribution of ocular biometry in 7- and 14-year-old Chinese children. Optom Vis Sci. 2015;92:566–72.
60. Richter GM, Wang M, Jiang X, et al. Ocular determinants of refractive error and its age- and sex-related variations in the Chinese American Eye Study. JAMA Ophthalmol. 2017;135:724–32.
61. Zadnik K, Mutti DO, Mitchell GL, Jones LA, Burr D, Moeschberger ML. Normal eye growth in emmetropic schoolchildren. Optom Vis Sci. 2004;81:819–28.
62. Gwiazda J, Hyman L, Hussein M, et al. A randomized clinical trial of progressive addition lenses versus single vision lenses on the progression of myopia in children. Invest Ophthalmol Vis Sci. 2003;44:1492–500.
63. Lau JK, Vincent SJ, Collins MJ, Cheung SW, Cho P. Ocular higher-order aberrations and axial eye growth in young Hong Kong children. Sci Rep. 2018;8:6726.
64. Huang J, Wen D, Wang Q, et al. Efficacy comparison of 16 interventions for myopia control in children: a network meta-analysis. Ophthalmology. 2016;123:697–708.

65. Read SA, Collins MJ, Vincent SJ, Alonso-Caneiro D. Choroidal thickness in myopic and non-myopic children assessed with enhanced depth imaging optical coherence tomography. Invest Ophthalmol Vis Sci. 2013;54:7578–86.
66. Xiong S, He X, Deng J, et al. Choroidal thickness in 3001 Chinese children aged 6 to 19 years using swept-source OCT. Sci Rep. 2017;7:45059.
67. Chen FK, Yeoh J, Rahman W, Patel PJ, Tufail A, Da Cruz L. Topographic variation and interocular symmetry of macular choroidal thickness using enhanced depth imaging optical coherence tomography. Invest Ophthalmol Vis Sci. 2012;53:975–85.
68. Esmaeelpour M, Povazay B, Hermann B, et al. Three-dimensional 1060-nm OCT: choroidal thickness maps in normal subjects and improved posterior segment visualization in cataract patients. Invest Ophthalmol Vis Sci. 2010;51:5260–6.
69. Gupta P, Jing T, Marziliano P, et al. Distribution and determinants of choroidal thickness and volume using automated segmentation software in a population-based study. Am J Ophthalmol. 2015;159:293–301.e293.
70. Li XQ, Munkholm A, Larsen M, Munch IC. Choroidal thickness in relation to birth parameters in 11- to 12-year-old children: the Copenhagen Child Cohort 2000 Eye Study. Invest Ophthalmol Vis Sci. 2014;56:617–24.
71. Ouyang Y, Heussen FM, Mokwa N, et al. Spatial distribution of posterior pole choroidal thickness by spectral domain optical coherence tomography. Invest Ophthalmol Vis Sci. 2011;52:7019–26.
72. Tan CS, Cheong KX. Macular choroidal thicknesses in healthy adultsDOUBLEHYPHENrelationship with ocular and demographic factors. Invest Ophthalmol Vis Sci. 2014;55:6452–8.
73. Wei WB, Xu L, Jonas JB, et al. Subfoveal choroidal thickness: the Beijing Eye Study. Ophthalmology. 2013;120:175–80.
74. Sanchez-Cano A, Orduna E, Segura F, et al. Choroidal thickness and volume in healthy young white adults and the relationships between them and axial length, ammetropy and sex. Am J Ophthalmol. 2014;158:574–83.
75. He X, Jin P, Zou H, et al. Choroidal thickness in healthy Chinese children aged 6 to 12: The Shanghai Children Eye Study. Retina. 2017;37:368–75.
76. Jin P, Zou H, Zhu J, et al. Choroidal and retinal thickness in children with different refractive status measured by swept-source optical coherence tomography. Am J Ophthalmol. 2016;168:164–76.
77. Zhang JM, Wu JF, Chen JH, et al. Macular choroidal thickness in children: the Shandong Children Eye Study. Invest Ophthalmol Vis Sci. 2015;56:7646–52.
78. Zhou LX, Shao L, Xu L, Wei WB, Wang YX, You QS. The relationship between scleral staphyloma and choroidal thinning in highly myopic eyes: the Beijing Eye Study. Sci Rep. 2017;7:9825.
79. Wang NK, Lai CC, Chou CL, et al. Choroidal thickness and biometric markers for the screening of lacquer cracks in patients with high myopia. PLoS One. 2013;8:e53660.
80. Ikuno Y, Jo Y, Hamasaki T, Tano Y. Ocular risk factors for choroidal neovascularization in pathologic myopia. Invest Ophthalmol Vis Sci. 2010;51:3721–5.
81. Nishida Y, Fujiwara T, Imamura Y, Lima LH, Kurosaka D, Spaide RF. Choroidal thickness and visual acuity in highly myopic eyes. Retina. 2012;32:1229–36.
82. Read SA, Alonso-Caneiro D, Vincent SJ, Collins MJ. Longitudinal changes in choroidal thickness and eye growth in childhood. Invest Ophthalmol Vis Sci. 2015;56:3103–12.
83. Fontaine M, Gaucher D, Sauer A, Speeg-Schatz C. Choroidal thickness and ametropia in children: a longitudinal study. Eur J Ophthalmol. 2017;27:730–4.
84. Jin P, Zou H, Xu X, et al. Longitudinal changes in choroidal and retinal thicknesses in children with myopic shift. Retina. 2019;39:1091–9.
85. Chen Z, Xue F, Zhou J, Qu X, Zhou X. Effects of orthokeratology on choroidal thickness and axial length. Optom Vis Sci. 2016;93:1064–71.
86. Li Z, Cui D, Hu Y, Ao S, Zeng J, Yang X. Choroidal thickness and axial length changes in myopic children treated with orthokeratology. Cont Lens Anterior Eye. 2017;40:417–23.

87. Sander BP, Collins MJ, Read SA. The effect of topical adrenergic and anticholinergic agents on the choroidal thickness of young healthy adults. Exp Eye Res. 2014;128:181–9.
88. Zhang Z, Zhou Y, Xie Z, et al. The effect of topical atropine on the choroidal thickness of healthy children. Sci Rep. 2016;6:34936.
89. Read SA. Ocular and environmental factors associated with eye growth in childhood. Optom Vis Sci. 2016;93:1031–41.
90. Elsheikh A, Geraghty B, Alhasso D, Knappett J, Campanelli M, Rama P. Regional variation in the biomechanical properties of the human sclera. Exp Eye Res. 2010;90:624–33.
91. Norman RE, Flanagan JG, Rausch SM, et al. Dimensions of the human sclera: thickness measurement and regional changes with axial length. Exp Eye Res. 2010;90:277–84.
92. Vurgese S, Panda-Jonas S, Jonas JB. Scleral thickness in human eyes. PLoS One. 2012;7:e29692.
93. McBrien NA, Gentle A. Role of the sclera in the development and pathological complications of myopia. Prog Retin Eye Res. 2003;22:307–38.
94. Downs JC, Ensor ME, Bellezza AJ, Thompson HW, Hart RT, Burgoyne CF. Posterior scleral thickness in perfusion-fixed normal and early-glaucoma monkey eyes. Invest Ophthalmol Vis Sci. 2001;42:3202–8.
95. Nemeth J. The posterior coats of the eye in glaucoma. An echobiometric study. Graefes Arch Clin Exp Ophthalmol. 1990;228:33–5.
96. Xue A, Bao F, Zheng L, Wang Q, Cheng L, Qu J. Posterior scleral reinforcement on progressive high myopic young patients. Optom Vis Sci. 2014;91:412–8.
97. Xue A, Zheng L, Tan G, et al. Genipin-crosslinked donor sclera for posterior scleral contraction/reinforcement to fight progressive myopia. Invest Ophthalmol Vis Sci. 2018;59:3564–73.
98. Read SA, Alonso-Caneiro D, Vincent SJ, et al. Anterior eye tissue morphology: scleral and conjunctival thickness in children and young adults. Sci Rep. 2016;6:33796.
99. Buckhurst HD, Gilmartin B, Cubbidge RP, Logan NS. Measurement of scleral thickness in humans using anterior segment optical coherent tomography. PLoS One. 2015;10:e0132902.
100. Pekel G, Yagci R, Acer S, Ongun GT, Cetin EN, Simavli H. Comparison of corneal layers and anterior sclera in emmetropic and myopic eyes. Cornea. 2015;34:786–90.
101. Consejo A, Radhakrishnan H, Iskander DR. Scleral changes with accommodation. Ophthalmic Physiol Opt. 2017;37:263–74.
102. Woodman-Pieterse EC, Read SA, Collins MJ, Alonso-Caneiro D. Anterior scleral thickness changes with accommodation in myopes and emmetropes. Exp Eye Res. 2018;177:96–103.
103. Bailey MD, Sinnott LT, Mutti DO. Ciliary body thickness and refractive error in children. Invest Ophthalmol Vis Sci. 2008;49:4353–60.
104. Kuchem MK, Sinnott LT, Kao CY, Bailey MD. Ciliary muscle thickness in anisometropia. Optom Vis Sci. 2013;90:1312–20.
105. Muftuoglu O, Hosal BM, Zilelioglu G. Ciliary body thickness in unilateral high axial myopia. Eye. 2009;23:1176–81.
106. Phillips JR, Khalaj M, McBrien NA. Induced myopia associated with increased scleral creep in chick and tree shrew eyes. Invest Ophthalmol Vis Sci. 2000;41:2028–34.
107. Siegwart JT Jr, Norton TT. Regulation of the mechanical properties of tree shrew sclera by the visual environment. Vis Res. 1999;39:387–407.
108. Sherman SM, Norton TT, Casagrande VA. Myopia in the lid-sutured tree shrew (Tupaia glis). Brain Res. 1977;124:154–7.
109. Wallman J, Turkel J, Trachtman J. Extreme myopia produced by modest change in early visual experience. Science. 1978;201:1249–51.
110. Wilson J, Sherman S. Differential effects of early monocular deprivation on binocular and monocular segments of cat striate cortex. J Neurophysiol. 1977;40:891–903.
111. Hodos W, Kuenzel WJ. Retinal-image degradation produces ocular enlargement in chicks. Invest Ophthalmol Vis Sci. 1984;25:652–9.
112. Wallman J, Ledoux C, Friedman MB. Simple devices for restricting the visual fields of birds. Behav Res Methods Instrum. 1978;10:401–3.

113. Howlett MH, McFadden SA. Form-deprivation myopia in the guinea pig (Cavia porcellus). Vis Res. 2006;46:267–83.
114. Ashby R, Ohlendorf A, Schaeffel F. The effect of ambient illuminance on the development of deprivation myopia in chicks. Invest Ophthalmol Vis Sci. 2009;50:5348–54.
115. Schaeffel F, Howland HC. Properties of the feedback loops controlling eye growth and refractive state in the chicken. Vis Res. 1991;31:717–34.
116. Schmid KL, Wildsoe CF. Contrast and spatial-frequency requirements for emmetropization in chicks. Vis Res. 1997;37:2011–21.
117. Wiesel TN, Raviola E. Myopia and eye enlargement after neonatal lid fusion in monkeys. Nature. 1977;266(5597):66–8.
118. Wildsoet CF, Schmid KL. Optical correction of form deprivation myopia inhibits refractive recovery in chick eyes with intact or sectioned optic nerves. Vis Res. 2000;40:3273–82.
119. Siegwart JT Jr, Norton TT. The susceptible period for deprivation-induced myopia in tree shrew. Vis Res. 1998;38:3505–15.
120. Troilo D, Nickla DL. The response to visual form deprivation differs with age in marmosets. Invest Ophthalmol Vis Sci. 2005;46:1873–81.
121. Smith EL, Hung L-F, C-s K, Qiao Y. Effects of brief periods of unrestricted vision on the development of form-deprivation myopia in monkeys. Invest Ophthalmol Vis Sci. 2002;43:291–9.
122. Smith EL, Li-Fang H, Harwerth RS. Effects of optically induced blur on the refractive status of young monkeys. Vis Res. 1994;34:293–301.
123. Schaeffel F, Feldkaemper M. Animal models in myopia research. Clin Exp Optom. 2015;98:507–17.
124. McBrien NA, Lawlor P, Gentle A. Scleral remodeling during the development of and recovery from axial myopia in the tree shrew. Invest Ophthalmol Vis Sci. 2000;41:3713–9.
125. Troilo D, Nickla DL, Wildsoet CF. Choroidal thickness changes during altered eye growth and refractive state in a primate. Invest Ophthalmol Vis Sci. 2000;41:1249–58.
126. Gottlieb MD, Joshi HB, Nickla DL. Scleral changes in chicks with form-deprivation myopia. Curr Eye Res. 1990;9:1157–65.
127. Hung LF, Wallman J, Smith EL. Vision-dependent changes in the choroidal thickness of macaque monkeys. Invest Ophthalmol Vis Sci. 2000;41:1259–69.
128. Funata M, Tokoro T. Scleral change in experimentally myopic monkeys. Graefes Arch Clin Exp Ophthalmol. 1990;228:174–9.
129. Smith EL 3rd, Hung LF. Form-deprivation myopia in monkeys is a graded phenomenon. Vis Res. 2000;40:371–81.
130. Troilo D, Gottlieb MD, Wallman J. Visual deprivation causes myopia in chicks with optic nerve section. Curr Eye Res. 1987;6:993–9.
131. Norton TT, Rada JA. Reduced extracellular matrix in mammalian sclera with induced myopia. Vis Res. 1995;35:1271–81.
132. Gottlieb MD, Fugate-Wentzek LA, Wallman J. Different visual deprivations produce different ametropias and different eye shapes. Invest Ophthalmol Vis Sci. 1987;28:1225–35.
133. Troilo D, Li T, Glasser A, Howland HC. Differences in eye growth and the response to visual deprivation in different strains of chicken. Vis Res. 1995;35:1211–6.
134. McKanna JA, Casagrande VA. Reduced lens development in lid-suture myopia. Exp Eye Res. 1978;26:715–23.
135. Napper GA, Brennan NA, Barrington M, Squires MA, Vessey GA, Vingrys AJ. The duration of normal visual exposure necessary to prevent form deprivation myopia in chicks. Vis Res. 1995;35:1337–44.
136. O'Leary D, Millodot M. Eyelid closure causes myopia in humans. Experientia. 1979;35:1478–9.
137. von Noorden GK, Lewis RA. Ocular axial length in unilateral congenital cataracts and blepharoptosis. Invest Ophthalmol Vis Sci. 1987;28:750–2.
138. Gee SS, Tabbara KF. Increase in ocular axial length in patients with corneal opacification. Ophthalmology. 1988;95:1276–8.
139. Miller-Meeks MJ, Bennett SR, Keech RV, Blodi CF. Myopia induced by vitreous hemorrhage. Am J Ophthalmol. 1990;109:199–203.

140. Bartmann M, Schaeffel F. A simple mechanism for emmetropization without cues from accommodation or colour. Vis Res. 1994;34:873–6.
141. Papastergiou GI, Schmid GF, Laties AM, Pendrak K, Lin T, Stone RA. Induction of axial eye elongation and myopic refractive shift in one-year-old chickens. Vis Res. 1998;38:1883–8.
142. Wildsoet C, Anchong R, Manasse J, Troilo D. Susceptibility to experimental myopia declines with age in the chick. Optom Vis Sci. 1998;75:265.
143. Bradley D, Fernandes A, Boothe R. Form deprivation myopia in adolescent monkeys. Optom Vis Sci. 1999;76:428–32.
144. Troilo D, Nickla DL, Wildsoet CF. Form deprivation myopia in mature common marmosets (Callithrix jacchus). Invest Ophthalmol Vis Sci. 2000;41:2043–9.
145. Schaeffel F, Glasser A, Howland HC. Accommodation, refractive error and eye growth in chickens. Vis Res. 1988;28:639–57.
146. Irving EL, Callender MG, Sivak JG. Inducing myopia, hyperopia, and astigmatism in chicks. Optom Vis Sci. 1991;68:364–8.
147. Irving EL, Sivak JG, Callender MG. Refractive plasticity of the developing chick eye. Ophthalmic Physiol Opt. 1992;12:448–56.
148. Schmid KL, Wildsoet CF. Effects on the compensatory responses to positive and negative lenses of intermittent lens wear and ciliary nerve section in chicks. Vis Res. 1996;36:1023–36.
149. Siegwart J, Norton T. Refractive and ocular changes in tree shrews raised with plus or minus lenses. Invest Ophthalmol Vis Sci. 1993;34:1208.
150. Hung LF, Crawford ML, Smith EL. Spectacle lenses alter eye growth and the refractive status of young monkeys. Nat Med. 1995;1:761–5.
151. Graham B, Judge SJ. The effects of spectacle wear in infancy on eye growth and refractive error in the marmoset (Callithrix jacchus). Vis Res. 1999;39:189–206.
152. Howlett MH, McFadden SA. Spectacle lens compensation in the pigmented guinea pig. Vis Res. 2009;49:219–27.
153. McFadden SA, Howlett MH, Mertz JR. Retinoic acid signals the direction of ocular elongation in the guinea pig eye. Vis Res. 2004;44:643–53.
154. Barathi VA, Boopathi VG, Yap EP, Beuerman RW. Two models of experimental myopia in the mouse. Vis Res. 2008;48:904–16.
155. Metlapally S, McBrien NA. The effect of positive lens defocus on ocular growth and emmetropization in the tree shrew. J Vis. 2008;8:1–12.
156. McFadden S, Wallman J. Guinea-pig eye growth compensates for spectacle lenses. Invest Ophthalmol Vis Sci. 1995;19106:S758.
157. Schaeffel F, Howland HC, Farkas L. Natural accommodation in the growing chicken. Vis Res. 1986;26:1977–93.
158. Whatham AR, Judge SJ. Compensatory changes in eye growth and refraction induced by daily wear of soft contact lenses in young marmosets. Vis Res. 2001;41:267–73.
159. Zhu X, Winawer JA, Wallman J. Potency of myopic defocus in spectacle lens compensation. Invest Ophthalmol Vis Sci. 2003;44:2818–27.
160. Chiang ST, Phillips JR, Backhouse S. Effect of retinal image defocus on the thickness of the human choroid. Ophthalmic Physiol Opt. 2015;35:405–13.
161. Read SA, Collins MJ, Sander BP. Human optical axial length and defocus. Invest Ophthalmol Vis Sci. 2010;51:6262–9.
162. Wang D, Chun RKM, Liu M, et al. Optical defocus rapidly changes choroidal thickness in school children. PLoS One. 2016;11:e0161535.
163. Chakraborty R, Read SA, Collins MJ. Hyperopic defocus and diurnal changes in human choroid and axial length. Optom Vis Sci. 2013;90:1187–98.
164. Chakraborty R, Read SA, Collins MJ. Monocular myopic defocus and daily changes in axial length and choroidal thickness of human eyes. Exp Eye Res. 2012;103:47–54.
165. Moderiano D, Do M, Hobbs S, et al. Influence of the time of day on axial length and choroidal thickness changes to hyperopic and myopic defocus in human eyes. Exp Eye Res. 2019;182:125–36.
166. Zhu X, Wallman J. Temporal properties of compensation for positive and negative spectacle lenses in chicks. Invest Ophthalmol Vis Sci. 2009;50:37–46.

167. Zhu X. Temporal integration of visual signals in lens compensation (a review). Exp Eye Res. 2013;114:69–76.
168. Winawer J, Wallman J. Temporal constraints on lens compensation in chicks. Vis Res. 2002;42:2651–68.
169. Zhu X, Park TW, Winawer J, Wallman J. In a matter of minutes, the eye can know which way to grow. Invest Ophthalmol Vis Sci. 2005;46:2238–41.
170. Wallman J, Adams JI. Developmental aspects of experimental myopia in chicks: susceptibility, recovery and relation to emmetropization. Vis Res. 1987;27:1139–63.
171. Norton TT. Experimental myopia in tree shrews. Ciba Found Symp. 1990;155:178–94.
172. Nickla DL, Wildsoet C, Wallman J. Visual influences on diurnal rhythms in ocular length and choroidal thickness in chick eyes. Exp Eye Res. 1998;66:163–81.
173. Troilo D, Wallman J. The regulation of eye growth and refractive state: an experimental study of emmetropization. Vis Res. 1991;31:1237–50.
174. Schaeffel F, Troilo D, Wallman J, Howland HC. Developing eyes that lack accommodation grow to compensate for imposed defocus. Vis Neurosci. 1990;4:177–83.
175. Schwahn HN, Schaeffel F. Chick eyes under cycloplegia compensate for spectacle lenses despite six-hydroxy dopamine treatment. Invest Ophthalmol Vis Sci. 1994;35:3516–24.
176. Chung KM. Critical review: effects of optical defocus on refractive development and ocular growth and relation to accommodation. Optom Vis Sci. 1993;70:228–33.
177. Morgan IG, Ashby RS, Nickla DL. Form deprivation and lens-induced myopia: are they different? Ophthalmic Physiol Opt. 2013;33:355–61.
178. C-S K, Marzani D, Wallman J. Differences in time course and visual requirements of ocular responses to lenses and diffusers. Invest Ophthalmol Vis Sci. 2001;42:575–83.
179. Bartmann M, Schaeffel F, Hagel G, Zrenner E. Constant light affects retinal dopamine levels and blocks deprivation myopia but not lens-induced refractive errors in chickens. Vis Neurosci. 1994;11:199–208.
180. Padmanabhan V, Shih J, Wildsoet CF. Constant light rearing disrupts compensation to imposed- but not induced-hyperopia and facilitates compensation to imposed myopia in chicks. Vis Res. 2007;47:1855–68.
181. Smith EL, Hung LF, Huang J. Protective effects of high ambient lighting on the development of form-deprivation myopia in rhesus monkeys. Invest Ophthalmol Vis Sci. 2012;53:421–8.
182. Ashby RS, Schaeffel F. The effect of bright light on lens compensation in chicks. Invest Ophthalmol Vis Sci. 2010;51:5247–53.
183. Feldkaemper M, Schaeffel F. An updated view on the role of dopamine in myopia. Exp Eye Res. 2013;114:106–19.
184. Dong F, Zhi Z, Pan M, et al. Inhibition of experimental myopia by a dopamine agonist: different effectiveness between form deprivation and hyperopic defocus in guinea pigs. Mol Vis. 2011;17:2824–34.
185. Harper AR, Summers JA. The dynamic sclera: extracellular matrix remodeling in normal ocular growth and myopia development. Exp Eye Res. 2015;133:100–11.
186. Crewther DP. The role of photoreceptors in the control of refractive state. Prog Retin Eye Res. 2000;19:421–57.
187. Wildsoet CF. Neural pathways subserving negative lens-induced emmetropization in chicks-insights from selective lesions of the optic nerve and ciliary nerve. Curr Eye Res. 2003;27:371–85.
188. Wallman J, Gottlieb MD, Rajaram V, Fugate-Wentzek LA. Local retinal regions control local eye growth and myopia. Science. 1987;237:73–7.
189. Diether S, Schaeffel F. Local changes in eye growth induced by imposed local refractive error despite active accommodation. Vis Res. 1997;37:659–68.
190. Smith EL, Huang J, Hung LF, Blasdel TL, Humbird TL, Bockhorst KH. Hemiretinal form deprivation: evidence for local control of eye growth and refractive development in infant monkeys. Invest Ophthalmol Vis Sci. 2009;50:5057–69.
191. Stone RA, Lin T, Laties AM, Iuvone PM. Retinal dopamine and form-deprivation myopia. Proc Natl Acad Sci U S A. 1989;86:704–6.

192. Iuvone PM, Tigges M, Stone RA, Lambert S, Laties AM. Effects of apomorphine, a dopamine receptor agonist, on ocular refraction and axial elongation in a primate model of myopia. Invest Ophthalmol Vis Sci. 1991;32:1674–7.
193. Nickla DL, Wilken E, Lytle G, Yom S, Mertz J. Inhibiting the transient choroidal thickening response using the nitric oxide synthase inhibitor l-NAME prevents the ameliorative effects of visual experience on ocular growth in two different visual paradigms. Exp Eye Res. 2006;83:456–64.
194. Nickla DL, Wildsoet CF. The effect of the nonspecific nitric oxide synthase inhibitor NG-nitro-L-arginine methyl ester on the choroidal compensatory response to myopic defocus in chickens. Optom Vis Sci. 2004;81:111–8.
195. Feldkaemper MP, Schaeffel F. Evidence for a potential role of glucagon during eye growth regulation in chicks. Vis Neurosci. 2002;19:755–66.
196. Zhou X, Pardue MT, Iuvone PM, Qu J. Dopamine signaling and myopia development: what are the key challenges. Prog Retin Eye Res. 2017;61:60–71.
197. Pendrak K, Nguyen T, Lin T, Capehart C, Zhu X, Stone RA. Retinal dopamine in the recovery from experimental myopia. Curr Eye Res. 1997;16:152–7.
198. Iuvone PM, Tigges M, Fernandes A, Tigges J. Dopamine synthesis and metabolism in rhesus monkey retina: development, aging, and the effects of monocular visual deprivation. Vis Neurosci. 1989;2:465–71.
199. Crewther DP, Crewther SG, Xie RZ. Changes in eye growth produced by drugs which affect retinal ON or OFF responses to light. J Ocul Pharmacol Ther. 1996;12:193–208.
200. Crewther DP, Crewther SG. Pharmacological modification of eye growth in normally reared and visually deprived chicks. Curr Eye Res. 1990;9:733–40.
201. Chakraborty R, Park H, Aung MH, et al. Comparison of refractive development and retinal dopamine in OFF pathway mutant and C57BL/6J wild-type mice. Mol Vis. 2014;20:1318–27.
202. Chakraborty R, Pardue MT. Molecular and biochemical aspects of the retina on refraction. Prog Mol Biol Transl Sci. 2015;134:249–67.
203. Chakraborty R, Park HN, Hanif AM, Sidhu CS, Iuvone PM, Pardue MT. ON pathway mutations increase susceptibility to form-deprivation myopia. Exp Eye Res. 2015;137:79–83.
204. Bergen MA, Chakraborty R, Landis EG, Sidhu C, He L, Iuvone PM, Pardue MT. Altered refractive development in mice with reduced levels of retinal dopamine. Invest Ophthalmol Vis Sci. 2016;57(10):4412–9.
205. Pardue MT, Faulkner AE, Fernandes A, et al. High susceptibility to experimental myopia in a mouse model with a retinal on pathway defect. Invest Ophthalmol Vis Sci. 2008;49:706–12.
206. Markand S, Baskin NL, Chakraborty R, et al. IRBP deficiency permits precocious ocular development and myopia. Mol Vis. 2016;22:1291–308.
207. Zhang Q, Xiao X, Li S, et al. Mutations in NYX of individuals with high myopia, but without night blindness. Mol Vis. 2007;13:330–6.
208. Xu X, Li S, Xiao X, Wang P, Guo X, Zhang Q. Sequence variations of GRM6 in patients with high myopia. Mol Vis. 2009;15:2094–100.
209. Pras E, Abu A, Rotenstreich Y, et al. Cone-rod dystrophy and a frameshift mutation in the PROM1 gene. Mol Vis. 2009;15:1709.
210. Sieving PA, Fishman GA. Refractive errors of retinitis pigmentosa patients. Br J Ophthalmol. 1978;62:163–7.
211. Charman WN. Aberrations and myopia. Ophthalmic Physiol Opt. 2005;25:285–301.
212. Wildsoet CF, Atchison DA, Collins MJ. Longitudinal chromatic aberration as a function of refractive error. Clin Exp Optom. 1993;76:119–22.
213. Little JA, McCullough SJ, Breslin KM, Saunders KJ. Higher order ocular aberrations and their relation to refractive error and ocular biometry in children. Invest Ophthalmol Vis Sci. 2014;55:4791–800.
214. Buehren T, Collins MJ, Carney LG. Near work induced wavefront aberrations in myopia. Vis Res. 2005;45:1297–312.
215. Vincent SJ, Collins MJ, Read SA, Carney LG, Yap MK. Corneal changes following near work in myopic anisometropia. Ophthalmic Physiol Opt. 2013;33:15–25.

216. Hiraoka T, Kotsuka J, Kakita T, Okamoto F, Oshika T. Relationship between higher-order wavefront aberrations and natural progression of myopia in schoolchildren. Sci Rep. 2017;7:7876.
217. Atchison DA, Li SM, Li H, et al. Relative peripheral hyperopia does not predict development and progression of myopia in children. Invest Ophthalmol Vis Sci. 2015;56:6162–70.
218. Lee TT, Cho P. Relative peripheral refraction in children: twelve-month changes in eyes with different ametropias. Ophthalmic Physiol Opt. 2013;33:283–93.
219. Cheng X, Xu J, Chehab K, Exford J, Brennan N. Soft contact lenses with positive spherical aberration for myopia control. Optom Vis Sci. 2016;93:353–66.
220. Hiraoka T, Okamoto C, Ishii Y, Kakita T, Oshika T. Contrast sensitivity function and ocular higher-order aberrations following overnight orthokeratology. Invest Ophthalmol Vis Sci. 2007;48:550–6.
221. Hiraoka T, Miyata K, Nakamura Y, et al. Influences of cycloplegia with topical atropine on ocular higher-order aberrations. Ophthalmology. 2013;120:8–13.
222. Huang HM, Chang DS, Wu PC. The association between near work activities and myopia in children-a systematic review and meta-analysis. PLoS One. 2015;10:e0140419.
223. Rosenfield M, Gilmartin B. Disparity-induced accommodation in late-onset myopia. Ophthalmic Physiol Opt. 1988;8:353–5.
224. Gwiazda J, Thorn F, Bauer J, Held R. Myopic children show insufficient accommodative response to blur. Invest Ophthalmol Vis Sci. 1993;34:690–4.
225. McBrien NA, Millodot M. The effect of refractive error on the accommodative response gradient. Ophthalmic Physiol Opt. 1986;6:145–9.
226. Gwiazda J, Bauer J, Thorn F, Held R. A dynamic relationship between myopia and blur-driven accommodation in school-aged children. Vis Res. 1995;35:1299–304.
227. Abbott ML, Schmid KL, Strang NC. Differences in the accommodation stimulus response curves of adult myopes and emmetropes. Ophthalmic Physiol Opt. 1998;18:13–20.
228. Cheng D, Schmid KL, Woo GC, Drobe B. Randomized trial of effect of bifocal and prismatic bifocal spectacles on myopic progression: two-year results. Arch Ophthalmol. 2010;128:12–9.
229. Berntsen DA, Barr CD, Mutti DO, Zadnik K. Peripheral defocus and myopia progression in myopic children randomly assigned to wear single vision and progressive addition lenses. Invest Ophthalmol Vis Sci. 2013;54:5761–70.
230. Mutti DO, Mitchell GL, Jones LA, et al. Accommodation, acuity, and their relationship to emmetropization in infants. Optom Vis Sci. 2009;86:666–76.
231. Weiss S, Schaeffel F. Diurnal growth rhythms in the chicken eye: relation to myopia development and retinal dopamine levels. J Comp Physiol A. 1993;172:263–70.
232. Chakraborty R, Read SA, Collins MJ. Diurnal variations in axial length, choroidal thickness, intraocular pressure, and ocular biometrics. Invest Ophthalmol Vis Sci. 2011;52:5121–9.
233. Brown JS, Flitcroft DI, Ying GS, et al. In vivo human choroidal thickness measurements: evidence for diurnal fluctuations. Invest Ophthalmol Vis Sci. 2009;50:5–12.
234. Stone RA, Quinn GE, Francis EL, et al. Diurnal axial length fluctuations in human eyes. Invest Ophthalmol Vis Sci. 2004;45:63–70.
235. Li T, Troilo D, Glasser A, Howland HC. Constant light produces severe corneal flattening and hyperopia in chickens. Vis Res. 1995;35:1203–9.
236. Guyton DL, Greene PR, Scholz RT. Dark-rearing interference with emmetropization in the rhesus monkey. Invest Ophthalmol Vis Sci. 1989;30:761–4.
237. Nickla DL, Totonelly K. Brief light exposure at night disrupts the circadian rhythms in eye growth and choroidal thickness in chicks. Exp Eye Res. 2016;146:189–95.
238. Nickla DL. The phase relationships between the diurnal rhythms in axial length and choroidal thickness and the association with ocular growth rate in chicks. J Comp Physiol A. 2006;192:399–407.
239. Kearney S, O'Donoghue L, Pourshahidi LK, Cobice D, Saunders KJ. Myopes have significantly higher serum melatonin concentrations than non-myopes. Ophthalmic Physiol Opt. 2017;37:557–67.

240. Jee D, Morgan IG, Kim EC. Inverse relationship between sleep duration and myopia. Acta Ophthalmol. 2016;94:e204–10.
241. Mutti DO, Mitchell GL, Moeschberger ML, Jones LA, Zadnik K. Parental myopia, near work, school achievement, and children's refractive error. Invest Ophthalmol Vis Sci. 2002;43:3633–40.
242. Morgan IG. The biological basis of myopic refractive error. Clin Exp Optom. 2003;86:276–88.
243. Au Eong KG, Tay TH, Lim MK. Education and myopia in 110,236 young Singaporean males. Singap Med J. 1993;34:489–92.
244. Williams KM, Bertelsen G, Cumberland P, et al. Increasing prevalence of myopia in Europe and the impact of education. Ophthalmology. 2015;122:1489–97.
245. Mirshahi A, Ponto KA, Hoehn R, et al. Myopia and level of education: results from the Gutenberg Health Study. Ophthalmology. 2014;121:2047–52.
246. Read SA, Collins MJ, Woodman EC, Cheong SH. Axial length changes during accommodation in myopes and emmetropes. Optom Vis Sci. 2010;87:656–62.
247. Woodman-Pieterse EC, Read SA, Collins MJ, Alonso-Caneiro D. Regional changes in choroidal thickness associated with accommodation. Invest Ophthalmol Vis Sci. 2015;56:6414–22.
248. Hepsen IF, Evereklioglu C, Bayramlar H. The effect of reading and near-work on the development of myopia in emmetropic boys: a prospective, controlled, three-year follow-up study. Vis Res. 2001;41:2511–20.
249. Jones LA, Sinnott LT, Mutti DO, Mitchell GL, Moeschberger ML, Zadnik K. Parental history of myopia, sports and outdoor activities, and future myopia. Invest Ophthalmol Vis Sci. 2007;48:3524–32.
250. He M, Zheng Y, Xiang F. Prevalence of myopia in urban and rural children in mainland China. Optom Vis Sci. 2009;86:40–4.
251. He M, Huang W, Zheng Y, Huang L, Ellwein LB. Refractive error and visual impairment in school children in rural southern China. Ophthalmology. 2007;114:374–82.
252. Zhang M, Li L, Chen L, et al. Population density and refractive error among Chinese children. Invest Ophthalmol Vis Sci. 2010;51:4969–76.
253. Ip JM, Rose KA, Morgan IG, Burlutsky G, Mitchell P. Myopia and the urban environment: findings in a sample of 12-year-old Australian school children. Invest Ophthalmol Vis Sci. 2008;49:3858–63.
254. Choi KY, Yu WY, Lam CHI, et al. Childhood exposure to constricted living space: a possible environmental threat for myopia development. Ophthalmic Physiol Opt. 2017;37:568–75.
255. Parssinen O, Lyyra AL. Myopia and myopic progression among schoolchildren: a three-year follow-up study. Invest Ophthalmol Vis Sci. 1993;34:2794–802.
256. Rose KA, Morgan IG, Ip J, et al. Outdoor activity reduces the prevalence of myopia in children. Ophthalmology. 2008;115:1279–85.
257. Guo Y, Liu LJ, Tang P, et al. Outdoor activity and myopia progression in 4-year follow-up of Chinese primary school children: The Beijing Children Eye Study. PLoS One. 2017;12:e0175921.
258. Guggenheim JA, Northstone K, McMahon G, et al. Time outdoors and physical activity as predictors of incident myopia in childhood: a prospective cohort study. Invest Ophthalmol Vis Sci. 2012;53:2856–65.
259. Parssinen O, Kauppinen M, Viljanen A. The progression of myopia from its onset at age 8-12 to adulthood and the influence of heredity and external factors on myopic progression. A 23-year follow-up study. Acta Ophthalmol. 2014;92:730–9.
260. Jones-Jordan LA, Sinnott LT, Cotter SA, et al. Time outdoors, visual activity, and myopia progression in juvenile-onset myopes. Invest Ophthalmol Vis Sci. 2012;53:7169–75.
261. Sherwin JC, Reacher MH, Keogh RH, Khawaja AP, Mackey DA, Foster PJ. The association between time spent outdoors and myopia in children and adolescents: a systematic review and meta-analysis. Ophthalmology. 2012;119:2141–51.
262. Flitcroft DI. The complex interactions of retinal, optical and environmental factors in myopia aetiology. Prog Retin Eye Res. 2012;31:622–60.
263. Cohen Y, Belkin M, Yehezkel O, Solomon AS, Polat U. Dependency between light intensity and refractive development under light-dark cycles. Exp Eye Res. 2011;92:40–6.

264. Karouta C, Ashby RS. Correlation between light levels and the development of deprivation myopia. Invest Ophthalmol Vis Sci. 2014;56:299–309.
265. Smith EL, Hung LF, Arumugam B, Huang J. Negative lens-induced myopia in infant monkeys: effects of high ambient lighting. Invest Ophthalmol Vis Sci. 2013;54:2959–69.
266. Read SA, Collins MJ, Vincent SJ. Light exposure and eye growth in childhood. Invest Ophthalmol Vis Sci. 2015;56:6779–87.
267. Ostrin LA, Sajjadi A, Benoit JS. Objectively measured light exposure during school and summer in children. Optom Vis Sci. 2018;95:332–42.
268. Wu PC, Chen CT, Lin KK, et al. Myopia prevention and outdoor light intensity in a school-based cluster randomized trial. Ophthalmology. 2018;125(8):1239–50.
269. Rudnicka AR, Kapetanakis VV, Wathern AK, et al. Global variations and time trends in the prevalence of childhood myopia, a systematic review and quantitative meta-analysis: implications for aetiology and early prevention. Br J Ophthalmol. 2016;100:882–90.
270. French AN, Morgan IG, Burlutsky G, Mitchell P, Rose KA. Prevalence and 5- to 6-year incidence and progression of myopia and hyperopia in Australian school children. Ophthalmology. 2013;120:1482–91.
271. Read SA, Vincent SJ, Tan CS, Ngo C, Collins MJ, Saw SM. Patterns of daily outdoor light exposure in Australian and Singaporean children. Transl Vis Sci Technol. 2018;7:8.
272. Lan W, Feldkaemper M, Schaeffel F. Intermittent episodes of bright light suppress myopia in the chicken more than continuous bright light. PLoS One. 2014;9:e110906.
273. He M, Xiang F, Zeng Y, et al. Effect of time spent outdoors at school on the development of myopia among children in China: a randomized clinical trial. JAMA. 2015;314:1142–8.
274. Wu PC, Tsai CL, Wu HL, Yang YH, Kuo HK. Outdoor activity during class recess reduces myopia onset and progression in school children. Ophthalmology. 2013;120:1080–5.
275. Torii H, Kurihara T, Seko Y, et al. Violet light exposure can be a preventive strategy against myopia progression. EBioMedicine. 2017;15:210–9.
276. Foulds WS, Barathi VA, Luu CD. Progressive myopia or hyperopia can be induced in chicks and reversed by manipulation of the chromaticity of ambient light. Invest Ophthalmol Vis Sci. 2013;54:8004–12.
277. Smith EL, Hung LF, Arumugam B, Holden BA, Neitz M, Neitz J. Effects of long-wavelength lighting on refractive development in infant rhesus monkeys. Invest Ophthalmol Vis Sci. 2015;56:6490–500.
278. Gawne TJ, Ward AH, Norton TT. Long-wavelength (red) light produces hyperopia in juvenile and adolescent tree shrews. Vis Res. 2017;140:55–65.
279. Jiang L, Zhang S, Schaeffel F, et al. Interactions of chromatic and lens-induced defocus during visual control of eye growth in guinea pigs (Cavia porcellus). Vis Res. 2014;94:24–32.

The Genetics of Myopia

5

Milly S. Tedja, Annechien E. G. Haarman, Magda A. Meester-Smoor, Virginie J. M. Verhoeven, Caroline C. W. Klaver, and Stuart MacGregor

Key Points

- While the recent global rise of myopia prevalence is primarily attributable to environmental changes, within populations inherited factors play a large role in explaining why some individuals are affected by myopia while others are not.
- Early efforts to identify the specific genes underlying the heritability of refractive error used linkage and candidate gene designs to identify up to 50 loci and genes, although most remain unconfirmed.

M. S. Tedja · A. E. G. Haarman · M. A. Meester-Smoor
Department of Ophthalmology, Erasmus Medical Center, Rotterdam, The Netherlands

Department of Epidemiology, Erasmus Medical Center, Rotterdam, The Netherlands

V. J. M. Verhoeven
Department of Ophthalmology, Erasmus Medical Center, Rotterdam, The Netherlands

Department of Epidemiology, Erasmus Medical Center, Rotterdam, The Netherlands

Department of Clinical Genetics, Erasmus Medical Center, Rotterdam, The Netherlands

C. C. W. Klaver
Department of Ophthalmology, Erasmus Medical Center, Rotterdam, The Netherlands

Department of Epidemiology, Erasmus Medical Center, Rotterdam, The Netherlands

Department of Ophthalmology, Radboud University Medical Center, Nijmegen, The Netherlands

S. MacGregor (✉)
Statistical Genetics, QIMR Berghofer Medical Research Institute, Brisbane, QLD, Australia
e-mail: stuart.macgregor@qimrberghofer.edu.au

M. Ang, T. Y. Wong (eds.), *Updates on Myopia*,
https://doi.org/10.1007/978-981-13-8491-2_5

- As the sample size in genome-wide association studies (GWAS) has increased, the number of implicated loci has risen steadily, with 161 variants reported in the latest meta-analysis.
- Interrogation of loci uncovered by GWAS offers insight into the molecular basis of myopia—for example, pathway analysis implicates the light induced retina-to-sclera signaling pathway in myopia development.
- Although many loci have been uncovered by GWAS, statistical modelling shows there are many more genes to find—identifying these will further illuminate the molecular pathways leading to myopia and open up new avenues for intervention.

5.1 Introduction

This chapter addresses the scientific exploration of the genetic architecture of myopia. Myopia is the most common eye condition worldwide and its prevalence is increasing. Changes in environmental conditions where time spent outdoors has reduced relative to previous generations are the main hypothesized culprit. Despite these environmental trends, within populations, myopia is highly heritable; genes explain up to 80% of the variance in refractive error. Initial attempts to identify myopia genes relied on family studies using linkage analysis or candidate gene approaches with limited progress. For the last decade, genome-wide association study (GWAS) approaches have predominated, ultimately resulting in the identification of hundreds of genes for refractive error and myopia, providing new insights into its molecular machinery. Thanks to these studies, it was revealed that myopia is a complex trait, with many genetic variants of small effect influencing retinal signaling, eye growth and the normal process of emmetropization. However, the genetic architecture and its molecular mechanisms are still to be clarified and while genetic risk score prediction models are improving, this knowledge must be expanded to have impact on clinical practice.

Some sections of this report follow the framework described in a recent International Myopia Institute Genetics report by Tedja et al. [1]

5.2 Heritability

The tendency for myopia to run in families has long been noted, suggesting genetic factors play a role in determining risk [2]. While family studies show familial aggregation, twin studies are required to reliably separate the effects of genes and familial environment [3–6]. Benchmarking of the relative contribution of genetics and environment is done by computation of heritability, the proportion of the total trait variance (here, spherical equivalent) due to additive genetic factors. Since the contributions of genes and environment can vary across human populations, heritabilities are population and even time specific [7, 8]. The influence of environmental variance is well illustrated in the case of the heritability study in Alaskan Eskimos, where the rapid introduction of the American school system dramatically increased the contribution of the environment. As a result heritability estimates, computed based on families where the parents are less educated relative to their offspring, were very low at this time (10%) [7].

Across most human populations, environment is fairly constant and the estimates of spherical equivalent heritability are usually high (~80%) [9–11]. Although the aggregate contribution of genetic factors to variation in refractive error is high, initial studies were unable to determine the genetic architecture of myopia—that is, is myopia caused by rare mutations of large effect? Or is most variation driven by common variants, each with individually small effect on risk? With the advent of genotyping arrays, it became possible to estimate the aggregate effect of all common variants, with "array heritability" estimates of 35% from the ALSPAC study. Such estimates place a lower bound on the proportion of the heritability that is attributable to genetic variants which are common in the population. The remaining 45% (80%–35%) is likely attributable to rare genetic variants, to variants not covered by genotyping arrays or to non-additive genetic effects.

5.3 Syndromic Myopia

Syndromic myopia is generally monogenic and can occur within a wide spectrum of clinical presentations. This type of myopia is usually accompanied by other systemic or ocular disorders. Table 5.1 summarizes all syndromic and ocular conditions that present with myopia [12]. We are able to learn about myopia development by investigating these syndromes. For instance, several types of heritable syndromes result in extreme axial elongation, due to abnormalities in the development of connective tissue (i.e. Marfan syndrome, OMIM #154700; Stickler syndrome, OMIM #,108300 #604841, #614134, #614284 and Ehlers–Danlos syndrome, OMIM #225400, #601776). Similarly, inherited retinal dystrophies lead to myopia due to defects in photoreceptors, for instance, in X-linked retinitis pigmentosa (mutations in *RPGR*-gene) and congenital stationary night blindness [13].

Interestingly, several syndromic myopia genes were found in association to other ocular traits, such as CCT (*ADAMTS2*, *COL4A3*, *COL5A1*, *FBN1*) [14], and Fuchs's dystrophy (*TCF4*) [15]. However, the majority of the genes causing syndromic myopia have not been linked to common forms of myopia, except for *COL2A1* [16, 17] and *FBN1* [18, 19]. Nevertheless, a recent study found an overrepresentation for syndromic myopia genes in GWAS studies on refractive error and myopia [20], implying their important role in myopia development.

5.4 Linkage Studies

Linkage studies have been successfully applied for many Mendelian disorders, although the success has been much more limited in complex traits. The linkage approach searches for cosegregation of genetic markers with the trait of interest in

Table 5.1 Overview of syndromic forms of myopia

Syndrome	Gene and inheritance pattern	Ocular phenotype other than myopia
(A) Syndromes associated with myopia and associated ocular phenotype		
Acromelic frontonasal dysostosis	*ZSWIM6* (*AD*)	Telecanthus, ptosis (some patients), corneal dermoid cyst (rare), glaucoma (rare), segmental optic nerve hypoplasia (rare), persistent primary vitreous (rare)
Alagille syndrome	*JAG1* (*AD*)	Deep-set eyes, hypertelorism, upslanting palpebral fissures, posterior embryotoxon, anterior chamber anomalies, eccentric or ectopic pupils, chorioretinal atrophy, band keratopathy, cataracts, retinal pigment clumping, Axenfeld anomaly, microcornea, choroidal folds, strabismus, anomalous optic disc
Alport syndrome	*COL4A5* (*XLD*); *COL4A3* (*AR/AD*)	Anterior lenticonus, lens opacities, cataracts, pigmentary changes ("flecks") in the perimacular region, corneal endothelial vesicles, corneal erosions
Angelman syndrome	*UBE3A* (*IP*); *CH*	Strabismus (most frequently exotropia), ocular hypopigmentation, refractive errors (astigmatism, hyperopia, myopia)
Bardet–Biedl syndrome	*ARL6*; *BBS1*; *BBS2*; *BBS4*; *BBS5*; *BBS7*; *BBS9*; *BBS10*; *BBS12*; *CEP290*; *LZTFL1*; *MKKS*; *MKS1*; *SDCCAG8*; *TMEM67*; *TRIM32*; *TTC8*; *WDPCP* (*AR*)	Rod-cone dystrophy onset by end of 2nd decade, retinitis pigmentosa, retinal degeneration, strabismus, cataracts
Beals syndrome	*FBN2* (*AD*)	Ectopia lentis
Beaulieu–Boycott–Innes syndrome	*THOC6* (*AR*)	Deep-set eyes, short palpebral fissures, upslanting palpebral fissures
Bohring–Opitz syndrome	*ASXL1* (*AD*)	Prominent eyes, hypoplastic orbital ridges, hypertelorism, upslanting palpebral fissures, strabismus, retinal abnormalities, optic nerve abnormalities
Bone fragility and contractures; arterial rupture and deafness	*PLOD3* (*AR*)	Shallow orbits, cataracts
Branchiooculofacial syndrome	*TFAP2A* (*AD*)	Lacrimal sac fistula, orbital dermoid cyst, iris pigment epithelial cyst, combined hamartoma of the retina and retinal pigment epithelium, upslanting palpebral fissures, telecanthus, hypertelorism, ptosis, lacrimal duct obstruction, iris coloboma, retinal coloboma, microphthalmia, anophthalmia, cataract, strabismus

Table 5.1 (continued)

Syndrome	Gene and inheritance pattern	Ocular phenotype other than myopia
Cardiofaciocutaneous syndrome	*MAP2K2* (*AD*)	Ptosis, nystagmus, strabismus, downslanting palpebral fissures, hypertelorism, exophthalmos, epicanthal folds, optic nerve dysplasia, oculomotor apraxia, loss of visual acuity, absence of eyebrows, absence of eyelashes
Cohen syndrome	*VPS13B* (*AR*)	Downslanting palpebral fissures, almond-shaped eyes, chorioretinal dystrophy, decreased visual acuity, optic atrophy
Cornelia de Lange syndrome	*NIPBL* (*AD*); *HDAC8* (*XLD*)	Synophrys, long curly eyelashes, ptosis
Cowden syndrome	*PTEN* (*AD*)	Cataract, angioid streaks
Cranioectodermal dysplasia	*IFT122* (*AR*)	Telecanthus, hypotelorism, epicanthal folds, myopia (1 patient), nystagmus (1 patient), retinal dystrophy (1 patient)
Cutis laxa	*ATP6V0A2*; *ALDH18A1* (*AR*)	Downslanting palpebral fissures, strabismus
Danon disease	*LAMP2* (*XLD*)	Moderate central loss of visual acuity in males, normal to near-normal visual acuity in carrier females, fine lamellar white opacities on slit lamp exam in carrier females, near complete loss of peripheral retinal pigment in males, peppered pigmentary mottling of peripheral retinal pigment in carrier females, nonspecific changes on electroretinogram in carrier females
Deafness and myopia	*SLITRK6* (*AR*)	High myopia
Desanto–Shinawi syndrome	*WAC* (*AD*)	Hypertelorism, downslanting palpebral issues, synophrys, deep-set eyes, astigmatism, strabismus
Desbuquois dysplasia	*CANT1* (*AR*)	Prominent eyes, bulging eyes, congenital glaucoma
Donnai–Barrow syndrome	*LRP2* (*AR*)	Hypertelorism, high myopia, loss of vision, iris coloboma, iris hypoplasia, cataract, enlarged globes, downslanting palpebral fissures, underorbital skin creases, retinal detachment, retinal dystrophy, prominent eyes
DOORS	*TBC1D24* (*AR*)	Optic atrophy, blindness, high myopia, cataracts
Ehlers–Danlos syndrome	*COL5A1* (*AD*); *PLOD1* (*AR*); *CHST14* (*AR*); *ADAMTS2* (*AR*); *B3GALT6* (*AR*); *FKBP14* (*AR*)	Blue sclerae, ectopia lentis, epicanthal folds

(continued)

Table 5.1 (continued)

Syndrome	Gene and inheritance pattern	Ocular phenotype other than myopia
Emanuel syndrome	CH	Hooded eyelids, deep-set eyes, upslanting palpebral fissures, strabismus
Fibrochondrogenesis	*COL11A1* (*AR*)	–
Gyrate atrophy of choroid and retina with/without ornithinemia	*OAT* (*AR*)	Progressive chorioretinal degeneration, night blindness (onset in first decade, progressive loss of peripheral vision, blindness (onset in fourth or fifth decade), posterior subcapsular cataracts (onset in second or third decade)
Hamamy syndrome	*IRX5* (*AR*)	Severe hypertelorism, laterally sparse eyebrows, myopia (progressive severe)
Homocystinuria	*CBS* (*AR*)	Ectopia lentis, glaucoma
Joint laxity; short stature; myopia	*GZF1* (*AR*)	Exophthalmos, severe myopia, retinal detachment (some patients), iris coloboma (some patients), chorioretinal coloboma (some patients), glaucoma (1 patient)
Kaufman oculocerebrofacial syndrome	*UBE3B* (*AR*)	Blepharophimosis, ptosis, upward-slanting palpebral fissures, telecanthus, hypertelorism, astigmatism, strabismus, mild
Kenny–Caffey syndrome	*FAM111A* (*AD*)	Hyperopia (not myopia), microphthalmia, papilledema, corneal and retinal calcification, congenital cataracts (rare)
Kniest dysplasia	*COL2A1* (*AD*)	Retinal detachment, cataracts, prominent eyes
Knobloch syndrome	*COL18A1* (*AR*)	High myopia, vitreoretinal degeneration, retinal detachment (childhood), congenital cataract, syneresis, vitreous attachment at the disc, persistent foetal hyaloid vasculature, peripapillary atrophy, phthisis bulbi, band keratopathy, macular hypoplasia, irregular white dots at the vitreoretinal interface, visual loss, nystagmus
Lamb–Shaffer syndrome	*SOX5* (*AD*)	Downslanting palpebral fissures, epicanthal folds, strabismus
Lethal congenital contracture syndrome	*ERBB3* (*AR*)	High myopia, degenerative vitreoretinopathy
Leukodystrophy	*POLR1C*; *POLR3A*; *POLR3B*; *GJC2* (*AR*)	–
Linear skin defects with multiple congenital anomalies	*NDUFB11*; *COX7B* (*XLD*)	Lacrimal duct atresia, nystagmus, strabismus
Loeys–Dietz syndrome	*TGFBR1*; *TGFBR2* (*AD*)	Hypertelorism, exotropia, blue sclerae, proptosis

Table 5.1 (continued)

Syndrome	Gene and inheritance pattern	Ocular phenotype other than myopia
Macrocephaly/ megalencephaly syndrome	*TBC1D7* (*AR*)	Astigmatism
Marfan syndrome	*FBN1* (*AD*)	Enophthalmos, ectopia lentis increased axial globe length, corneal flatness, retinal detachment, iris hypoplasia, early glaucoma, early cataracts, downslanting palpebral fissures, trabeculodysgenesis, primary (some patients), strabismus (some patients), exotropia (some patients), esotropia (rare), hypertropia (rare)
Marshall syndrome	*COL11A1* (*AD*)	congenital cataracts, esotropia, retinal detachment, glaucoma, lens dislocation, vitreoretinal degeneration, hypertelorism, epicanthal folds
Microcephaly with/ without chorioretinopathy; lymphedema; and/or mental retardation	*KIF11* (*AD*)	Upslanting palpebral fissures, downslanting palpebral fissures (some patients), epicanthal folds (some patients), nystagmus, reduced visual acuity, hypermetropia, myopic astigmatism, hypermetropic astigmatism, corneal opacity, microcornea, microphthalmia, cataract, retrolenticular fibrotic mass, chorioretinopathy, retinal folds, falciform retinal folds, retinal detachment, temporal dragging of optic disc, retinal pigment changes (some patients), optic atrophy (uncommon)
Mohr–Tranebjaerg syndrome	*TIMM8A* (*XLR*)	Photophobia, cortical blindness, decreased visual acuity, constricted visual fields, abnormal electroretinogram
Mucolipidosis	*GNPTAG* (*AR*)	Fine corneal opacities
Muscular dystrophy	*TRAPPC11*; *POMT*; *POMT1*; *POMT2*; *POMGNT1*; *B3GALNT2*; *FKRP*; *DAG1*; *FKTN*(*AR*)	Cataracts, strabismus, alacrima (some patients)
Nephrotic syndrome	*LAMB2* (*AR*)	Nystagmus, strabismus, microcoria, aplasia/atrophy of the dilatator pupillae muscle, hypoplasia of the iris and ciliary body, lenticonus posterior, blindness, decreased or absent laminin beta-2 immunoreactivity in tissues of the anterior eye

(continued)

Table 5.1 (continued)

Syndrome	Gene and inheritance pattern	Ocular phenotype other than myopia
Noonan syndrome	*A2ML1*; *BRAF*; *CBL*; *HRAS*; *KRAS*; *MAP2K1*; *MAP2K2*; *NRAS*; *PTPN11*; *RAF1*; *RIT1*; *SOS1*; *SHOC2*; *SPRED1* (*AD*)	Ptosis, hypertelorism, downslanting palpebral fissures, epicanthal folds, blue-green irides
Oculocutaneous albinism	*TYR* (*AR*)	Absent pigment in iris and retina, translucent iris, pink irides (childhood), blue-gray irides (adult), choroidal vessels visible, foveal hypoplasia, decreased visual acuity, strabismus, nystagmus, photophobia, high refractive errors (hyperopia, myopia, with-the-rule astigmatism), albinotic optic disc, misrouting of the optic nerves at the chiasm, absent stereopsis due to anomalous decussation at the optic chiasm, positive angle kappa (appearance of exotropia but no shift on cover test), asymmetric visual evoked potentials
Oculodentodigital dysplasia	*GJA1* (*AR*)	Hypoplastic eyebrows, sparse eyelashes, telecanthus, short palpebral fissures, downslanting palpebral fissures, microphthalmia, microcornea, cataract, persistent pupillary membrane
Pallister–Killian syndrome	CH	Sparse eyebrows, sparse eyelashes, upslanting palpebral fissures, hypertelorism, ptosis, strabismus, epicanthal folds, cataracts, exophthalmos
Papillorenal syndrome	*PAX2* (*AD*)	Retinal coloboma, optic nerve anomalies (coloboma, gliosis, absent optic nerve head), optic disc anomalies (dysplasia, excavation, hyperplasia, morning glory optic disc, hypoplasia), orbital cysts, microphthalmia, abnormal retinal pigment epithelium, abnormal retinal vessels, chorioretinal degeneration, retinal detachment (rare). retinal staphyloma (rare), retinal edema (rare), macular degeneration (rare), papillomacular detachment (rare), hyperpigmentation of the macula (rare), cystic degeneration of the macula (rare), posterior lens luxation (rare), lens opacity (rare)

Table 5.1 (continued)

Syndrome	Gene and inheritance pattern	Ocular phenotype other than myopia
Peters-plus syndrome	*B3GLCT* (*AR*)	Hypertelorism, Peter's anomaly, anterior chamber cleavage disorder, nystagmus, ptosis, glaucoma, upslanting palpebral fissures, cataract, iris coloboma, retinal coloboma
Pitt–Hopkins syndrome	*TCF4* (*AD*)	Deep-set eyes, strabismus, astigmatism, upslanting palpebral fissures
Pontocerebellar hypoplasia	*CHMP1A* (*AR*)	Astigmatism, esotropia, strabismus, hyperopia, nystagmus (some patients), cortical visual impairment (some patients), poor visual tracking (some patients)
Poretti–Boltshauser syndrome	*LAMA1* (*AR*)	Strabismus, amblyopia, oculomotor apraxia, nystagmus, retinal atrophy, retinal dystrophy, retinal dysfunction, macular heterotopia
Prader–Willi syndrome	*NDN* (PC); *SNRPN* (IP); CH	Almond-shaped eyes, strabismus, upslanting palpebral fissures, hyperopia
Pseudoxanthoma elasticum	*ABCC6* (*AR*)	Peau d'orange retinal changes (yellow-mottled retinal hyperpigmentation), angioid streaks of the retina (85% of patients), macular degeneration, visual impairment (50–70% of patients), central vision loss, colloid bodies, retinal haemorrhage, choroidal neovascularization, optic head drusen (yellowish-white irregularities of optic disc), owl's eyes (paired hyperpigmented spots)
Renal hypomagnesemia	*CLDN16*; *CLDN19* (*AR*)	Strabismus, nystagmus, hyperopia, astigmatism
SADDAN	*FGFR3* (*AD*)	High myopia, exotropia
Schaaf–Yang syndrome	*MAGEL2* (*AD*)	Esotropia, strabismus, almond-shaped eyes, short palpebral fissures, bushy eyebrows
Schimke immunoosseous dysplasia	*SMARCAL1* (*AR*)	Corneal opacities, astigmatism
Schuurs–Hoeijmakers syndrome	*PACS1* (*AD*)	Full, arched eyebrows, long eyelashes, hypertelorism, downslanting palpebral fissures, ptosis, nystagmus, strabismus
Schwartz–Jampel syndrome	*HSPG2* (*AR*)	Narrow palpebral fissures, blepharophimosis, cataract, microcornea, long eyelashes in irregular rows, ptosis
Sengers syndrome	*AGK* (*AR*)	Cataracts (infantile), strabismus, glaucoma
Short stature; hearing loss; retinitis pigmentosa and distinctive facies	*EXOSC2* (*AR*)	Deep-set eyes, short palpebral fissures, upslanting palpebral fissures, retinitis pigmentosa (2 patients), corneal dystrophy (2 patients, young-adult onset), glaucoma (1 patient), nystagmus (1 patient), strabismus (1 patient)

(continued)

Table 5.1 (continued)

Syndrome	Gene and inheritance pattern	Ocular phenotype other than myopia
Short stature; optic nerve atrophy; and Pelger–Huet anomaly	*NBAS* (*AR*)	Thick and bush eyebrows, small orbits, bilateral exophthalmos, epicanthus, bilateral optic nerve atrophy, non-progressive decreased visual acuity, (in) complete achromatopsia, strabismus (some patients), hypertelorism (some patients), hypermetropia (rare), pigmented nevus (rare)
SHORT syndrome	*PIK3R1* (*AD*)	Deep-set eyes, Rieger anomaly, telecanthus, glaucoma, megalocornea, cataracts
Short-rib thoracic dysplasia with/without polydactyly	*WDR19* (*AR*)	Cataracts, attenuated arteries, macular anomalies
Shprintzen–Goldberg syndrome	*SKI* (*AD*)	Telecanthus, hypertelorism, proptosis, strabismus, downslanting palpebral fissures, ptosis, shallow orbits
Singleton–Merten syndrome	*IFIH1* (*AD*)	Glaucoma
Small vessel brain disease with/without ocular anomalies	*COL4A1* (*AD*)	Retinal arteriolar tortuosity, hypopigmentation of the fundus, episodic scotomas, episodic blurred vision, amblyopia (1 family), strabismus (1 family), high intraocular pressure (1 family). *Reported in some patients*: astigmatism, hyperopia, congenital cataracts, prominent or irregular Schwalbe line, iridocorneal synechiae, Axenfeld–Rieger anomalies, corneal opacities, microphthalmia, microcornea, iris hypoplasia, corectopia. *Rare*: decreased visual acuity, glaucoma, corneal neovascularization, polycoria, iridogoniodysgenesis, macular haemorrhage and Fuchs spots, peripapillary atrophy, choroidal atrophy
Smith–Magenis syndrome	*RAI1* (*AD*)	–
Spastic paraplegia and psychomotor retardation with or without seizures	*HACE1* (*AR*)	Strabismus, retinal dystrophy (some patients)
Split hand/foot malformation	CH	–
Stickler syndrome	*COL2A1* (*AD*); *COL11A1* (*AD*); *COL9A1* (*AR*); *COL9A2* (*AR*)	Retinal detachment, blindness, occasional cataracts, glaucoma, membranous (type I) vitreous phenotype

Table 5.1 (continued)

Syndrome	Gene and inheritance pattern	Ocular phenotype other than myopia
Syndromic mental retardation	*SETD5* (AD); *MBD5* (AD); *USP9X* (XLD); *NONO* (XLR); *RPL10* (XLR); *SMS* (XLR); *ELOVL4* (AR); *KDM5C* (XLR)	Synophrys, eyebrow abnormalities, upslanting and short palpebral fissures, epicanthal folds, mild hypertelorism, strabismus, cataracts, hypermetropia, astigmatism, poor vision
Syndromic microphthalmia	*OTX2*; *BMP4* (*AD*)	Uni- or bilateral microphthalmia, uni- or bilateral anophthalmia, coloboma, microcornea, cataract, retinal dystrophy, optic nerve hypoplasia or agenesis
Temtamy syndrome	*C12orf57* (*AR*)	Hypertelorism. "key-hole" iris, retina and choroid coloboma, dislocated lens (upward), downslanting palpebral fissures, arched eyebrows
White–Sutton syndrome	*POGZ* (*AD*)	Visual abnormalities, strabismus, astigmatism, hyperopia, optic atrophy, rod-cone dystrophy, cortical blindness
Zimmermann–Laband syndrome	*KCNH1* (*AD*)	Thick eyebrows, synophrys, cataracts

AD autosomal dominant, *AR* autosomal recessive, *XLR* X linked recessive, *XLD* X linked dominant, *CH* chromosomal, *IP* imprinting defect

Table 5.1A Ocular conditions associated with myopia

Ocular condition	Gene and inheritance pattern
Achromatopsia	*CNGB3* (*AR*)
Aland Island eye disease	*GPR143* (*XLR*)
Anterior segment dysgenesis	*PITX3* (*AD*)
Bietti crystalline corneoretinal dystrophy	*CYP4V2* (*AD*)
Blue cone monochromacy	*OPN1LW*; *OPN1MW* (*XLR*)
Brittle cornea syndrome	*ZNF469*; *PRDM5* (*AR*)
Cataract	*BFSP2*; *CRYBA2*; *EPHA2* (*AD*)
Colobomatous macrophthalmia with microcornea	CH
Cone dystrophy	*KCNV2* (*AD*)
Cone rod dystrophy	*C8orf37* (*AR*); *RAB28* (*AR*); *RPGR* (*XLR*); *CACNA1F* (*XLR*)
Congenital microcoria	CH
Congenital stationary night blindness	*NYX* (*XLR*); *CACNA1F* (*XLR*); *GRM6* (*AR*); *SLC24A1* (*AR*); *LRIT3* (*AR*); *GNB3* (*AR*); *GPR179* (*AR*)
Ectopia lentis et pupillae	*ADAMTSL4* (*AR*)

(continued)

Ocular condition	Gene and inheritance pattern
High myopia with cataract and vitreoretinal degeneration	*P3H2* (*AR*)
Keratoconus	*VSX1* (*AD*)
Leber congenital amaurosis	*TULP1* (*AR*)
Microcornea, myopic chorioretinal atrophy, and telecanthus	*ADAMTS18* (*AR*)
Microspherophakia and/or megalocornea, with ectopia lentis and/or secondary glaucoma	*LTBP2* (*AR*)
Ocular albinism	*OCA2* (*AR*)
Primary open angle glaucoma	*MYOC*; *OPTN* (*AD*)
Retinal cone dystrophy	*KCNV2* (*AR*)
Retinal dystrophy	*C21orf2* (*AR*); *TUB* (*AR*)
Retinitis pigmentosa	*RP1* (*AD*); *RP2* (*XLR*); *RPGR* (*XLR*); *TTC8* (*AR*)
Sveinsson chorioretinal atrophy	*TEAD1* (*AD*)
Vitreoretinopathy	*ZNF408* (*AD*)
Wagner vitreoretinopathy	*VCAN* (*AD*)
Weill–Marchesani syndrome	*ADAMTS10* (*AR*); *FBN1*(*AD*); *LTBP2* (*AR*); *ADAMTS17* (*AR*)

AD autosomal dominant, *AR* autosomal recessive, *XLR* X linked recessive, *CH* chromosomal

pedigrees [21]. Families with genetic variants which show an autosomal dominant inheritance pattern were also most successful for myopia linkage studies. Up to now, 20 MYP loci [22–25] and several other loci [26–31] are identified for (high) myopia. Fine mapping led to candidate genes, such as the *IGF1* gene located in the MYP3 locus [32]. Linkage using a complex inheritance design found five additional loci [33–37].

Validation of candidate genes often resulted in no association, but other variants appeared associated with the non-Mendelian, common form of myopia. This hints towards a genetic overlap between Mendelian and common myopia [38]. As the GWAS era progressed, linkage studies fell by the wayside. Nevertheless, segregation analyses combined with linkage and next generation sequencing (i.e. whole exome sequencing) of regions in pedigrees with high myopia are, in theory, expected to facilitate the discovery of rare variants with large effects; an aspect which cannot be distilled from GWAS.

5.5 Candidate Gene Studies

In candidate gene studies the focus is on a gene with suspected biological, physiological or functional relevance to myopia, in particular high myopia. Although sometimes effective, candidate gene studies are limited by their reliance on this existing knowledge. Table 5.2 summarizes candidate gene studies on (high) myopia. Particularly

Table 5.2 Summary of candidate gene studies reporting positive association results with myopia

Gene symbol	Gene name	Hypothesized gene function	Associated phenotype	Ethnicity	Confirmation type (PMID)	Study (PMID)	Year
APLP2	Amyloid beta precursor like protein 2	Amacrine cell function modulation	Refractive error	Caucasian	n/a	Tkatchenko et al. [39] (26313004)	2015
BMP2K	Bone morphogenic protein-2-inducible protein kinase	Ocular development (embryogenesis) and retinal tissue remodelling	High myopia	Chinese	n/a	Liu et al. [40] (19927351)	2009
CHRM1	Cholinergic receptor muscarinic 1	Target of atropine	High myopia (−6.5 dpt)	Han Chinese	Expression study found no association with CHRM1 (19262686) and finding has been debated (20414262)	Lin et al. [41, 42] (19753311)	2010
CHRM1	Cholinergic receptor muscarinic 1	Target of atropine	High myopia (−6.5 dpt)	Han Chinese	Expression study found no association with CHRM1 (19262686) and finding has been debated (20414262)	Lin et al. [43, 44] (19753311)	2009
cMET (*alias HGFR*)	Tyrosine-protein kinase met	Hepatocyte growth factor and its receptor	Paediatric myopia (<−0.5 dpt)	Chinese	Replication independent high myopia cohort (24766640)	Khor et al. [45] (19500853)	2009
COL1A1	Collagen type I alpha 1 chain	Extracellular matrix	High myopia (<−9.25 dpt)	Japanese	Multiple systemic meta-analyses with contradicting results (27162737; 26131177; 27588274)	Inamori et al. [46] (17557158)	2007
COL2A1	Collagen type II alpha 1 chain	Extracellular matrix	High myopia (−5 dpt)	Caucasian	No replication independent high myopia cohort (21993774)	Metlapally et al. [47] (19387081)	2009
COL2A1	Collagen type II alpha 1 chain	Extracellular matrix	Paediatric myopia (<−0.75 dpt)	Caucasian	No replication independent high myopia cohort (21993774)	Mutti et al. [48] (17653045)	2007

(continued)

Table 5.2 (continued)

Gene symbol	Gene name	Hypothesized gene function	Associated phenotype	Ethnicity	Confirmation type (PMID)	Study (PMID)	Year
CRYBA4	Crystallin beta A4	Retinal and scleral remodelling	High myopia (<−8 dpt)	Chinese	No replication independent high myopia cohort (29263643)	Ho et al. [49] (22792142)	2012
HGF	Hepatocyte growth factor	Hepatocyte growth factor and its receptor	High myopia	Han Chinese	No replication independent high myopia cohort (19060265)	Han et al. [50] (16723436)	2006
HGF	Hepatocyte growth factor	Hepatocyte growth factor and its receptor	Refractive error	Caucasian	No replication independent high myopia cohort (19060265)	Veerappan et al. [51] (20005573)	2010
HGF	Hepatocyte growth factor	Hepatocyte growth factor and its receptor	High Myopia (−5 dpt)	Caucasian	No replication independent high myopia cohort (19060265)	Yanovitch et al. [52] (19471602)	2009
IGF1	Insulin-like growth factor 1	Hepatocyte growth factor and its receptor	High myopia (−5 dpt)	Caucasian	Systematic review and meta-analysis of studies in high myopics resulted in no association (28135889)	Metlapally et al. [53] (20435602)	2010
LAMA1	Laminin subunit alpha 1	Extracellular matrix	High myopia (<−6 dpt and axial length >26 mm)	Chinese	No replication independent high myopia cohort (29805427; 19668483)	Zhao et al. [54] (21541277)	2011
LUM	Lumican	Scleral and extracellular matrix remodelling	Extreme high myopia	Han Chinese	Meta-analysis of studies in high myopics resulted in no association (24927138)	Chen et al. [55] (19616852)	2009
LUM	Lumican	Scleral and extracellular matrix remodelling	High myopia	Han Chinese	Meta-analysis of studies in high myopics resulted in no association (24927138) and finding has been debated (20414262)	Lin et al. [41, 42] (19643966)	2010
LUM	Lumican	Scleral and extracellular matrix remodelling	High myopia (<−6.5 dpt)	Han Chinese	Meta-analysis of studies in high myopics resulted in no association (24927138)	Lin et al. [41, 42] (20010793)	2010

LUM	Lumican	Scleral and extracellular matrix remodelling	Extreme high myopia	Han Chinese	Meta-analysis of studies in high myopics resulted in no association (24927138)	Wang et al. [56] (16902402)	2006
MFN1	Mitofusin 1	Mitochondrial remodelling and apoptosis	Myopia	Caucasian	Expression study found association with myopia (27609161) and replication independent myopia cohort (26682159)	Andrew et al. [57] (18846214)	2008
MMP1	Matrix metallopeptidase 1	Extracellular matrix	Refractive error	Amish	No replication independent high myopia cohort (20435584; 23077567)	Wojciechowski et al. [58] (20484597)	2010
MMP1	Matrix metallopeptidase 1	Extracellular matrix	Refractive error	Caucasian	No replication independent high myopia cohort (20435584; 23077567)	Wojciechowski et al. [59] (23098370)	2013
MMP10	Matrix metallopeptidase 10	Extracellular matrix	Refractive error	Caucasian	No replication independent high myopia cohort (23077567)	Wojciechowski et al. [59] (23098370)	2013
MMP2	Matrix metallopeptidase 2	Extracellular matrix	Refractive error	Amish	Expression study found association with myopia (28402202; 29803830; 28900109; 24876280); no replication independent high myopia cohort (20435584; 23378725)	Wojciechowski et al. [58] (20484597)	2010
MMP2	Matrix metallopeptidase 2	Extracellular matrix	Refractive error	Caucasian	Expression study found association with myopia (28402202; 29803830; 28900109; 24876280); no replication independent high myopia cohort (20435584; 23378725)	Wojciechowski et al. [59] (23098370)	2013

(continued)

Table 5.2 (continued)

Gene symbol	Gene name	Hypothesized gene function	Associated phenotype	Ethnicity	Confirmation type (PMID)	Study (PMID)	Year
MMP3	Matrix metallopeptidase 3	Extracellular matrix	Refractive error	Caucasian	Expression study found no association with myopia (24876280); No replication independent high myopia cohort (20435584; 23077567; 16935611)	Hall et al. [60] (19279308)	2009
MMP9	Matrix metallopeptidase 9	Extracellular matrix	Refractive error	Caucasian	No replication independent high myopia cohort (23077567)	Hall et al. [60] (19279308)	2009
MYOC	Myocilin	Cytoskeletal function	High myopia	Chinese	No replication independent high myopia cohort (22809227; 24766640)	Tang et al. [61] (17438518)	2007
MYOC	Myocilin	Cytoskeletal function	High myopia	Caucasian	No replication independent high myopia cohort (22809227; 24766640)	Vatavuk et al. [62] (19260140)	2009
MYOC	Myocilin	Cytoskeletal function	High myopia	Caucasian	No replication independent high myopia cohort (22809227; 24766640)	Zayats et al. [63] (19180258)	2009
PAX6	Paired box 6	Ocular development (embryogenesis)	High myopia	Han Chinese	Systemic review and meta-analysis of studies in high and extreme myopics resulted in replication (24637479)	Han et al. [64] (19124844)	2009
PAX6	Paired box 6	Ocular development (embryogenesis)	High myopia (<−9 dpt)	Japanese	Systemic review and meta-analysis of studies in high and extreme myopics resulted in replication (24637479)	Kanemaki et al. [65] (26604670)	2015
PAX6	Paired box 6	Ocular development (embryogenesis)	High myopia (axial length >26 mm)	Japanese	Systemic review and meta-analysis of studies in high and extreme myopics resulted in replication (24637479)	Miyake et al. [66] (23213273)	2012

PAX6	Paired box 6	Ocular development (embryogenesis)	High myopia (<−6 dpt and axial length >26 mm)	Han Chinese	Systemic review and meta-analysis of studies in high and extreme myopics resulted in replication (24637479)	Ng et al. [67] (19907666)	2009
PAX6	Paired box 6	Ocular development (embryogenesis)	Extreme high myopia	Chinese	Systemic review and meta-analysis of studies in high and extreme myopics resulted in replication (24637479)	Tsai et al. [68] (17948041)	2008
PSARL	Presenilins-associated rhomboid-like protein	Mitochondrial remodelling and apoptosis	Myopia	Caucasian	n/a	Andrew et al. [57] (18846214)	2008
SOX2OT	Sex-determining region Y-box 2 overlapping transcript	Neurogenesis and vertebrate development (embryogenesis)	Myopia	Caucasian	n/a	Andrew et al. [57] (18846214)	2008
TGFβ1	Transforming growth factor beta 1	Extracellular matrix remodelling	High myopia (<−8 dpt)	Chinese	Replication GWAS-meta-analysis on refractive error (29808027)	Khor et al. [69] (20697017)	2010
TGFβ1	Transforming growth factor beta 1	Extracellular matrix remodelling	High myopia	Chinese	Replication GWAS-meta-analysis on refractive error (29808027)	Lin et al. [70] (16807529)	2006
TGFβ1	Transforming growth factor beta 1	Extracellular matrix remodelling	High myopia	Indian	Replication GWAS-meta-analysis on refractive error (29808027)	Rasool et al. [71] (23325483)	2013
TGFβ1	Transforming growth factor beta 1	Extracellular matrix remodelling	High myopia (<−8 dpt)	Chinese	Replication GWAS-meta-analysis on refractive error (29808027)	Zha et al. [72] (19365037)	2009

(continued)

Table 5.2 (continued)

Gene symbol	Gene name	Hypothesized gene function	Associated phenotype	Ethnicity	Confirmation type (PMID)	Study (PMID)	Year
TGFβ2	Transforming growth factor beta 2	Extracellular matrix remodelling	High myopia (<−6.5 dpt)	Han Chinese	Expression study found association with myopia (28900109; 29188062; 27214233; 24967344); expression study found no association with myopia (25112847)	Lin et al. [43, 44] (19710942)	2009
TGIF (*alias TGIF1*)	TGFB induced factor homeobox 1	Extracellular matrix remodelling	High myopia	Chinese	No replication independent high myopia cohort (19060265; 18172074; 17048038; 15223781)	Lam et al. [73] (12601022)	2003
TGIF1	TGFB induced factor homeobox 1	Extracellular matrix remodelling	High myopia	Indian	No replication independent high myopia cohort (19060265; 18172074; 17048038; 15223781)	Ahmed et al. [74] (24215395)	2014
UMODL1	Uromodulin like 1	Extracellular matrix	High myopia (<−9.25 dpt)	Japanese	No replication independent high myopia cohort (22857148)	Nishizaki et al. [75] (18535602)	2009

notable are genes encoding extracellular matrix-related proteins (*COL1A1*, *COL2A1* [16, 17] and *MMP1*, *MMP2*, *MMP3*, *MMP9*, *MMP10* [59, 60]). For candidates such as *PAX6* and *TGFB1*, the results were replicated in multiple independent extreme/high myopia studies and validated in a large GWAS meta-analysis in 2018, respectively [18, 76]. However in most other cases, the results were not independently validated: *LUM* and *IGF1* failed to confirm an association [77, 78]. Interestingly, in a few cases the candidates were subsequently implicated in GWAS of other ocular traits: *TGFβ2* and *LUM* for central corneal thickness (CCT), a glaucoma and keratoconus endophenotype [14], *PAX6* with optic disc area [79] and *HGF* [80].

5.6 Genome-Wide Association Studies

Generally, linkage studies are limited to identification of genetic variants with a large effect on myopia [81]. Given the limited number of genes identified by linkage, it became apparent in the 2000s that identifying large numbers of additional myopia genes was more practical with genome-wide association studies (GWASes), since it has dramatically higher statistical power. GWASes have greatly enhanced our knowledge of the genetic architecture of (complex) diseases [82]. Most of the variants found via GWAS reside in non-exonic regions and their effect sizes are typically small [82, 83]. For GWAS, 200 k–500 k genetic markers are usually genotyped and a further >10 million "imputed", taking advantage of the correlation structure of the genome. This approach is most effective for common variants (allele frequencies >0.01 in the population, although with larger reference panels, rarer alleles can also be detected).

Initially, GWASes for myopia were performed as a dichotomous outcome (i.e. case-control, Table 5.3). Since myopia constitutes a dichotomization of the quantitative trait spherical equivalent, considering the quantitative trait should be more informative for gene mapping. The first GWASes for spherical equivalent were conducted in 2010 [96, 97], with ~4000 individuals required to identify the first loci. The first loci to reach the genome-wide significance threshold ($P < 5 \times 10^{-8}$, the threshold reflecting the large number of statistical tests conducted genome-wide) were markers near the *RASGFR1* gene on 15q25.1 ($P = 2.70 \times 10^{-9}$) and markers near *GJD2* on 15q14 ($P = 2.21 \times 10^{-14}$). A subsequent analysis combining five cohorts ($N = 7000$) identified another locus at the *RBFOX1* gene on chromosome 16 ($P = 3.9 \times 10^{-9}$) [98].

These early efforts made it clear that individual groups would have difficulty in mapping many genes for spherical equivalent, motivating the formation of the Consortium for Refractive Error and Myopia (CREAM) in 2010, which included researchers and cohorts from the USA, Europe, Asia and Australia. They replicated SNPs in the 15q14 loci [99], which was further affirmed by other studies on both spherical equivalent and axial length alongside with the replication of the 15q25 locus [100, 101].

In 2013, two major GWAS meta-analyses on refractive error traits (spherical equivalent and age of spectacle wear) identified 37 novel loci (Table 5.4), with robust replication of *GJD2*, *RFBOX1* and *RASGFR1* in both meta-analyses. The first was the collaborative work of CREAM based on a GWAS meta-analysis on spherical equivalent, comprising 35 individual cohorts ($N_{European} = 37{,}382$; $N_{SoutheastAsian} = 12{,}332$) [108]. 23andMe, a direct-to-consumer genetic testing company, performed the second major GWAS, replicating 8 of the novel loci found by CREAM and identifying another 11 novel loci based on a GWAS survival analysis

Table 5.3 Summary of case-control design GWASs and their highest associations with myopia

Authors (year)	Study description	Associations	Ethnicity	PMID
Nakanishi et al. (2009) [84]	Genome-wide association study (GWAS) 830 cases (pathologic myopia; AL >26 mm) 1911 controls	Strongest association with 11q24.1, 44kb upstream of the *BLID* gene and in the second intron of *LOC399959*	Japanese	19779542
Li et al. (2011) [85]	GWAS 287 cases (high myopia; SE ≤ −6D) 673 controls	Strongest suggestive association ($P = 1.51 \times 10^{-5}$) with 5p15.2 for an intronic SNP within the *CTNND2* gene, but with replication in Japanese independent cohort (959 cases and 2128 controls; $P = 0.035$)	Chinese Japanese	21095009
Lu et al. (2011) [86]	GWAS 1203 cases (high myopia; SE ≤ −6D) 955 controls (SE -0.50 D to +1.00 D)	Replication ($P = 2.17 \times 10^{-5}$) with a SNP in *CTNND2* region	Chinese	21911587
Wang et al. [87] (2011)	SNP ($n = 3$) look-up in 11q24.1 and 21q22.3 regions 1255 cases (complex myopia; SE < −10.00 D <SE ≤−4.00 D) 563 cases (high myopia; SE ≤-6.00 D) 1052 controls (−0.50 D ≤ SE ≤ +2.00 D)	No statistically significant differences found for the genotype or allele frequencies of the three SNPs between the myopia cases and controls	Chinese	22194655
Yu et al. (2012) [88]	SNP ($n = 27$) look-up in 5p15 and 11q24 regions 321 cases (pathologic myopia; SE ≤ −6 D and AL > 26 mm) 310 control	Significantly associated SNPs in the *CTNND2* gene and 11q24.1 region ($P = 0.0126$ and 0.0293, respectively) with pathological myopia, replicating previous findings for these loci	Chinese	22759899
Liu et al. (2014) [89]	Meta-analysis comprising the SNPs of all 5 previously published data on the *CTNND2* gene and 11q24.1 region association with myopia 6954 cases 9346 controls	Significant association of 11q24.1 region with myopia ($P = 0.013$). No significant association with myopia for the *CTNND2* gene (two SNPs tested: $P = 0.725$, $P = 0.065$)	Chinese Japanese	24672220
Li et al. (2011) [85]	GWAS 102 cases (high myopia; SE ≤ −8 D with retinal degeneration) 335 controls	The strongest association ($P = 7.70 \times 10^{-13}$) was in a gene desert within the *MYP11* region on 4q25	Chinese	21505071

Shi et al. (2011) [90]	GWAS 419 high myopia cases (≤−6D) 669 controls	The strongest association ($P = 1.91 \times 10^{-16}$) was in an intron within the *MIPEP* gene on 13q12	Han Chinese	21640322
Shi et al. (2013) [91]	GWAS 665 cases (high myopia; SE ≤ −6D) 960 controls	The strongest association ($P = 8.95 \times 10^{-14}$) was in the *VIPR2* gene within the MYP4 locus, followed by three other variants in LD of the *SNTB1* gene region ($P = 1.13 \times 10^{-8}$ to 2.13×10^{-11})	Han Chinese	23406873
Khor et al. (2013) [92]	GWAS meta-analysis of 4 Asian studies 1603 cases ("severe" myopia; SE ≤−6 D and AL ≥26 mm) 3427 controls	The *SNTB1* gene was confirmed and a novel variant within the *ZFHX1B* gene (also known as *ZEB2*) reached genome-wide significance ($P = 5.79 \times 10^{-10}$)	East-Asian	23933737
Hosada et al. (2018) [93]	GWAS meta-analysis of 5 Asian studies 828 cases 3624 controls	Discovery ($P = 1.46 \times 10^{-10}$) and replication ($P = 2.40 \times 10^{-6}$) of the CCDC102B locus.	East-Asian	29725004
Meng et al. (2012) [94]	GWAS 192 cases (high myopia; SE ≤−6 D) 1064 controls	Confirmation of SNPs 3kb downstream of *PPP1R3B* in vicinity of MYP10 on 8p23 ($P = 6.32 \times 10^{-7}$) and MYP15 on 10q21.1 ($P = 2.17 \times 10^{-5}$)	European	23049088
Pickrell et al. (2016) [95]	GWAS 106,086 cases (Myopia "yes"; questionnaire) 85,757 controls (Myopia "no"; questionnaire)	More than 100 novel loci associated with myopia	European	27182965

Table 5.4 Overview of the 37 novel loci found in 2013 by CREAM and 23andMe and subsequent replication

Locus #	Locus name	Discovery—*P* value HapMapII CREAM (2013)	Replication—*P* value HapMapII 23andMe (2013)	Replication—individual cohort (PMID)	Replication—*P* value 1000G CREAM&23 and Me (2018)
2	*BICC1*	2.06×10^{-13}	n/a	Simpson et al. (2014) [102] (25233373), Yoshikawa et al. (2014) [103] (25335978)	1.07×10^{-18}
3	*LAMA2*	1.79×10^{-12}	6.80×10^{-53}	Cheng et al. (2013) [104] (24144296), Simpson et al. (2014) [102] (25233373)	1.91×10^{-57}
4	*CD55*	3.05×10^{-12}	n/a	Cheng et al. (2013) [104] (24144296), Yoshikawa et al. (2014) [103] (25335978)	4.42×10^{-13}
5	*TOX/CA8*	3.99×10^{-12}	4.00×10^{-22}	Simpson et al. (2014) [102] (25233373)	4.64×10^{-31}
6	*RDH5*	4.44×10^{-12}	1.30×10^{-23}		4.06×10^{-43}
7	*CYP26A1*	1.03×10^{-11}	n/a	Yoshikawa et al. (2014) [103] (25335978)	7.49×10^{-10}
8	*RASGRF1*	4.25×10^{-11}	8.20×10^{-13}	Oishi et al. (2013) [105] (24150758), Yoshikawa et al. (2014) [103] (25335978)	4.24×10^{-23}
9	*CHRNG*	5.15×10^{-11}	n/a	Tideman et al. (2016) [106] (27611182)	1.16×10^{-24}
10	*SHISA6*	7.29×10^{-11}	5.20×10^{-15}		9.46×10^{-29}
11	*PRSS56*	7.86×10^{-11}	5.80×10^{-18}	Simpson et al. (2014) [102] (25233373)	2.25×10^{-29}
12	*MYO1D*	9.66×10^{-11}	n/a		2.91×10^{-16}
13	*ZMAT4/SFRP1*	3.69×10^{-10}	1.80×10^{-18}	Simpson et al. (2014) [102] (25233373), Yoshikawa et al. (2014) [103] (25335978)	1.02×10^{-27}
14	*A2BP/RBFOX1*	5.64×10^{-10}	4.10×10^{-26}	Simpson et al. (2014) [102] (25233373), Tideman et al. (2016) [106] (27611182)	1.13×10^{-42}
15	*KCNQ5*	4.18×10^{-9}	2.70×10^{-25}	Liao et al. (2017) [107] (28884119), Yoshikawa et al. (2014) [103] (25335978), Tideman et al. (2016) [106] (27611182)	5.43×10^{-48}
16	*PTPRR*	5.47×10^{-9}	n/a		1.81×10^{-13}
17	*GRIA4*	5.92×10^{-9}	n/a	Tideman et al. (2016) [106] (27611182), Yoshikawa et al. (2014) [103] (25335978)	8.84×10^{-12}

18	*TJP2*	7.26×10^{-9}	5.20×10^{-13}		1.35×10^{-21}
19	*SIX6*	1.00×10^{-8}	n/a		2.12×10^{-8}
20	*LOC100506035*	1.09×10^{-8}	n/a		1.56×10^{-15}
21	*BMP2*	1.57×10^{-8}	n/a	Tideman et al. (2016) [106] (27611182), Yoshikawa et al. (2014) [103] (25335978)	3.11×10^{-9}
22	*CHD7*	1.82×10^{-8}	n/a		1.94×10^{-7}
23	*PCCA*	2.11×10^{-8}	n/a		1.68×10^{-7}
24	*CACNA1D*	2.14×10^{-8}	n/a	Tideman et al. (2016) [106] (27611182)	4.10×10^{-10}
25	*KCNJ2*	2.79×10^{-8}	n/a		5.53×10^{-13}
26	*RORB*	4.15×10^{-8}	n/a		1.07×10^{-11}
27	*LRRC4C*	n/a	2.30×10^{-30}	Tideman et al. (2016) [106] (27611182), Yoshikawa et al. (2014) [103] (25335978)	4.43×10^{-42}
28	*PABPCP2*	n/a	1.50×10^{-14}		1.05×10^{-17}
29	*BMP3*	n/a	4.20×10^{-12}	Simpson et al. (2014) [102] (25233373)	2.08×10^{-20}
30	*RGR*	n/a	8.00×10^{-12}		9.26×10^{-17}
31	*DLG2*	n/a	1.70×10^{-11}		8.85×10^{-15}
32	*ZBTB38*	n/a	3.60×10^{-11}		1.23×10^{-15}
33	*PDE11A*	n/a	8.70×10^{-11}		1.30×10^{-15}
34	*DLX1*	n/a	1.40×10^{-10}		2.77×10^{-16}
35	*KCNMA1*	n/a	7.30×10^{-10}		2.36×10^{-16}
36	*BMP4*	n/a	1.10×10^{-9}	Yoshikawa et al. (2014) [103] (25335978)	1.09×10^{-12}
37	*ZIC2*	n/a	2.10×10^{-8}	Oishi et al. (2013) [105] (24150758), Simpson et al. (2014) [102] (25233373), Tideman et al. (2016) [106] (27611182)	2.80×10^{-15}
S-38[*]	*B4GALNT2*	n/a	8.30×10^{-7}	Yoshikawa et al. (2014) [103] (25335978)	2.68×10^{-10}
S-39[*]	*EHBP1L1*	n/a	2.10×10^{-7}	Yoshikawa et al. (2014) [103] (25335978)	1.07×10^{-9}

[*]These two loci were subthreshold (S) in the analysis in 2013, but exceeded genome-wide significance in 2018 using a larger sample size

of age of spectacle wear in 55,177 participants of European ancestry. To the surprise of some in the field, the effect sizes and direction of the effects of the loci found by these two groups were concordant despite the difference in phenotype definition and in scale: dioptres for CREAM and hazard ratios for 23andMe [109]. Subsequently, replication studies provided validation for the associated loci and highlighted two other suggestive associations. At this point, the implicated loci explained 3% of the phenotypic variance in refractive error [108, 110].

The CREAM and 23andMe studies represented a large increase in sample size over the initial GWASs. Their meta-analysis approach was very effective in discovering new loci. This motivated joined efforts of CREAM and 23andMe, which resulted in a GWAS meta-analysis including 160,420 participants. Moreover, a denser imputation reference set was used (1000G phase 1 version 3), enabling better characterization of genetic variations. Although CREAM and 23andMe used different phenotypes (spherical equivalent and age at first spectacle wear, respectively) again the results were concordant and the new findings were replicated in an independent cohort with refractive error available (UK biobank, comprising 95,505 participants). Overall, this GWAS increased the number of risk loci to 161, explaining 7.8% of the phenotypic variance in refractive error. Very large sample sizes (millions) will be required to identify all of the loci contributing to myopia risk.

The genetic correlation was estimated to be 0.78 between European and Asian ancestry, suggesting that despite (1) large differences in the rate of myopia between these groups and (2) differences in the genetic ancestry of these groups, most of the genetic variation is in common. Figure 5.1 provides the chronological discovery of all associated loci and Fig. 5.2 shows the effect sizes of the established 161 loci.

Several "endophenotypes" have been considered for myopia: spherical equivalent, axial length, corneal curvature and age of diagnosis of myopia. Axial length is a well-studied "endophenotype" which correlates strongly with refractive error. The first GWAS of axial length considered 4944 Asian ancestry individuals and identified a locus at 1q41. A subsequent meta-analysis combining data on 12,531 European and 8216 Asian ancestry individuals uncovered a further eight genome-wide significant loci at *RSPO1*, *C3orf26*, *LAMA2*, *GJD2*, *ZNRF3*, *CD55*, *MIP*, *ALPPL2*, as well as confirming the 1q41 locus. Five of the axial length loci were also associated loci for refractive error. GWASs performed for corneal curvature [104, 111–114] identified the loci *FRAP1*, *CMPK1*, *RBP3* and *PDGFRA*; in the case of *PDGFRA*, associations have also been found with eye size. A study in 9804 Japanese individuals and replication in Chinese and European ancestry cohorts analysed three myopia-related traits (refractive error, axial length and corneal curvature). They replicated the association of *GJD2* and refractive error as well as the association of SNPs in *WNT7B* for axial length and corneal curvature [114, 115]

5.7 Pathway Analysis Approaches

GWAS approaches improve our understanding of the molecular basis of traits by mapping individual loci. However, it is possible to place such loci into a broader context by applying pathway analysis approaches. In myopia, a retina-to-sclera signaling cascade has been postulated, but the specific molecular components were unclear. Recent GWASs have uncovered genes which lie along this pathway [108, 110, 116]—genetic changes at individual loci only make small changes to phenotype but collectively these

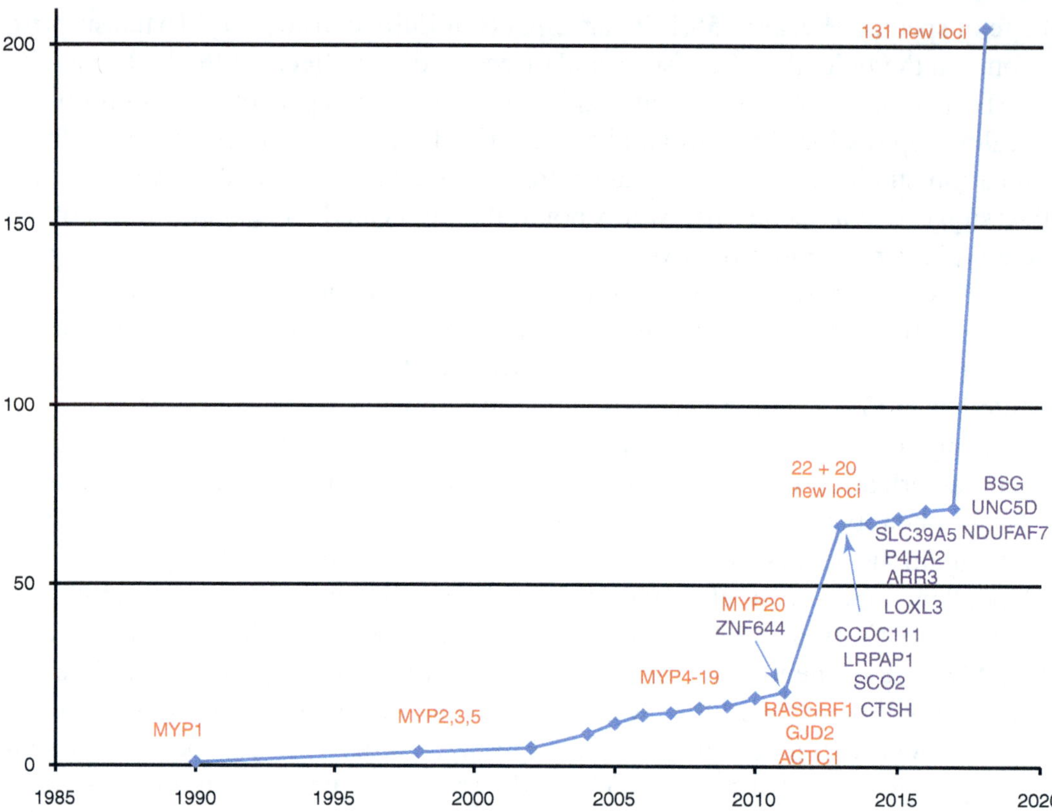

Fig. 5.1 Historic overview of myopia gene finding. Overview of myopia gene finding in historic perspective. Genes identified using whole exome sequencing are marked as purple. Other loci (linkage studies, GWAS) are marked as red

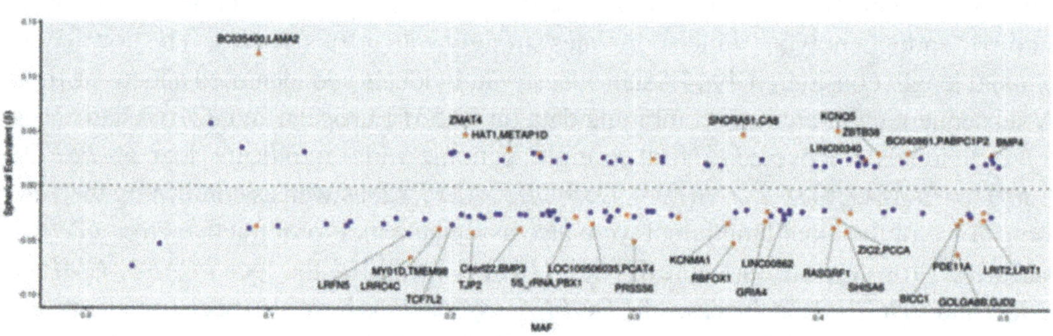

Fig. 5.2 Effect sizes of common and rare variants for myopia and refractive error. Overview of SNPs and annotated genes found in the most recent GWAS meta-analysis [18]. X-axis displays the minor allele frequency of each SNP; y-axis displays the effect size of per individual SNP. The blue dots represent the novel loci discovered by Tedja et al. [18] and the pink dots represent the loci found by Verhoeven et al. [108], which now have been replicated

perturbations are responsible for larger changes in the retina-to-sclera signaling cascade, ultimately explaining differences in refractive error from individual to individual.

Pathways inferred from the first large-scale CREAM GWAS [108, 110] included neurotransmission (*GRIA4*), ion transport (*KCNQ5*), retinoic acid metabolism (*RDH5*), extracellular matrix remodelling (*LAMA2*, *BMP2*) and eye development (*SIX6*, *PRSS56*). The 23andMe GWAS identified an overlapping set of pathways: neuronal development (*KCNMA1*, *RBFOX1*, *LRRC4C*, *NGL-1*, *DLG2*, *TJP2*),

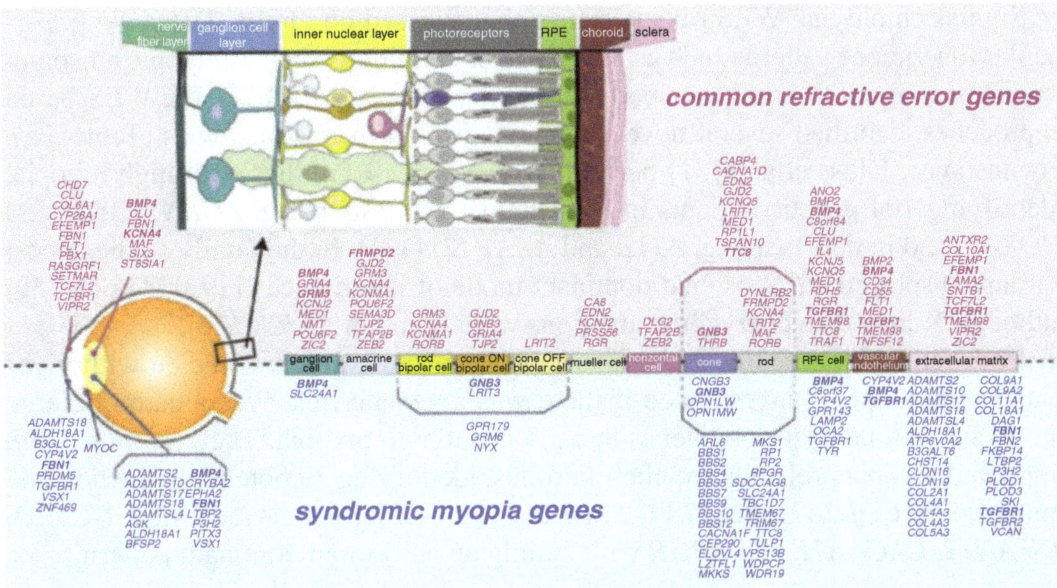

Fig. 5.3 Schematic overview of known function in retinal cell types of refractive error and syndromic myopia genes according to literature. Bold: genes identified for both common refractive error and in syndromic myopia

extracellular matrix remodelling (*ANTXR2*, *LAMA2*), the visual cycle (*RDH5*, *RGR*, *KCNQ5*), eye and body growth (*PRSS56*, *BMP4*, *ZBTB38*, *DLX1*) and retinal ganglion cell (*ZIC2*, *SFRP1*) [117]. When considered in the context of known protein–protein interactions, many genes in these pathways are related to growth and cell cycle pathways, such as the TGF-beta/SMAD and MAPK pathways [118].

The most recent meta-analysis combining data from CREAM and 23andMe data taken together confirmed previous findings and offered additional insights [18]. In a gene-set analysis, several pathways were highlighted including “abnormal photoreceptor inner segment morphology” (Mammalian Phenotype Ontology (MP) 0003730); “thin retinal outer nuclear layer” (MP 0008515); “nonmotile primary cilium” (Gene Ontology (GO) 0031513); “abnormal anterior-eye-segment morphology” (MP 0005193) and “detection of light stimulus” (GO 0009583). The genes implicated in this large-scale GWAS were distributed across all cell types in the retina-to-sclera signaling cascade (neurosensory retina, RPE, vascular endothelium and extracellular matrix, Fig. 5.3). The larger GWAS also suggested novel mechanisms, including angiogenesis, rod-and-cone bipolar synaptic neurotransmission and anterior-segment morphology. Interestingly, a novel association was found at the *DRD1* gene, supporting previous work linking the dopamine pathway to myopia.

5.8 Next Generation Sequencing

GWAS approaches have been highly effective in assessing the role of common variants in myopia but such methods cannot effectively characterize very rare genomic variants. Whole exome sequencing (WES) allows investigation of rare variants in exonic regions; due to cost, applications to date have primarily been in family studies or studies of early onset high myopia.

Studies employing WES to date have either focused on family designs (e.g. particular inheritance patterns such as X-linkage or conditions such as myopic anisometropia) or case-control studies of early onset high myopia [119–122]. The WES-based approaches identified several novel mutations in known myopia genes (Table 5.5). For instance, Kloss et al. [131] performed WES on 14 families with high myopia, identifying 104 genetic variants in both known MYP loci (e.g. *AGRN*, *EME1* and *HOXA2*) and in new loci (e.g. *ATL3* and *AKAP12*) [131]. In the family studies, most variants displayed an autosomal dominant mode of inheritance [119, 123, 124, 130] although X-linked heterozygous mutations were found in *ARR3* [126].

Both retinal dystrophies and ocular development disorders coincide with myopia. Sun et al. [132] investigated if there was a genetic link by evaluating a large number of retinal dystrophy genes in early onset high myopia. They examined 298 unrelated myopia probands and their families, identifying 29 potentially pathogenic mutations in *COL2A1*, *COL11A1*, *PRPH2*, *FBN1*, *GNAT1*, *OPA1*, *PAX2*, *GUCY2D*, *TSPAN12*, *CACNA1F* and *RPGR* with mainly an autosomal dominant pattern.

5.9 Environmental Influences Through Genetics

Although myopia is highly heritable within specific cohorts, dramatic changes in environment across many human populations have led to large changes in prevalence over time [133–136]. The role of changes in socioeconomic status, time spent outdoors, education and near-work are now well established as risk factors for myopia, based on observational studies [137–139]. Education has proven the most influential and consistent factor, with a doubling in myopia prevalence when attending higher education compared to finishing only primary education [140–142]. There are two main areas where genetic studies can inform our understanding of the role of environment. Firstly, gene–environment studies can highlight where interactions exist. Secondly, observational studies only establish association and not causation—in some circumstances genetic data can be used to strengthen the case for an environmental risk factor causally (or not) influencing myopia risk (Mendelian randomization).

Gene–environment (GxE) interaction analyses examine whether genes operate differently across varying environments. GxE studies in myopia have focused primarily on education. An early study in North American samples examined GxE for myopia and the matrix metalloproteinases genes (*MMP1-MMP10*): a subset of SNPs were only associated with refraction in the lower education level [58, 59]. A subsequent study in five Singapore cohorts found variants in *DNAH9*, *GJD2* and *ZMAT4*, which had a larger effect on myopia in a high education subset [143]. Subsequent efforts to examine GxE considered the aggregate effects of many SNPs together. A study in Europeans found that a genetic risk score comprising 26 genetic variants was most strongly associated with myopia in individuals with a university level education [144]. A study examining GxE in children considered near work and time outdoors in association with 39 SNPs and found weak evidence for an interaction with near work [144, 145]. Finally, a CREAM study was able to identify additional myopia risk loci by allowing for a GxE approach [19].

Mendelian randomization (MR) infers whether a risk factor is causally associated with a disease. MR exploits the fact that germline genotypes are randomly

Table 5.5 Overview of genes and their mutations found by next generation sequencing

Gene	Pathway	Method	Inheritance Pattern	Mutation type	Mutation	Author (Year)	PMID
CCDC111	DNA transcription	Targeted sequencing and exome sequencing	Autosomal dominant	Missense	c.265T>G:p.Y89D in *CCDC111*	Zhao et al. (2013) [120]	23579484
NDUFAF7	Mitochondrial function	Genotyping and WES	Autosomal dominant	Missense	c.798C>G:p.D266E in *NDUFAF7*	Wang et al. (2017) [121]	28837730
P4HA2	Collagen synthesis	WES	Autosomal dominant	Missense	c.1147A>G:p.(K383E) in *P4HA2*	Napolitano et al. (2018) [119]	29364500
SCO2	Mitochondrial function	WES	Autosomal dominant	Missense	c.334C>T:p.R112W; c.358C>T:p.R120W in *SCO2*	Jiang et al. (2014) [123]	25525168
SCO2	Mitochondrial function	WES	Autosomal dominant	Nonsense Missense	c.157C>T:p.Q53* in SCO2; c.341G>A:p.R114H; c.418G>A:p.E140K and c.776C>T:p.A259V) in *SCO2*	Tran-Viet et al. (2013) [124]	23643385
UNC5D	Cell signaling	WES	Autosomal dominant	Missense	c.1297C>T:p.R433C in *UNC5D*	Feng et al. (2017) [122]	28614238
BSG	Cell signaling	WES	Autosomal dominant	Missense Splicing Nonsense	c.889G>A:p.G297S; c.661C>T:p.P221S in *BSG* c.205C>T:p.Q69X in *BSG* c.415+1G>A in *BSG*	Jin et al. [125] (2017)	28373534
ARR3	Retina-specific signal transduction	WES	X-linked female-limited	Missense	c.893C>A:p.A298D; c.298C>T:p.R100* and c.239T>C:p.L80P in *ARR3*	Xiao et al. (2016) [126]	27829781

LOXL3	Transforming growth factor-beta pathway	WES	Autosomal recessive	Frameshift	c.39dup:p.L14Afs*21; c.39dup:p.L14Afs*21 and c.594delG:p.Q199Kfs*35 in *LOXL3*	Li et al. [127] (2016)	26957899
SLC39A5	Transforming growth factor-beta pathway	WES	Autosome dominant Autosome dominant	Nonsense Missense	c.141C>G:p.Y47* in *SLC39A5* c.911T>C:p.M304T in *SLC39A5*	Guo et al. [128] (2014)	24891338
SLC39A5	Transforming growth factor-beta pathway	WES	Autosome dominant	Missense	c.1238G>C:p.G413A in *SLC39A5*	Jiang et al. (2014) [123]	25525168
LRPAP1	Transforming growth factor-beta pathway	WES	Autosomal recessive	Frameshift, truncating	N202Tfs*8 and I288Rfs*118 in *LRPAP1*	Aldahmesh [129] et al. (2013)	23830514
LRPAP1	Transforming growth factor-beta pathway	WES	Autosomal recessive	Truncating	c.199delC:p.Q67Sfs*8 in *LRPAP1*	Jiang et al. (2014) [123]	25525168
CTSH	Degradation of proteins in lysosomes	WES	Autosomal recessive	Frameshift, truncating	c.485_488del in *CTSH*	Aldahmesh [129] et al. (2013)	23830514
ZNF644	DNA transcription	WES	Autosomal dominant	Missense	I587V, R680G, C699Y, 3′UTR+12 C>G, and 3′UTR+592 G>A in ZNF644	Shi et al. [130] (2011)	21695231
ZNF644	DNA transcription	WES	Autosomal dominant	Missense	c.2014A>G:p.S672G; c.2048G>C:p.R683T and c.2551G>C:p.D851H	Jiang et al. (2014) [123]	25525168
104 novel genetic variants (73 rare)	–	WES in 14 families	Autosomal dominant	Non synonymous	–	Kloss et al. (2017) [131]	28384719

assigned at meiosis, to enable a “natural” randomized controlled trial. Since the assigned genotypes are independent of non-genetic confounding and are unmodified by disease processes, MR offers a better assessment of causality than that available from observational studies [146, 147].

Two MR studies found a causal effect of education on the development of myopia. One of the MR studies tested for causality bi-directionally [148]. Both found a larger effect through MR than that estimated from observational studies suggesting that confounding in observational studies may have been obscuring the true relationship [149]. As expected, there was little evidence of myopia affecting education (−0.008 years/dioptre, $P = 0.6$). Another study focused on the causality of low vitamin D on myopia due to controversy in the literature [150]. The estimated effects of vitamin D on refractive error were so small (Caucasians: −0.02 [95% CI −0.09, 0.04] dioptres (D) per 10 nmol/l increase in vitamin D concentration; Asians: 0.01 [95% CI −0.17, 0.19] D per 10 nmol/l increase) that the authors concluded that the true contribution of vitamin D levels to degree of myopia is probably zero and that previous observational findings were likely confounded by the effects of time spent outdoors.

5.10 Epigenetics

Epigenetics in refractive error and myopia is postulated to be important due to the known effects of environmental factors on refractive error and myopia development. Nevertheless, this field is still developing and some characteristics of epigenetics render it a difficult issue to unravel. Epigenetic features can be influenced by environmental factors and are time dependent and tissue specific. This complicates the study of these effects, since myopia and refractive errors develop during childhood and young adolescence and obtaining eye tissue, preferably retinal and scleral would be unethical. Furthermore, although some epigenetic processes are conserved across species, this is not always the case: making animal studies not always translational to humans.

Non-Coding RNAs and Myopia The latest GWAS meta-analysis found 31 of 161 loci residing in or near regions transcribing (small) noncoding RNAs, thus hinting towards the importance of epigenetics [18, 151]. MicroRNAs, or miRNAs, are the best-characterized family of small non-coding RNAs. They are approximately 19–24 nucleotides in length in their mature form. They are able to bind to 3′ UTR regions on RNA polymers by sequence-specific post-transcriptional gene silencing; one miRNA can regulate the translation of many genes. MiRNAs have been a hot topic in the last years due to their potential clinical application: the accessibility of the retina for miRNA-based therapeutic delivery has great potential for the prevention and treatment of retinal pathologies [152]. Up to now, there have only been a handful of studies on miRNA and its role in myopiagenesis in humans, these are summarized in Table 5.6.

5.11 Implications for Clinical Management

Due to the high polygenicity of myopia and low explained phenotypic variance by genetic factors (7.8%), clinical applications derived from genetic analyses of myopia are currently limited. Risk predictions for myopia in children are based on family history, education level of the parents, the amount of outdoor exposure and the easily measurable refractive error and axial length.

Currently, we are able to make a distinction between high myopes and high hyperopes based on the polygenic risk scores derived from CREAM studies: persons in the highest decile for the polygenic risk score had a 40-fold-greater risk of myopia relative to those in the lowest decile.

A prediction model including age, sex and polygenic risk score achieved an AUC of 0.77 (95% CI = 0.75–0.79) for myopia versus hyperopia in adults (Rotterdam Study I–III) [18]. This AUC is similar to that achieved by modelling environmental factors only; the AUC for myopia incidence in a European child cohort was 0.78 considering parental myopia, 1 or more books read per week, time spent reading, no participation in sports, non-European ethnicity, less time spent outdoors and baseline AL-to-CR ratio [156]. To date, one study has assessed both environmental and

Table 5.6 Overview of microRNAs associated with myopia

MiRNA	SNP	Study design	Outcome	Author
MiR-328 binding site in 3′UTR of PAX6 gene	rs662702	High myopia case-control study (Ncase = 1083, ≤−6 D; Ncontrol 1096 ≥−1.5 D)	Down regulation effect on PAX6 expression with C allele, relative to T allele. OR for CC genotype 2.1 ($P = 0.007$). This effect was significant for extreme myopia (<−10 D) and not for high myopia	Liang et al. (2011) [153]
MiR-184	n.a.	MiR-184 region sequenced in 780 unrelated keratoconus patients and 96 unrelated Han southern Chinese patients with axial myopia under the hypothesis that axial myopia is associated with keratoconus, possibly under regulation of MiR-184	No miR-184 mutations were detected in the axial myopia cohort	Lechner et al. (2013) [154]
MiR-29a	rs157907	High myopia case-control study (Ncases = 254, ≤−6 D; Ncontrols = 300, −0.5 to 0.5 D). COL1A1 is possibly targeted by MiR-29a	The G allele of the rs157907 locus was significantly associated with decreased risk of severe myopia (<10 D; $P = 0.04$), compared to the A allele. rs157907 A/G might regulate miR-29a expression levels, but no functional studies have been conducted to confirm this hypothesis	Xie et al. (2016) [155]
Let-7i	rs10877885	High myopia case-control study (Ncases = 254, ≤−6 D; Ncontrols = 300, −0.5 to 0.5 D). COL1A1 is possibly targeted by Let-7i	No significant association with rs10877885 (C/T) was found with myopia risk	Xie et al. (2016) [155]

genetic factors together and showed that modelling both genes and environment improved prediction accuracy [157]. Although these efforts to improve prediction are promising, a prediction-based approach will only be beneficial if randomized controlled trials of atropine therapy show that children with persistent myopic progression benefit from an earlier and higher dose of atropine administration. The additional costs of genetic testing and potentially invasive regime (collecting blood from children) also need to be taken into account.

5.12 Concluding Remarks

The scientific community has discovered more than 200 loci associated with myopia and its endophenotypes with a variety of approaches (linkage, candidate gene, GWAS, post-GWAS gene-based associations, next generation sequencing approaches, gene environment interactions and epigenetic approaches). With the rise of large biobanks, such as the UK Biobank [158], further GWAS meta-analyses between large consortia and companies will enable identification of many more genes. This will allow full elucidation of the molecular mechanism of myopiagenesis. Whole genome sequencing approaches will replace both GWAS and WES, and will elucidate the genetic structure which regulates the function of the myopia risk variants.

To fully understand the underlying mechanisms, the focus should lie on unraveling the genetic and epigenetic architecture of myopia by exploring interactions and effects of other "omics" in relevant tissue, i.e. multi-omics. This concept includes incorporation of methylomics, transcriptomics, proteomics and metabolomics. Future projects should focus on gathering more omics data on eye tissue. Next to the multi-omics approach, modelling gene–environment effects will tell us more about the genetic key players which are also susceptible to the environment. Furthermore, future functional studies interrogating the candidate genes and loci will point us to therapeutic solutions for myopia management.

References

1. Tedja MS, et al. International Myopia Institute (IMI) - myopia genetics report. Investig Ophthalmol Vis Sci. 2019;60:M31–88.
2. Duke-Elder SS. The practice of refraction. Philadelphia: Blakiston; 1943.
3. Guggenheim JA. The heritability of high myopia: a reanalysis of Goldschmidt's data. J Med Genet. 2000;37:227–31.
4. Sorsby A, Sheridan M, Leary GA. Refraction and its components in twins. Medical Research Council, Special Report Series No. 303; 1962.
5. Lin LL, Chen CJ. A twin study on myopia in Chinese school children. Acta Ophthalmol Suppl. 1988;185:51–3.
6. Wojciechowski R, et al. Heritability of refractive error and familial aggregation of myopia in an elderly American population. Invest Ophthalmol Vis Sci. 2005;46:1588–92.
7. Young FA, et al. The transmission of refractive errors within Eskimo families. Am J Optom Arch Am Acad Optom. 1969;46:676–85.
8. Angi MR, Clementi M, Sardei C, Piattelli E, Bisantis C. Heritability of myopic refractive errors in identical and fraternal twins. Graefes Arch Clin Exp Ophthalmol. 1993;231:580–5.
9. Teikari JM, Kaprio J, Koskenvuo MK, Vannas A. Heritability estimate for refractive errorsDOUBLEHYPHENa population-based sample of adult twins. Genet Epidemiol. 1988;5:171–81.

10. Lyhne N, Sjølie AK, Kyvik KO, Green A. The importance of genes and environment for ocular refraction and its determiners: a population based study among 20-45 year old twins. Br J Ophthalmol. 2001;85:1470–6.
11. Sanfilippo PG, Hewitt AW, Hammond CJ, Mackey DA. The heritability of ocular traits. Surv Ophthalmol. 2010;55:561–83.
12. OMIM - Online Mendelian Inheritance in Man. Available at https://www.omim.org/. Accessed 27 June 2018.
13. Hendriks M, et al. Development of refractive errors-what can we learn from inherited retinal dystrophies? Am J Ophthalmol. 2017;182:81–9.
14. Iglesias AI, et al. Cross-ancestry genome-wide association analysis of corneal thickness strengthens link between complex and Mendelian eye diseases. Nat Commun. 2018;9:1864.
15. Baratz KH, et al. E2-2 protein and Fuchs's corneal dystrophy. N Engl J Med. 2010;363:1016–24.
16. Mutti DO, et al. Candidate gene and locus analysis of myopia. Mol Vis. 2007;13:1012–9.
17. Metlapally R, et al. COL1A1 and COL2A1 genes and myopia susceptibility: evidence of association and suggestive linkage to the COL2A1 locus. Invest Ophthalmol Vis Sci. 2009;50:4080–6.
18. Tedja MS, et al. Genome-wide association meta-analysis highlights light-induced signaling as a driver for refractive error. Nat Genet. 2018;50:834–48.
19. Fan Q, et al. Meta-analysis of gene-environment-wide association scans accounting for education level identifies additional loci for refractive error. Nat Commun. 2016;7:11008.
20. Flitcroft DI, et al. Novel myopia genes and pathways identified from syndromic forms of myopia. Invest Ophthalmol Vis Sci. 2018;59:338–48.
21. Dawn Teare M, Barrett JH. Genetic linkage studies. Lancet. 2005;366:1036–44.
22. Wojciechowski R. Nature and nurture: the complex genetics of myopia and refractive error. Clin Genet. 2011;79:301–20.
23. Baird PN, Schäche M, Dirani M. The GEnes in Myopia (GEM) study in understanding the aetiology of refractive errors. Prog Retin Eye Res. 2010;29:520–42.
24. Hornbeak DM, Young TL. Myopia genetics: a review of current research and emerging trends. Curr Opin Ophthalmol. 2009;20:356–62.
25. Jacobi FK, Pusch CM. A decade in search of myopia genes. Front Biosci. 2010;15:359–72.
26. Zhang Q, et al. A new locus for autosomal dominant high myopia maps to 4q22-q27 between D4S1578 and D4S1612. Mol Vis. 2005;11:554–60.
27. Young TL, et al. A second locus for familial high myopia maps to chromosome 12q. Am J Hum Genet. 1998;63:1419–24.
28. Naiglin L, et al. A genome wide scan for familial high myopia suggests a novel locus on chromosome 7q36. J Med Genet. 2002;39:118–24.
29. Paluru P, et al. New locus for autosomal dominant high myopia maps to the long arm of chromosome 17. Invest Ophthalmol Vis Sci. 2003;44:1830–6.
30. Nallasamy S, et al. Genetic linkage study of high-grade myopia in a Hutterite population from South Dakota. Mol Vis. 2007;13:229–36.
31. Lam CY, et al. A genome-wide scan maps a novel high myopia locus to 5p15. Invest Ophthalmol Vis Sci. 2008;49:3768–78.
32. Stambolian D. Genetic susceptibility and mechanisms for refractive error. Clin Genet. 2013;84:102–8.
33. Stambolian D, et al. Genomewide linkage scan for myopia susceptibility loci among Ashkenazi Jewish families shows evidence of linkage on chromosome 22q12. Am J Hum Genet. 2004;75:448–59.
34. Wojciechowski R, et al. Genomewide scan in Ashkenazi Jewish families demonstrates evidence of linkage of ocular refraction to a QTL on chromosome 1p36. Hum Genet. 2006;119:389–99.
35. Wojciechowski R, et al. Genomewide linkage scans for ocular refraction and meta-analysis of four populations in the Myopia Family Study. Invest Ophthalmol Vis Sci. 2009;50:2024–32.
36. Hammond CJ, Andrew T, Mak YT, Spector TD. A susceptibility locus for myopia in the normal population is linked to the PAX6 gene region on chromosome 11: a genomewide scan of dizygotic twins. Am J Hum Genet. 2004;75:294–304.
37. Ciner E, et al. Genome-wide scan of African-American and white families for linkage to myopia. Am J Ophthalmol. 2009;147:512–517.e2.

38. Hawthorne FA, Young TL. Genetic contributions to myopic refractive error: insights from human studies and supporting evidence from animal models. Exp Eye Res. 2013;114:141–9.
39. Tkatchenko AV, Tkatchenko TV, Guggenheim JA, Verhoeven VJM, Hysi PG, Wojciechowski R, et al. APLP2 regulates refractive error and myopia development in mice and humans. PLoS Genet. 2015;11:e1005432.
40. Liu H-P, Lin Y-J, Lin W-Y, Wan L, Sheu JJ-C, Lin H-J, et al. A novel genetic variant of BMP2K contributes to high myopia. J Clin Lab Anal. 2009;23:362–7.
41. Lin H-J, Kung Y-J, Lin Y-J, Sheu JJC, Chen B-H, Lan Y-C, et al. Association of the lumican gene functional 3'-UTR polymorphism with high myopia. Invest Ophthalmol Vis Sci. 2010;51:96–102.
42. Lin H-J, Wan L, Tsai Y, Chen W-C, Tsai S-W, Tsai F-J. The association between lumican gene polymorphisms and high myopia. Eye. 2010;24:1093–101.
43. Lin H-J, Wan L, Tsai Y, Chen W-C, Tsai S-W, Tsai F-J. Muscarinic acetylcholine receptor 1 gene polymorphisms associated with high myopia. Mol Vis. 2009;15:1774–80.
44. Lin H-J, Wan L, Tsai Y, Liu S-C, Chen W-C, Tsai S-W, et al. Sclera-related gene polymorphisms in high myopia. Mol Vis. 2009;15:1655–63.
45. Khor CC, Grignani R, Ng DPK, Toh KY, Chia K-S, Tan D, et al. cMET and refractive error progression in children. Ophthalmology. 2009;116:1469–74. 1474.e1
46. Inamori Y, Ota M, Inoko H, Okada E, Nishizaki R, Shiota T, et al. The COL1A1 gene and high myopia susceptibility in Japanese. Hum Genet. 2007;122:151–7.
47. Metlapally R, Li Y-J, Tran-Viet K-N, Abbott D, Czaja GR, Malecaze F, et al. COL1A1 and COL2A1 genes and myopia susceptibility: evidence of association and suggestive linkage to the COL2A1 locus. Invest Ophthalmol Vis Sci. 2009;50:4080–6.
48. Mutti DO, Cooper ME, O'Brien S, Jones LA, Marazita ML, Murray JC, et al. Candidate gene and locus analysis of myopia. Mol Vis. 2007;13:1012–9.
49. Ho DWH, Yap MKH, Ng PW, Fung WY, Yip SP. Association of high myopia with crystallin beta A4 (CRYBA4) gene polymorphisms in the linkage-identified MYP6 locus. PLoS One. 2012;7:e40238.
50. Han W, Yap MKH, Wang J, Yip SP. Family-based association analysis of hepatocyte growth factor (HGF) gene polymorphisms in high myopia. Invest Ophthalmol Vis Sci. 2006;47:2291–9.
51. Veerappan S, Pertile KK, Islam AFM, Schäche M, Chen CY, Mitchell P, et al. Role of the hepatocyte growth factor gene in refractive error. Ophthalmology. 2010;117:239–45.e1–2.
52. Yanovitch T, Li Y-J, Metlapally R, Abbott D, Viet K-NT, Young TL. Hepatocyte growth factor and myopia: genetic association analyses in a Caucasian population. Mol Vis. 2009;15:1028–35.
53. Metlapally R, Ki C-S, Li Y-J, Tran-Viet K-N, Abbott D, Malecaze F, et al. Genetic association of insulin-like growth factor-1 polymorphisms with high-grade myopia in an international family cohort. Invest Ophthalmol Vis Sci. 2010;51:4476–9.
54. Zhao YY, Zhang FJ, Zhu SQ, Duan H, Li Y, Zhou ZJ, et al. The association of a single nucleotide polymorphism in the promoter region of the LAMA1 gene with susceptibility to Chinese high myopia. Mol Vis. 2011;17:1003–10.
55. Chen ZT-Y, Wang I-J, Shih Y-F, Lin LL-K. The association of haplotype at the lumican gene with high myopia susceptibility in Taiwanese patients. Ophthalmology. 2009;116:1920–7.
56. Wang I-J, Chiang T-H, Shih Y-F, Hsiao CK, Lu S-C, Hou Y-C, et al. The association of single nucleotide polymorphisms in the 5'-regulatory region of the lumican gene with susceptibility to high myopia in Taiwan. Mol Vis. 2006;12:852–7.
57. Andrew T, Maniatis N, Carbonaro F, Liew SHM, Lau W, Spector TD, et al. Identification and replication of three novel myopia common susceptibility gene loci on chromosome 3q26 using linkage and linkage disequilibrium mapping. PLoS Genet. 2008;4:e1000220.
58. Wojciechowski R, Bailey-Wilson JE, Stambolian D. Association of matrix metalloproteinase gene polymorphisms with refractive error in Amish and Ashkenazi families. Invest Ophthalmol Vis Sci. 2010;51:4989–95.
59. Wojciechowski R, Yee SS, Simpson CL, Bailey-Wilson JE, Stambolian D. Matrix metalloproteinases and educational attainment in refractive error: evidence of gene-environment interactions in the Age-Related Eye Disease Study. Ophthalmology. 2013;120:298–305.
60. Hall NF, Gale CR, Ye S, Martyn CN. Myopia and polymorphisms in genes for matrix metalloproteinases. Invest Ophthalmol Vis Sci. 2009;50:2632–6.

61. Tang WC, Yip SP, Lo KK, Ng PW, Choi PS, Lee SY, et al. Linkage and association of myocilin (MYOC) polymorphisms with high myopia in a Chinese population. Mol Vis. 2007;13:534–44.
62. Vatavuk Z, Skunca Herman J, Bencić G, Andrijević Derk B, Lacmanović Loncar V, Petric Vicković I, et al. Common variant in myocilin gene is associated with high myopia in isolated population of Korcula Island, Croatia. Croat Med J. 2009;50:17–22.
63. Zayats T, Yanovitch T, Creer RC, McMahon G, Li Y-J, Young TL, et al. Myocilin polymorphisms and high myopia in subjects of European origin. Mol Vis. 2009;15:213–22.
64. Han W, Leung KH, Fung WY, Mak JYY, Li YM, Yap MKH, et al. Association of PAX6 polymorphisms with high myopia in Han Chinese nuclear families. Invest Ophthalmol Vis Sci. 2009;50:47–56.
65. Kanemaki N, Meguro A, Yamane T, Takeuchi M, Okada E, Iijima Y, et al. Study of association of PAX6 polymorphisms with susceptibility to high myopia in a Japanese population. Clin Ophthalmol. 2015;9:2005–11.
66. Miyake M, Yamashiro K, Nakanishi H, Nakata I, Akagi-Kurashige Y, Tsujikawa A, et al. Association of paired box 6 with high myopia in Japanese. Mol Vis. 2012;18:2726–35.
67. Ng TK, Lam CY, Lam DSC, Chiang SWY, Tam POS, Wang DY, et al. AC and AG dinucleotide repeats in the PAX6 P1 promoter are associated with high myopia. Mol Vis. 2009;15:2239–48.
68. Tsai Y-Y, Chiang C-C, Lin H-J, Lin J-M, Wan L, Tsai F-J. A PAX6 gene polymorphism is associated with genetic predisposition to extreme myopia. Eye. 2008;22:576–81.
69. Khor CC, Fan Q, Goh L, Tan D, Young TL, Li Y-J, et al. Support for TGFB1 as a susceptibility gene for high myopia in individuals of Chinese descent. Arch Ophthalmol. 2010;128:1081–4.
70. Lin H-J, Wan L, Tsai Y, Tsai Y-Y, Fan S-S, Tsai C-H, et al. The TGFbeta1 gene codon 10 polymorphism contributes to the genetic predisposition to high myopia. Mol Vis. 2006;12:698–703.
71. Rasool S, Ahmed I, Dar R, Ayub SG, Rashid S, Jan T, et al. Contribution of TGFβ1 codon 10 polymorphism to high myopia in an ethnic Kashmiri population from India. Biochem Genet. 2013;51:323–33.
72. Zha Y, Leung KH, Lo KK, Fung WY, Ng PW, Shi M-G, et al. TGFB1 as a susceptibility gene for high myopia: a replication study with new findings. Arch Ophthalmol. 2009;127:541–8.
73. Lam DSC, Lee WS, Leung YF, Tam POS, Fan DSP, Fan BJ, et al. TGFbeta-induced factor: a candidate gene for high myopia. Invest Ophthalmol Vis Sci. 2003;44:1012–5.
74. Ahmed I, Rasool S, Jan T, Qureshi T, Naykoo NA, Andrabi KI. TGIF1 is a potential candidate gene for high myopia in ethnic Kashmiri population. Curr Eye Res. 2014;39:282–90.
75. Nishizaki R, Ota M, Inoko H, Meguro A, Shiota T, Okada E, et al. New susceptibility locus for high myopia is linked to the uromodulin-like 1 (UMODL1) gene region on chromosome 21q22.3. Eye. 2009;23:222–9.
76. Tang SM, et al. PAX6 gene associated with high myopia: a meta-analysis. Optom Vis Sci. 2014;91:419–29.
77. Li M, et al. Lack of association between LUM rs3759223 polymorphism and high myopia. Optom Vis Sci. 2014;91:707–12.
78. Zhang D, et al. Association of IGF1 polymorphism rs6214 with high myopia: a systematic review and meta-analysis. Ophthalmic Genet. 2017;38:434–9.
79. Springelkamp H, et al. New insights into the genetics of primary open-angle glaucoma based on meta-analyses of intraocular pressure and optic disc characteristics. Hum Mol Genet. 2017;26:438–53.
80. Burdon KP, et al. Association of polymorphisms in the hepatocyte growth factor gene promoter with keratoconus. Invest Ophthalmol Vis Sci. 2011;52:8514–9.
81. Risch N, Merikangas K. The future of genetic studies of complex human diseases. Science. 1996;273:1516–7.
82. Ku CS, Loy EY, Pawitan Y, Chia KS. The pursuit of genome-wide association studies: where are we now? J Hum Genet. 2010;55:195–206.
83. Cordell HJ, Clayton DG. Genetic association studies. Lancet. 2005;366:1121–31.
84. Nakanishi H, et al. A genome-wide association analysis identified a novel susceptible locus for pathological myopia at 11q24.1. PLoS Genet. 2009;5:e1000660.
85. Li Y-J, et al. Genome-wide association studies reveal genetic variants in CTNND2 for high myopia in Singapore Chinese. Ophthalmology. 2011;118:368–75.

86. Lu B, et al. Replication study supports CTNND2 as a susceptibility gene for high myopia. Invest Ophthalmol Vis Sci. 2011;52:8258–61.
87. Wang Q, et al. Replication study of significant single nucleotide polymorphisms associated with myopia from two genome-wide association studies. Mol Vis. 2011;17:3290–9.
88. Yu Z, et al. Polymorphisms in theCTNND2Gene and 11q24.1 genomic region are associated with pathological myopia in a Chinese population. Ophthalmologica. 2012;228:123–9.
89. Liu J, Zhang H-X. Polymorphism in the 11q24.1 genomic region is associated with myopia: a comprehensive genetic study in Chinese and Japanese populations. Mol Vis. 2014;20:352–8.
90. Shi Y, et al. Genetic variants at 13q12.12 are associated with high myopia in the Han Chinese population. Am J Hum Genet. 2011;88:805–13.
91. Shi Y, et al. A genome-wide meta-analysis identifies two novel loci associated with high myopia in the Han Chinese population. Hum Mol Genet. 2013;22:2325–33.
92. Khor CC, et al. Genome-wide association study identifies ZFHX1B as a susceptibility locus for severe myopia. Hum Mol Genet. 2013;22:5288–94.
93. Hosoda Y, et al. CCDC102B confers risk of low vision and blindness in high myopia. Nat Commun. 2018;9:1782.
94. Meng W, et al. A genome-wide association study provides evidence for association of chromosome 8p23 (MYP10) and 10q21.1 (MYP15) with high myopia in the French population. Invest Ophthalmol Vis Sci. 2012;53:7983–8.
95. Pickrell JK, et al. Detection and interpretation of shared genetic influences on 42 human traits. Nat Genet. 2016;48:709–17.
96. Solouki AM, et al. A genome-wide association study identifies a susceptibility locus for refractive errors and myopia at 15q14. Nat Genet. 2010;42:897–901.
97. Hysi PG, et al. A genome-wide association study for myopia and refractive error identifies a susceptibility locus at 15q25. Nat Genet. 2010;42:902–5.
98. Stambolian D, et al. Meta-analysis of genome-wide association studies in five cohorts reveals common variants in RBFOX1, a regulator of tissue-specific splicing, associated with refractive error. Hum Mol Genet. 2013;22:2754–64.
99. Verhoeven VJM, et al. Large scale international replication and meta-analysis study confirms association of the 15q14 locus with myopia. The CREAM consortium. Hum Genet. 2012;131:1467–80.
100. Schache M, et al. Genetic association of refractive error and axial length with 15q14 but Not 15q25 in the Blue Mountains Eye Study cohort. Ophthalmology. 2013;120:292–7.
101. Simpson CL, et al. Regional replication of association with refractive error on 15q14 and 15q25 in the Age-Related Eye Disease Study cohort. Mol Vis. 2013;19:2173–86.
102. Simpson CL, Wojciechowski R, Oexle K, Murgia F, Portas L, Li X, et al. Genome-wide meta-analysis of myopia and hyperopia provides evidence for replication of 11 loci. PLoS One. 2014;9:e107110.
103. Yoshikawa M, Yamashiro K, Miyake M, Oishi M, Akagi-Kurashige Y, Kumagai K, et al. Comprehensive replication of the relationship between myopia-related genes and refractive errors in a large Japanese cohort. Invest Ophthalmol Vis Sci. 2014;55:7343–54.
104. Cheng C-Y, Schache M, Ikram MK, Young TL, Guggenheim JA, Vitart V, et al. Nine loci for ocular axial length identified through genome-wide association studies, including shared loci with refractive error. Am J Hum Genet. 2013;93:264–77.
105. Oishi M, Yamashiro K, Miyake M, Akagi-Kurashige Y, Kumagai K, Nakata I, et al. Association between ZIC2, RASGRF1, and SHISA6 genes and high myopia in Japanese subjects. Invest Ophthalmol Vis Sci. 2013;54:7492–7.
106. Tideman JWL, Fan Q, Polling JR, Guo X, Yazar S, Khawaja A, et al. When do myopia genes have their effect? Comparison of genetic risks between children and adults. Genet Epidemiol. 2016;40:756–66.
107. Liao X, Yap MKH, Leung KH, Kao PYP, Liu LQ, Yip SP. Genetic association study of KCNQ5 polymorphisms with high myopia. Biomed Res Int. 2017;2017:3024156.
108. Verhoeven VJM, et al. Genome-wide meta-analyses of multiancestry cohorts identify multiple new susceptibility loci for refractive error and myopia. Nat Genet. 2013;45:314–8.
109. Wojciechowski R, Hysi PG. Focusing in on the complex genetics of myopia. PLoS Genet. 2013;9:e1003442.
110. Kiefer AK, et al. Genome-wide analysis points to roles for extracellular matrix remodeling, the visual cycle, and neuronal development in myopia. PLoS Genet. 2013;9:e1003299.

111. Mishra A, et al. Genetic variants near PDGFRA are associated with corneal curvature in Australians. Invest Ophthalmol Vis Sci. 2012;53:7131–6.
112. Guggenheim JA, et al. A genome-wide association study for corneal curvature identifies the platelet-derived growth factor receptor α gene as a quantitative trait locus for eye size in white Europeans. Mol Vis. 2013;19:243–53.
113. Han S, et al. Association of variants in FRAP1 and PDGFRA with corneal curvature in Asian populations from Singapore. Hum Mol Genet. 2011;20:3693–8.
114. Chen P, et al. CMPK1 and RBP3 are associated with corneal curvature in Asian populations. Hum Mol Genet. 2014;23:6129–36.
115. Miyake M, et al. Identification of myopia-associated WNT7B polymorphisms provides insights into the mechanism underlying the development of myopia. Nat Commun. 2015;6:6689.
116. Hysi PG, et al. Common mechanisms underlying refractive error identified in functional analysis of gene lists from genome-wide association study results in 2 European British cohorts. JAMA Ophthalmol. 2014;132:50–6.
117. Chandra A, Mitry D, Wright A, Campbell H, Charteris DG. Genome-wide association studies: applications and insights gained in ophthalmology. Eye. 2014;28:1066–79.
118. Hysi PG, Wojciechowski R, Rahi JS, Hammond CJ. Genome-wide association studies of refractive error and myopia, lessons learned, and implications for the future. Invest Ophthalmol Vis Sci. 2014;55:3344–51.
119. Napolitano F, et al. Autosomal-dominant myopia associated to a novel P4HA2 missense variant and defective collagen hydroxylation. Clin Genet. 2018;93:982–91.
120. Zhao F, et al. Exome sequencing reveals CCDC111 mutation associated with high myopia. Hum Genet. 2013;132:913–21.
121. Wang B, et al. A novel potentially causative variant of NDUFAF7 revealed by mutation screening in a Chinese family with pathologic myopia. Invest Ophthalmol Vis Sci. 2017;58:4182–92.
122. Feng L, et al. Exome sequencing identifies a novel UNC5D mutation in a severe myopic anisometropia family: a case report. Medicine. 2017;96:e7138.
123. Jiang D, et al. Detection of mutations in LRPAP1, CTSH, LEPREL1, ZNF644, SLC39A5, and SCO2 in 298 families with early-onset high myopia by exome sequencing. Invest Ophthalmol Vis Sci. 2014;56:339–45.
124. Tran-Viet K-N, et al. Mutations in SCO2 are associated with autosomal-dominant high-grade myopia. Am J Hum Genet. 2013;92:820–6.
125. Jin ZB, et al. Trio-based exome sequencing arrests de novo mutations in early-onset high myopia. Proc Natl Acad Sci U S A. 2017;114:4219–24.
126. Xiao X, Li S, Jia X, Guo X, Zhang Q. X-linked heterozygous mutations in cause female-limited early onset high myopia. Mol Vis. 2016;22:1257–66.
127. Li J, et al. Exome sequencing identified null mutations in LOXL3 associated with early-onset high myopia. Mol Vis. 2016;22:161–7.
128. Guo H, et al. SLC39A5 mutations interfering with the BMP/TGF-β1 pathway in non-syndromic high myopia. J Med Genet. 2014;51:518–25.
129. Aldahmesh MA, et al. Mutations in LRPAP1 are associated with severe myopia in humans. Am J Hum Genet. 2013;93:313–20.
130. Shi Y, et al. Exome sequencing identifies ZNF644 mutations in high myopia. PLoS Genet. 2011;7:e1002084.
131. Kloss BA, et al. Exome sequence analysis of 14 families with high myopia. Invest Ophthalmol Vis Sci. 2017;58:1982–90.
132. Sun W, et al. Exome sequencing on 298 probands with early-onset high myopia: approximately one-fourth show potential pathogenic mutations in RetNet genes. Invest Ophthalmol Vis Sci. 2015;56:8365–72.
133. Morgan I, Rose K. How genetic is school myopia? Prog Retin Eye Res. 2005;24:1–38.
134. Morgan IG, Ohno-Matsui K, Saw S-M. Myopia. Lancet. 2012;379:1739–48.
135. Dolgin E. The myopia boom. Nature. 2015;519:276–8.
136. Williams KM, et al. Increasing prevalence of myopia in europe and the impact of education. Ophthalmology. 2015;122:1489–97.
137. Dirani M, Shekar SN, Baird PN. The role of educational attainment in refraction: the Genes in Myopia (GEM) twin study. Invest Ophthalmol Vis Sci. 2008;49:534–8.
138. Foster PJ, Jiang Y. Epidemiology of myopia. Eye. 2014;28:202–8.

139. Pan C-W, Ramamurthy D, Saw S-M. Worldwide prevalence and risk factors for myopia. Ophthalmic Physiol Opt. 2012;32:3–16.
140. Mirshahi A, et al. Myopia and level of education: results from the Gutenberg Health Study. Ophthalmology. 2014;121:2047–52.
141. Morgan IG, Rose KA. Myopia and international educational performance. Ophthalmic Physiol Opt. 2013;33:329–38.
142. Ramessur R, Williams KM, Hammond CJ. Risk factors for myopia in a discordant monozygotic twin study. Ophthalmic Physiol Opt. 2015;35:643–51.
143. Fan Q, et al. Education influences the association between genetic variants and refractive error: a meta-analysis of five Singapore studies. Hum Mol Genet. 2014;23:546–54.
144. Verhoeven VJM, et al. Education influences the role of genetics in myopia. Eur J Epidemiol. 2013;28:973–80.
145. Fan Q, et al. Childhood gene-environment interactions and age-dependent effects of genetic variants associated with refractive error and myopia: The CREAM Consortium. Sci Rep. 2016;6:25853.
146. Ebrahim S, Davey Smith G. Mendelian randomization: can genetic epidemiology help redress the failures of observational epidemiology? Hum Genet. 2008;123:15–33.
147. Smith GD, Ebrahim S. Mendelian randomization: prospects, potentials, and limitations. Int J Epidemiol. 2004;33:30–42.
148. Mountjoy E, et al. Education and myopia: assessing the direction of causality by mendelian randomisation. BMJ. 2018;362:k2932.
149. Cuellar-Partida G, et al. Assessing the genetic predisposition of education on myopia: A Mendelian Randomization Study. Genet Epidemiol. 2016;40:66–72.
150. Cuellar-Partida G, et al. Genetically low vitamin D concentrations and myopic refractive error: a Mendelian randomization study. Int J Epidemiol. 2017;46:1882–90.
151. Teperino R, Lempradl A, Pospisilik JA. Bridging epigenomics and complex disease: the basics. Cell Mol Life Sci. 2013;70:1609–21.
152. Jiang B, Huo Y, Gu Y, Wang J. The role of microRNAs in myopia. Graefes Arch Clin Exp Ophthalmol. 2017;255:7–13.
153. Liang CL, et al. A functional polymorphism at 3'UTR of the PAX6 gene may confer risk for extreme myopia in the Chinese. Invest Ophthalmol Vis Sci. 2011;52:3500–5.
154. Lechner J, et al. Mutational analysis of MIR184 in sporadic keratoconus and myopia. Invest Ophthalmol Vis Sci. 2013;54:5266–72.
155. Xie M, et al. Genetic variants in MiR-29a associated with high myopia. Ophthalmic Genet. 2016;37:456–8.
156. Tideman JWL, et al. Environmental factors explain socioeconomic prevalence differences in myopia in 6-year-old children. Br J Ophthalmol. 2018;102:243–7.
157. Ghorbani Mojarrad N, Williams C, Guggenheim JA. A genetic risk score and number of myopic parents independently predict myopia. Ophthalmic Physiol Opt. 2018;38(5):492–502. https://doi.org/10.1111/opo.12579.
158. Sudlow C, et al. UK biobank: an open access resource for identifying the causes of a wide range of complex diseases of middle and old age. PLoS Med. 2015;12:e1001779.

Risk Factors for Myopia: Putting Causal Pathways into a Social Context

6

Ian G. Morgan, Amanda N. French, and Kathryn A. Rose

Key Points

- Myopia commencing school myopia is found mainly is found mainly in developed societies, with only around 1% of any population affected by predominantly genetic forms of myopia.
- Exposure to environmental risk factors plays a significant role in the development of "school myopia" myopia, both within and between populations.
- Within populations, changes in exposure to environmental risk factors are primarily responsible for the emergence of an increasing prevalence of myopia.
- The major environmental risk factors identified are educational pressures, perhaps best characterized in terms of near work, and limited time outdoors during daylight hours.
- These risk factors suggest that strategies based on decreases in the amount of near work and increases in the amount of time spent outdoors during school hours are likely to be useful in the controlling the epidemic of myopia.

I. G. Morgan (✉)
Research School of Biological Science, Australian National University,
Canberra, ACT, Australia
e-mail: ian.morgan@anu.edu.au

A. N. French · K. A. Rose
Discipline of Orthoptics, Graduate School of Health, University of Technology Sydney,
Ultimo, NSW, Australia

M. Ang, T. Y. Wong (eds.), *Updates on Myopia*,
https://doi.org/10.1007/978-981-13-8491-2_6

It is now generally accepted that there is an environmental epidemic of myopia in several parts of East and Southeast Asia, namely Singapore, Japan, South Korea, China, including Hong Kong and Macau, as well as in Taiwan [1–8]. In these parts of the world, the prevalence of myopia in young adults who have completed 12 years of schooling, as most do, is now 70–90%, up from 20 to 30% two or three generations ago. In addition, the prevalence of high and potentially pathological myopia (more than 5 D or 6 D of myopia) is of the order of 10–20% [9–12]. The simple argument that the speed at which the prevalence of myopia has increased in these locations is not compatible with a predominant role for genetic determination of myopia [1, 2] has generally been accepted, even though genetic variation associated with myopia has been conclusively demonstrated [13]. This emphasizes the need to define the environmental exposures responsible for the rapid increases in prevalence, in order to design preventive interventions.

The term "an epidemic of myopia" covers two distinct, but related, issues. The first is an increase in the prevalence of myopia overall, with a characteristic increase in onset of myopia in children in the early school years, leading to a need to provide optical correction for a significant proportion of the population from an early age. The high prevalence of myopia observed in young adults will gradually become the norm for the entire adult population, as younger more myopic generations replace those who are older and less myopic.

The second issue is an increase in the prevalence of high myopia, which is associated with a higher prevalence of pathological outcomes. The cutoff values used to define high myopia are somewhat arbitrary (generally −5 D or −6 D), since the prevalence of pathological complications rises steeply with severity of myopia. The best cutoff to define high and potentially pathological myopia is one which distinguishes, as effectively as possible, between lower and higher risks of pathology, but no cutoff will do this perfectly [14]. The increase in more severe levels of myopia seems to arise from the fact that myopia has appeared at increasingly early ages as the epidemic has developed [11]. With subsequent progression, the myopic refractive error will increase toward the cutoff for high myopia, a tendency exacerbated by rapid progression in younger children [15]. In these circumstances, slowing the onset of myopia should lead to a disproportionate reduction in high myopia. An important question in this area is whether the risk factors for increased prevalence of myopia are similar to the risk factors for progression, or in practical terms whether increased time outdoors would help to limit progression directly, as well as by delaying the onset of myopia. It is certainly possible to slow the development of high myopia by clinically slowing progression rates, using optical or pharmaceutical interventions, and many of these interventions are now available [16].

This chapter reviews the scientific evidence on risk factors in all these areas, and relates this evidence to strategies for slowing the onset and progression of myopia. We will also mention a number of commonly believed risk factors for myopia that may not have a substantial scientific basis. Myopia is such a common condition in societies with well-developed education systems that there are many popular beliefs about the causes of myopia. These often remain influential, sometimes even when the scientific evidence is against them.

6.1 Key Issues When Studying Risk Factors for Myopia

In assessing the literature on risk factors for myopia, it is essential to be clear about a number of fundamental issues.

6.1.1 Myopia Is Etiologically Heterogeneous

It is now generally accepted that environmental factors have a major role to play in the development of myopia. Nevertheless, there are 100–200 clearly genetic forms of myopia documented in the Online Mendelian Inheritance in Man (OMIM) database (https://www.omim.org/, accessed Jan 30, 2019) that clearly run in families [17]. These are individually quite rare, but account collectively for myopia in around 1% of any population. In a recent detailed analysis, 119 genes were associated specifically with myopia, generally in association with other clinical features [17]. Most of these forms are therefore called syndromic, although in some, myopia seems to be the major clinical feature. The latter cases are often called nonsyndromic [18]. Environmental factors appear to play a rather limited role in these diseases, but their existence does not mean that all forms of myopia are similarly genetic—This issue is further discussed in Chapter 5 etc.

In addition to these genetic forms, in modern societies, myopia generally appears in association with schooling, as "school myopia." It is this form that has increased in the epidemics of myopia. Genetic variation has some role to play in this form of myopia, with the most recent genetic data identifying variants in over 160 genes associated with spherical equivalent refraction (SER). Many of these variants are associated with the genes involved in the more clearly genetic forms, suggesting that mutations in coding regions of the same genes can lead to highly genetic forms of myopia, or to more modest effects if the mutations affect regulatory regions [17].

Identified single nucleotide polymorphisms (SNPs) in samples of European ancestry account for less than 10% of the variance in refraction [13]. Measured as SNP-heritability, they may account for 20–35% of the phenotypic variance [19]. These values fall well short of the twin study heritability of 80–90% [20–22]—an example of the missing heritability seen with many complex traits [23]. The estimated SNP-heritability in East Asian samples is much lower at around 5% [13], as would be expected if the amount of phenotypic variation due to genetic variation had remained constant, but that induced by environmental factors had increased substantially in populations severely affected by the environmentally induced epidemic of myopia. We have recently reviewed this area, and readers can consult these reviews for more details [2, 24].

Given this picture, genetic variation may have little, if any, role to play in the rapid changes that have produced the current epidemic of myopia, but this does not mean that it has no role to play in the determination of variations in refractive error within a population. In fact, some myopia geneticists have argued that environmental factors are important between populations, but within populations, genetic factors are the primary determinants [5, 6, 8]. However, this argument does

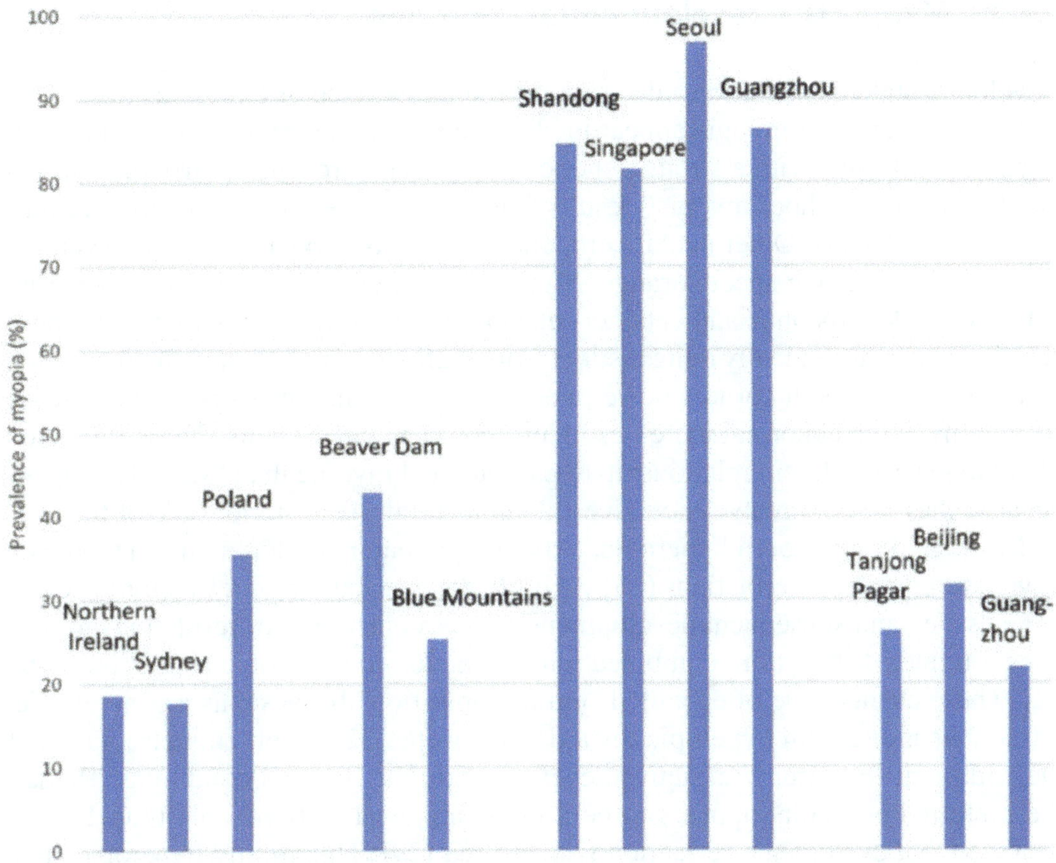

Fig. 6.1 Prevalence of myopia in older and more recent cohorts in older and more recent younger cohorts. Data taken from cohorts closest in age to 20 from Breslin et al. [66], French et al. [96], Czepita et al. [71] Wang et al. [58], Attebo et al. [59], Wu et al. [12], Koh et al. [10], Jung et al. [9], Wong et al. [60]. Xu et al. [198], and He et al. [140]

not make sense, because between-population differences have largely emerged due to selective changes within populations of the kind seen in East and Southeast Asia (Fig. 6.1). The key to understanding lies in the recognition that the balance between genetic and environmental factors is population-specific. In the case of myopia, the evidence suggests that there is little difference between ethnic groups in the levels of SNPs associated with myopia [13], although studies on a wider range of ethnic groups are required. However, environmental exposures can differ substantially between ethnic groups, and can change rapidly. Environmental factors are therefore far more likely to be involved in rapid intergenerational change, or in the rapid emergence of differences between societies—both features of the current epidemic.

This has an important implication; key insights into the epidemics are most likely to come from comparisons of societies with different prevalence of myopia, rather than from detailed studies within populations. Many epidemiologists are wary of this ecological approach, because of what is known as the "ecological fallacy"—the error that can be made if conclusions are based only upon ecological comparisons. But in the case of myopia, this is not an issue, because education and time outdoors clearly play a role both within and between populations.

6.1.2 Myopia Is a Developmental Condition

Developmental considerations also support the importance of etiological heterogeneity. Some forms of myopia appear in children before they start school. These are often severe forms, with a strong genetic etiology, and are called early onset myopia. In contrast, "school myopia" results from excessive elongation of the eye during the school years. Other ocular components, such as corneal and lens power, are within the normal age-specific range. Myopic refractions are also seen in two other conditions—keratoconus and cataract-related myopic shifts in older people. These conditions are etiologically quite distinct from "school myopia"—the first involving abnormal increases in corneal power, generally during the teen-age years, and the second involving abnormal increases in lens power in older adults. These forms are likely to have a different relationship to pathological myopia than "school myopia," because they do not involve excessive enlargement of the posterior pole of the eye.

Most children are born hyperopic, although premature children have a tendency toward more myopic refractions [25]. At birth, the distribution of refractions is close to Gaussian, and subsequent development involves clustering of refractions to produce a tighter distribution, combined with reduction in hyperopic refractions [26–28]. These changes are often called "emmetropisation" because, as a general rule, refractions move from hyperopic toward emmetropic. However, emmetropia is not the end point for human refractive development under normal conditions. Rather, the preferred end point appears to be a moderate level of hyperopia (1.0–1.3 D), provided that cycloplegic refraction is measured [29]. This mildly hyperopic state can be maintained even in adults in some environments [30]. However, in populations where the prevalence of myopia becomes high, the hyperopic clustering of refractions disappears.

This part of refractive development is consistent with animal studies on experimental myopia that suggest that hyperopic defocus induces faster axial elongation, thus reducing hyperopic refractive error, while myopic defocus can slow axial elongation, and thus might be expected to affect the progression of myopia [31]. Simple expectations from the animal models, namely that myopia would be a self-limiting condition, or that it would be dangerous to correct myopia since it would reduce the error signal, are not consistent with current evidence [32–34]. However, there is some evidence that early myopic errors can be cleared [35], and contact lenses designed to impose myopic appear to slow the progression of myopia [36]. Thus, these mechanisms can come into play in particular circumstances, but what these circumstances are is currently unclear.

6.1.3 Cycloplegia and Definitions of Myopia: Important Methodological Issues

It is now generally accepted that cycloplegia is the gold standard for studies with children, with the use of up to three drops of 1% cyclopentolate as a common practice, with monitoring of pupil diameter and the light reflex to assess adequacy of cycloplegia [37]. This issue is particularly important in young children, where the prevalence of myopia is low, and a small amount of pseudomyopia can significantly increase prevalence estimates. It is also important when comparing ethnic groups, because it is harder to achieve cycloplegia in children with darkly pigmented irises. Without cycloplegia, hyperopia is substantially underestimated, emmetropia may be overestimated, with a smaller but significant overestimation of the prevalence of myopia. Suboptimal cycloplegia is likely to lead to errors of lesser magnitude, but in the same direction.

In contrast to studies on children, cycloplegia has generally not been used in studies on adults. Adults over the age of 50 show minimal differences between cycloplegic and noncycloplegic refractions [37, 38], consistent with the evidence that by this age, accommodative capacity has essentially disappeared, resulting in the need for some form of correction for reading. However, in younger adults, cycloplegia is required for accurate refraction, yet it generally has not been used in the larger studies on adults, even if they included young adults.

This emphasis on cycloplegia poses problems, because gaining informed consent for cycloplegia appears to be becoming more difficult. It is worth considering alternatives, and biometric variables like axial length and the ratio of the axial length to corneal radius of curvature (AL/CR ratio) could be used [39–41]. Both correlate highly with myopia [42, 43]. Changes in lens power also play a major role in refractive development, but they do not correlate highly with refraction and cannot be measured directly [44]. The advantage of the first two parameters is that they can be measured noninvasively. Their disadvantage is that measurement requires relatively expensive modern equipment, and that there is only a very limited set of data for comparison. But where repeated measures of cycloplegic refraction are envisaged, the highly correlated biometric variables may provide a useful alternative.

It is also important to note that a range of definitions is used in the literature for both myopia and high myopia. Cutoff values for myopia range from −0.25 D to −1.0 D, with some variation in the use of less than, or less than or equal to. Results are sometimes reported in relation to the better eye, worse eye, either eye, or both eyes, depending, to some extent, on the aims of the study. The most common standard for epidemiology is at least −0.5 D in the right eye. Similarly, the prevalence of high myopia is sometimes reported in relation to a cutoff of −5 D or −6 D. Sometimes more stringent cutoffs (−8 D, −10 D or −12 D) are used, which is likely to concentrate more genetic forms of myopia in the sample. Cumberland et al. [45] have therefore called for the development of an approach that "serves research, policy and practice," but made no specific recommendations. However, standard definitions will be of little use without standardization of cycloplegia. While awaiting agreement in both these areas, if it ever comes, we suggest a pragmatic approach is to publish a distribution of refraction in all studies in sufficient detail that others can apply the cutoff they think is most relevant. Cumberland et al. [45] also emphasized the sensitivity of risk factor analysis to different definitions of myopia, and where appropriate, sensitivity analysis should be used to establish that conclusions are robust [46].

These issues are very relevant to several major studies on risk factors for myopia. Studies on childhood and adolescence, the period during which myopia develops, and on young adults, when myopia stabilizes, are particularly important, since exposures over this period can be most directly related to the development of myopia. In addition, studies on young adults give estimates of prevalence that can be most directly compared to assess whether and to what extent there is an epidemic of myopia. Table 6.1 lists some of the most important studies that used cycloplegia. In general, there is a dearth of systematic evidence on the prevalence of myopia in most populations, particularly in the critical period

Table 6.1 Major studies on childhood refraction that measured cycloplegic refraction

Detailed studies of risk factors for refractive errors in school-aged children using cycloplegic refraction	
Australia	
Study name	*Sydney Myopia Study (SMS) and Sydney Adolescent Vascular and Eye Disease Study (SAVES)*
Location	Sydney, Australia
Design	School based, with stratified randomized selection of schools. Large cohorts at baseline in Year 1 (1765, 6–7 year olds) and Year 7 (2353, 12–13 year olds), with 4–5 year follow-up
Methodology	Cycloplegic refraction (cyclopentolate plus tropicamide). Risk factor questionnaire, including near work and time outdoors
Europe	
Study name	*Northern Ireland Childhood Errors of Refraction (NICER)*
Location	Northern Ireland
Design	Stratified, random-cluster design with school-based assessment. Cohorts 6–7 years old (392) and 12–13 years old (661) at baseline, with 6 year follow-up
Methodology	Cycloplegic refraction (cyclopentolate). Risk factor questionnaire, not including near work and time outdoors
Study name	*Ireland Eye Study*
Location	Republic of Ireland
Design	School based with stratified randomized selection of schools. Cohorts of 6–7 year olds (681) and 12–13 year olds (745) at baseline
Methodology	Cycloplegic refraction (cyclopentolate). Lifestyle questionnaire
Study name	*Generation R Study*
Location	Rotterdam, The Netherlands
Design	Birth Cohort Study, with 4734 children examined at the age of 6 and 9
Methodology	Cycloplegic refraction (cyclopentolate) introduced for a large subsample at age 9. Risk factor questionnaire including near work and time outdoors
United States	
Study name	*Orinda Longitudinal Study of Myopia (OLSM)*
Location	Orinda, California
Design	Volunteer sample of 1246 children from the Orinda Union School District followed up longitudinally
Methodology	Cycloplegic refraction (tropicamide). Annual parent questionnaire on risk factors including education and time outdoors or on sports

(continued)

Table 6.1 (continued)

Study name	*Collaborative Longitudinal Evaluation of Ethnicity and Refractive Error (CLEERE)*
Location	Multi-Centre Study, with centers at Orinda (California), Eutaw (Alabama), Houston (Texas), Irvine (California), and Tucson (Arizona)
Design	Volunteer sample of 2583 with selective recruitment of children of different ethnicities from different centers, followed up longitudinally
Methodology	Cycloplegic refraction (tropicamide or cyclopentolate plus tropicamide). Risk factor questionnaire
Singapore	
Study name	*Singapore Cohort Study of the Risk Factors for Myopia (SCORM)*
Location	Singapore
Design	1979 children aged 7–9 recruited from three schools in Singapore, with longitudinal follow-up
Methodology	Cycloplegic refraction (cyclopentolate). Risk factor questionnaire, including near work and time outdoors
China	
Study name	*Anyang Childhood Eye Study*
Location	Anyang City, Hebei Province
Design	At baseline, cohorts recruited from Year 1 (2283) and Year 7 (1453), with longitudinal follow-up for 5 and 3 years respectively
Methodology	Cycloplegic refraction (cyclopentolate). Risk factor questionnaire including near work and time outdoors
Study name	*Guangzhou Twin Eye Study*
Location	Guangzhou City, Guangdong Province
Design	Population-based recruitment of over 1000 twin pairs aged from 7 to 15 at baseline from Guangzhou City, with annual longitudinal follow-up
Methodology	Cycloplegic refraction (cyclopentolate). Risk factor questionnaire including near work and time outdoors
Study name	*Mojiang Eye Study*
Location	Mojiang County, Yunnan Province
Design	At baseline, cohorts recruited from all students in Year 1 (2432) and Year 7 (1453), with annual follow-up for 5 and 3 years respectively
Methodology	Cycloplegic refraction (cyclopentolate). Risk factor questionnaire including near work and time outdoors
Study name	*Jiading Eye Study*
Location	Jiading District, Shanghai
Design	Cross-sectional study of 8267 students from randomly selected preschools and primary schools
Methodology	Cycloplegic refraction (cyclopentolate) and risk factor questionnaire

up to the emergence of young adults. Large studies have rarely been designed to look at refractive errors, and studies reporting on refractive errors from the 1958 British Birth Cohort Study [47], the Avon Longitudinal Study of Parents and Children (ALSPAC) [48–50], the British Twins Early Development Study (TEDS) [51], the US-based National Health and Nutrition Evaluation Survey (NHANES) [52], the Korean NHANES [53], the Gutenberg Health Survey [54], and the UK Biobank Study [55] measured noncycloplegic refractions. Data from the European Eye Epidemiology (E3) consortium suffers from the same bias [56,

57]. Major studies of eye diseases, including refractive errors, such as the Beaver Dam Eye Study [58], the Blue Mountains Eye Study [59], and the Tanjong Pagar Eye Study [60] also measured noncycloplegic refractions. However, the Tehran Eye Study measured both cycloplegic and noncycloplegic refractions over a wide age range [61].

In general, studies designed to look specifically at refractive errors in school age children, such as the pioneering studies from Taiwan [11], the RESC (Refractive Error Study in Children) Studies [62], the Singapore Cohort Study of the Risk Factors for Myopia (SCORM) Study [63], the Orinda [64] and Collaborative Longitudinal Evaluation of Ethnicity and Refractive Error (CLEERE) [34] Studies in the United States, the Sydney Myopia Study and the Sydney Adolescent Vascular and Eye Study (SMS and SAVES) [65], the Northern Ireland Childhood Errors of Refraction Study [66], the Ireland Eye Study [67], several studies from China [12, 58, 68, 69] and Poland [70, 71], have measured cycloplegic refractions. The Generation R birth cohort study [72] introduced cycloplegic refractions at an early stage, but after the initial data collection. Studies on pediatric and preschool samples are more limited, but cycloplegia has generally been used [27, 28, 35, 73–77]. Cycloplegia needs to be carefully controlled in these studies, because when the prevalence of myopia is low, even a small amount of pseudomyopia may have a significant effect on the apparent prevalence.

6.1.4 Myopia: The Importance of Causal Pathways

The aim of identifying risk factors is to generate preventive interventions. This requires identification of modifiable causal risk factors, not just associations. Observational epidemiological studies can only establish associations, but far too often, papers on cross-sectional associations conclude with a limitation that conclusions about causality cannot be drawn. This seems to imply that longitudinal data can establish causality, but this is not correct. Parallel longitudinal changes are equally ambiguous, and this makes understanding the epidemic of myopia difficult since many parameters, such as industrialization, urbanization, pollution, incomes, nutrition, and education, have changed over the same period.

Strictly, randomized intervention studies are required to establish causality, but often studies of this kind would be regarded as unethical. In many cases, we therefore have to rely on the nonrandomized trials that occur as a part of social development. For example, it would be unethical to offer differential educational opportunities to children in a randomly selected fashion, but social differences often lead to differential educational opportunities, and these can be highly informative, although they lack randomization. The high prevalence of myopia seen in Jewish males who received an intensive religious education, compared to their sisters who received a less intensive religious education, as well as boys and girls who received a less intensive secular education [78], provides rather compelling evidence of causality. In some cases, Mendelian randomization analysis can be used. Although there are strict limitations on its use [79, 80], it has already been usefully applied to the problem of myopia [81–83].

While the limitations of cross-sectional or longitudinal data are clear, avoiding discussing causality misses the point, because whether the association is potentially causal is crucial. Causality is therefore an important issue to discuss. Unfortunately, journals often discourage speculation, both explicitly and through tight word and reference limits. We recognize that wild speculation is not useful—Curtin's description of the ophthalmologist waking after a sleepless night with "a new and usually more bizarre" hypothesis often rings true [84]. But evidence-based speculation should be encouraged, and subjected to critical review.

A related issue is the distinction between proximal and distal risk factors. Proximal risk factors are those closest to having a direct impact on eye growth, whereas distal factors will modulate the magnitude of more proximal factors. A plausible causal chain leads from education (excessive near work and limited time outdoors) to control of dopamine release and changes in axial elongation. Parental socioeconomic status, increases in the accessibility to education, and social attitudes to education may all increase involvement in education and/or result in reduced time outdoors, changing the prevalence of myopia through a common pathway that probably involves regulation of dopamine release and certainly involves regulation of axial elongation.

6.1.5 Statistical Analysis

There are also some associated considerations in relation to statistical analysis. A very common approach in analysis of risk factors is to identify significant associations in univariate analysis, then put the significant associations into multivariate regression analysis, labeling those factors that remain significant as "independent" risk factors. Often this appears to be done without serious consideration of whether the risk factors make sense in terms of causal pathways, whether they are modifiable, whether they are accurately measureable, whether they are likely to be collinear, whether they could result from reverse causality, and how complete the list of variables is. All these considerations can affect the validity of regression analysis.

Statistical analysis can be used more scientifically to address specific hypotheses about mediation by associated factors [85]. For example, in considering the relationship between myopia, education, and socioeconomic status (SES), it is possible to include SES and then the SES and education to see if there is a reduction in the strength of the association. This would be a sign that education mediates the influence of SES. In general, stepwise procedures need to be increasingly used in analysis. The quality of the variables is also important—whether they are continuous or categorical variables, and whether they can be accurately measured. Even if one factor is entirely mediated by another, if either variable is poorly measured, adjustment may only reduce rather than largely eliminate the effect of the other variable. Thus, the concept of independent risk factors is somewhat problematic [86].

Some of the variables are intrinsically complex. Education, for example, can be assessed in adults as a set of categories (primary school, high school, and university completed) or as a continuous variable (years of education). But intensity of education is also important, since children who obtain higher academic grades at a given level of schooling are more likely to be myopic. No variable captures both duration and intensity effectively. Myopia is associated with both intelligence quotient (IQ) [87] and school results [88]. Both are sometimes included in analyses to measure "innate" potential. But this approach is problematic since IQ shows complex changes over time [89, 90], and like myopia, combines significant twin heritability, considerable missing heritability, and social malleability [91]. There are both phenotypic and genetic correlations between myopia and IQ [92], as well as strong environmental effects. Inclusion of past performance or IQ in analyses as indicators of "innate potential," may, if these measures are influenced by the same environmental factors that influence myopia, obscure their role.

Regression analyses that combine variables that are more or less proximal also pose a problem. It is well known that axial elongation is the biological basis of myopic shifts in refraction, and thus it correlates highly with SER. If axial length is included in a regression analysis with more distal factors, it will tend to obscure the associations of these more distal factors with refraction.

In summary, there are a number of conceptual and methodological issues that need careful consideration in seeking to tease out the risk factors for myopia. Further progress in the analysis of risk factors for myopia requires more critical approaches in several areas.

6.2 The Main Risk Factors for "School Myopia": Education and Time Outdoors

We have recently reviewed this topic in detail, and these reviews can be consulted for more detailed references [1, 2, 4, 24]. In one of them, we distinguish between societies where the provision of education is limited and the prevalence of myopia is low (operationally, less than 10% myopia in young adults), at an age when 12 years of schooling would be the norm in the developed world, societies with western style education where the prevalence is between 10 and 60%, and developed countries in East and Southeast Asia, where education is intense, time outdoors is low, and the prevalence of myopia is high at 70–90%, particularly in urban areas.

It seems likely that the gradual transition from a very low prevalence in societies with little formal education to that typical of modern western societies with widespread education is predominantly due to the expansion of educational provision to cover all children, combined with increases in educational standards. Many of the countries in the first group are currently well short of the UN Sustainable Development Goals in Education for 2030 (https://sustainabledevelopment.un.org/sdg4, accessed January 30, 2019). The prevalence of myopia is unlikely to increase in these countries until progress is made in achieving these goals. In contrast, the very high prevalence rates now typical of developed countries in East and Southeast Asia compared to the much more moderate prevalence rates observed in western countries cannot be attributed to more years of education, but are probably related to more intense education, early onset of high homework loads, and much less time outdoors.

Because of the common observation in societies with significant educational provision that the prevalence of myopia increases with age, there is now a widespread assumption that myopia is affected by chronological age. However, the low prevalence of myopia in societies where educational opportunities are limited, suggests that it is not chronological age, but cumulative experience of schooling that is important, because without schooling most children do not become myopic. For this reason, it is often a useful sampling strategy to obtain a large sample of a given age, rather than smaller age-specific samples over a range of ages.

In adults, years of schooling is often used as a variable to look at associations with myopia. Consistent with the preceding arguments, those who have completed university education are more likely to be myopic than those who have completed secondary education, or primary education [55, 93]. Data from the UK Biobank dataset was recently used to address the issue of causality in relation to years of schooling and myopia [83]. The authors used two sets of genetic data—one on SNPs that associated with years of education, the other on SNPs associated with myopia. It was found that people with SNPs associated with more years of education were more likely to be myopic, whereas those with SNPs associated with more myopia did not have more years of education. This provides a clear direction of causation from years of education to myopia. It is important to note that this does not mean that variables such as years of education or myopia are predominantly genetically determined. The percentage of variation in the two parameters explained by identified SNPs was low in both cases.

Rapid historical increases in years of schooling cannot be explained by genetic change but must depend on more distal social changes that made mass education more available, and linked employment and salary to increased skill levels, creating a strong incentive for parents to extend the education of their children. In the west, the expansion of mass education paralleled industrialization and the rise of modern capitalism, and later the introduction of new technologies. Data suggesting that the prevalence of myopia has increased can in fact be traced back to the early years of last century in the United States [94]. In contrast, the rapid economic development of countries in East and Southeast Asia has been based on industrialization supported by rapid development of a skilled work force. This, combined with recent experiences of rural poverty and Confucian concepts of familial obligation and work ethic, appears to have taken educational intensity to a much higher level, producing the epidemic of myopia.

Intensity of schooling shows up in measures of achievements during schooling. There is a general association of higher school performance with more myopia, for a given number of years of schooling [88], with associations of more myopia with involvement in accelerated learning streams within or between schools [95–97], and use of after-school tutoring [98]. These factors seem to be associated with the strong international performance of school systems in the countries with high prevalence of myopia [99], and may point to possible control measures. For example, if involvement in accelerated learning streams starts early, this provides an incentive for parents to impose intensive study regimes on children early in life so that they get into the higher level streams, leading to early onset myopia and rapid progression. A possible reform would therefore be to delay the onset of myopia with policies designed to control the early introduction of accelerated or elite streams within or between schools, while controlling intensive academic streams in private schools, private tutorial colleges, or cram schools.

Analysis of the results of the E3 consortium suggested that education was not the whole story [56]. This is not surprising, since the role of time outdoors, discussed below, has been demonstrated. But the analysis rests on an implicit assumption that completion of primary education (defined in this paper as 16 years) posed the same educational load across the many decades of development of education systems. Putting to one side the rather unusual definition of primary school education, it is very unlikely that this is the case. Educational standards at the end of primary school when most children completed schooling to work as unskilled laborers or homemakers were almost certainly lower than they are today, when most children complete many further years of education, and a significant percentage engage in tertiary studies.

Two potentially more proximal factors that may be related to educational intensity have also been considered—reading distance and reading duration without breaks [100]. The first has a long history, dating back to Cohn, who supported the use of headrests to maintain head position while reading. These were abandoned, but it is not clear if that was because they were not effective, or because children refused to use with them. Some studies report a strong independent association of reading distance with myopia, but it is not clear whether the relationship is causal, or whether children decrease their reading distance as they become myopic. The use of headrests has been reintroduced in some schools in China, and many products are available online to control head position. Longitudinal studies are required to establish if close reading positions are adopted prior to, or in parallel with the development of myopia, and randomized trials are required to assess whether controlling reading position does reduce myopia. Reading without breaks has also often been regarded as a risk factor, and the rule of a 10 min break every 30 min forms part of myopia prevention in both Taiwan and mainland China. An intervention study is also important in this area.

6.2.1 The Search for Causal Mechanisms for Education

While there can be no doubt about the causal relationship between education and myopia, the causal pathways are less clear. Near work was generally considered to be a likely mediating factor; however, the evidence on near work has been rather inconsistent, although meta-analyses indicate that there is a relatively small effect [101]. Part of the problem may be that near work is generally estimated from questionnaire responses which are intrinsically not particularly reliable. It is also difficult because the slow development of myopia means that near work estimates need to cover periods of at least some months if not years to be related to significant changes in axial length or refraction. Recent development of instruments for objectively measuring near work may provide better estimates, although considerable thought will need to be given to the sampling frames, given the marked daily, weekly, and seasonal variations in near work demands.

Initial thinking about the causal connection invoked accommodation as the probable driver, but this idea has been increasingly called into question. Some of the important negative evidence came from animal experimentation, which showed that refractive development was not drastically affected by cutting the ciliary nerve [102], and that animals that had no accommodative capacity showed normal patterns of refractive development [103, 104]. The ability of atropine to block axial elongation was initially interpreted as supporting the hypothesis, but this judgment had to be reevaluated, since atropine was effective, even in animals such as chickens where control of accommodation involves nicotinic rather than muscarinic pathways.

Attention therefore shifted to the possibility of control by defocus on the retina, given the clear role for defocus signals in controlling axial elongation demonstrated in animal models [31]. The link to education was provided by the hypothesis that lags in accommodation would result in residual hyperopia, which could stimulate axial elongation. Testing this hypothesis has led to inconsistent results, and Mutti et al. have shown that accommodative lag may be a consequence rather than a cause [105]. There is thus no clear pattern of support for the hypothesis.

It has also been suggested that peripheral rather than central defocus may play the dominant role in controlling eye growth [106]. This hypothesis developed from evidence that trainee pilots with eye shapes that created peripheral hyperopia were more likely to become myopic [107], leading to the idea that peripheral hyperopia leads to the development of myopia. Elegant animal experiments then demonstrated that eyes could normally regulate eye growth, even if the central retina was ablated [108]. However, this hypothesis has not been supported by several lines of evidence. The interpretation of the original evidence on development of myopia has been questioned [109], and while there is a general trend for eyes to develop from more oblate to more prolate, the relationship between eye shape and refraction has been quite variable tend to appear [110]. It remains possible that peripheral hyperopic defocus might drive myopic progression but attempts to control myopic correction by reducing peripheral hyperopic have not been particularly successful. However, selective imposition of myopic defocus in the periphery may provide a method for controlling myopia [111].

A clear causal mechanism linking education to myopia has therefore not been identified, but the causal relationship nevertheless appears to be solid. A recent hypothesis is that the problem may be associated with the predominant use of black text on white background [112]. This hypothesis proposes that the problem lies in the balance of stimulation of ON and OFF visual pathways, with natural scenes leading to balanced stimulation, with black text on white heavily overstimulating OFF pathways. Given that ON-bipolar pathways stimulate release of dopamine from amacrine cells [113], and dopamine agonists can inhibit axial elongation in animal models [114, 115], this is a promising link.

6.2.2 Protection by Time Outdoors

In contrast to the long history of speculation and research about near work, solid evidence that time outdoors was an important factor only became available about 10 years ago. However, since the first presentation of the evidence at the 2006 ARVO meeting, a large amount of evidence supporting the idea has been accumulated [2, 116], and a recent meta-analysis has confirmed the association [117]. Two key pieces of evidence are shown in Figs. 6.2 and 6.3 [118, 119]. The first shows that increased time outdoors can override the impact of increased near work, the second that increased time outdoors can override the impact of parental myopia. There are some reports that have failed to find this association, but these have generally been in situations where the amount of time spent outdoors is low and may be subthreshold for protection. The evidence now includes successful school-based intervention trials that have shown that increases in time outdoors of 40–80 min per day produced significant reductions in incident myopia [46, 120, 121], consistent with expectations from the epidemiological data.

Rose et al. [118] postulated that the mechanism was probably that the brighter light outdoors during daylight hours led to more dopamine release, which in turn inhibited axial elongation. This hypothesis was confirmed by laboratory experiments that demonstrated the inhibitory effects of bright light on myopia, and the protective effect was shown to involve D2-dopamine receptors [122–126]. The plausible possibility that lower vitamin D levels, observed in children who spend less time outdoors, played a causal role has not been supported by further analysis [81, 82, 127]. The hypothesis that the protective effects might be due to a different balance of hyperopic and myopia defocus outdoors as compared to indoors [14], while plausible in terms of the results of animal experimentation, also seems unlikely, given that increasing light intensity alone blocks experimental myopia.

The question of causality has been settled with the randomized intervention trials in children. However, some issues are still unclear. The initial studies were based on distinctions between time spent outdoors and indoors, and were later linked to an operational definition of outdoors as involving light intensities over 1000 lux.

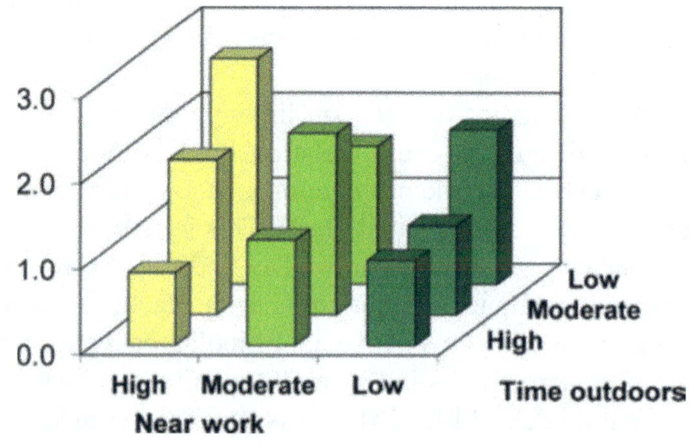

Fig. 6.2 Impacts of tertiles of near work and time outdoors on the odds ratio for myopia. Figure reproduced from Rose et al. [118]

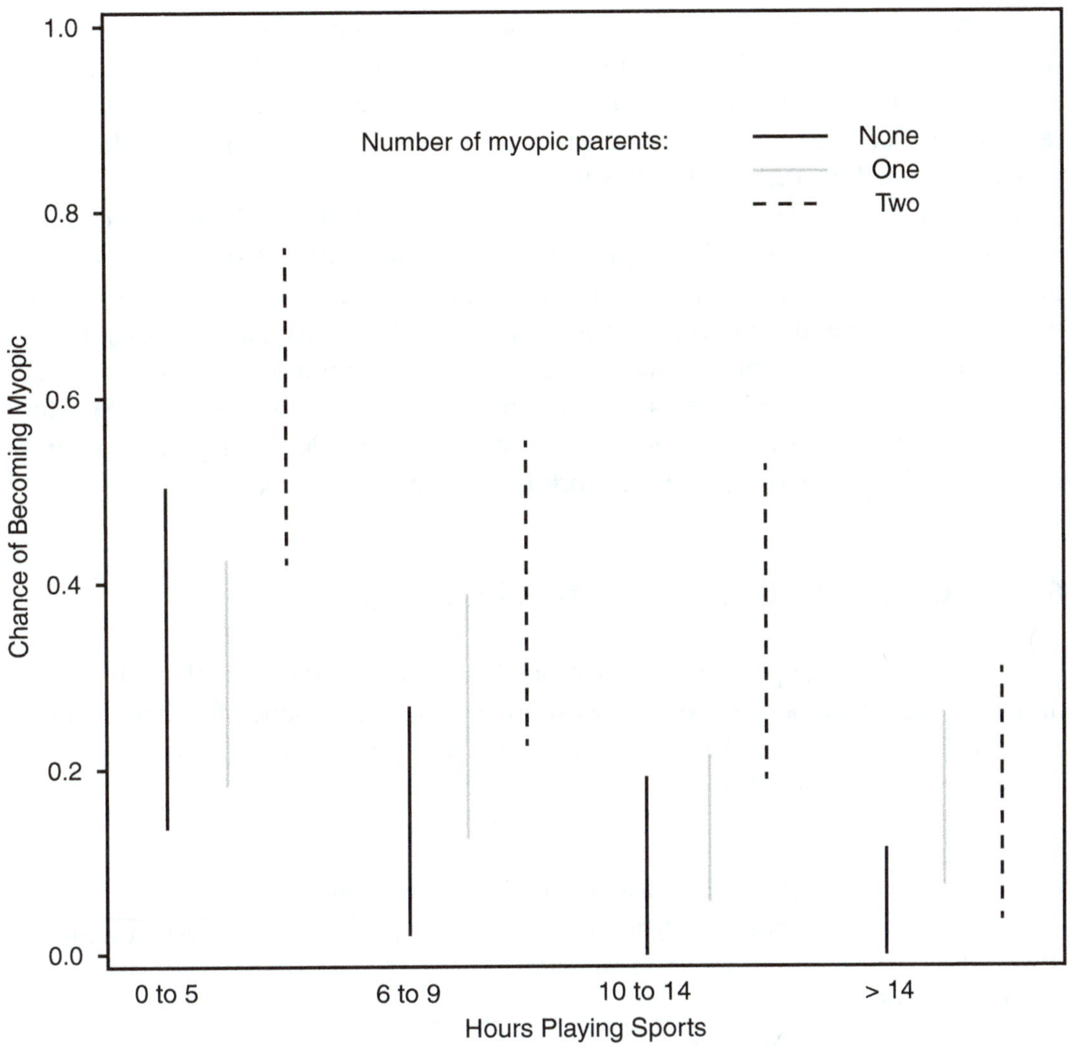

Fig. 6.3 Impact of hours playing sport (and outdoor activity) on the risk of myopia against number of myopic parents. Figure reproduced with permission from Jones et al. [119]

Animal studies suggested that light intensities considerably higher, at least 10,000 lux, might be required to produce significant effects, but there is suggestive evidence that lower light intensities might be effective in humans [120, 128]. One intervention trial has even suggested that modest increases in classroom lighting strongly inhibit the development of myopia [129], and this study requires urgent replication. A school-based intervention trial in Taiwan has reported that more modest outdoor light exposures might also reduce incident myopia and, in fact, some research using objective measurements of light suggests that effective exposures of over a few thousand lux are rare outdoors, even though light appears to be regulating axial elongation. It would not be surprising if animal experimentation overestimated the light exposures required for protection, given that the stimulus for eye growth is strong and constant, whereas signals in humans may be more intermittent. It has also been suggested that the timing of the exposures, or their frequency, and parameters such as spectral composition may be important. There is limited and so far inconsistent support for these ideas, but the uncertainty around them does not matter when the simple intervention, increased time outdoors, is considered. These factors may become important if increased time outdoors needs to be supplemented or even replaced by artificial light exposures.

There is also controversy over whether increased time outdoors reduces progression as well as onset of myopia. The initial work did not support this possibility [118, 119, 130], but even at that time, there was considerable evidence that there were seasonal differences in progression that suggested that progression rates were slower in summer than in winter, suggesting regulation of progression consistent with the documented effects of near work and time outdoors [131–135]. More recent reports have provided evidence that more time outdoors may slow progression [120, 136], but more definitive work in this area is required.

6.3 Other Possible Risk Factors for Myopia

A range of other "independent" risk factors that are less obviously related to education have been documented. As well as summarizing the evidence for them, we will discuss whether they are likely to be mediated by exposures associated with education and time outdoors (Table 6.2).

Table 6.2 Summary of probable mechanisms for risk factors for myopia

Risk factor	Possibly mediated by environmental exposures	Independent biological pathways	Genetic basis
Digital screen time	X		
Ethnicity	X		
Sex	X		
Parental myopia	X		
Urban/rural differences	X		
Pollution	X		
Housing	X		
Height	X		
Diet	X		
Sleep	X		
Smoking		X	
Birth order	X	X	
Season of birth	X		
Allergic rhinoconjunctivitis		X	X
Childhood febrile diseases		X	X

While the evidence is not conclusive, most of the reported independent risk factors for myopia might be mediated by environmental exposure to educational pressures and limited time outdoors. Systematic use of mediation analysis is required to test independence

6.3.1 Use of Computers and Smart Phones

In the last few years, use of computers and smart phones has become a routine part of daily life, with digital devices integrated into schooling in advanced countries. Increased digital screen time is often invoked to explain claimed continuing increases in the prevalence and severity of myopia, or at least as explanations for the increasingly early onset of myopia. Somewhat in advance of the available evidence, Taiwan has introduced laws controlling the amount of digital screen time that children of preschool age are allowed, although how regulations of this kind could be enforced is not clear. Dirani et al. [137] have recently asked whether increased digital screen time might be "the single modifiable risk factor for myopia," accounting for "increased near-work activity and decreased outdoor activity."

We suggest that this is unlikely, since the epidemic of myopia appeared well before the common use of these electronic devices. The prevalence of myopia was already high in Taiwan and Singapore for children born in the early 1960s, whereas the internet did not become available to the general public until 1993. Early analysis in the Sydney Myopia Study found that use of devices such as Nintendos and Game Boys was associated with less myopia, perhaps because they were predominantly used by academically underperforming boys. It is certainly possible that digital devices have now come to constitute a significant form of near work, and will correlate more closely with education and myopia, and some recent studies have documented significant associations between myopia and digital screen time [51, 138].

However, the historical perspective is important in considering preventive interventions. If limits are placed on the use of digital devices, children may simply revert to older forms of near work, such as reading books. And if digital devices encourage even more time indoors, active steps may need to be taken to get children to break with established behavior patterns and spend more time outdoors. We believe overemphasis on digital screen time may in fact have negative consequences if it leads to neglect of the other important factors. There is currently no evidence that time using digital devices is more dangerous than a similar amount of time reading. However, digital devices may make near work more pervasive and favor indoor lifestyles.

6.3.2 Sex

Many studies have compared the prevalence of myopia in males and females. Older studies have some tendency to report higher prevalence in males, whereas more recent studies more commonly report higher prevalence in females. For example, the Blue Mountains Eye Study reported that older male adults were more myopic than females [59], but the situation was reversed in the Sydney Myopia Study on children [42, 43, 96, 139]. Similarly, the Liwan Eye Study reported that sex differences in older adults were marginal [140], but in younger cohorts, girls were more likely to be myopic than boys [141]. The massive difference between the prevalence of myopia in girls and boys in Orthodox Jewish communities in Israel, where the boys undergo very intensive education from an early age, provides an extreme inverted example of this trend [78]. This variability does not suggest a direct biological link between sex and myopia, but rather suggests that the links may be mediated by social factors such as access to education for girls, which have changed considerably in many places in recent decades.

6.3.3 Ethnicity

Ethnicity or race has often been proposed as a risk factor for myopia, and indeed as evidence for genetic determination of myopia. It is however important to note that ethnicity and race covers both genetic differences, which are small in magnitude compared to the commonalities that make us human, and cultural differences that are often hard to quantify. Epidemiological evidence clearly shows major differences between ethnic groups in the prevalence of myopia, but more detailed analysis shows that these are predominantly due to environmental exposures. For example, the prevalence of myopia is high in the three major ethnic groups in Singapore, Chinese, Indian, and Malay, but in India and Malaysia, the prevalence is much lower [1, 4, 24]. This suggests that it is the environment of Singapore, perhaps most of all the education system and the limited time spent outdoors, that is crucial.

6.3.4 Parental Myopia

One of the best documented risk factors for myopia that is not directly linked to education is having myopic parents. Although shared attitudes to education are just as plausible, it is often assumed that this must be a genetic phenomenon, which is clearly true for the very genetic, highly familial forms of myopia. But the impact of parental myopia is also seen for "school myopia." Consistently, studies covering a range of different ethnic groups have shown that having one or two myopic parents increases the risk of myopia [142–147], although the risk is inevitably lower in populations with a high prevalence of myopia. Wu and Edwards have shown the impact of parental myopia over three generations in China [148].

The effect of parental myopia is often cited as evidence for a genetic contribution to myopia, on the grounds that parents and children share genes. But they also share environments, and the possibility that myopic parents provide their children with environments more conducive for developing myopia, perhaps by placing more emphasis on education, has not been excluded, although early analyses did not support this hypothesis. However, recent studies have shown that children with myopic parents do not have a significantly greater level of myopia-associated SNPs [149], undermining the genetic argument. A more detailed analysis of environmental risk factors with objective measures of near work and time outdoors may be required to explain this association.

6.3.5 Intelligence

Higher intelligence or IQ, and some other cognitive measures, are generally associated with myopia. However, whether they are factors independent of education and time outdoors is not clear. While there are some genetic influences on these factors, as noted previously, like myopia, they are socially malleable, rather than genetically determined [89, 90]. In the SCORM Study, both academic grades and IQ scores appear to be independently associated with myopia [87, 88], and the same result has been obtained in a very large study of Israeli conscripts [150]. But the causal chains are very obscure, with a number of questions to be answered. For example, Are the links explained by the genetic correlations of the phenotypes? Do people with high IQs do more near work? Or is part of their high IQ achieved by more time reading and indoors? Do people with higher IQs need less effort to achieve high grades? Whatever the answer to these questions, reducing intelligence does not provide a route to prevention.

6.3.6 Urban/Rural Differences

Another consistent association of myopia is with urban residence, with children growing up in more rural areas generally being less myopic. In general, educational outcomes for children from rural areas are lower, and they often report less near work and more time outdoors. It is hard to see a direct link between axial elongation and postcode, and we suggest that urban/rural differences are likely to be based on differences in near work and time outdoors.

Population density has been invoked as one factor [151], but a major study in China has found that while there was a positive association of myopia with increased population density [152], even in the area with the lowest population density studied, the prevalence of myopia was still very high. This suggests other factors were more important. Access to green space has also been linked to lower use of spectacles [153].

6.3.7 Pollution

Pollution is one of the factors that has increased markedly since the Second World War in parts of East and Southeast Asia. There are many forms of pollution. Speculation about this factor has been fueled by the high levels of air pollution seem in some parts of China, but in fact, in international terms, Chinese cities rank well behind many cities in South Asia and the Middle East, where the prevalence of myopia is much lower than in Chinese cities (https://www.who.int/airpollution/data/cities/en/, accessed Jan 30, 2019). Increased use of spectacles, presumably for myopia, has been associated with traffic-related pollution [154], but this may in fact be related to the association between urban residence and more myopia, as well as links to socioeconomic status, area of residence, and education [153].

6.3.8 Housing

Nature of housing has also been invoked as a factor. However, the results in this area are currently quite contradictory. In Singapore, more spacious housing was associated with more myopia, possibly because of a causal chain involving socioeconomic status and its associations with education [60, 95]. In contrast, in both Sydney [151] and Hong Kong [155], small apartment dwelling has been associated with more myopia. A causal chain is not as obvious in this case and more complex pathways may need to be considered.

6.3.9 Height

Height has often been considered as a potential risk factor for myopia, and indeed, there have been substantial increases in height in populations over the last 150 years. These increases in height have been generally attributed to more adequate nutrition. It has also been argued that associations between height and myopia might be expected, given that taller people have longer axial lengths, but this argument does not take into account the "emmetropisation" mechanisms that produce substantial convergence of refractive status, despite differences in body stature. While several papers have reported that height is a risk factor for myopia [9, 156], the evidence on this is very inconsistent. Rosner et al. [157] reported that Israeli male military conscripts, who were not myopic, were taller and weighed more than those who were not myopic—the reverse of expectations. Another inconsistency lies in the difference in prevalence of myopia between males and females, with a higher prevalence of myopia being commonly reported in girls in recent studies. If there were a tight biological link between height and refraction, a more consistent relationship would be expected. Social factors affecting nutrition and education may therefore be important. Given the differences in height between the sexes, studies need to be carried out with population stratification wherever possible.

Rahi and colleagues reported that maternal height (and age) was associated with more myopia [47]. In the United Kingdom, height differs by socioeconomic status, with greater heights (and also maternal age) in higher SES groups [158]. Since children from higher SES groups are generally more myopic, these associations need to be tested for mediation by social factors.

6.3.10 Diet

Diets in East and Southeast Asia have changed significantly since the Second World War, and Cordain et al. argued that dietary change could have contributed to the increased prevalence of myopia, backed up by a plausible hypothesis linking insulin resistance, chronic hyperinsulinemia, increased circulating insulin-like growth factor (IGF-1), decreased circulating growth hormone, and decreased retinoid receptor signaling to increases in scleral growth [159]. But in other ways, this hypothesis has gained little support, and expected associations of height, weight, body mass index (BMI) and obesity with myopia have not been consistently observed. Improved diet is associated with greater height and axial length, but it does not appear to have produced increased refraction, consistent with the powerful eye growth control mechanisms that have been reported. It is also worth noting that international variations in overweight and obesity do not parallel the international distribution of myopia, with none of the countries with a high prevalence of myopia making the list of the top 20 countries ranked by percentage of obesity (https://www.who.int/gho/ncd/risk_factors/overweight/en/, accessed Jan 30, 2019) and thus there is little support for a tight biological link between diet and myopia.

6.3.11 Sleep

Associations between sleep and myopia have also been reported, but the evidence is quite inconsistent [160–162]. It is clear that children who have heavy study loads after school are likely to get less sleep, both because there is less time available, but also because mental activity close to bed time can disrupt sleep. Lack of sleep is more likely to be a problem in the senior years of school, when homework loads in many parts of East and Southeast Asia are very high. However, sleep deprivation is likely to be less common in the early primary years, when myopia first appears, which reduces the likelihood that it is a major risk factor. Kearney et al. [163] have recently reported that myopes in the Northern Ireland Childhood Errors of Refraction (NICER) Study have lower levels of serum melatonin, which could be linked to disruption of circadian rhythms, which have sometimes been linked to myopia [164], or could be linked to reduced light exposures and dopaminergic function.

6.3.12 Smoking

Maternal smoking was associated with a lower risk of myopia in the SCORM Study from Singapore, but there was no association with paternal smoking, and the number of mothers who smoked was small [165]. In the subsequent Strabismus, Amblyopia and Refractive Error in young Singaporean Children Study (STARS) Study, a stronger negative association with maternal and paternal smoking was reported [166]. A similar protective relationship was reported in a sample from a pediatric ophthalmology clinic, which largely persisted after adjustment for a range of factors including child's near work activity and parental myopia and education [167]. A detailed study from South Korea reported consistent results for exposure to passive smoke estimated from urinary cotinine level [168], supporting the suggestion that nicotinic pathways are involved in the regulation of eye growth. In contrast, Rahi et al. reported a positive association between maternal smoking in early pregnancy and more myopia [47]. Although some of the associations reported are substantial, given the associations of smoking with SES and education, and lower gestational weight, these studies need to be carefully controlled for confounding.

6.3.13 Birth Order

Associations between myopia and birth order were reported with first-born children tending to be more myopic [49]. However, in educational studies, it is well documented that first-born children generally get more education [169]. A subsequent study on the UK Biobank dataset, adjusted for education, showed that the association between myopia and birth order was reduced but not eliminated [170]. In addition, in China, children from one child families are also more myopic than other children with siblings, and this was attributed to greater parental support for their child's education [171]. However, the sociology of these differences is very complex, and more work needs to be done to establish that birth order is an independent risk factor.

6.3.14 Season of Birth

Season of birth has also been associated with myopia in several studies, with children born in summer tending to be more myopic [51, 172, 173]. No plausible pathway has been suggested for a direct link. Instead, it has been suggested that children born in summer often start school up to a year younger than their peers born in spring. This could mean first exposure to education and less time outdoors at an age when myopic shifts in refraction, including myopic progression, are larger, resulting in more myopia.

6.3.15 Allergic Conjunctivitis: Hay Fever and Kawasaki Disease

In 2011, Herbort et al. proposed a general association of myopia with inflammatory conditions affecting the choriocapillaris [174]. An association between ocular inflammatory conditions such as uveitis was subsequently demonstrated [175]. Later, a higher risk of myopia was associated with allergic conjunctivitis, and less so allergic rhinitis, atopic dermatitis, and asthma [176]. A large population-based study using the NHANES dataset showed that hay fever was also associated with a higher prevalence of high myopia [177]. A recent report has also associated increased myopia with Kawasaki disease [178], which has conjunctivitis as one of its core diagnostic criteria. This association needs further study.

These studies provide a persuasive case for some link between ocular allergic responses and the development of myopia, and using an animal model. Wei et al. have proposed a mechanism involving increased tumor necrosis factor (TNF)-alpha and interleukins. It does not seem likely that a link between ocular inflammation and myopia can explain the epidemic of myopia in East and Southeast Asia, since there is no parallel between the international distribution myopia and that of allergic rhinoconjunctivitis in children [179]. One possibility is that eye rubbing may lead to myopic refractions through corneal changes, as may be the case with keratoconus [180], but the US study on hay fever ruled out a role for them. The possibility that children with these conditions tend to spend less time outside should be examined. It also seems possible that allergic conditions might add to the incidence and progression of myopia, without being the primary determinant.

6.3.16 Febrile Diseases

Using data from the UK Biobank, Guggenheim et al. reported associations between several childhood diseases and myopia. From a list including pneumonia, encephalitis, meningitis, rheumatic fever, measles, rubella, mumps, diphtheria, and pertussis, rubella, mumps and pertussis were associated with myopia, while measles, rubella, and pertussis were associated with high myopia [181]. The authors argued against a link to educational disruption or limited time outdoors, since not all serious childhood diseases were linked to myopia, but this link, whatever its causes, cannot explain the emergence of the epidemic of myopia. But these findings may have clinical implications that need to be explored.

6.3.17 Fertility Treatment

The British TEDS Study has documented a standard range of social variables, with level of maternal education, summer birth, hours spent playing computer games surviving full multivariate regression analysis, with associations with socioeconomic status, educational attainment, reading enjoyment, and cognitive variables showing associations at multiple stages in the life-course analysis. A unique feature of the analysis was the protective associations of fertility treatment detected in the final analysis [51]. The authors ruled out associations with parental education, and the causes are currently obscure.

6.4 Popular Beliefs About the Causes of Myopia

There are many popular beliefs in the causes of myopia around the world, which have presumably arisen because the development of myopia and its progression is often observed by parents, who naturally seek explanations. In the western world, a common belief is that reading in dim light, or under the bed clothes causes vision to deteriorate, but this outcome, and these behaviors might indeed be common in those who like reading books, and there is some evidence that reading for pleasure is a risk factor for myopia. We have not attempted a systematic survey in this area, but in China, there seem to be many beliefs of this kind, perhaps because the prevalence of myopia has increased so conspicuously. One commonly encountered belief is that myopia is associated with reading and writing postures that violate the "foot, fist, inch" rule, that is the eyes should be one foot from the book, the chest should be one fist from the desk, and the fingers should be 1 inch from the nib of the pen. This is a variant on the idea that bad posture while reading leads to the development of myopia, which has widespread currency, but has never been proven. A similar common belief is that reading while riding on public transport is dangerous, but again this has never been tested. Other, intuitively unlikely ideas include the development of myopia in children who read on their back, or their front, or who read extracurricular books with font sizes greater than standard textbooks. These have occasionally been looked at in scientific papers, and associations have sometimes been reported. These proposed factors need to be rigorously tested epidemiologically, and if they survive that sort of testing, they need to be subjected to standard Randomised Control Trial (RCT) testing. Unfortunately, without any positive evidence, two of these have been written into China's National Myopia Prevention Plan.

6.5 Comparing Genetic and Environmental Effects

Comparing the impact of genetic to environmental effects is difficult, because they are often quantified in different ways, with genetic effects generally determined in relation to variation in refraction, while evidence on the impact of environmental effects is generally related to prevalence of myopia. Genetic studies have identified myopia-associated SNPs that account for slightly less than 10% of the variance in refraction, although these factors are very precisely measured [13]. Compared to the possibly misplaced expectations from twin studies with heritability estimates in the range of 80–90%, there is obviously a large amount of what has come to be called missing heritability, although it is actually the identified genetic variation which is missing. Use of the SNP-heritability approach suggests that Genome-Wide Association Study (GWAS) has the potential to explain more like 20–35% of the variance [19]. It is often suggested that improvements in methodology and increases in sample size may help to close the gap, although there is a law of diminishing returns with increased sample sizes. There is little evidence that other forms of genetic variation such as copy number variations or rare genetic effects of large size have a role to play.

In contrast, the measurement of risk factor exposures is much less precise, largely involving estimates derived from questionnaires. These questionnaires not only suffer from the general problem of recall bias, but in relation to near work and time outdoors, they also ask for a very difficult task to be performed, namely estimating average exposures. Not surprisingly, such questionnaires are more accurate when estimates of recent exposures over a limited time frame are compared to measurements obtained using objective instruments, but even then, discrepancies are significant. We are therefore not yet in a position to calculate individual environmental risk factor effect sizes. This may explain why attempts to quantify the associations between estimates of near work and time outdoors on the one hand and myopia on the other explain only low percentages of the variance [19], despite the evidence that changes in them appear to be responsible for the major increases in prevalence of myopia seen recently.

We suggest that while awaiting more quantitative data on environmental risk exposures, the change in mean SER from the age of 5–6 to the end of schooling may be taken to represent the cumulative effect of relevant environmental exposures over this time. This assumption seems reasonable, given that children exposed to only limited schooling generally develop little myopia. The only exception that we have found to this statement is the increase in prevalence of myopia in Eskimo and Inuit children after exposure to rudimentary schooling in extreme northern latitudes [182–184]. This may be an exception due to the limited light exposures available during winter, combined with reductions in the amount of time spent outdoors.

The data from the RESC Study in Nepal, where there is little development of myopia and limited schooling, appears to be an average shift of −0.02 D/year with minimal schooling [185]. This figure is about −0.16 D/year of schooling in the Sydney Myopia Study. East Asian studies suggest a total change that is much greater. In the Guangzhou RESC Study, refraction changed by at least −3.00 D over 10 years, or a change of −0.3 D/year [141]. In the Shandong Eye Study [12], the change was closer to −4.00 D over 10 years, or −0.4 D/year. One limitation of this simple analysis is that it assumes linear changes across the years of schooling, which may not be the case. These values compare with estimates from the UK Biobank Study on refractive shifts associated with years of schooling, which suggest shifts from epidemiological analysis of −0.16 D/year, while the Mendelian randomization analysis gives a change of −0.28 D/year [83]. It is encouraging that these figures are in the same ballpark when children have been exposed to schooling, but it needs to be recognized that these figures are only first approximations.

Accepting these estimates as the best currently available, we can then attempt to use them to understand the onset of myopia. Age of onset may be a very significant parameter, since it has decreased markedly during the emergence of the myopia epidemics [11], appears to have similar genetic associations to the final level of myopia in adults [13, 186], and appears to be a good predictor of final myopia [187].

In several studies that have used rigorous cycloplegia, refractions at the age of 5–7 are concentrated in the range of 1.0–1.3 D. This range has been documented for children in East Asia [12, 46, 75, 188] and in western societies [43, 76, 96]. The similarity of the values reported for children of East Asian and European backgrounds is striking, given the massively different prevalence rates that emerge later. In other reports, mean SER has been lower, and we suggest that, in many of these cases, inadequate cycloplegia may be involved. This means that the challenge is to explain how genetic factors and environmental factors can produce myopic shifts of 1.5 D or more to reach the threshold for myopia of −0.5 D. The steps involved in moving from this baseline value to the threshold for myopia and onto final SER at the age of 20 are summarized in Fig. 6.4.

In the ALSPAC Study [149] on average, participants carried around 130 risk alleles, with most of the distribution fitting within ±15 alleles [149]. If the average number of risk alleles corresponds to a mean SER of +1.0 to 1.3 D, with an average effect size of −0.1 D/risk allele, few participants would reach the myopia cutoff of −0.5 D on purely genetic grounds, and several years of schooling would be required to reach the threshold. Modeling by Ghorbani-Mojarrad et al. [149] also suggests that additive genetic effects are unlikely to produce "school myopia," without additional contributions from environmental factors. In contrast, in East Asian environments, 2–4 years of schooling would bring many children past the myopia cutoff. This is likely to happen more rapidly for those who are already at risk genetically.

This picture is based on a number of assumptions and needs extensive further development in relation to the size and linearity of effects, but it provides a

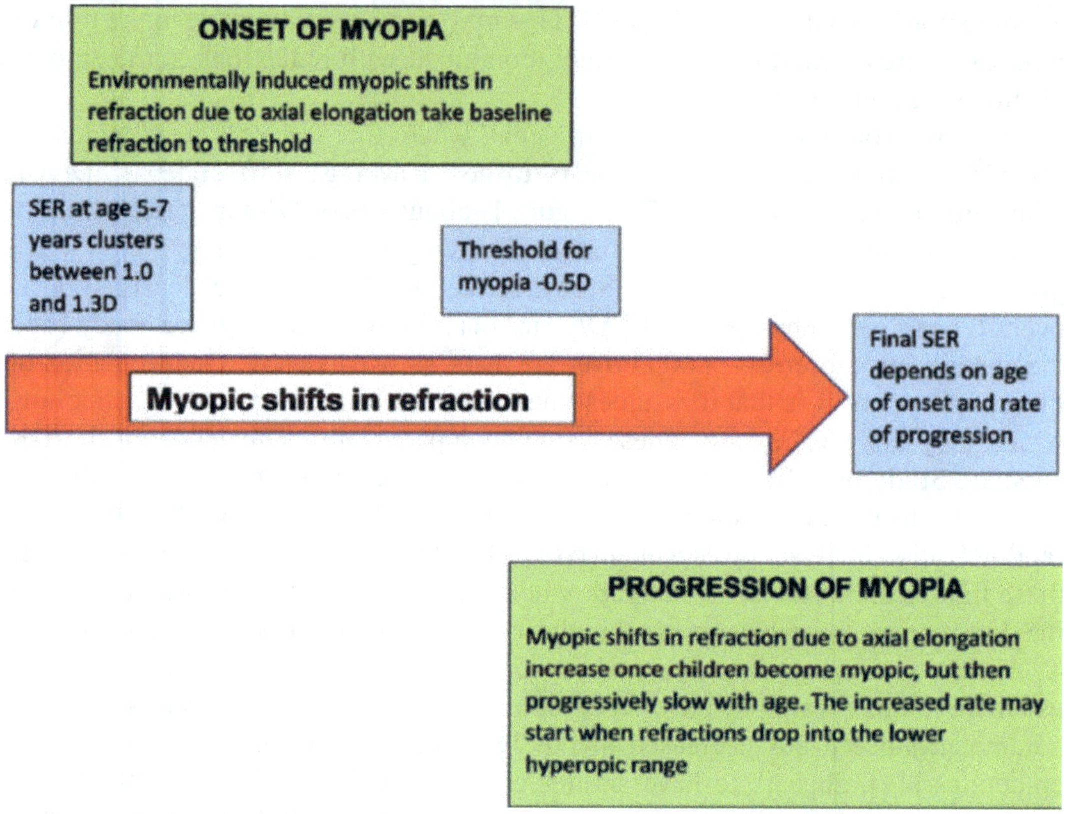

Fig. 6.4 Environmentally driven axial elongation and myopic shifts in refraction lead to final refraction. Rate of axial elongation and myopia shifts in refraction increase prior to the onset of myopia, and remain elevated but decline with age [199, 200]. This increase may begin when SER reaches the low hyperopic range [201]. The earlier the onset, the greater the progression

framework for understanding one of the distinctive characteristics of the current epidemic of "school myopia," the importance of environmental exposures and the modest impact of genetic risk. It also suggests that more work needs to be done on the determinants of spherical equivalent at the age of 5–7 years, and determinants of the age of onset of myopia, because the latter is a significant predictor of subsequent progression and final myopia [187].

Gene–environment interactions also need to be taken into account. It must be remembered that simple environmental regulation of gene expression is not an example of gene–environment interactions. Gene–environment interactions are characterized by situations in which genetic risk and environmental risk combine to produce impacts which are greater or less than expected from their individual effects—or in other words that expression of different alleles of a given gene are differentially affected by different environments. Verhoeven et al. [189] have examined the specific case of the interaction of genetic risk and educational risk, reporting major interactions, with the combination of high genetic risk and high educational risk producing very high risk greater than the arithmetic sum of the individual risks, using the synergy analyses of Rothman [190–192]. Cortina-Borjas et al. [193] have argued that this method produces many false cases of gene–environment interactions, in part because when using odds ratios, risks are more likely to be multiplicative. From our analysis of the data in the paper by Verhoeven et al., the interactions in this paper are close to multiplicative, and we suggest that a more detailed analysis is required. A search for more specific cases has produced some more specific examples of gene–environment interactions [194–197], but the cases reported appear to be rare. More work is clearly needed in this complex area.

6.6 Conclusions

Our overview of risk factors for myopia has identified education and limited time outdoors as the major risk factors for myopia. We suggest that the evidence on these two risk factors is now very strong. These two factors both suggest evidence-based approaches to control of myopia, such as increased time outdoors and decreased near work time. These two factors then appear to converge to regulate eye growth, through cellular and biological pathways that require further definition, but appear to involve regulation of the rate of dopamine release as one component, and axial elongation as another.

Many other risk factors for myopia have been proposed. Many of them may be more distal social factors such as parental and social attitudes to education, provision of educational opportunities, and organization of school systems and schools, and may be mediated by the educational and time outdoor exposures that children receive.

We suggest that future studies in this area need to become more rigorous in several ways. Cycloplegia needs to the required standard in new studies. Mediation analysis needs to become a standard part of risk factor analysis, used to define causal pathways. As a minimum, new studies also need to collect data on educational exposures and time outdoors, increasingly using the new methods for collection of objective data that are becoming available. These higher standards need to be enforced by more rigorous review and publication processes.

While there are many aspects of the risk factors for myopia that require further analysis, the picture that we currently have provides important insight into the characteristics of the current epidemics. In particular, we can now see why genetic effects on "school myopia" are so slight, despite the evidence for a large number of SNPs of small effect size associated with myopia.

The evidence for a major role of education and time outdoors has given us insight into effective means of control, some of which are currently being implemented in myopia control rather than school myopia programs, such as programs aimed to increase time outdoors. Many other interventions at more distal levels also can be envisaged that might reduce early competition for privileged places in schools. When these are combined with clinical interventions to control myopia progression, and there are now many available, in principle, we now understand how to turn back the epidemic of myopia.

But understanding does not automatically lead to success in prevention; after all we have known how to correct refractive errors for some time, but uncorrected refractive error is still a major cause of visual impairment. Research into more effective means of preventing the onset and progression of myopia needs to, and will undoubtedly continue. But the next big challenge may already be to identify and overcome the barriers to implementation, so that we can ensure that we achieve what increasingly appears to be a realizable goal—the prevention of "school myopia."

References

1. Morgan I, Rose K. How genetic is 'school myopia'? Prog Retin Eye Res. 2005;24:1–38.
2. Morgan IG, French AN, Ashby RS, Guo X, Ding X, He M, et al. The epidemics of myopia: aetiology and prevention. Prog Retin Eye Res. 2018;62:134–49.
3. Morgan IG, He M, Rose KA. Epidemic of pathological myopia: what can laboratory studies and epidemiology tell us? Retina. 2017;37:989–97.
4. Morgan IG, Ohno-Matsui K, Saw SM. Myopia. Lancet. 2012;379:1739–48.
5. Hysi PG, Wojciechowski R, Rahi JS, Hammond CJ. Genome-wide association studies of refractive error and myopia, lessons learned, and implications for the future. Invest Ophthalmol Vis Sci. 2014;55:3344–51.
6. Wojciechowski R. Nature and nurture: the complex genetics of myopia and refractive error. Clin Genet. 2011;79:301–20.
7. Wojciechowski R, Cheng CY. Involvement of multiple molecular pathways in the genetics of ocular refraction and myopia. Retina. 2017;38:91–101.
8. Wojciechowski R, Hysi PG. Focusing in on the complex genetics of myopia. PLoS Genet. 2013;9:e1003442.
9. Jung SK, Lee JH, Kakizaki H, Jee D. Prevalence of myopia and its association with body stature and educational level in 19-year-old male conscripts in Seoul, South Korea. Invest Ophthalmol Vis Sci. 2012;53:5579–83.
10. Koh V, Yang A, Saw SM, Chan YH, Lin ST, Tan MM, et al. Differences in prevalence of refractive errors in young Asian males in Singapore between 1996-1997 and 2009-2010. Ophthalmic Epidemiol. 2014;21:247–55.
11. Lin LL, Shih YF, Hsiao CK, Chen CJ. Prevalence of myopia in Taiwanese schoolchildren: 1983 to 2000. Ann Acad Med Singap. 2004;33:27–33.
12. Wu JF, Bi HS, Wang SM, Hu YY, Wu H, Sun W, et al. Refractive error, visual acuity and causes of vision loss in children in Shandong, China. The Shandong Children Eye Study. PLoS One. 2013;8:e82763.
13. Tedja MS, Wojciechowski R, Hysi PG, Eriksson N, Furlotte NA, Verhoeven VJM, et al. Genome-wide association meta-analysis highlights light-induced signaling as a driver for refractive error. Nat Genet. 2018;50:834–48.
14. Flitcroft DI. The complex interactions of retinal, optical and environmental factors in myopia aetiology. Prog Retin Eye Res. 2012;31:622–60.
15. Sankaridurg PR, Holden BA. Practical applications to modify and control the development of ametropia. Eye. 2014;28:134–41.
16. Huang J, Wen D, Wang Q, McAlinden C, Flitcroft I, Chen H, et al. Efficacy comparison of 16 interventions for myopia control in children: a network meta-analysis. Ophthalmology. 2016;123:697–708.
17. Flitcroft DI, Loughman J, Wildsoet CF, Williams C, Guggenheim JA, Consortium C. Novel myopia genes and pathways identified from syndromic forms of myopia. Invest Ophthalmol Vis Sci. 2018;59:338–48.
18. Young TL. Molecular genetics of human myopia: an update. Optom Vis Sci. 2009;86:E8–E22.
19. Guggenheim JA, St Pourcain B, McMahon G, Timpson NJ, Evans DM, Williams C. Assumption-free estimation of the genetic contribution to refractive error across childhood. Mol Vis. 2015;21:621–32.

20. Baird PN, Schache M, Dirani M. The GEnes in Myopia (GEM) study in understanding the aetiology of refractive errors. Prog Retin Eye Res. 2010;29:520–42.
21. Hammond CJ, Snieder H, Gilbert CE, Spector TD. Genes and environment in refractive error: the twin eye study. Invest Ophthalmol Vis Sci. 2001;42:1232–6.
22. Lyhne N, Sjolie AK, Kyvik KO, Green A. The importance of genes and environment for ocular refraction and its determiners: a population based study among 20-45 year old twins. Br J Ophthalmol. 2001;85:1470–6.
23. Manolio TA, Collins FS, Cox NJ, Goldstein DB, Hindorff LA, Hunter DJ, et al. Finding the missing heritability of complex diseases. Nature. 2009;461:747–53.
24. Morgan IG, Rose KA. Myopia: is the nature-nurture debate finally over? Clin Exp Optom. 2019;102:3–17.
25. Varughese S, Varghese RM, Gupta N, Ojha R, Sreenivas V, Puliyel JM. Refractive error at birth and its relation to gestational age. Curr Eye Res. 2005;30:423–8.
26. Cook RC, Glasscock RE. Refractive and ocular findings in the newborn. Am J Ophthalmol. 1951;34:1407–13.
27. Mayer DL, Hansen RM, Moore BD, Kim S, Fulton AB. Cycloplegic refractions in healthy children aged 1 through 48 months. Arch Ophthalmol. 2001;119:1625–8.
28. Mutti DO, Mitchell GL, Jones LA, Friedman NE, Frane SL, Lin WK, et al. Axial growth and changes in lenticular and corneal power during emmetropization in infants. Invest Ophthalmol Vis Sci. 2005;46:3074–80.
29. Morgan IG, Rose KA, Ellwein LB, Refractive Error Study in Children Survey G. Is emmetropia the natural endpoint for human refractive development? An analysis of population-based data from the refractive error study in children (RESC). Acta Ophthalmol. 2010;88:877–84.
30. Sorsby A, Sheridan M, Leary GA, Benjamin B. Vision, visual acuity, and ocular refraction of young men: findings in a sample of 1,033 subjects. Br Med J. 1960;1:1394–8.
31. Wallman J, Winawer J. Homeostasis of eye growth and the question of myopia. Neuron. 2004;43:447–68.
32. French AN, Morgan IG, Mitchell P, Rose KA. Risk factors for incident myopia in Australian schoolchildren: the Sydney adolescent vascular and eye study. Ophthalmology. 2013;120:2100–8.
33. Ma X, Congdon N, Yi H, Zhou Z, Pang X, Meltzer ME, et al. Safety of spectacles for children's vision: a cluster-randomized controlled trial. Am J Ophthalmol. 2015;160:897–904.
34. Zadnik K, Sinnott LT, Cotter SA, Jones-Jordan LA, Kleinstein RN, Manny RE, et al. Prediction of juvenile-onset myopia. JAMA Ophthalmol. 2015;133:683–9.
35. Ehrlich DL, Atkinson J, Braddick O, Bobier W, Durden K. Reduction of infant myopia: a longitudinal cycloplegic study. Vis Res. 1995;35:1313–24.
36. Lam CS, Tang WC, Tse DY, Tang YY, To CH. Defocus incorporated soft contact (DISC) lens slows myopia progression in Hong Kong Chinese schoolchildren: a 2-year randomised clinical trial. Br J Ophthalmol. 2014;98:40–5.
37. Morgan IG, Iribarren R, Fotouhi A, Grzybowski A. Cycloplegic refraction is the gold standard for epidemiological studies. Acta Ophthalmol. 2015;93:581–5.
38. Fotouhi A, Morgan IG, Iribarren R, Khabazkhoob M, Hashemi H. Validity of noncycloplegic refraction in the assessment of refractive errors: the Tehran Eye Study. Acta Ophthalmol. 2012;90:380–6.
39. He X, Zou H, Lu L, Zhao R, Zhao H, Li Q, et al. Axial length/corneal radius ratio: association with refractive state and role on myopia detection combined with visual acuity in Chinese school children. PLoS One. 2015;10:e0111766.
40. Tideman JWL, Polling JR, Vingerling JR, Jaddoe VWV, Williams C, Guggenheim JA, et al. Axial length growth and the risk of developing myopia in European children. Acta Ophthalmol. 2018;96:301–9.
41. Guo Y, Liu LJ, Tang P, Lv YY, Feng Y, Xu L, et al. Outdoor activity and myopia progression in 4-year follow-up of Chinese primary school children: The Beijing Children Eye Study. PLoS One. 2017;12:e0175921.

42. Ip JM, Huynh SC, Robaei D, Kifley A, Rose KA, Morgan IG, et al. Ethnic differences in refraction and ocular biometry in a population-based sample of 11-15-year-old Australian children. Eye. 2008;22:649–56.
43. Ojaimi E, Rose KA, Morgan IG, Smith W, Martin FJ, Kifley A, et al. Distribution of ocular biometric parameters and refraction in a population-based study of Australian children. Invest Ophthalmol Vis Sci. 2005;46:2748–54.
44. Iribarren R. Crystalline lens and refractive development. Prog Retin Eye Res. 2015;47:86–106.
45. Cumberland PM, Bountziouka V, Rahi JS. Impact of varying the definition of myopia on estimates of prevalence and associations with risk factors: time for an approach that serves research, practice and policy. Br J Ophthalmol. 2018;102:1407–12.
46. He M, Xiang F, Zeng Y, Mai J, Chen Q, Zhang J, et al. Effect of time spent outdoors at school on the development of myopia among children in China: a randomized clinical trial. JAMA. 2015;314:1142–8.
47. Rahi JS, Cumberland PM, Peckham CS. Myopia over the lifecourse: prevalence and early life influences in the 1958 British birth cohort. Ophthalmology. 2011;118:797–804.
48. Deere K, Williams C, Leary S, Mattocks C, Ness A, Blair SN, et al. Myopia and later physical activity in adolescence: a prospective study. Br J Sports Med. 2009;43:542–4.
49. Guggenheim JA, McMahon G, Northstone K, Mandel Y, Kaiserman I, Stone RA, et al. Birth order and myopia. Ophthalmic Epidemiol. 2013;20:375–84.
50. Guggenheim JA, Northstone K, McMahon G, Ness AR, Deere K, Mattocks C, et al. Time outdoors and physical activity as predictors of incident myopia in childhood: a prospective cohort study. Invest Ophthalmol Vis Sci. 2012;53:2856–65.
51. Williams KM, Kraphol E, Yonova-Doing E, Hysi PG, Plomin R, Hammond CJ. Early life factors for myopia in the British Twins Early Development Study. Br J Ophthalmol. 2019. https://doi.org/10.1136/bjophthalmol-2018-312439.
52. Vitale S, Ellwein L, Cotch MF, Ferris FL, Sperduto R. Prevalence of refractive error in the United States, 1999-2004. Arch Ophthalmol. 2008;126:1111–9.
53. Kim EC, Morgan IG, Kakizaki H, Kang S, Jee D. Prevalence and risk factors for refractive errors: Korean National Health and Nutrition Examination Survey 2008-2011. PLoS One. 2013;8:e80361.
54. Wolfram C, Hohn R, Kottler U, Wild P, Blettner M, Buhren J, et al. Prevalence of refractive errors in the European adult population: the Gutenberg Health Study (GHS). Br J Ophthalmol. 2014;98:857–61.
55. Cumberland PM, Bao Y, Hysi PG, Foster PJ, Hammond CJ, Rahi JS, et al. Frequency and distribution of refractive error in adult life: methodology and findings of the UK Biobank Study. PLoS One. 2015;10:e0139780.
56. Williams KM, Bertelsen G, Cumberland P, Wolfram C, Verhoeven VJ, Anastasopoulos E, et al. Increasing prevalence of myopia in Europe and the impact of education. Ophthalmology. 2015;122:1489–97.
57. Williams KM, Verhoeven VJ, Cumberland P, Bertelsen G, Wolfram C, Buitendijk GH, et al. Prevalence of refractive error in Europe: the European Eye Epidemiology (E(3)) Consortium. Eur J Epidemiol. 2015;30:305–15.
58. Wang Q, Klein BE, Klein R, Moss SE. Refractive status in the Beaver Dam Eye Study. Invest Ophthalmol Vis Sci. 1994;35:4344–7.
59. Attebo K, Ivers RQ, Mitchell P. Refractive errors in an older population: the Blue Mountains Eye Study. Ophthalmology. 1999;106:1066–72.
60. Wong TY, Foster PJ, Hee J, Ng TP, Tielsch JM, Chew SJ, et al. Prevalence and risk factors for refractive errors in adult Chinese in Singapore. Invest Ophthalmol Vis Sci. 2000;41:2486–94.
61. Hashemi H, Fotouhi A, Mohammad K. The age- and gender-specific prevalences of refractive errors in Tehran: the Tehran Eye Study. Ophthalmic Epidemiol. 2004;11:213–25.
62. Negrel AD, Maul E, Pokharel GP, Zhao J, Ellwein LB. Refractive error study in children: sampling and measurement methods for a multi-country survey. Am J Ophthalmol. 2000;129:421–6.

63. Saw SM, Carkeet A, Chia KS, Stone RA, Tan DT. Component dependent risk factors for ocular parameters in Singapore Chinese children. Ophthalmology. 2002;109:2065–71.
64. Zadnik K. The Glenn A. Fry Award Lecture (1995). Myopia development in childhood. Optom Vis Sci. 1997;74:603–8.
65. Ojaimi E, Rose KA, Smith W, Morgan IG, Martin FJ, Mitchell P. Methods for a population-based study of myopia and other eye conditions in school children: the Sydney Myopia Study. Ophthalmic Epidemiol. 2005;12:59–69.
66. Breslin KM, O'Donoghue L, Saunders KJ. A prospective study of spherical refractive error and ocular components among Northern Irish schoolchildren (the NICER study). Invest Ophthalmol Vis Sci. 2013;54:4843–50.
67. Harrington SC, Stack J, Saunders K, O'Dwyer V. Refractive error and visual impairment in Ireland school children. Br J Ophthalmol. 2019. https://doi.org/10.1136/bjophthalmol-2018-312573.
68. Li SM, Liu LR, Li SY, Ji YZ, Fu J, Wang Y, et al. Design, methodology and baseline data of a school-based cohort study in Central China: the Anyang Childhood Eye Study. Ophthalmic Epidemiol. 2013;20:348–59.
69. Zheng Y, Ding X, Chen Y, He M. The Guangzhou twin project: an update. Twin Res Hum Genet. 2013;16:73–8.
70. Czepita D, Mojsa A, Zejmo M. Prevalence of myopia and hyperopia among urban and rural schoolchildren in Poland. Ann Acad Med Stetin. 2008;54:17–21.
71. Czepita D, Zejmo M, Mojsa A. Prevalence of myopia and hyperopia in a population of Polish school children. Ophthalmic Physiol Opt. 2007;27:60–5.
72. Tideman JWL, Polling JR, Jaddoe VWV, Vingerling JR, Klaver CCW. Environmental risk factors can reduce axial length elongation and myopia incidence in 6- to 9-year-old children. Ophthalmology. 2019;126:127–36.
73. Ehrlich DL, Braddick OJ, Atkinson J, Anker S, Weeks F, Hartley T, et al. Infant emmetropization: longitudinal changes in refraction components from nine to twenty months of age. Optom Vis Sci. 1997;74:822–43.
74. Giordano L, Friedman DS, Repka MX, Katz J, Ibironke J, Hawes P, et al. Prevalence of refractive error among preschool children in an urban population: the Baltimore Pediatric Eye Disease Study. Ophthalmology. 2009;116:739–46.
75. Guo X, Fu M, Ding X, Morgan IG, Zeng Y, He M. Significant axial elongation with minimal change in refraction in 3- to 6-year-old chinese preschoolers: the Shenzhen Kindergarten Eye Study. Ophthalmology. 2017;124:1826–38.
76. Mutti DO, Sinnott LT, Lynn Mitchell G, Jordan LA, Friedman NE, Frane SL, et al. Ocular component development during infancy and early childhood. Optom Vis Sci. 2018;95:976–85.
77. Wen G, Tarczy-Hornoch K, McKean-Cowdin R, Cotter SA, Borchert M, Lin J, et al. Prevalence of myopia, hyperopia, and astigmatism in non-Hispanic white and Asian children: multi-ethnic pediatric eye disease study. Ophthalmology. 2013;120:2109–16.
78. Zylbermann R, Landau D, Berson D. The influence of study habits on myopia in Jewish teenagers. J Pediatr Ophthalmol Strabismus. 1993;30:319–22.
79. Paternoster L, Tilling K, Smith GD. Genetic epidemiology and Mendelian randomization for informing disease therapeutics: conceptual and methodological challenges. PLoS Genet. 2017;13:e1006944.
80. Smith GD, Ebrahim S. Mendelian randomization: prospects, potentials, and limitations. Int J Epidemiol. 2004;33:30–42.
81. Cuellar-Partida G, Lu Y, Kho PF, Hewitt AW, Wichmann HE, Yazar S, et al. Assessing the genetic predisposition of education on myopia: a Mendelian randomization study. Genet Epidemiol. 2016;40:66–72.
82. Cuellar-Partida G, Williams KM, Yazar S, Guggenheim JA, Hewitt AW, Williams C, et al. Genetically low vitamin D concentrations and myopic refractive error: a Mendelian randomization study. Int J Epidemiol. 2017;46:1882–90.
83. Mountjoy E, Davies N, Plotnikov D, Davey Smith G, Rodriguez S, Williams C, Guggenheim J, Atan D. Education and myopia: a Mendelian randomisation study. BMJ. 2018;361:k2022.

84. Curtin BJ. The myopias: basic science and clinical management. Philadelphia: Harper and Row; 1985.
85. Lee H, Herbert RD, McAuley JH. Mediation analysis. JAMA. 2019;321(7):697–8.
86. Brotman DJ, Walker E, Lauer MS, O'Brien RG. In search of fewer independent risk factors. Arch Intern Med. 2005;165:138–45.
87. Saw SM, Tan SB, Fung D, Chia KS, Koh D, Tan DT, et al. IQ and the association with myopia in children. Invest Ophthalmol Vis Sci. 2004;45:2943–8.
88. Saw SM, Cheng A, Fong A, Gazzard G, Tan DT, Morgan I. School grades and myopia. Ophthalmic Physiol Opt. 2007;27:126–9.
89. Shayer M, Ginsburg D. Thirty years on--a large anti-Flynn effect? (II): 13- and 14-year-olds. Piagetian tests of formal operations norms 1976-2006/7. Br J Educ Psychol. 2009;79: 409–18.
90. Shayer M, Ginsburg D, Coe R. Thirty years on - a large anti-Flynn effect? The Piagetian test volume & heaviness norms 1975-2003. Br J Educ Psychol. 2007;77:25–41.
91. Sauce B, Matzel LD. The paradox of intelligence: heritability and malleability coexist in hidden gene-environment interplay. Psychol Bull. 2018;144:26–47.
92. Williams KM, Hysi PG, Yonova-Doing E, Mahroo OA, Snieder H, Hammond CJ. Phenotypic and genotypic correlation between myopia and intelligence. Sci Rep. 2017;7:45977.
93. Au Eong KG, Tay TH, Lim MK. Education and myopia in 110,236 young Singaporean males. Singap Med J. 1993;34:489–92.
94. Lee KE, Klein BE, Klein R, Wong TY. Changes in refraction over 10 years in an adult population: the Beaver Dam Eye study. Invest Ophthalmol Vis Sci. 2002;43:2566–71.
95. Quek TP, Chua CG, Chong CS, Chong JH, Hey HW, Lee J, et al. Prevalence of refractive errors in teenage high school students in Singapore. Ophthalmic Physiol Opt. 2004;24:47–55.
96. French AN, Morgan IG, Burlutsky G, Mitchell P, Rose KA. Prevalence and 5- to 6-year incidence and progression of myopia and hyperopia in Australian schoolchildren. Ophthalmology. 2013;120:1482–91.
97. Ma Y, Qu X, Zhu X, Xu X, Zhu J, Sankaridurg P, et al. Age-specific prevalence of visual impairment and refractive error in children aged 3-10 years in Shanghai, China. Invest Ophthalmol Vis Sci. 2016;57:6188–96.
98. Tsai DC, Fang SY, Huang N, Hsu CC, Chen SY, Chiu AW, et al. Myopia development among young schoolchildren: the myopia investigation study in Taipei. Invest Ophthalmol Vis Sci. 2016;57:6852–60.
99. Morgan IG, Rose KA. Myopia and international educational performance. Ophthalmic Physiol Opt. 2013;33:329–38.
100. Ip JM, Saw SM, Rose KA, Morgan IG, Kifley A, Wang JJ, et al. Role of near work in myopia: findings in a sample of Australian school children. Invest Ophthalmol Vis Sci. 2008;49:2903–10.
101. Huang HM, Chang DS, Wu PC. The association between near work activities and myopia in children-a systematic review and meta-analysis. PLoS One. 2015;10:e0140419.
102. Wildsoet C. Neural pathways subserving negative lens-induced emmetropization in chicks--insights from selective lesions of the optic nerve and ciliary nerve. Curr Eye Res. 2003;27:371–85.
103. McBrien NA, Moghaddam HO, New R, Williams LR. Experimental myopia in a diurnal mammal (Sciurus carolinensis) with no accommodative ability. J Physiol. 1993;469: 427–41.
104. McBrien NA, Moghaddam HO, Reeder AP. Atropine reduces experimental myopia and eye enlargement via a nonaccommodative mechanism. Invest Ophthalmol Vis Sci. 1993;34:205–15.
105. Mutti DO, Mitchell GL, Hayes JR, Jones LA, Moeschberger ML, Cotter SA, et al. Accommodative lag before and after the onset of myopia. Invest Ophthalmol Vis Sci. 2006;47:837–46.
106. Smith EL. Prentice award lecture 2010: a case for peripheral optical treatment strategies for myopia. Optom Vis Sci. 2011;88:1029–44.

107. Hoogerheide J, Rempt F, Hoogenboom WP. Acquired myopia in young pilots. Ophthalmologica. 1971;163:209–15.
108. Smith EL, Hung LF, Huang J. Relative peripheral hyperopic defocus alters central refractive development in infant monkeys. Vis Res. 2009;49:2386–92.
109. Atchison DA, Rosen R. The possible role of peripheral refraction in development of myopia. Optom Vis Sci. 2016;93:1042–4.
110. Sng CC, Lin XY, Gazzard G, Chang B, Dirani M, Lim L, et al. Change in peripheral refraction over time in Singapore Chinese children. Invest Ophthalmol Vis Sci. 2011;52:7880–7.
111. Smith EL, Hung LF, Huang J, Arumugam B. Effects of local myopic defocus on refractive development in monkeys. Optom Vis Sci. 2013;90:1176–86.
112. Aleman AC, Wang M, Schaeffel F. Reading and myopia: contrast polarity matters. Sci Rep. 2018;8:10840.
113. Boelen MK, Boelen MG, Marshak DW. Light-stimulated release of dopamine from the primate retina is blocked by 1-2-amino-4-phosphonobutyric acid (APB). Vis Neurosci. 1998;15:97–103.
114. Iuvone PM, Tigges M, Stone RA, Lambert S, Laties AM. Effects of apomorphine, a dopamine receptor agonist, on ocular refraction and axial elongation in a primate model of myopia. Invest Ophthalmol Vis Sci. 1991;32:1674–7.
115. McCarthy CS, Megaw P, Devadas M, Morgan IG. Dopaminergic agents affect the ability of brief periods of normal vision to prevent form-deprivation myopia. Exp Eye Res. 2007;84:100–7.
116. French AN, Ashby RS, Morgan IG, Rose KA. Time outdoors and the prevention of myopia. Exp Eye Res. 2013;114:58–68.
117. Xiong S, Sankaridurg P, Naduvilath T, Zang J, Zou H, Zhu J, et al. Time spent in outdoor activities in relation to myopia prevention and control: a meta-analysis and systematic review. Acta Ophthalmol. 2017;95:551–66.
118. Rose KA, Morgan IG, Ip J, Kifley A, Huynh S, Smith W, et al. Outdoor activity reduces the prevalence of myopia in children. Ophthalmology. 2008;115:1279–85.
119. Jones LA, Sinnott LT, Mutti DO, Mitchell GL, Moeschberger ML, Zadnik K. Parental history of myopia, sports and outdoor activities, and future myopia. Invest Ophthalmol Vis Sci. 2007;48:3524–32.
120. Wu PC, Chen CT, Lin KK, Sun CC, Kuo CN, Huang HM, et al. Myopia prevention and outdoor light intensity in a school-based cluster randomized trial. Ophthalmology. 2018;125:1239–50.
121. Wu PC, Tsai CL, Hu CH, Yang YH. Effects of outdoor activities on myopia among rural school children in Taiwan. Ophthalmic Epidemiol. 2010;17:338–42.
122. Ashby R, Ohlendorf A, Schaeffel F. The effect of ambient illuminance on the development of deprivation myopia in chicks. Invest Ophthalmol Vis Sci. 2009;50:5348–54.
123. Ashby RS, Schaeffel F. The effect of bright light on lens compensation in chicks. Invest Ophthalmol Vis Sci. 2010;51:5247–53.
124. Karouta C, Ashby RS. Correlation between light levels and the development of deprivation myopia. Invest Ophthalmol Vis Sci. 2015;56:299–309.
125. Smith EL, Hung LF, Arumugam B, Huang J. Negative lens-induced myopia in infant monkeys: effects of high ambient lighting. Invest Ophthalmol Vis Sci. 2013;54:2959–69.
126. Smith EL, Hung LF, Huang J. Protective effects of high ambient lighting on the development of form-deprivation myopia in rhesus monkeys. Invest Ophthalmol Vis Sci. 2012;53:421–8.
127. Guggenheim JA, Williams C, Northstone K, Howe LD, Tilling K, St Pourcain B, et al. Does vitamin D mediate the protective effects of time outdoors on myopia? Findings from a prospective birth cohort. Invest Ophthalmol Vis Sci. 2014;55:8550–8.
128. Read SA, Collins MJ, Vincent SJ. Light exposure and eye growth in childhood. Invest Ophthalmol Vis Sci. 2015;56:6779–87.
129. Hua WJ, Jin JX, Wu XY, Yang JW, Jiang X, Gao GP, et al. Elevated light levels in schools have a protective effect on myopia. Ophthalmic Physiol Opt. 2015;35:252–62.

130. Jones-Jordan LA, Sinnott LT, Cotter SA, Kleinstein RN, Manny RE, Mutti DO, et al. Time outdoors, visual activity, and myopia progression in juvenile-onset myopes. Invest Ophthalmol Vis Sci. 2012;53:7169–75.
131. Cui D, Trier K, Munk R-MS. Effect of day length on eye growth, myopia progression, and change of corneal power in myopic children. Ophthalmology. 2013;120:1074–9.
132. Deng L, Gwiazda J, Thorn F. Children's refractions and visual activities in the school year and summer. Optom Vis Sci. 2010;87:406–13.
133. Deng L, Pang Y. The role of outdoor activity in myopia prevention. Eye Sci. 2015;30: 137–9.
134. Donovan L, Sankaridurg P, Ho A, Chen X, Lin Z, Thomas V, et al. Myopia progression in Chinese children is slower in summer than in winter. Optom Vis Sci. 2012;89:1196–202.
135. Gwiazda J, Deng L, Manny R, Norton TT, Group CS. Seasonal variations in the progression of myopia in children enrolled in the correction of myopia evaluation trial. Invest Ophthalmol Vis Sci. 2014;55:752–8.
136. Sanchez-Tocino H, Villanueva Gomez A, Gordon Bolanos C, Alonso Alonso I, Vallelado Alvarez A, Garcia Zamora M, et al. The effect of light and outdoor activity in natural lighting on the progression of myopia in children. J Fr Ophtalmol. 2019;42:2–10.
137. Dirani M, Crowston JG, Wong TY. From reading books to increased smart device screen time. Br J Ophthalmol. 2019;103:1–2.
138. Saxena R, Vashist P, Tandon R, Pandey RM, Bhardawaj A, Gupta V, et al. Incidence and progression of myopia and associated factors in urban school children in Delhi: The North India Myopia Study (NIM Study). PLoS One. 2017;12:e0189774.
139. Ojaimi E, Robaei D, Rochtchina E, Rose KA, Morgan IG, Mitchell P. Impact of birth parameters on eye size in a population-based study of 6-year-old Australian children. Am J Ophthalmol. 2005;140:535–7.
140. He M, Huang W, Li Y, Zheng Y, Yin Q, Foster PJ. Refractive error and biometry in older Chinese adults: the Liwan eye study. Invest Ophthalmol Vis Sci. 2009;50:5130–6.
141. He M, Zeng J, Liu Y, Xu J, Pokharel GP, Ellwein LB. Refractive error and visual impairment in urban children in Southern China. Invest Ophthalmol Vis Sci. 2004;45:793–9.
142. Edwards MH. Effect of parental myopia on the development of myopia in Hong Kong Chinese. Ophthalmic Physiol Opt. 1998;18:477–83.
143. Ip JM, Huynh SC, Robaei D, Rose KA, Morgan IG, Smith W, et al. Ethnic differences in the impact of parental myopia: findings from a population-based study of 12-year-old Australian children. Invest Ophthalmol Vis Sci. 2007;48:2520–8.
144. Liang CL, Yen E, Su JY, Liu C, Chang TY, Park N, et al. Impact of family history of high myopia on level and onset of myopia. Invest Ophthalmol Vis Sci. 2004;45:3446–52.
145. Mutti DO, Mitchell GL, Moeschberger ML, Jones LA, Zadnik K. Parental myopia, near work, school achievement, and children's refractive error. Invest Ophthalmol Vis Sci. 2002;43:3633–40.
146. Xiang F, He M, Morgan IG. The impact of parental myopia on myopia in Chinese children: population-based evidence. Optom Vis Sci. 2012;89:1487–96.
147. Xiang F, He M, Morgan IG. The impact of severity of parental myopia on myopia in Chinese children. Optom Vis Sci. 2012;89:884–91.
148. Wu MM, Edwards MH. The effect of having myopic parents: an analysis of myopia in three generations. Optom Vis Sci. 1999;76:387–92.
149. Ghorbani Mojarrad N, Williams C, Guggenheim JA. A genetic risk score and number of myopic parents independently predict myopia. Ophthalmic Physiol Opt. 2018;38:492–502.
150. Rosner M, Belkin M. Intelligence, education, and myopia in males. Arch Ophthalmol. 1987;105:1508–11.
151. Ip JM, Rose KA, Morgan IG, Burlutsky G, Mitchell P. Myopia and the urban environment: findings in a sample of 12-year-old Australian school children. Invest Ophthalmol Vis Sci. 2008;49:3858–63.
152. Zhang M, Li L, Chen L, Lee J, Wu J, Yang A, et al. Population density and refractive error among Chinese children. Invest Ophthalmol Vis Sci. 2010;51:4969–76.

153. Dadvand P, Sunyer J, Alvarez-Pedrerol M, Dalmau-Bueno A, Esnaola M, Gascon M, et al. Green spaces and spectacles use in schoolchildren in Barcelona. Environ Res. 2017;152:256–62.
154. Dadvand P, Nieuwenhuijsen MJ, Basagana X, Alvarez-Pedrerol M, Dalmau-Bueno A, Cirach M, et al. Traffic-related air pollution and spectacles use in schoolchildren. PLoS One. 2017;12:e0167046.
155. Choi KY, Yu WY, Lam CHI, Li ZC, Chin MP, Lakshmanan Y, et al. Childhood exposure to constricted living space: a possible environmental threat for myopia development. Ophthalmic Physiol Opt. 2017;37:568–75.
156. Saw SM, Chua WH, Hong CY, Wu HM, Chia KS, Stone RA, et al. Height and its relationship to refraction and biometry parameters in Singapore Chinese children. Invest Ophthalmol Vis Sci. 2002;43:1408–13.
157. Rosner M, Laor A, Belkin M. Myopia and stature: findings in a population of 106,926 males. Eur J Ophthalmol. 1995;5:1–6.
158. Bann D, Johnson W, Li L, Kuh D, Hardy R. Socioeconomic inequalities in childhood and adolescent body-mass index, weight, and height from 1953 to 2015: an analysis of four longitudinal, observational, British birth cohort studies. Lancet Public Health. 2018;3: e194–203.
159. Cordain L, Eaton SB, Brand Miller J, Lindeberg S, Jensen C. An evolutionary analysis of the aetiology and pathogenesis of juvenile-onset myopia. Acta Ophthalmol Scand. 2002;80:125–35.
160. Jee D, Morgan IG, Kim EC. Inverse relationship between sleep duration and myopia. Acta Ophthalmol. 2016;94:e204–10.
161. Zhou Z, Morgan IG, Chen Q, Jin L, He M, Congdon N. Disordered sleep and myopia risk among Chinese children. PLoS One. 2015;10:e0121796.
162. Ayaki M, Torii H, Tsubota K, Negishi K. Decreased sleep quality in high myopia children. Sci Rep. 2016;6:33902.
163. Kearney S, O'Donoghue L, Pourshahidi LK, Cobice D, Saunders KJ. Myopes have significantly higher serum melatonin concentrations than non-myopes. Ophthalmic Physiol Opt. 2017;37:557–67.
164. Chakraborty R, Ostrin LA, Nickla DL, Iuvone PM, Pardue MT, Stone RA. Circadian rhythms, refractive development, and myopia. Ophthalmic Physiol Opt. 2018;38:217–45.
165. Saw SM, Chia KS, Lindstrom JM, Tan DT, Stone RA. Childhood myopia and parental smoking. Br J Ophthalmol. 2004;88:934–7.
166. Iyer JV, Low WC, Dirani M, Saw SM. Parental smoking and childhood refractive error: the STARS study. Eye. 2012;26:1324–8.
167. Stone RA, Wilson LB, Ying GS, Liu C, Criss JS, Orlow J, et al. Associations between childhood refraction and parental smoking. Invest Ophthalmol Vis Sci. 2006;47:4277–87.
168. Nam GE, Hwang BE, Lee YC, Paik JS, Yang SW, Chun YH, et al. Lower urinary cotinine level is associated with a trend toward more myopic refractive errors in Korean adolescents. Eye. 2017;31:1060–7.
169. Booth AJ, Kee HJ. Birth order matters. The effect of family size and birth order on educational attainment. J Popul Econ. 2009;22:367–97.
170. Guggenheim JA, Williams C, UK Biobank Eye and Vision Consortium. Role of educational exposure in the association between myopia and birth order. JAMA Ophthalmol. 2015;133:1408–14.
171. Zhao L, Zhou M. Do only children have poor vision? Evidence from China's one-child policy. Health Econ. 2018;27:1131–46.
172. Mandel Y, Grotto I, El-Yaniv R, Belkin M, Israeli E, Polat U, et al. Season of birth, natural light, and myopia. Ophthalmology. 2008;115:686–92.
173. McMahon G, Zayats T, Chen YP, Prashar A, Williams C, Guggenheim JA. Season of birth, daylight hours at birth, and high myopia. Ophthalmology. 2009;116:468–73.
174. Herbort CP, Papadia M, Neri P. Myopia and inflammation. J Ophthalmic Vis Res. 2011;6:270–83.

175. Lin HJ, Wei CC, Chang CY, Chen TH, Hsu YA, Hsieh YC, et al. Role of chronic inflammation in myopia progression: clinical evidence and experimental validation. EBioMedicine. 2016;10:269–81.
176. Wei CC, Kung YJ, Chen CS, Chang CY, Lin CJ, Tien PT, et al. Allergic conjunctivitis-induced retinal inflammation promotes myopia progression. EBioMedicine. 2018;28:274–86.
177. Shafer BM, Qiu M, Rapuano CJ, Shields CL. Association between hay fever and high myopia in United States adolescents and adults. Eye Contact Lens. 2017;43:186–91.
178. Kung YJ, Wei CC, Chen LA, Chen JY, Chang CY, Lin CJ, et al. Kawasaki disease increases the incidence of myopia. Biomed Res Int. 2017;2017:2657913.
179. Ait-Khaled N, Pearce N, Anderson HR, Ellwood P, Montefort S, Shah J, et al. Global map of the prevalence of symptoms of rhinoconjunctivitis in children: The International Study of Asthma and Allergies in Childhood (ISAAC) phase three. Allergy. 2009;64:123–48.
180. Gordon-Shaag A, Millodot M, Kaiserman I, Sela T, Barnett Itzhaki G, Zerbib Y, et al. Risk factors for keratoconus in Israel: a case-control study. Ophthalmic Physiol Opt. 2015;35:673–81.
181. Guggenheim JA, Williams C, Eye UKB, Vision C. Childhood febrile illness and the risk of myopia in UK Biobank participants. Eye. 2016;30:608–14.
182. Morgan RW, Munro M. Refractive problems in Northern natives. Can J Ophthalmol. 1973;8:226–8.
183. Morgan RW, Speakman JS, Grimshaw SE. Inuit myopia: an environmentally induced "epidemic"? Can Med Assoc J. 1975;112:575–7.
184. Young FA, Leary GA, Baldwin WR, West DC, Box RA, Harris E, et al. The transmission of refractive errors within eskimo families. Am J Optom Arch Am Acad Optom. 1969;46:676–85.
185. Pokharel GP, Negrel AD, Munoz SR, Ellwein LB. Refractive error study in children: results from Mechi zone, Nepal. Am J Ophthalmol. 2000;129:436–44.
186. Verhoeven VJ, Hysi PG, Wojciechowski R, Fan Q, Guggenheim JA, Hohn R, et al. Genome-wide meta-analyses of multiancestry cohorts identify multiple new susceptibility loci for refractive error and myopia. Nat Genet. 2013;45:314–8.
187. Chua SY, Sabanayagam C, Cheung YB, Chia A, Valenzuela RK, Tan D, et al. Age of onset of myopia predicts risk of high myopia in later childhood in myopic Singapore children. Ophthalmic Physiol Opt. 2016;36:388–94.
188. Lan W, Zhao F, Lin L, Li Z, Zeng J, Yang Z, et al. Refractive errors in 3-6 year-old Chinese children: a very low prevalence of myopia? PLoS One. 2013;8:e78003.
189. Verhoeven VJ, Buitendijk GH, Consortium for Refractive E, Myopia, Rivadeneira F, Uitterlinden AG, et al. Education influences the role of genetics in myopia. Eur J Epidemiol. 2013;28:973–80.
190. Rothman KJ. Synergy and antagonism in cause-effect relationships. Am J Epidemiol. 1974;99:385–8.
191. Rothman KJ. The estimation of synergy or antagonism. Am J Epidemiol. 1976;103:506–11.
192. Rothman KJ. Estimation versus detection in the assessment of synergy. Am J Epidemiol. 1978;108:9–11.
193. Cortina-Borja M, Smith AD, Combarros O, Lehmann DJ. The synergy factor: a statistic to measure interactions in complex diseases. BMC Res Notes. 2009;2:105.
194. Fan Q, Guo X, Tideman JW, Williams KM, Yazar S, Hosseini SM, et al. Childhood gene-environment interactions and age-dependent effects of genetic variants associated with refractive error and myopia: The CREAM Consortium. Sci Rep. 2016;6:25853.
195. Fan Q, Verhoeven VJ, Wojciechowski R, Barathi VA, Hysi PG, Guggenheim JA, et al. Meta-analysis of gene-environment-wide association scans accounting for education level identifies additional loci for refractive error. Nat Commun. 2016;7:11008.
196. Fan Q, Wojciechowski R, Kamran Ikram M, Cheng CY, Chen P, Zhou X, et al. Education influences the association between genetic variants and refractive error: a meta-analysis of five Singapore studies. Hum Mol Genet. 2014;23:546–54.
197. Tkatchenko AV, Tkatchenko TV, Guggenheim JA, Verhoeven VJ, Hysi PG, Wojciechowski R, et al. APLP2 regulates refractive error and myopia development in mice and humans. PLoS Genet. 2015;11:e1005432.

198. Xu L, Li J, Cui T, Hu A, Fan G, Zhang R, et al. Refractive error in urban and rural adult Chinese in Beijing. Ophthalmology. 2005;112(10):1676–83.
199. Mutti DO, Sinnott LT, Mitchell GL, Jones-Jordan LA, Moeschberger ML, Cotter SA, et al. Relative peripheral refractive error and the risk of onset and progression of myopia in children. Invest Ophthalmol Vis Sci. 2011;52(1):199–205.
200. Xiang F, He M, Morgan IG. Annual changes in refractive errors and ocular components before and after the onset of myopia in Chinese children. Ophthalmology. 2012;119(7):1478–84.
201. Thorn F, Gwiazda J, Held R. Myopia progression is specified by a double exponential growth function. Optom Vis Sci. 2005;82(4):286–97.

Prevention of Myopia Onset

7

Mingguang He, Yanxian Chen, and Yin Hu

Key Points

- Time spent outdoors is well recognized as a factor preventing the development of myopia onset, and measures including adding an outdoor class, locking classroom doors during class recess, or glassed roof and walls incorporated in a classroom have been developed. But promotion to increase time spent outdoors as a school-based intervention program remains challenging especially in East Asia.
- Near work activity has been suggested as a risk factor for myopia although the evidence is not entirely consistent. The total duration of near work activity may not be as important as the type of near work activity. Core techniques to implementing interventions of near work activities include effective measures of near work-related parameters, real-time data analyses, and alert systems.

M. He (✉)
Centre for Eye Research Australia, Royal Victorian Eye and Ear Hospital, Melbourne, VIC, Australia

Ophthalmology, Department of Surgery, University of Melbourne, Melbourne, VIC, Australia

State Key Laboratory of Ophthalmology, National Clinical Research Center, Zhongshan Ophthalmic Center, Sun Yat-sen University, Guangzhou, China

Y. Chen
Shenzhen Key Laboratory of Ophthalmology, Shenzhen Eye Hospital, Shenzhen University, School of Medicine, Shenzhen, China

Y. Hu
State Key Laboratory of Ophthalmology, National Clinical Research Center, Zhongshan Ophthalmic Center, Sun Yat-sen University, Guangzhou, China

M. Ang, T. Y. Wong (eds.), *Updates on Myopia*,
https://doi.org/10.1007/978-981-13-8491-2_7

- School children growing up in myopigenic environments are likely to benefit from optical interventions designed to induce myopic defocus. The lens with multiple segments of defocus showed promising effect on slowing progression of myopia.
- The Chinese eye exercises of acupoints advocated in mainland China and Taiwan were designed to relieve ocular fatigue and reduce the development and progression of myopia. But clinical significance of its efficacy has not been established according to available data.
- Maximizing the utility of time outdoors is still the priority in the prevention of myopia onset. The role of screen time in myopia development is still ambiguous, the restriction may enable more time for children to go outdoors. Other approaches to prevent myopia onset still require further investigations, such as imposed myopic defocus, low-dose atropine, or some novel pharmacological agents for non-myopes.

7.1 Introduction

Over recent decades, the prevalence of myopia in school-aged children has been increasing significantly in East Asia. Up to 80% of junior high school students have myopia, of which 20% have high myopia in mainland China [1, 2], Hong Kong [3], Taiwan [4], South Korea [5], Japan [6], and Singapore [7]. Longitudinal data suggests that the incidence of myopia is around 10–20% per year among school-aged children [8–11]. If the onset of myopia can be delayed, the prevalence of myopia as well as high myopia in school-aged children will likely reduce. This chapter focuses on the clinical strategy to prevent or delay the onset of myopia among school-aged children, summarizing the interventions currently available, and takes a glance at future perspectives.

7.2 Onset of Myopia

The vast majority of literature suggests that most cases of myopia develop during the school-going age in children. The prevalence of myopia among preschool children is relatively low [12–15]; furthermore, a longitudinal study in Shunyi Beijing demonstrates that the annual incidence of myopia among 5-year-old children is below 5% [16]. After the age of 6 years, the prevalence of myopia starts to rise [6, 16–19]. The highest annual incidence of myopia is reported among school children from urban mainland China [18] and Taiwan [20], ranging from 20% to 30% through ages 7–14 years with earlier onset of myopia also being identified [6]. A study in Japan showed that while the prevalence of myopia has been increasing from 1984 to 1996, the prevalence among children aged 6 or younger has remained unchanged. This suggests that the majority of increased myopia onset is secondary to increased educational intensity and develops when children reach school age (Fig. 7.1) [6].

A long-term longitudinal study has demonstrated that there is a steady shift in refraction toward myopia, before the actual onset of myopia. Rates of progression increase dramatically the year of onset and this has been suggested by spherical equivalent refraction and axial length (Fig. 7.2) [21]. After the first detection of

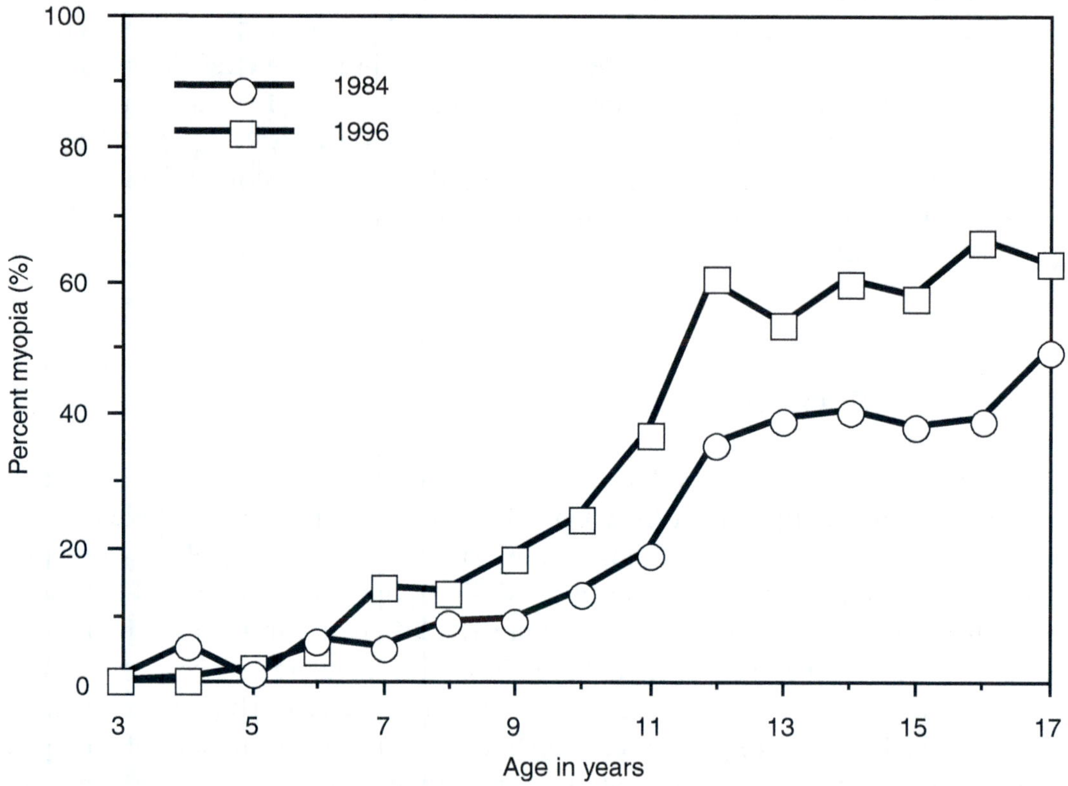

Fig. 7.1 Age-specific prevalence of myopia in Japan in 1984 and 1996. © Matsumura et al. [6]

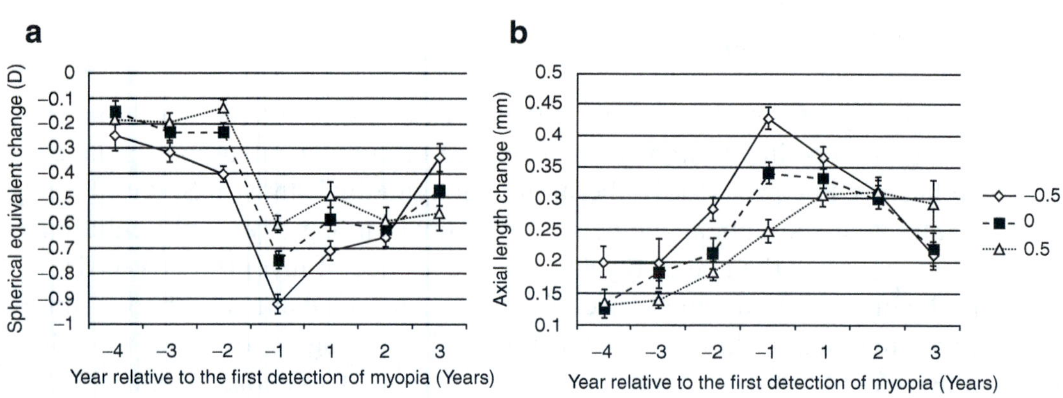

Fig. 7.2 Changes in spherical equivalent refractions (**a**) and axial lengths (**b**) before and after myopia onset. © Xiang et al. [21]

myopia, this acceleration is reduced (Fig. 7.2) [21, 22]. Myopic refractions tend to stabilize in late adolescent but can remain progressive until adulthood. The mean age at myopia stabilization is 15.6 years but this can vary among children of different ethnicities [23].

Several factors have been found to be associated with the development of incident myopia in school. Asian ethnicity [19, 24], parental history of myopia [25, 26], reduced time outdoors [26], and level of near work activity [27, 28] are risk factors for incident myopia, although the evidence can be seen as controversial in some instances. Some studies have also suggested that non-myopic children with less hyperopic refractions and greater axial length/corneal radius of curvature ratios are more predisposed to develop myopia [18, 19]. The impact of gender to the development of myopia varies among populations. In Chinese school children, females have a greater chance of progressing to myopia [18]; while in multiethnic populations, gender seems to be less impactful [19, 24, 27].

Attempts have been made to establish tools to identify children at risk of developing myopia or high myopia. Among numerous associated factors, spherical equivalent refraction is the most promising predictor. By using a single measurement of refraction alone, future myopia onset of non-myopic children can be accurately predicted [29]. Moreover, children at risk of developing high myopia in adulthood can also be identified, with reasonably good sensitivity and specificity, when using an age-specific 5th percentile curve of refraction of the population (Fig. 7.3) as a cutoff [30]. Other promising tools for the prediction of future high myopia include the age of myopia onset [31] and age-specific annual refraction progression of children with myopia (Fig. 7.4) [32]. Information on age of myopia onset alone can predict high myopia with 85% accuracy using a receiver operating curve (ROC) [31].

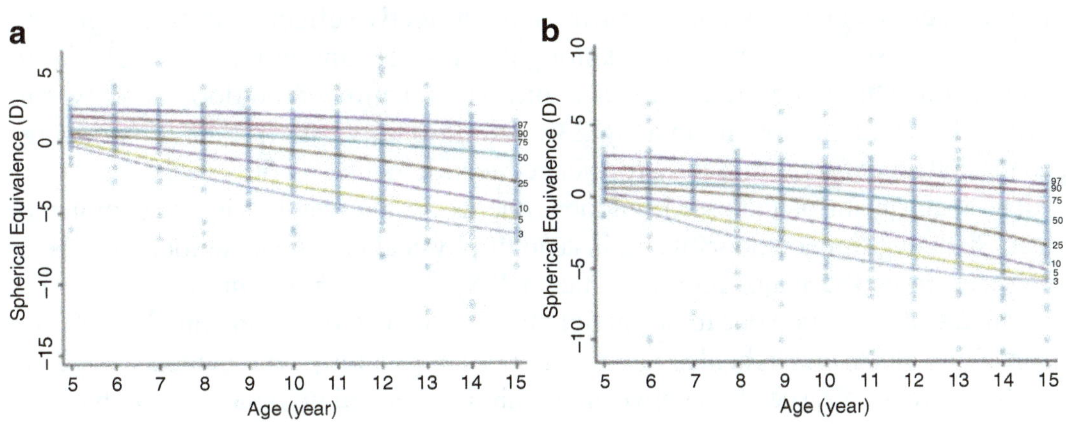

Fig. 7.3 Percentile curves of refractions for urban Chinese boys (**a**) and girls (**b**). © Chen et al. [30]

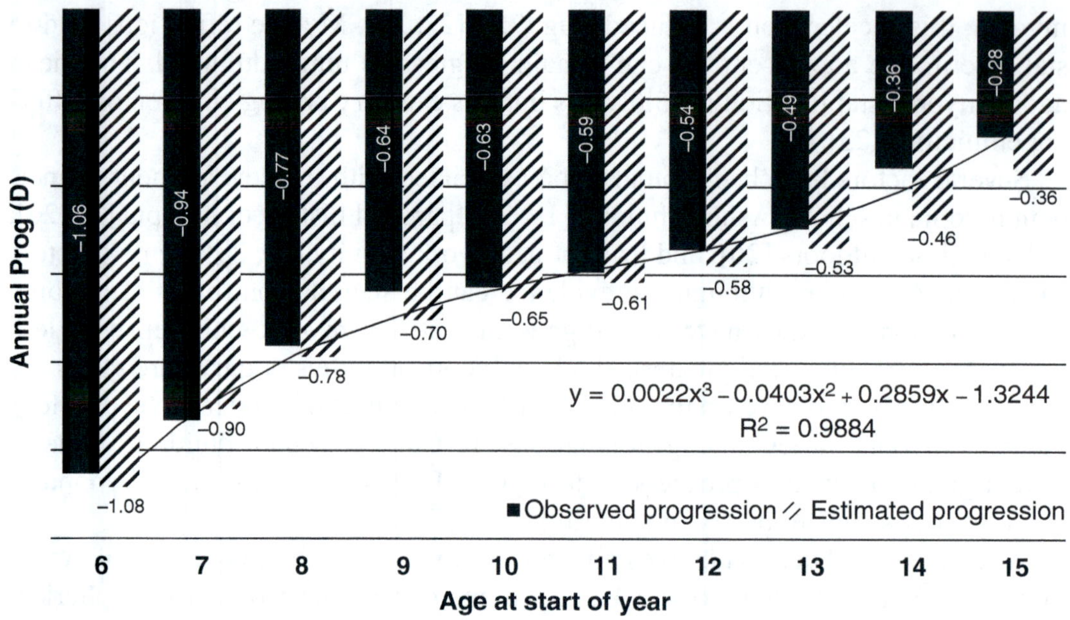

Fig. 7.4 Age-specific annual progression of refraction in children with myopia. © Sankaridurg et al. [32]

7.3 Increased Time Outdoors as an Intervention

Time spent outdoors is well recognized as a factor preventing the development of myopia onset. Evidence of this was first presented in a three-year follow-up study of myopia in school children, showing that those who spent more time outdoors were less likely to progress [33]. Consistent results were reported in various studies, such as the Sydney Myopia Study, Orinda study as well as the Singapore Cohort Study of Risk Factors for Myopia [34–36]. This led to the commencement of several clinical trials, which confirmed the protective effect against myopia and indicated a dose-dependent effect, among them is the randomized clinical trial in Guangzhou which reported that an additional 40 min of outdoor activity can reduce the incidence of myopia by 23%. Additionally, the trial in Taiwan suggested that an extra 80 min may further reduce incidence by 50% [10, 37].

The mechanism of increased outdoor time as an intervention is not completely clear. Spending time outdoors itself, instead of physical activities outdoors, has been suggested to be the major protective factor [38]. Results from animal experiments indicated that protection due to bright light may be mediated by dopamine [39]. Some believe that ultraviolet light also plays an important role [40], with evidence suggesting that there is an association between vitamin D level and myopia [41–43], but data from a population-based cohort did not support this idea [44]. Alternatively, patterns of defocus on the retina by three-dimensional structures of the environment have also been proposed as a possible mechanism of protection from outdoor activities [45].

As an economically feasible intervention, getting children outside the classroom has been promoted in many public health programs such as Taiwan's "Daily 120." However, promotion to increase time spent outdoors as a school-based intervention program remains challenging. First, what is an effective amount of time outdoors? Population-based data suggest that 2–3 h a day would be beneficial [26, 35], however, this is difficult to achieve in some East Asian countries where the education system is very intensive. Some programs recommend adding an outdoor class into the curriculum, while others recommend prohibiting being inside during recess by locking classroom doors. Another group of researchers proposed a classroom design that incorporates a glassed roof and walls that enable maximize light intensity while students study indoors (Fig. 7.5) [46]. The protective effect of this bright classroom is now under investigation. Second, what is the appropriate location for outdoor activities? The ideal location appears to be in an area with bright light more than 10,000 lux, suggested by evidence from animal experiments [47, 48]. But the most recent results from Wu et al.'s study indicated that less bright light exposure, 1000-lux or 3000-lux for instance, is sufficient enough to generate a protective effect (Fig. 7.6) [49]. These findings seem to suggest that an environment such as the shade of a tree or building, the hallway, or playground could still work with an advantage to avoid sunburn or other side effects from UV exposure.

Another concern is how do we measure outdoor activities? Traditionally, questionnaires have been commonly used to measure time outdoors but are less accurate due to recall bias. Objective measures can provide more precise real-time data. Wearable detectors have been developed to record light intensity and time outdoors, and even track the patterns of outdoor activities, including HOBO light meters, Nike+ Fuel Band, and others. Other measures have been used to estimate exposure to natural light such as conjunctival ultraviolet autofluorescence and skin photodamage, but these are more appropriate when measuring the cumulative light dosage or UV exposure [50, 51].

If increased time spent outdoors can prevent or delay the onset of myopia, it would ultimately reduce the prevalence of myopia or even high myopia among

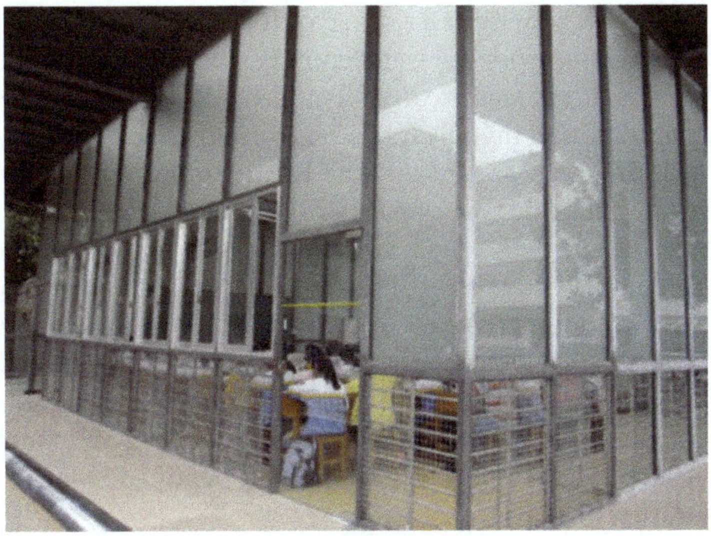

Fig. 7.5 Classroom constructed with glass in China. ©Zhou et al. [46]

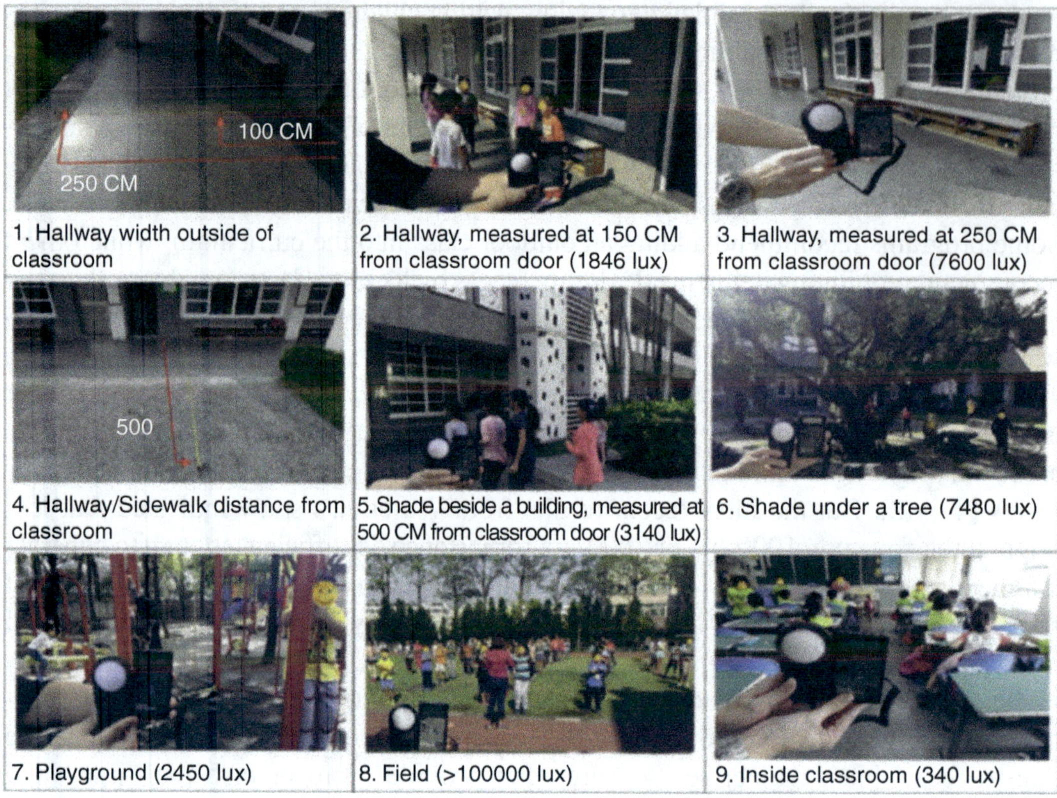
100 CM
250 CM
1. Hallway width outside of classroom
2. Hallway, measured at 150 CM from classroom door (1846 lux)
3. Hallway, measured at 250 CM from classroom door (7600 lux)
500
4. Hallway/Sidewalk distance from classroom
5. Shade beside a building, measured at 500 CM from classroom door (3140 lux)
6. Shade under a tree (7480 lux)
7. Playground (2450 lux)
8. Field (>100000 lux)
9. Inside classroom (340 lux)

Fig. 7.6 Light intensity of different locations in the school. ©Wu et al. [49]

school-aged children. Documentation on the impact of time spent outdoors on the prevalence of myopia is of public health importance.

7.4 Reduced Near Work Intensity as an Intervention

Near work activity as a risk factor for myopia has been documented in some studies, although the evidence is not entirely consistent. A recent meta-analysis has reported a modest, but statistically significant, association between time spent performing near work and myopia (odds ratio, 1.14) [28].

It has been argued that the total duration of near work activity may not be as important as the type of near work activity. Studies have found that continuous reading of more than 30–45 min is associated with the presence of myopia and greater myopic refractive errors [52, 53]. Interestingly, after prolonged continuous reading, children are more likely to take up their preferred relaxed postures [54], such as close reading distance [53] and head tilt [52], both of which have been reported to be associated with the presence of myopia. Other factors that have been proposed to potentially contribute to the development of myopia include close nib-to-finger distance [52], downward angle of gaze [55, 56] and inadequate desk [52], or classroom lighting [56].

Efforts have been dedicated to developing novel devices to detect and correct inadequate near work behaviors. In mainland China, pens for myopia prevention has been invented. The pens are capable of detecting close reading distances (China Invention Patent, 200620010200.6) or nib-to-finger distances (China Invention Patent, 201020640746.6). Real-time retraction of the nib will occur when the eyes are too close to the reading materials or the nib-to-finger distance is inadequate, compelling children to adopt correct postures. The effect of the pens on preventing myopia onset is to be examined by future clinical trials.

Core techniques to implementing interventions of near work activities include effective measures of near work-related parameters, real-time data analyses, and alert systems. Wearable devices that possess these techniques have emerged in the last decade. A head-mounted instrument (Fig. 7.7) was built in Hong Kong for continuous logging of near work distance [57]. Measurements have proved to be accurate and repeatable over a range of distances and angles [57]. The Clouclip (Fig. 7.8) is another novel device developed in mainland China, primarily for the use of

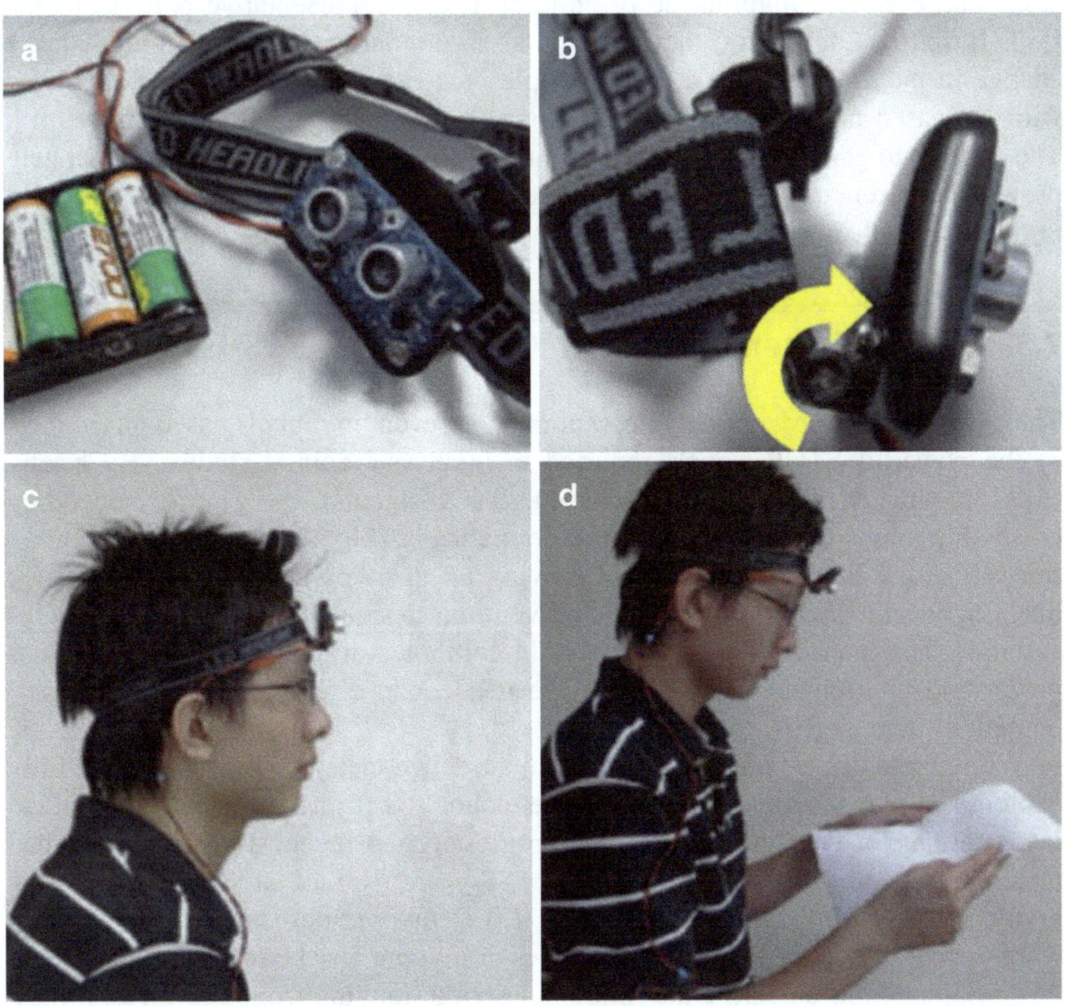

Fig. 7.7 Front view (**a**) and side view (**b**) of the near work analyzer for logging near work distance and its alignment in a straight-ahead position (**c**) and reading position (**d**). © Leung et al. [57]

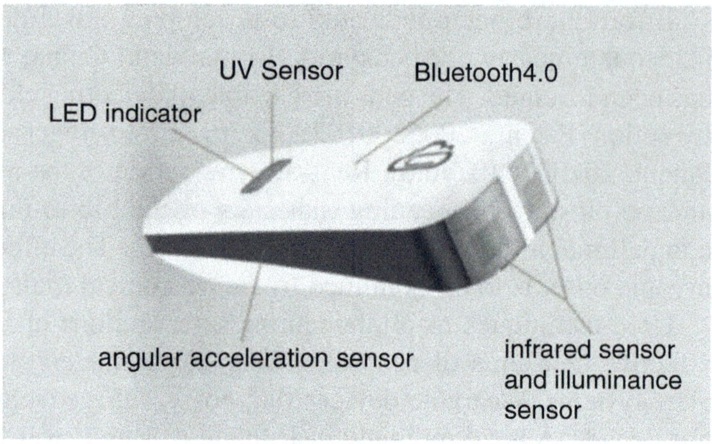

Fig. 7.8 Clouclip to monitor near work time. © Wen et al. [58]

myopic children [58]. The device can measure reading distances and ambient illuminance, perform real-time data analyses, and feedback to children and parents (www.clouclip.com). This group of researchers used Clouclip to track reading distance and eye-level illuminance of children over a representative period of time [59]. Based on these data, they developed a summative index and found that a change in the index toward a more myopic behavior was significantly associated with increased myopic refractive errors in a preliminary longitudinal study [59]. The attempt to generate a simplified, summative index for risk estimation will help provide comprehensive information on near work-related behaviors and may help improve the efficacy of interventions.

7.5 Optical Interventions

The use of noninvasive optical interventions to prevent myopia is based on findings of the powerful STOP signals reported in numerous animal studies. By briefly exposing chickens to myopic defocus (the STOP signals), eye growth induced by presenting minus lenses can be slowed dramatically (Fig. 7.9) [60, 61]. It is therefore suggested that school children growing up in myopigenic environments are likely to benefit from routine optical interventions designed to induce myopic defocus [62]. The intervention regimen should combine variables including age, lens power, and duration of exposure to achieve an adequate effect on delaying the development of myopia [62].

While these optical interventions are an attractive idea, they have not been fully explored in human subjects—this will be elaborated further in Chap. 13 (Optical interventions for Prevention of Myopia Progression). A recent study has prescribed plus lenses to non-myopic children aged 5–8 years who are at risk of developing myopia [63]. The plus lenses imposed a 1.0 D myopic defocus and the children wore the correction the entire day. No cases of myopia onset have been observed in this group of children during the follow-up period (ranging from 3 to 9 years) [63]. The robustness of these study findings needs to be examined by future investigations.

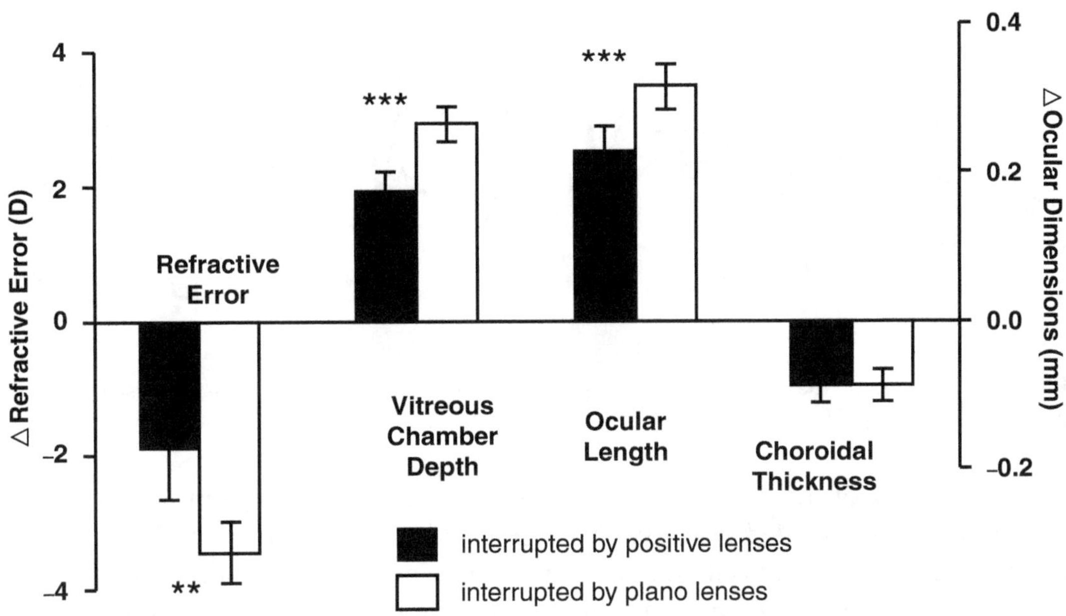

Fig. 7.9 Changes in refractions and ocular biometric parameters over 3 days of binocular negative lens wear interrupted by brief periods of positive lens wear on one eye and plano lens wear on the other eye. $^{**}P < 0.01$; $^{***}P < 0.001$. © Zhu et al. [61]

The Defocus Incorporated Multiple Segments Lens (DIMS Lens) is a novel spectacle lens primarily designed for use in myopic children. The lens is composed of a central zone for optical correction of refractive error and an annular peripheral zone to induce myopic defocus. Interestingly, the lens peripheral zone contains numerous well-arranged small plus lenses, separated by small non-defocus areas. By using this design, myopic defocus is induced and visual quality is well reserved at the same time (presentation at the 16th International Myopia Conference [IMC]). In a pilot study conducted among school children, the DIMS lens slowed progression of myopia by 59% (presentation at the 16th IMC). The lens may also be promising for preventing myopia onset if adaptation can be successfully made for non-myopic children.

7.6 Eye Exercises of Acupoints

The eye exercises of acupoints are a set of bilateral acupoint self-massages designed to relieve ocular fatigue and reduce the development and progression of myopia. These eye exercises were introduced by the Chinese National Education Commission and have been advocated since the 1960s in mainland China and Taiwan. Children in primary and junior middle schools are required to perform the eye exercises twice a day. The 5-min exercises include: (1) knead Tianying (Ashi); (2) press and squeeze Jingming (BL1); (3) press and knead Sibai (ST2); and (4) press Taiyang (EX-HN5) and scrape Cuanzhu (BL2), Yuyao (EX-HN4), Sizhukong (TE23), Tongziliao (GB1), Chengqi (ST1) (Fig. 7.10).

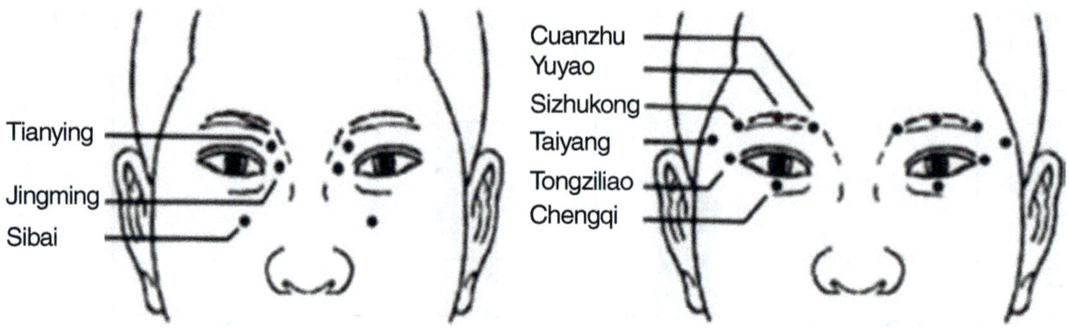

Fig. 7.10 Schematic diagram demonstrating the positions of acupoints used in Chinese eye exercises. © Lin et al. [67]

The efficacy of the Chinese eye exercises is believed to be from the theory of Traditional Chinese Medicine. By massaging the acupoints, Chi can be achieved and help relieve eye strain and recover ocular functions. Peak systolic velocity in the central retinal and ophthalmic arteries is observed after the eye exercises [64], which might provide some evidences to support this theory. Accommodative lag decreases significantly by 0.1 D after 5 min of performing the eye exercises [65].

Clinical significance has never been established in the published literature thus far. Cross-sectional studies have assessed the association between Chinese eye exercises and myopia with varied results [66–69]. The inconsistency can be explained by the different settings studied (rural vs. urban), failure to adjust for potential confounders (including parental myopia, time outdoors, and near work) and the lack of representative populations in some studies. In a recent study, the impact of Chinese eye exercises on the development of myopia has been examined using a longitudinal design [70]. No association between eye exercises and myopia onset has been found [70]. However, due to the limited sample size, low level of intervention time, and performance qualities of the exercises in the study, the actual impact is still not conclusive and needs to be justified by further studies.

7.7 Future Prospects

It has been estimated that without any effective controls or interventions the proportion of myopes in the population will reach up to 50% and 10% for high myopes by 2050 [71]. Approaches that have produced a reduction of at least 50% in incidence, such as time outdoors, have the potential to make a significant difference on the impending myopia epidemic. But the level of impact of the full utility of available interventions needs to be evaluated by further studies.

Another critical issue is how to implement both education intensity and outdoor time interventions in East Asia. There needs to be a balance between educational achievement and interventions delivered, which don't exacerbate the prevalence of myopia in East Asia. This balance can be seen in Australia [72], with some of the highest educational ranks in the world (PISA, https://www.oecd.org/pisa/data/) but

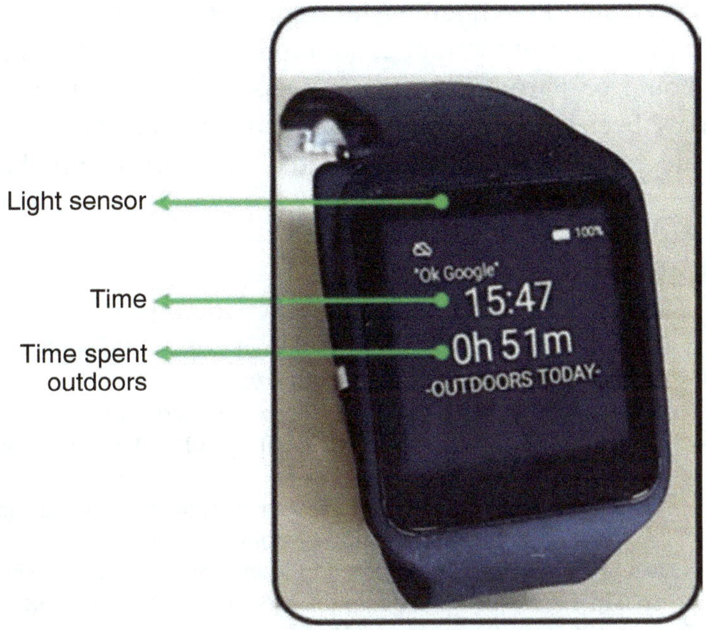

Fig. 7.11 FitSight fitness tracker to record time outdoors. ©Verkicharla et al. [73]

also high levels of outdoor activity and light intensity. Preventing the onset of myopia is certainly challenging in the East Asian population and requires a collaborative effort among clinics, schools, parents, and the entire society.

Nonetheless, maximizing the utility of time outdoors is still the priority in the prevention of myopia onset. The implementation of outdoor activities in school programs and daily life necessitates further propagation and feedback from parents and children. Novel devices combined with the internet and even social networks are a potential direction. An example is FitSight, which was developed by Saw et al. (Fig. 7.11) and comprises of a smartwatch with a light sensor and smartphone app that records time outdoors and sends feedback to parents and children [73]. This kind of devices needs to be proven to be useful by undertaking field study and determining wearability. Additionally, the price of the device should be considered in the design.

Another behavior control method focuses on limiting the screen time on computers, tablets, and smart phones. Though the role of screen time in myopia development is still ambiguous, the restriction may enable more time for children to go outdoors. Applications to provide screen distance and time monitoring, alerts to rest eyes, blue light filters, and remote locking capability for parents are available in some countries (plano, https://www.plano.co/). The effect of this technology on myopia prevention remains to be seen.

Other approaches to prevent myopia onset still require further investigations, such as imposed myopic defocus, low-dose atropine, or some novel pharmacological agents for non-myopes. They may help to prevent myopia in those who are rapidly progressing or have high-risk genetic forms. Thus, a question is raised: how do we identify children that have an increased risk of becoming myopic or highly myopic? Risk estimation is therefore critical to achieve personalized treatment for individuals. For children who are non-myopic but at an increased risk of developing high myopia in the future, additional outdoor activities and aggressive approaches should be introduced with frequent follow-up visits. Tools of myopia prediction have been developed as mentioned before, and we expect to see the outcomes of the integration of risk prediction and clinical practice in the near future.

References

1. Wu LJ, et al. Prevalence and associated factors of myopia in high-school students in Beijing. PLoS One. 2015;10:e0120764. https://doi.org/10.1371/journal.pone.0120764.
2. Wu JF, et al. Refractive error, visual acuity and causes of vision loss in children in Shandong, China. The Shandong Children Eye Study. PLoS One. 2013;8:e82763. https://doi.org/10.1371/journal.pone.0082763.
3. Goh WS, Lam CS. Changes in refractive trends and optical components of Hong Kong Chinese aged 19-39 years. Ophthalmic Physiol Opt. 1994;14:378–82.
4. Lin LL, et al. Epidemiologic study of the prevalence and severity of myopia among schoolchildren in Taiwan in 2000. J Formos Med Assoc. 2001;100:684–91.
5. Jung SK, Lee JH, Kakizaki H, Jee D. Prevalence of myopia and its association with body stature and educational level in 19-year-old male conscripts in Seoul, South Korea. Invest Ophthalmol Vis Sci. 2012;53:5579–83. https://doi.org/10.1167/iovs.12-10106.
6. Matsumura H, Hirai H. Prevalence of myopia and refractive changes in students from 3 to 17 years of age. Surv Ophthalmol. 1999;44(Suppl 1):S109–15.
7. Wu HM, et al. Does education explain ethnic differences in myopia prevalence? A population-based study of young adult males in Singapore. Optom Vis Sci. 2001;78:234–9.
8. Shah RL, Huang Y, Guggenheim JA, Williams C. Time outdoors at specific ages during early childhood and the risk of incident myopia. Invest Ophthalmol Vis Sci. 2017;58:1158–66. https://doi.org/10.1167/iovs.16-20894.
9. Ku P.-W. et al. The associations between near visual activity and incident myopia in children. Ophthalmology. https://doi.org/10.1016/j.ophtha.2018.05.010.
10. He M, et al. Effect of time spent outdoors at school on the development of myopia among children in China: a randomized clinical trial. JAMA. 2015;314:1142–8. https://doi.org/10.1001/jama.2015.10803.
11. Lin LL, Shih YF, Hsiao CK, Chen CJ. Prevalence of myopia in Taiwanese schoolchildren: 1983 to 2000. Ann Acad Med Singap. 2004;33:27–33.
12. Guo X, et al. Significant axial elongation with minimal change in refraction in 3- to 6-year-old Chinese preschoolers: The Shenzhen Kindergarten Eye Study. Ophthalmology. 2017;124:1826–38. https://doi.org/10.1016/j.ophtha.2017.05.030.
13. Giordano L, et al. Prevalence of refractive error among preschool children in an urban population: the Baltimore Pediatric Eye Disease Study. Ophthalmology. 2009;116:739–46. https://doi.org/10.1016/j.ophtha.2008.12.030.
14. Multi-Ethnic Pediatric Eye Disease Study Group. Prevalence of myopia and hyperopia in 6- to 72-month-old african american and Hispanic children: the multi-ethnic pediatric eye disease study. Ophthalmology. 2010;117:140–147.e143. https://doi.org/10.1016/j.ophtha.2009.06.009.
15. Dirani M, et al. Prevalence of refractive error in Singaporean Chinese children: the strabismus, amblyopia, and refractive error in young Singaporean Children (STARS) study. Invest Ophthalmol Vis Sci. 2010;51:1348–55. https://doi.org/10.1167/iovs.09-3587.
16. Zhao J, et al. The progression of refractive error in school-age children: Shunyi district, China. Am J Ophthalmol. 2002;134:735–43.
17. Xiang F, et al. Increases in the prevalence of reduced visual acuity and myopia in Chinese children in Guangzhou over the past 20 years. Eye. 2013;27:1353–8. https://doi.org/10.1038/eye.2013.194.

18. Wang SK, et al. Incidence of and factors associated with myopia and high myopia in Chinese children, based on refraction without cycloplegia. JAMA Ophthalmol. 2018;136:1017–24. https://doi.org/10.1001/jamaophthalmol.2018.2658.
19. Saw SM, et al. Incidence and progression of myopia in Singaporean school children. Invest Ophthalmol Vis Sci. 2005;46:51–7. https://doi.org/10.1167/iovs.04-0565.
20. Tsai DC, et al. Myopia development among young schoolchildren: The Myopia Investigation Study in Taipei. Invest Ophthalmol Vis Sci. 2016;57:6852–60. https://doi.org/10.1167/iovs.16-20288.
21. Xiang F, He M, Morgan IG. Annual changes in refractive errors and ocular components before and after the onset of myopia in Chinese children. Ophthalmology. 2012;119:1478–84. https://doi.org/10.1016/j.ophtha.2012.01.017.
22. Mutti DO, et al. Refractive error, axial length, and relative peripheral refractive error before and after the onset of myopia. Invest Ophthalmol Vis Sci. 2007;48:2510–9. https://doi.org/10.1167/iovs.06-0562.
23. COMET Group. Myopia stabilization and associated factors among participants in the Correction of Myopia Evaluation Trial (COMET). Invest Ophthalmol Vis Sci. 2013;54:7871–84. https://doi.org/10.1167/iovs.13-12403.
24. French AN, Morgan IG, Burlutsky G, Mitchell P, Rose KA. Prevalence and 5- to 6-year incidence and progression of myopia and hyperopia in Australian schoolchildren. Ophthalmology. 2013;120:1482–91. https://doi.org/10.1016/j.ophtha.2012.12.018.
25. Jones-Jordan LA, et al. Early childhood refractive error and parental history of myopia as predictors of myopia. Invest Ophthalmol Vis Sci. 2010;51:115–21. https://doi.org/10.1167/iovs.08-3210.
26. Jones LA, et al. Parental history of myopia, sports and outdoor activities, and future myopia. Invest Ophthalmol Vis Sci. 2007;48:3524–32. https://doi.org/10.1167/iovs.06-1118.
27. Williams C, Miller LL, Gazzard G, Saw SM. A comparison of measures of reading and intelligence as risk factors for the development of myopia in a UK cohort of children. Br J Ophthalmol. 2008;92:1117–21. https://doi.org/10.1136/bjo.2007.128256.
28. Huang HM, Chang DS, Wu PC. The association between near work activities and myopia in children-a systematic review and meta-analysis. PLoS One. 2015;10:e0140419. https://doi.org/10.1371/journal.pone.0140419.
29. Zadnik K, et al. Prediction of juvenile-onset myopia. JAMA Ophthalmol. 2015;133:683–9. https://doi.org/10.1001/jamaophthalmol.2015.0471.
30. Chen Y, Zhang J, Morgan IG, He M. Identifying children at risk of high myopia using population centile curves of refraction. PLoS One. 2016;11:e0167642. https://doi.org/10.1371/journal.pone.0167642.
31. Chua SY, et al. Age of onset of myopia predicts risk of high myopia in later childhood in myopic Singapore children. Ophthalmic Physiol Opt. 2016;36:388–94. https://doi.org/10.1111/opo.12305.
32. Sankaridurg PR, Holden BA. Practical applications to modify and control the development of ametropia. Eye. 2014;28:134–41. https://doi.org/10.1038/eye.2013.255.
33. Parssinen O, Lyyra AL. Myopia and myopic progression among school children: a three-year follow-up study. Invest Ophthalmol Vis Sci. 1993;34:2794–802.
34. Mutti DO, Mitchell GL, Moeschberger ML, Jones LA, Zadnik K. Parental myopia, near work, school achievement, and children's refractive error. Invest Ophthalmol Vis Sci. 2002;43:3633–40.
35. Rose KA, et al. Outdoor activity reduces the prevalence of myopia in children. Ophthalmology. 2008;115:1279–85. https://doi.org/10.1016/j.ophtha.2007.12.019.
36. Dirani M, et al. Outdoor activity and myopia in Singapore teenage children. Br J Ophthalmol. 2009;93:997.
37. Wu PC, Tsai CL, Wu HL, Yang YH, Kuo HK. Outdoor activity during class recess reduces myopia onset and progression in school children. Ophthalmology. 2013;120:1080–5. https://doi.org/10.1016/j.ophtha.2012.11.009.

38. Nina J, Hanne J, Ernst G. Does the level of physical activity in university students influence development and progression of myopia?--a 2-year prospective cohort study. Invest Ophthalmol Vis Sci. 2008;49:1322.
39. Feldkaemper M, Schaeffel F. An updated view on the role of dopamine in myopia. Exp Eye Res. 2013;114:106–19.
40. Prepas SB. Light, literacy and the absence of ultraviolet radiation in the development of myopia. Med Hypotheses. 2008;70:635–7.
41. Jeremy AG, et al. Does vitamin D mediate the protective effects of time outdoors on myopia? Findings from a prospective birth cohort. Invest Ophthalmol Vis Sci. 2015;55:8550–8.
42. Mutti DO, Marks AR. Blood levels of vitamin D in teens and young adults with myopia. Optom Vis Sci. 2011;88:377–82.
43. Tideman JWL, et al. Low serum vitamin D is associated with axial length and risk of myopia in young children. Eur J Epidemiol. 2016;31:491–9.
44. Hammond DS, Josh W, Wildsoet CF. Dynamics of active emmetropisation in young chicks--influence of sign and magnitude of imposed defocus. Ophthalmic Physiol Opt. 2013;33: 215–26.
45. Flitcroft DI. The complex interactions of retinal, optical and environmental factors in myopia aetiology. Prog Retin Eye Res. 2012;31:622–60.
46. Zhou Z, et al. Pilot study of a novel classroom designed to prevent myopia by increasing children's exposure to outdoor light. PLoS One. 2017;12:e0181772. https://doi.org/10.1371/journal.pone.0181772.
47. Cindy K, Regan Scott A. Correlation between light levels and the development of deprivation myopia. Invest Ophthalmol Vis Sci. 2015;56:299–309.
48. Lan W, Yang Z, Feldkaemper M, Schaeffel F. Changes in dopamine and ZENK during suppression of myopia in chicks by intense illuminance. Exp Eye Res. 2016;145:118–24.
49. Wu PC, et al. Myopia prevention and outdoor light intensity in a school-based cluster randomized trial. Ophthalmology. 2018;125(8):1239–50.
50. Mcknight CM, et al. Myopia in young adults is inversely related to an objective marker of ocular sun exposure: The Western Australian Raine Cohort Study. Am J Ophthalmol. 2014;158:1079–1085.e1072.
51. Lingham G, et al. Investigating the long-term impact of a childhood sun-exposure intervention, with a focus on eye health: protocol for the Kidskin-Young Adult Myopia Study. BMJ Open. 2018;8:e020868. https://doi.org/10.1136/bmjopen-2017-020868.
52. Li SM, et al. Near work related parameters and myopia in chinese children: the Anyang Childhood Eye Study. PLoS One. 2015;10:e0134514. https://doi.org/10.1371/journal.pone.0134514.
53. Ip JM, et al. Role of near work in myopia: findings in a sample of Australian school children. Invest Ophthalmol Vis Sci. 2008;49:2903–10. https://doi.org/10.1167/iovs.07-0804.
54. Charman WN. Myopia, posture and the visual environment. Ophthalmic Physiol Opt. 2011;31:494–501. https://doi.org/10.1111/j.1475-1313.2011.00825.x.
55. Vincent SJ, Collins MJ, Read SA, Carney LG, Yap MK. Corneal changes following near work in myopic anisometropia. Ophthalmic Physiol Opt. 2013;33:15–25. https://doi.org/10.1111/opo.12003.
56. Hua WJ, et al. Elevated light levels in schools have a protective effect on myopia. Ophthalmic Physiol Opt. 2015;35:252–62. https://doi.org/10.1111/opo.12207.
57. Leung TW, et al. A novel instrument for logging nearwork distance. Ophthalmic Physiol Opt. 2011;31:137–44. https://doi.org/10.1111/j.1475-1313.2010.00814.x.
58. Wen L, et al. A novel device to record the behavior related to myopia development— preliminary results in the lab. Invest Ophthalmol Vis Sci. 2016;57:2491.
59. Lan WZ, et al. The correlation between an objective index summarizing individual environmental risk factors and the change of refractive error. Invest Ophthalmol Vis Sci. 2018;41:59.
60. Winawer J, Wallman J. Temporal constraints on lens compensation in chicks. Vis Res. 2002;42:2651–68.

61. Zhu X, Winawer JA, Wallman J. Potency of myopic defocus in spectacle lens compensation. Invest Ophthalmol Vis Sci. 2003;44:2818–27.
62. Morgan I, Megaw P. Using natural STOP growth signals to prevent excessive axial elongation and the development of myopia. Ann Acad Med. 2004;33:16–20.
63. Tarutta E, Khodzhabekyan N, Filinova O, Milash S, Kruzhkova G. Long -term effects of optical defocus on eye growth and refractogenesis. Pomeranian J Life Sci. 2016;62:25–30.
64. Lin J. Observation of ocular haemodynamic change pre and post doing the eye exercises using color Doppler flood image. Chin J Ultrasound Diagn. 2004;5:446–7.
65. Li SM, et al. Efficacy of Chinese eye exercises on reducing accommodative lag in school-aged children: a randomized controlled trial. PLoS One. 2015;10:e0117552. https://doi.org/10.1371/journal.pone.0117552.
66. Changjun L, Wang J, Gou H, Jianzhou W. A survey on prevalence of myopia and its influential factors in middle school students. Mod Prev Med. 2010;37:3047–51.
67. Lin Z, et al. Eye exercises of acupoints: their impact on refractive error and visual symptoms in Chinese urban children. BMC Complement Altern Med. 2013;13:306. https://doi.org/10.1186/1472-6882-13-306.
68. Lin Z, et al. Eye exercises of acupoints: their impact on myopia and visual symptoms in Chinese rural children. BMC Complement Altern Med. 2016;16:349. https://doi.org/10.1186/s12906-016-1289-4.
69. Ping Z, Wang K, Chunhua Z, Bin Z. The epidemiological investigation of myopia in junior students. Prac J Med Pharm. 2004;21:543–5.
70. Kang MT, et al. Chinese eye exercises and myopia development in school age children: a Nested Case-Control Study. Sci Rep. 2016;6:28531. https://doi.org/10.1038/srep28531.
71. Holden BA, et al. Global prevalence of myopia and high myopia and temporal trends from 2000 through 2050. Ophthalmology. 2016;123:1036–42. https://doi.org/10.1016/j.ophtha.2016.01.006.
72. Morgan IG. New perspectives on the prevention of myopia. Eye Sci. 2011;26:3.
73. Verkicharla PK, et al. Development of the fitsight fitness tracker to increase time outdoors to prevent myopia. Transl Vis Sci Technol. 2017;6:20.

Clinical Management and Control of Myopia in Children

8

Audrey Chia and Su Ann Tay

Key Points

- Our understanding of the pathogenesis and etiology of myopia continues to evolve, and with it, various interventions that prevent or slow the progression of myopia. These include the use of bifocal spectacles, peripheral defocus spectacles and contact lenses, orthokeratology contact lenses, atropine and environmental interventions.
- With various interventions available for myopia control, understanding the effectiveness, safety profile and cost of each intervention can aid the clinician in making collective decisions with patients and their families on the most appropriate intervention for each child.
- An atropine-based protocol for the treatment of myopia developed based on evidence from studies collected thus far is discussed. This includes assessment of risk factors for myopia progression, factors to consider when starting atropine, monitoring response to atropine treatment and factors to consider before cessation of treatment.
- It is important that there is continued assessment of the long-term effect and value of these treatments in preventing high myopia and its associated complications.

A. Chia (✉) · S. A. Tay
Singapore National Eye Centre, Singapore, Singapore

Singapore Eye Research Institute, Singapore, Singapore
e-mail: audrey.chia.w.l@singhealth.com.sg; tay.su.ann@singhealth.com.sg

M. Ang, T. Y. Wong (eds.), *Updates on Myopia*,
https://doi.org/10.1007/978-981-13-8491-2_8

8.1 Introduction

The understanding of the pathogenesis of myopia and various interventions has evolved over time. The belief of an association between myopia and near work in the 1980s [1–5] led to interventions targeting accommodation such as bifocal glasses [6–8] and topical atropine [9–12]. The discovery of the importance of the peripheral retina [13–15], and how peripheral hyperopic defocus may aggravate eye growth and myopia [16–19] resulted in the exploration of peripheral defocus glasses and contact lenses as potential interventions in the 2000s. Induced peripheral myopic defocus is now thought to be how orthokeratology contact lenses slow myopia [16]. Research has moved on to novel contact lens designs, which also induce peripheral or dual defocus. More recently, it is hoped that with greater understanding of gene and molecular processes involved in eye growth, novel genetic and pharmacological treatments may be developed over time to control myopia.

8.2 Near Activity and Accommodation

8.2.1 Bifocal and Progressive Addition Spectacles

Progressive and bifocal glasses were introduced in the 1990s to try and slow myopia. However, studies with progressive addition lenses (PALs) showed a small and clinically insignificant or no effect on myopia progression [20–23]. One meta-analysis noted small reductions in myopia progression (0.25 D, 95% CI 0.13–0.38; nine trials) and axial length (−0.12 mm, 95% CI −0.18 to −0.05; six trials) [24]. This effect may be greater for children with a higher myopia (<−3.0 D), accommodative lag, or near esophoria [24–28].

In contrast, randomized controlled trials (RCTs) showed that executive bifocal lenses slowed myopia progression by 39% and up to 51% with base-in prisms incorporated [29]. It is possible that the larger near segment made it more likely for children to use the near add during near work, and may also induce more peripheral myopic defocus. However, because of the lack of collaborating evidence, meta-analysis across trials found data to be limited and inconsistent [20].

8.2.2 Atropine

Atropine is a non-specific muscarinic acetylcholine receptor antagonist and was initially thought to work by blocking accommodation. This theory has since been disproved in animal studies [30]. Its exact mechanism is still unknown but it is thought to work through muscarinic or non-muscarinic pathways either in the retina or in the sclera [31, 32]. Atropine has a strong dose-dependent inhibitory effect of myopia progression [30]. The initial high doses of atropine (i.e., 0.5% or 1.0%) slowed myopia progression by more than 70% over 1–2 years [33–36]. However, lower doses (0.1% or less) can also slow myopia by 30–60%, and may be associated with fewer side effects (pupil dilation, glare or blur) [36, 37]. Huang et al. in a review of the data, found that high-dose and low-dose atropine slowed spherical equivalent by 0.68 D

[0.52–0.84] and 0.53 D [0.21–0.85] respectively, and axial length by −0.21 mm [−0.28 to −0.16] and−0.15 mm [−0.25 to −0.05] respectively over 1 year [38].

Washout data from the Atropine Treatment of Myopia (ATOM) studies, however, showed that there was a myopic rebound if atropine was stopped suddenly, especially at higher doses and in younger children [39, 40]. Up to 12% of children may exhibit a poor response (i.e., progress >1.0 D over 1 year) even on high-dose atropine. A poorer response was associated with younger children, a higher degree of myopia at baseline and myopic parents [41]. Similarly, in the ATOM2 study, 9.3%, 6.4%, and 4.3% of children in the 0.01%, 0.1%, and 0.5% group, respectively, progressed by 1.5 D or more in the first 2 years of treatment [42].

More recently, in the Low-Concentration Atropine for Myopia Progression (LAMP) study involving children aged 4–12 years, those treated with 0.01%, 0.02%, and 0.05% atropine showed a reduction of SE progression of 27%, 43%, and 67%, and axial length growth of 12%, 29%, and 51%, respectively [37]. Overall, the effect on spherical equivalent was larger than that of axial length.

8.3 Peripheral Defocus

From animal studies, it is known that eyeball growth (i.e., hyperopia or myopia) could be induced by using positive and negative lenses, respectively [43, 44]. These studies also showed that peripheral refraction could influence eye growth, independent of central vision. Excessive near work could induce hyperopic defocus in the peripheral retina and promote eye growth [25, 45–48]. The increased prolate growth of the myopic eyeball and use of spherical glasses correcting for central vision may aggravate this effect [46, 49–52]. Based on this theory, optical interventions that induce a myopic defocus in the periphery should slow myopia.

8.3.1 Peripheral Myopic Defocus Glasses

In 2010, Sankaridurg et al. published their results of three novel spectacle lenses. All lenses had a central clear aperture with varying amounts of plus defocus in the periphery. Unfortunately, there was no significant effect on myopic progression with all three designs compared to single vision lenses (SVLs). In a subgroup of younger children with parental myopia, however, the prototype where the central aperture extended into the horizontal and inferior meridians with a peripheral power of +1.9 D did result in less myopia progression [53]. However, in a recent RCT conducted in Japanese children involving this design, no difference in myopia reduction was found [54].

8.3.2 Bifocal or Dual-Focus Contact Lenses

Bifocal contact lens designs often include a central distance focus, and peripheral rings with near add, creating a peripheral myopic defocus. Studies exploring the effect of these bifocal soft contact lenses indicate slowing of myopia progression by

30–38% and axial length by 31–51% over a period of 24 months [55–57]. Different studies suggest that efficacy may improve with increase in wear time, in children with faster rates of progression [58], near esophoria [59], and with designs possessing a higher hyperopic power in the mid-periphery (up to 6 D) [60]. With the myriad of lens designs possible, the challenge now is to develop the most effective design with the least compromise to visual quality, comfort, and safety [61].

8.3.3 Orthokeratology

Orthokeratology (Ortho-k) lenses optically correct myopia by flattening the central cornea, resulting in a relative peripheral myopic defocus [62, 63]. Individual studies and meta-analyses have shown a 40–60% reduction in the rate of myopia progression with ortho-k lenses compared with controls using SVL spectacles [64–69]. In a meta-analysis by Sun et al., the combined results showed a mean AL reduction of 0.27 mm (95% CI: 0.22, 0.32) after 2 years, corresponding to a 45% reduction in myopic progression [69]. Younger children (aged 7–8 years) with faster myopic progression (>1.0 D/year) might benefit more [66], and benefits were noted even in partially corrected children with high myopia [68]. However, studies show that the efficacy may decrease over time, especially after 4–5 years [70–72], and a potential "rebound" after discontinuation, especially in children under 14 years [73]. There is also a potential non-response rate of 7–12% [74, 75]. The risk of infective keratitis remains [76–81]; a recent systemic review suggested an infection rate similar to overnight wear of soft contact lenses, which is estimated at 13.9 per 10,000 [82, 83].

8.4 Time Spent Outdoors

While initial strategies were targeted at minimizing near work, it became apparent that increasing time spent outdoors could be more important [84, 85]. In the Sydney Myopia Study, exposure to more than 2 h of outdoor activity per day decreased the odds of myopia and countered the effects of near work [86]. Interventions involving increasing time outdoors appeared to reduce the onset of myopia and also its progression in myopic children [87, 88]. A meta-analysis has suggested a 2% reduced odds of myopia per additional hour of time spent outdoors per week [89]. Another meta-analysis showed that time outdoors protected children against incident myopia with a risk ratio (RR) of 0.536–0.574 in clinical trials and longitudinal cohort studies, and an odds ratio of 0.964 in cross-sectional studies, but had less effect in slowing progression in children who were already myopic [90].

8.4.1 Environmental Interventions

Based on new evidence, the advice has shifted from spending at least 2 h/day outdoors in addition to avoiding excessive near work. This has changed health and school messaging in many East Asian countries [88].

8.4.2 Higher Light Intensities and Dopamine

Potential reasons why time outdoors may be protective include higher light intensities [91, 92], differences in chromatic composition [93–95], the reduction in dioptric accommodative focus and psychometric influences encountered outdoors [96]. Higher light intensities increase retina dopamine production, which is believed to retard axial length elongation [97]. In animal studies, higher light levels greatly retarded form-deprivation myopia [91, 92, 98], a reaction which is abolished by dopamine antagonists [97]. The role of chromaticity (red and blue) and ultraviolet (UV) light is still uncertain [99–102], while that of higher vitamin D levels has been debunked [103, 104].

8.5 Inheritance and Genetics of Myopia

Epidemiology studies suggest that the risk of myopia is doubled if children had one myopic parent, and 3–5 times if they had two [105], with a possible additive effect with subsequent generations [106]. In addition, monozygous twins have a 75–90% chance of having a similar refraction compared to 30% in dizygous twins [107–109].

From pedigree analysis, multiple inheritance patterns (i.e., autosomal dominant, autosomal recessive, and X-linked) have been identified. Genome-wide sequencing analyses have identified more than 20 myopia and high myopia loci and over 130 potential genes (MYP1-3, 5–19) in different populations [107, 110]. These loci have been linked to neuronal signaling, retinoic acid synthesis, ion transport, channel activity, and membrane potential [110], which may influence ocular development, differentiation, and growth [111]. It is hoped that by understanding the genetics of myopia, it may be possible to predict who may develop high myopia or complications of myopia early, how people may respond to various interventions, and uncover novel interventions.

8.6 Application to Clinical Practice

In deciding on treatment regimes, questions on which children would benefit most from treatment in terms of age, baseline myopia, rate of progression, and family history remain. In addition, the appropriate duration of treatment and the best time to start, stop, and restart treatment need to be further studied. With the various interventions available for myopia control, decisions need to be made in conjunction with patients and their families on the most appropriate one, taking into consideration the effectiveness, safety profile, and cost of the each intervention (Table 8.1).

The following is an atropine-based protocol which has been developed, based on evidence collected thus far (Table 8.2 and Fig. 8.1). On presentation, the risk of the child developing myopia and its potential complications are assessed. Low-risk children may be older children (aged >11 years), those with little or no myopia progression in the last 1 year, and relatively low myopia. High-risk children may be those who have a strong family history of high myopia or myopic complications, are younger (<9 years), and with documented rapid progression of myopia over the last year. Parental and child

Table 8.1 Summary of interventions for myopia control efficacy, safety, and accessibility

	Effectiveness	Safety	Accessibility
Time outdoors	Decrease onset of myopia by 30%; and progression of myopia by 18% [87, 88]	Safe. Requires sun protection of eyes and skin	Available to all. Limited by social factors (academic expectations), weather, and seasonal variations
Executive bifocal spectacles	Decrease myopia progression by 39%; 51% with base-in prisms incorporated [29]	Safe although may result in some visual distortion	Moderately expensive Readily available in most spectacle shops
PAL spectacles	Decrease myopia progression 0–20% [24]		
Peripheral myopic defocus spectacles	No significant difference from SVL [53, 54]		
Bifocal or dual focus soft contact lenses	Decrease myopia progression 30–38% over 24 months [57] Better effect with near esophoria [59]	Possible risk of infective keratitis, contact lens intolerance No data on discontinuation and rebound effect	Moderately expensive although likely readily available in most spectacle shops
Orthokeratology contact lenses	40–50% reduction in myopia progression over 1–2 years Effect may wane over time Rebound noted if stopped suddenly [69, 70]	Risk of infective keratitis similar to overnight soft CL wear: 13.9 per 10,000 [83] Ocular surface problems, corneal staining [82]	Can be expensive Require clinical expertise to ensure proper fit
Atropine	Dose-related response for myopia control with 70–80% reduction with high dose (0.5–1%) [33–36] and 30–60% with low dose (0.01–0.05%) [36, 37] Rebound noted if stopped suddenly (esp. in younger children and at higher doses) [39, 40]	Glare and near blur with higher doses Allergy 1–4% Systemic effects rare Effect on spherical equivalent greater than axial length	Can be cost-effective if manufactured in bulk Lower doses not readily available in all communities

sentiments are also assessed (e.g., overall anxiety, willingness to administer eye drops every day, possibly till the child is in his/her mid-teens). Various options are discussed, ensuring that parents have realistic expectations of the outcome. The possibility of a poor response and need for a higher dose of atropine or alternative treatments are also carefully explained. Options would then include starting atropine or waiting another 6–12 months to monitor the natural progression of refraction.

In this protocol, children are first started on a lower dose of atropine with a plan to increase the dose as necessary. However, an alternative would be to start initially

Table 8.2 An atropine-based protocol for myopia treatment

A. Starting atropine – Assess child's risk of myopia – High risk: family history of high myopia or myopic complications, younger age, documented rapid progression of myopia, poor life-style profile (outdoor–near work) – Assess parents' and children's risk aversion to treatment, willingness to continue on treatment till at least teenage years – Age 4–13 years of age with documented progression of myopia of at least >0.5 D in the last year
B1: Not keen on treatment: monitor over next 6–12 months B2: Keen on treatment: commence atropine 0.01% daily for at least 2 years
C. Follow-up on treatment – Review child every 6 months – Monitor for compliance and side effects : near blur, glare, and allergy – Cycloplegic refraction and axial length measurements at least once per year
D1: Good or acceptable response to treatment (<0.5 D/year) Age <12 years old: consider continuing dose or slowly taper if no myopia progression noted in the past year Age >12 years old: consider taper of medication if no/little progression noted in the past year D2: Poor response to treatment (>0.5 D/year) – Particularly in younger children (<9 years), with strong family history, with baseline high myopia and rapid progression prior to starting atropine – Consider an increased dose (e.g., atropine 0.01% 2× per day, 0.1% daily or 1.0% 2–3× per week) – Consider tinted glasses with near add if required – Once stabilization of myopia is achieved, continue at that dose, and taper frequency of drops as child reaches teenage years D3: Poor response despite maximum atropine dose – Consider stopping and changing or adding different treatment options
E. Long-term follow-up – Continue to monitor child for at least 1 year after stopping treatment

on a higher dose, with an aim to taper medication over time. Once medication is started, progression (refraction and/or axial length) is monitored every 6 months, with an initial aim to continue children on medication (i.e., atropine 0.01% daily) for at least 2 years. Children may respond to treatment in three ways: well (with little or no progression); adequately (with acceptable amount of progression, e.g., <0.5 D/year); or poorly (>0.5 D/year).

If a good response is obtained, the next question is how long treatment should continue for and when treatment should be stopped. From the ATOM 2 study, we know that stopping atropine 0.01% between 8 and 10 years resulted in a 60% risk of a rebound effect, compared to 30% at age 10–12 years and 8% after the age of 12 years. In addition, children who did not demonstrate rebound tended to show little or no myopic progression within the last year [67]. This suggests that in children younger than 12 years who showed no progression in the past year, atropine 0.01% may be slowly tapered (e.g., by reducing drop frequency by 1–2 days/week each year). However, if children are older than 12 years, then the frequency of eye drops could be tapered more quickly (e.g., by 1–2 days/week every 6 months). Using this regime, most children will be off medication by about 14–15 years of age.

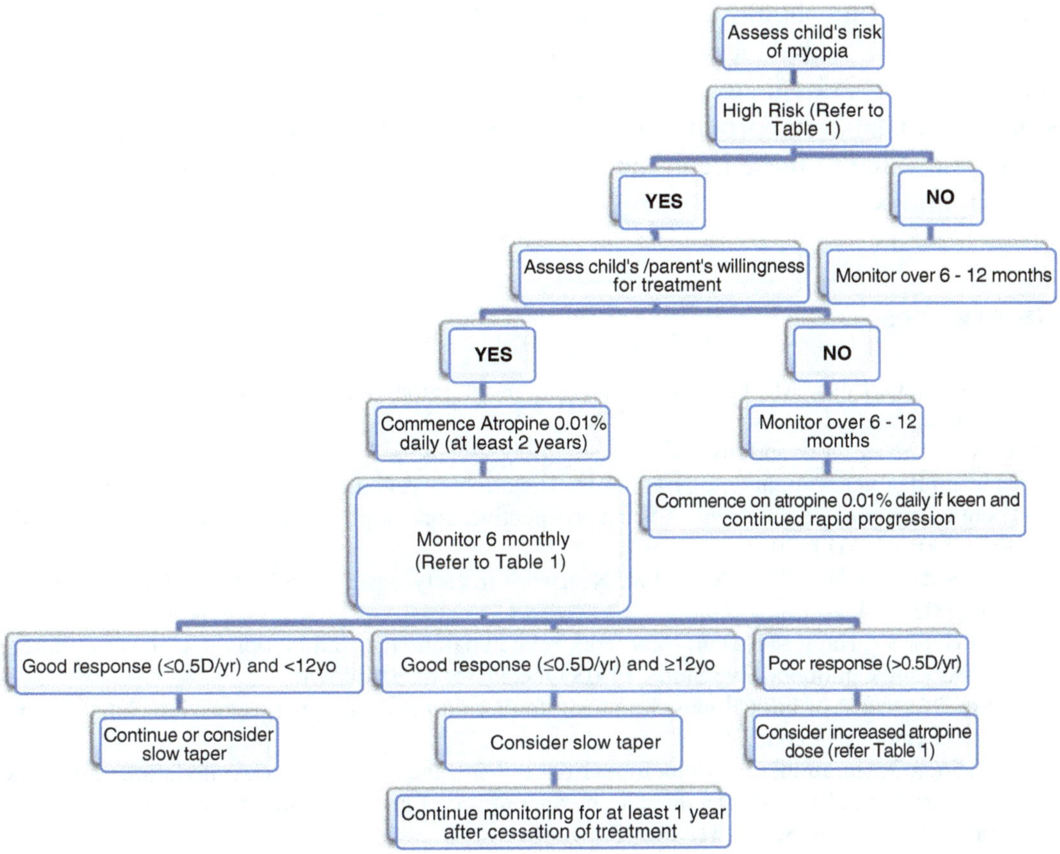

Fig. 8.1 Flow chart of atropine-based protocol for myopia treatment.

In children who progress on low-dose atropine, the frequency of application or dose could be increased (e.g., using atropine 0.01% twice a day; or using a higher concentration, e.g., 0.1% or 1%). Note that while using higher concentrations, a daily dose may not be necessary and children may require tinted glasses with near add to cope with any glare or near blur. Once an adequate control of myopia is achieved, medication can be continued till the child reaches teenage years and then tapered as required. There are some children (10%), however, who may progress rapidly even on higher doses of atropine [68]. If this occurs, then the possibility of stopping treatment or trying other treatment modalities should be discussed. Even after stopping treatment, it may be necessary to monitor children for a further 6–12 months to ensure that there is no further rebound.

Since our knowledge of how children respond to atropine and other interventions continues to increase over time, any protocol developed needs to be evaluated regularly, taking full advantage of our knowledge and accessibility to different treatment options.

8.7 Conclusion

Our management of myopia continues to evolve over time with a better understanding of the pathogenesis of myopia and its interventions. The challenge is to identify which individuals to treat, when to start treatment and which interventions one should use. There are differences in efficacy, safety, and cost which need to be balanced. More work is required to determine how to combine or time treatments to optimize outcome, and when treatments can be safely stopped. It is also important that there is continued assessment of the long-term effect and value of these treatments in preventing high myopia and its associated complications.

References

1. Parssinen O, Lyyra AL. Myopia and myopic progression among schoolchildren: a three-year follow-up study. Invest Ophthalmol Vis Sci. 1993;34:2794–802.
2. Goss DA. Nearwork and myopia. Lancet. 2000;356:1456–7.
3. Hepsen IF, Evereklioglu C, Bayramlar H. The effect of reading and near-work on the development of myopia in emmetropic boys: a prospective, controlled, three-year follow-up study. Vis Res. 2001;41:2511–20.
4. Saw SM, Chua WH, Hong CY, et al. Nearwork in early-onset myopia. Invest Ophthalmol Vis Sci. 2002;43:332–9.
5. Li SM, Li SY, Kang MT, et al. Near work related parameters and myopia in Chinese children: The Anyang Childhood Eye Study. PLoS One. 2015;10:e0134514.
6. Goss DA. Effect of bifocal lenses on the rate of childhood myopia progression. Am J Optom Physiol Optic. 1986;63:135–41.
7. Parssinen O, Hemminki E, Klemetti A. Effect of spectacle use and accommodation on myopic progression: final results of a three-year randomised clinical trial among schoolchildren. Br J Ophthalmol. 1989;73:547–51.
8. Grosvenor T, Perrigin DM, Perrigin J, Maslovitz B. Houston Myopia Control Study: a randomized clinical trial. Part II. Final report by the patient care team. Am J Optom Physiol Optic. 1987;64:482–98.
9. Bedrossian RH. The effect of atropine on myopia. Ann Ophthalmol. 1971;3:891–7.
10. Gimbel HV. The control of myopia with atropine. Can J Ophthalmol. 1973;8:527–32.
11. Bedrossian RH. The effect of atropine on myopia. Ophthalmology. 1979;86:713–9.
12. Brodstein RS, Brodstein DE, Olson RJ, et al. The treatment of myopia with atropine and bifocals. A long-term prospective study. Ophthalmology. 1984;91:1373–9.
13. Wallman J, Gottlieb MD, Rajaram V, et al. Local retinal regions control local eye growth and myopia. Science. 1987;237:73–8.
14. Diether S, Schaeffel F. Local changes in eye growth induced by imposed local refractive error despite active accommodation. Vis Res. 1997;37:659–68.
15. Miles FA, Wallman J. Local ocular compensation for imposed local refractive error. Vis Res. 1990;30:339–49.
16. Wallman J, Winawer J. Homeostasis of eye growth and the question of myopia. Neuron. 2004;43:447–68.
17. Smith EL III, Hung LF, Ramamirtham R, et al. Optically imposed hyperopic defocus in the periphery can produce central axial myopia in infant monkeys. Invest Ophthalmol Vis Sci. 2007;48(13):1533.
18. Smith EL, Hung LF, Huang J. Relative peripheral hyperopic defocus alters central refractive development in infant monkeys. Vis Res. 2009;49:2386–92.
19. Smith EL III, Hung LF, Huang J, et al. Effects of optical defocus on refractive development in monkeys: evidence for local, regionally selective mechanisms. Invest Ophthalmol Vis Sci. 2010;51:3864–73.
20. Walline JJ, Lindsley K, Vedula SS, et al. Interventions to slow progression of myopia in children. Cochrane Database Syst Rev. 2011;12:CD004916.
21. Gwiazda JE, Hyman L, Everett D, The COMET Group, et al. Five–year results from the correction of myopia evaluation trial (COMET). Invest Ophthalmol Vis Sci. 2006;47(13):1166.

22. Hasebe S, Ohtsuki H, Nonaka T, et al. Effect of progressive addition lenses on myopia progression in Japanese children: a prospective, randomized, double-masked, crossover trial. Invest Ophthalmol Vis Sci. 2008;49(7):2781–9.
23. Hasebe S, Jun J, Vamas SR, et al. Myopia control with positively aspherised progressive additional lenses: a 2 year, multicentre, randomized, controlled trial. Invest Ophthalmol Vi Sci. 2014;55(11):7177–88.
24. Li SM, Ji YZ, Wu SS, et al. Multifocal versus single vision lenses intervention to slow progression of myopia in school-age children: a meta-analysis. Surv Ophthalmol. 2011;56:451–60.
25. Gwiazda JE, Hyman L, Norton TT, COMET Group, et al. Accommodation and related risk factors associated with myopia progression and their interaction with treatment in COMET children. Invest Ophthalmol Vis Sci. 2004;45(7):2143–51.
26. Correction of Myopia Evaluation Trial 2 Study Group for the Pediatric Eye Disease Investigator Group. Progressive-addition lenses versus single-vision lenses for slowing progression of myopia in children with high accommodative lag and near esophoria. Invest Ophthalmol Vis Sci. 2011;52:2749–57.
27. Berntsen DA, Sinnott LT, Mutti DO, Zadnik K. A randomized trial using progressive addition lenses to evaluate theories of myopia progression in children with a high lag of accommodation. Invest Ophthalmol Vis Sci. 2012;53:640–9.
28. Yang Z, Lan W, Ge J, Liu W, Chen X, Chen L, Yu M. The effectiveness of progressive addition lenses on the progression of myopia in Chinese children. Ophthalmic Physiol Opt. 2009;29:41–8.
29. Cheng D, Woo GC, Drobe B, Schmid KL. Effect of bifocal and prismatic bifocal spectacles on myopia progression in children: three-year results of a randomized clinical trial. Ophthamology. 2014;132:258–64.
30. McBrien NA, Moghaddam HO, Reeder AP. Atropine reduces experimental myopia and eye enlargement via a nonaccommodative mechanism. Invest Ophthalmol Vis Sci. 1993;34:205–15.
31. McBrien NA, Stell WK, Carr B. How does atropine exert its anti-myopia effects? Ophthalmic Physiol Opt. 2013;33(3):373–8.
32. Lind GJ, Chew SJ, Marzani D, Wallman J. Muscarinic acetylcholine receptor antagonists inhibit chick scleral chondrocytes. Invest Ophthalmol Vis Sci. 1998;39:2217–31.
33. Yen MY, Liu JH, Kao SC, Shiao CH. Comparison of the effect of atropine and cyclopentolate on myopia. Ann Ophthalmol. 1989;21:180–2.
34. Shih YF, Chen CH, Chou AC, et al. Effects of different concentrations of atropine on controlling myopia in myopic children. J Ocul Pharmacol Ther. 1999;15:85–90.
35. Chua WH, Balakrishnan V, Chan YH, et al. Atropine for the treatment of childhood myopia. Ophthalmology. 2006;113(12):2285–91.
36. Chia A, Chua WH, Cheung YB, et al. Atropine for the treatment of childhood myopia: safety and efficacy of 0.5%, 0.1%, and 0.01% doses (Atropine for the Treatment of Myopia 2). Ophthalmology. 2012;119(2):347–54.
37. Yam JC, Jiang Y, Tang SM, et al. Low-concentration atropine for myopia progression (LAMP) study: a randomized, double-blinded, placebo-controlled trial of 0.05%, 0.025%, and 0.01% atropine eye drops in myopia control. Ophthalmology. 2019;126(1):113–24.
38. Huang J, Wen D, Wang Q, et al. Efficacy comparison of 16 interventions for myopia control in children: a network meta-analysis. Ophthalmology. 2016;123(4):697–708.
39. Tong L, Huang XL, Koh AL, et al. Atropine for the treatment of childhood myopia: effect on myopia progression after cessation of atropine. Ophthalmology. 2009;116:572–9.
40. Chia A, Chua WH, Wen L, et al. Atropine for the treatment of childhood myopia: changes after stopping atropine 0.01%, 0.1% and 0.5%. Am J Ophthalmol. 2014;157(2):451–457.e1.
41. Loh KL, Lu Q, Tan D, Chia A. Risk factors for progressive myopia in the atropine therapy for myopia study. Am J Ophthalmol. 2015;159:945–9.
42. Chia A, Lu QS, Tan D. Five-year clinical trial on atropine for the treatment of myopia 2: myopia control with atropine 0.01% eyedrops. Ophthalmology. 2016;123(2):391–9.
43. Troilo D, Wallman J. The regulation of eye growth and refractive state: an experimental study of emmetropization. Vis Res. 1991;31:1237–50.

44. Schaeffel F, Troilo D, Wallman J, Howland HC. Developing eyes that lack accommodation grow to compensate for imposed defocus. Vis Neurosci. 1990;4:177–83.
45. Seidemann A, Schaeffel F. An evaluation of the lag of accommodation using photorefraction. Vis Res. 2003;43:419–30.
46. Gwiazda J, Bauer J, Thorn F, et al. A dynamic relationship between myopia and blur-driven accommodation in school-aged children. Vis Res. 1995;35:1299–304.
47. Gwiazda J, Thorn F, Bauer J, et al. Myopic children show insufficient accommodative response to blur. Invest Ophthalmol Vis Sci. 1993;34:690–4.
48. Charman WN. Near vision, lags of accommodation and myopia. Ophthalmic Physiol Opt. 1999;19:126–33.
49. Mutti DO, Sinnott LT, Mitchell GL, CLEERE Study Group, et al. Relative peripheral refractive error and the risk of onset and progression of myopia in children. Invest Ophthalmol Vis Sci. 2011;52(1):199–205.
50. Atchison DA, Jones CE, Schmid KL, et al. Eye shape in emmetropia and myopia. Invest Ophthalmol Vis Sci. 2004;45(10):3380–6.
51. Schmid GF. Association between retinal steepness and central myopic shift in children. Optom Vis Sci. 2011;88(6):684–90.
52. Sng CCA, Lin XY, Gus G, et al. Change in peripheral refraction over time in Singapore Chinese children. Invest Ophthalmol Vis Sci. 2011;52(11):7880–7.
53. Sankaridurg P, Donovan L, Varnas S, et al. Spectacle lenses designed to reduce progression of myopia: 12-month results. Optom Vis Sci. 2010;87(9):631–41.
54. Kanda H, Oshika T, Hiraoka T, et al. Effect of spectacle lenses designed to reduce relative peripheral hyperopia on myopia progression in Japanese children: a 2-year multicenter randomized controlled trial. Jpn J Ophthalmol. 2018;62:537–43.
55. Benavente-Pérez A, Nour A, Troilo D. Axial eye growth and refractive error development can be modified by exposing the peripheral retina to relative myopic or hyperopic defocus. Invest Ophthalmol Vis Sci. 2014;55(10):6765–73.
56. Walline JJ. Myopia control: a review. Eye Contact Lens. 2016;42(1):3–8.
57. Li SM, Kang MT, Wu SS, et al. Studies using concentric ring bifocal and peripheral add multifocal contact lenses to slow myopia progression in school-aged children: a meta-analysis. Ophthalmic Physiol Opt. 2017;37(1):51–9.
58. Lam CSY, Tang WC, Tse DY-Y, Tang YY, To CH. Defocus incorporated soft contact (DISC) lens slows myopia progression in Hong Kong Chinese schoolchildren: a 2-year randomised clinical trial. Br J Ophthalmol. 2014;98:40–5.
59. Aller TA, Liu M, Wildsoet CF. Myopia control with bifocal contact lenses: a randomized clinical trial. Optom Vis Sci. 2016;93(4):344–52.
60. Paune J, Morales H, Armengol J, et al. Myopia control with a novel peripheral gradient soft lens and orthokeratology: a 2-year clinical trial. Biomed Res Int. 2015;2015:507572.
61. Anstice NS, Phillips JR. Effect of dual-focus soft contact lens wear on axial myopia progression in children. Ophthalmology. 2011;118:1152–61.
62. Charman WN, Mountford J, Atchison DA, et al. Peripheral refraction in orthokeratology patients. Optom Vis Sci. 2006;83:641–8.
63. Queirós A, González-Méijome JM, Jorge J, et al. Peripheral refraction in myopic patients after orthokeratology. Optom Vis Sci. 2010;87(5):323–9.
64. Wen D, Huang J, Chen H, et al. Efficacy and acceptability of orthokeratology for slowing myopic progression in children: a systematic review and meta-analysis. J Ophthalmol. 2015;2015:360806.
65. Si JK, Tang K, Bi HS, et al. Orthokeratology for myopia control: a meta-analysis. Optom Vis Sci. 2015;92:252–7.
66. Cho P, Cheung SW, Edwards M, et al. The longitudinal orthokeratology research in children (LORIC) in Hong Kong: a pilot study on refractive changes and myopic control. Curr Eye Res. 2005;30:71–80.
67. Santodomingo-Rubido J, Villa-Collar C, Gilmartin B, et al. Myopia control with orthokeratology contact lenses in Spain: refractive and biometric changes. Invest Ophthalmol Vis Sci. 2012;53:5060–5.

68. Charm J, Cho P. High myopia partial reduction ortho-k: a 2-year randomized study. Optom Vis Sci. 2013;90:530–9.
69. Sun Y, Xu F, Zhang T, Liu M, Wang D, Chen Y, Liu Q. Orthokeratology to control myopia progression: a meta-analysis. PLoS One. 2015;10(4):e0124535.
70. Hiraoka T, Kakita T, Okamoto F, et al. Long-term effect of overnight orthokeratology on axial length elongation in childhood myopia: a 5-year follow-up study. Invest Ophthalmol Vis Sci. 2012;53:3913–9.
71. Lee YC, Wang JH, Chiu CJ. Effect of Orthokeratology on myopia progression: twelve-year results of a retrospective cohort study. BMC Ophthalmol. 2017;17(1):243.
72. Santodomingo-Rubido J, Villa-Collar C, Gilmartin B, Gutiérrez-Ortega R, Sugimoto K. Long-term efficacy of orthokeratology contact lens wear in controlling the progression of childhood myopia. Curr Eye Res. 2017;42(5):713–20.
73. Cho P, Cheung SW. Discontinuation of orthokeratology on eyeball elongation (DOEE). Cont Lens Anterior Eye. 2017;40:82–7.
74. Cho P, Cheung SW. Retardation of myopia in orthokeratology (ROMIO) study: a 2-year randomized clinical trial. Invest Ophthalmol Vis Sci. 2012;53:7077–85.
75. Chen C, Cheung SW, Cho P. Myopia control using toric orthokeratology (TO-SEE Study). Invest Ophthalmol Vis Sci. 2013;54(10):6510–7.
76. Sun X, Zhao H, Deng S, et al. Infectious keratitis related to orthokeratology. Ophthalmic Physiol Opt. 2006;26:133–6.
77. Yepes N, Lee SB, Hill V, et al. Infectious keratitis after overnight orthokeratology in Canada. Cornea. 2005;24:857–60.
78. Tseng CH, Fong CF, Chen WL, et al. Overnight orthokeratology-associated microbial keratitis. Cornea. 2005;24:778–82.
79. Young AL, Leung AT, Cheng LL, et al. Orthokeratology lens–related corneal ulcers in children: a case series. Ophthalmology. 2004;111:590–5.
80. Xuguang S, Lin C, Yan Z, et al. Acanthamoeba keratitis as a complication of orthokeratology. Am J Ophthalmol. 2003;136:1159–61.
81. Chan TC, Li EY, Wong VW, Jhanji V. Orthokeratology-associated infectious keratitis in a tertiary care eye hospital in Hong Kong. Am J Ophthalmol. 2014;158:1130–5.
82. Liu YM, Xie P. The safety of orthokeratology—a systematic review. Eye Contact Lens. 2016;42:35–42.
83. Meter V, Woodford S, et al. Safety of overnight orthokeratology for myopia. Ophthalmology. 2008;115(12):2301–13.
84. Guggenheim JA, Northstone K, McMahon G, et al. Time outdoors and physical activity as predictors of incident myopia in childhood: a prospective cohort study. Invest Ophthalmol Vis Sci. 2012;53(6):2856–65.
85. Rose KA, Morgan IG, Smith W, Burlutsky G, Mitchell P, Saw SM. Myopia, lifestyle, and schooling in students of Chinese ethnicity in Singapore and Sydney. Arch Ophthalmol. 2008;126(4):527–30.
86. Rose KA, Morgan IG, Ip J, Kifley A, Huynh S, Smith W, Mitchell P. Outdoor activity reduces the prevalence of myopia in children. Ophthalmology. 2008;115(8):1279–85.
87. He M, Xiang F, Zeng Y, et al. Effect of time spent outdoors at school on the development of myopia among children in china a randomized clinical trial. JAMA. 2015;314(11):1142–8.
88. Wu PC, Chen CT, Lin KK, et al. Myopia prevention and outdoor light intensity in a school-based cluster randomized trial. Ophthalmology. 2018;125(8):1239–50.
89. Sherwin JC, Reacher MH, Keogh RH, et al. The association between time spent outdoors and myopia in children and adolescents: a systematic review and meta-analysis. Ophthalmology. 2012;119:2141–51.
90. Xiong S, Sankaridurg P, Naduvilath T, Zang J, Zou H, Zhu J, Lv M, He X, Xu X. Time spent in outdoor activities in relation to myopia prevention and control: a meta-analysis and systematic review. Acta Ophthalmol. 2017;95(6):551–66.
91. Ashby R, Ohlendorf A, Schaeffel F. The effect of ambient illuminance on the development of deprivation myopia in chicks. Invest Ophthalmol Vis Sci. 2009;50:5348–54.

92. Karouta C, Ashby RS. Correlation between light levels and the development of deprivation myopia. Invest Ophthalmol Vis Sci. 2015;56:299–309.
93. Rohrer B, Schaeffel F, Zrenner E. Longitudinal chromatic aberration and emmetropization: results from the chicken eye. J Physiol. 1992;449:363–76.
94. Seidemann A, Schaefel F. Effects of longitudinal chromatic aberration on accommodation and emmetropization. Vis Res. 2002;42:2409–17.
95. Rucker FJ, Wallman J. Chick eyes compensate for chromatic simulations of hyperopic and myopic defocus: evidence that the eye uses longitudinal chromatic aberration to guide eye growth. Vis Res. 2009;49:1775–83.
96. Flitcroft DI. The complex interactions of retinal, optical and environmental factors in myopia aetiology. Prog Retin Eye Res. 2012;31:622–60.
97. Feldkaemper M, Schaeffel F. An updated view on the role of dopamine in myopia. Exp Eye Res. 2013;114:106–19.
98. Smith EL 3rd, Hung LF, Huang J. Protective effects of high ambient lighting on the development of form-deprivation myopia in rhesus monkeys. Invest Ophthalmol Vis Sci. 2012;53:421–8.
99. Prepas SB. Light, literacy and the absence of ultraviolet radiation in the development of myopia. Med Hypotheses. 2008;70:635–7.
100. Foulds WS, Barathi VA, Luu CD. Progressive myopia or hyperopia can be induced in chicks and reversed by manipulation of the chromaticity of ambient light. Invest Ophthalmol Vis Sci. 2013;54(13):8004–12.
101. Smith EL, Hung LF, Arumugam B, et al. Effects of long-wavelength lighting on refractive development in infant rhesus monkeys. Invest Ophthalmol Vis Sci. 2015;56(11):6490–500.
102. Hung LF, Arumugam B, She Z, et al. Narrow-band, long-wavelength lighting promotes hyperopia and retards vision-induced myopia in infant rhesus monkeys. Exp Eye Res. 2018;4(176):147–60.
103. Guggenheim JA, Williams C, Northstone K, et al. Does vitamin D mediate the protective effects of time outdoors on myopia? Findings from a prospective birth cohort. Invest Ophthalmol Vis Sci. 2014;55:8550–8.
104. Cuellar-Partida G, Williams KM, Yazar S, et al. Genetically low vitamin D concentrations and myopic refractive error: a Mendelian randomization study. Int J Epidemiol. 2017;46:1882–90.
105. Wenbo L, Congxia B, Hui L. Genetic and environmental-genetic interaction rules for the myopia based on a family exposed to risk from a myopic environment. Gene. 2017;626:305–8.
106. Ahn H, Lyu IS, Rim TH. The influence of parental myopia on children's myopia in different generations of parent-offspring pairs in South Korea. Semin Ophthalmol. 2018;33(3):419–28.
107. Li J, Zhang Q. Insight into the molecular genetics of myopia. Mol Vis. 2017;23:1048–80.
108. Chen Y, Zhang J, Morgan IG, He M. Identifying children at risk of high myopia using population centile curves of refraction. PLoS One. 2016;11(12):e0167642.
109. Guggenheim JA, Ghorbani Mojarrad N, Williams C, et al. Genetic prediction of myopia: prospects and challenges. Ophthalmic Physiol Opt. 2017;37:549–56.
110. Rong SS, Chen LJ, Pang CP. Myopia Genetics-The Asia-Pacific Perspective. Asia Pac J Ophthalmol. 2016;5(4):236–44.
111. Flitcroft DI, Loughman J, Wildsoet CF, Williams C, Guggenheim JA, CREAM Consortium. Novel myopia genes and pathways identified from syndromic forms of myopia. Invest Ophthalmol Vis Sci. 2018;59(1):338–48.

Understanding Pathologic Myopia

9

Kyoko Ohno-Matsui and Jost B. Jonas

Key Points

- Pathologic myopia is defined by the presence of posterior staphylomas and/or the presence of myopic chorioretinal atrophy equal to or more serious than diffuse atrophy.
- Myopic CNV is the most frequent cause of central vision loss.
- Ultra wide-field OCT is a useful tool to detect posterior staphylomas.
- Anti-VEGF therapies have greatly improved the prognosis of myopic CNV.
- Vitreoretinal surgeries for myopic macular retinoschisis are useful.

9.1 Introduction

Pathologic myopia (PM) is a major cause of blindness in the world, especially in East Asian countries [1–5]. The cause of blindness in patients with PM includes myopic maculopathy with or without posterior staphyloma, myopic macular retinoschisis, and glaucoma or glaucoma-like optic neuropathy. In this chapter, the lesions of myopic fundus complications including posterior staphylomas are described.

K. Ohno-Matsui (✉)
Department of Ophthalmology and Visual Science, Tokyo Medical and Dental University, Tokyo, Japan
e-mail: k.ohno.oph@tmd.ac.jp

J. B. Jonas
Department of Ophthalmology, University of Heidelberg, Heidelberg, Germany

M. Ang, T. Y. Wong (eds.), *Updates on Myopia*,
https://doi.org/10.1007/978-981-13-8491-2_9

9.2 Definition of Pathologic Myopia

The terms "pathologic myopia," "high myopia," and "axial myopia" have long been used in a parallel manner in the literature. According to recent discussions, the term "high myopia" simply describes the status of a "high degree of myopia" and should be defined by a cut-off value of myopic refractive error. The term "axial myopia" may be used to describe the situation with an axial elongation as cause for the myopic refractive error. It is in contrast to the term refractive myopia, which is used for eyes with an abnormally high refractive power of their optical media. The term "pathologic myopia" describes the situation of pathologic consequences of a myopic axial elongation. According to a recent consensus article by Ohno-Matsui et al. [6], pathologic myopia was defined by myopic chorioretinal atrophy equal to or more serious than diffuse atrophy (by META-PM study group classification [7]) and/or the presence of posterior staphylomas.

9.3 Posterior Staphyloma

Posterior staphyloma has been considered a hallmark lesion of pathologic myopia. While axial elongation may primarily start in the equatorial and retro-equatorial region with secondary changes taking place at the posterior fundus, posterior staphylomas occur in the posterior segment of the eye and can be associated with, or lead to, vision-threatening complications in the macula as part of a myopic maculopathy [7–11] and myopic optic neuropathy/glaucoma [12, 13].

9.3.1 Definition of Staphyloma by Spaide (Fig. 9.1)

A posterior staphyloma is an outpouching of a circumscribed area of the posterior fundus, where the radius of curvature is less than the curvature radius of the surrounding eye wall [14].

9.3.2 Detection of Posterior Staphyloma

Moriyama et al. recently applied three-dimensional magnetic resonance imaging (3D-MRI) to analyze the shape of the entire eye from the corneal surface to the posterior pole including even large posterior staphylomas (Fig. 9.2) [15–17]. The technique allowed visualizing a staphyloma from any angle. The advantage of 3D-MRI of visualizing the shape of the whole eye including the anterior ocular segment is combined with its disadvantage of not being feasible as a screening technique. Instead, a new prototype of a wide-field swept-source optical coherence tomographic (OCT) system has been developed, which uses not only one but multiple scan lines and which generates scan maps allowing a three-dimensional

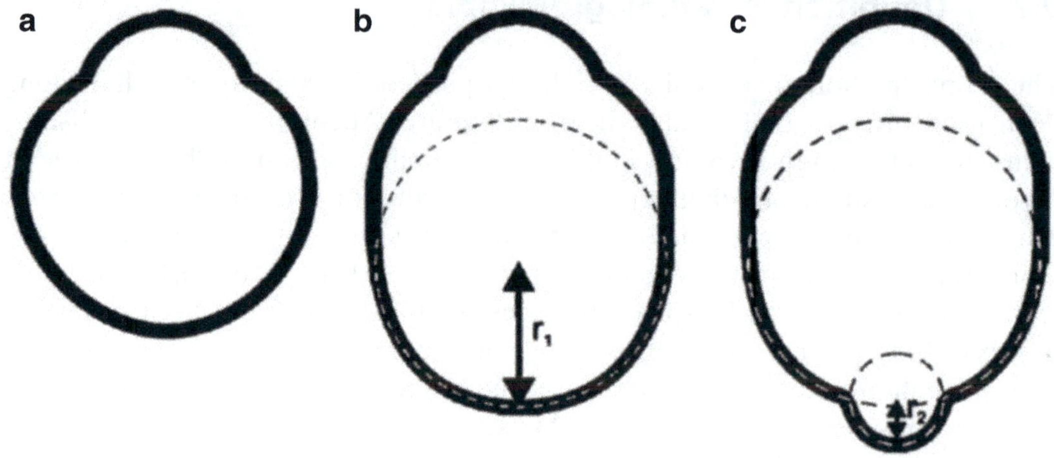

Fig. 9.1 Definition of posterior staphyloma (cited from the textbook *Pathologic Myopia* [14]). (**a**) Normal eye shape. (**b**) Axial expansion occurring in the equatorial region that does not induce any altered curvature in the posterior aspect of the eye. This eye would have axial myopia but no staphyloma. (**c**) Posterior staphyloma. A second curvature occurs in the posterior portion of the eye, and this second curvature has a small radius (r_2) than the surrounding eye wall (r_1). This secondary curve is a staphyloma. (This figure does not take into account changes in scleral thickness)

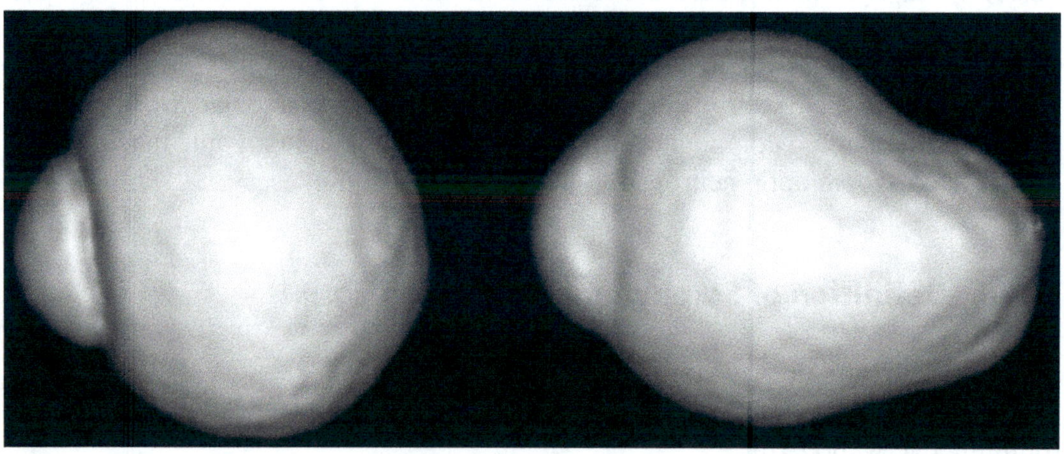

Fig. 9.2 Three-dimensional magnetic resonance images of eyes with emmetropia and posterior staphyloma. The shape of the emmetropic eye (left) is almost spherical and symmetrical, while the eye with a posterior staphyloma shows an outpouching of its posterior segment

reconstruction of posterior staphylomas in a region of interest of 23 × 20 mm with a depth of 5 mm. Applying a wide-field OCT (WF-OCT), Shinohara et al. [18] showed that WF-OCT could provide tomographic images of posterior staphylomas in a resolution and size unachievable up to that time, and that WF-OCT might replace 3D-MRI in examining posterior staphylomas. Upon WF-OCT, the edges of the staphylomas showed consistent features, consisting of a gradual thinning of the choroid from the periphery toward the staphyloma edge and a gradual re-thickening of the choroid from the staphyloma edge in direction to the posterior pole (Fig. 9.3).

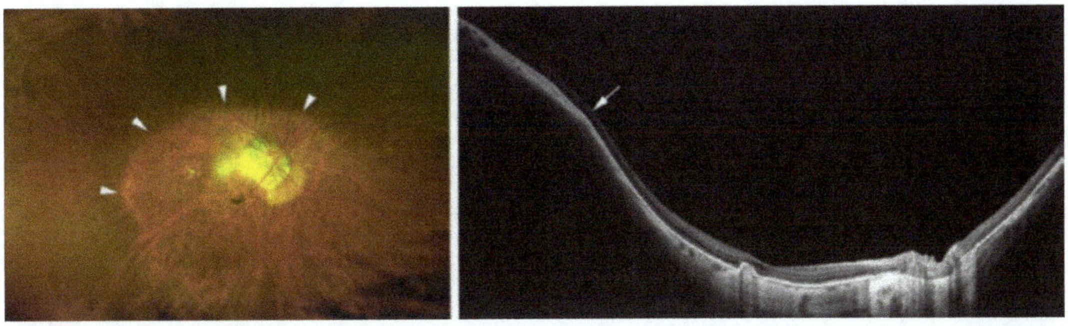

Fig. 9.3 Swept-source wide-field optical coherence tomographic (OCT) image of a posterior staphyloma. (Left) Right fundus shows a wide staphyloma (arrowheads). (Right) The wide-field OCT image shows the staphyloma edge (arrow) with a gradual thinning of the choroid from the periphery toward the staphyloma edge and a gradual re-thickening of the choroid toward the posterior pole. The white arrow indicates the change in the curvature radius of the sclera at the staphyloma edge

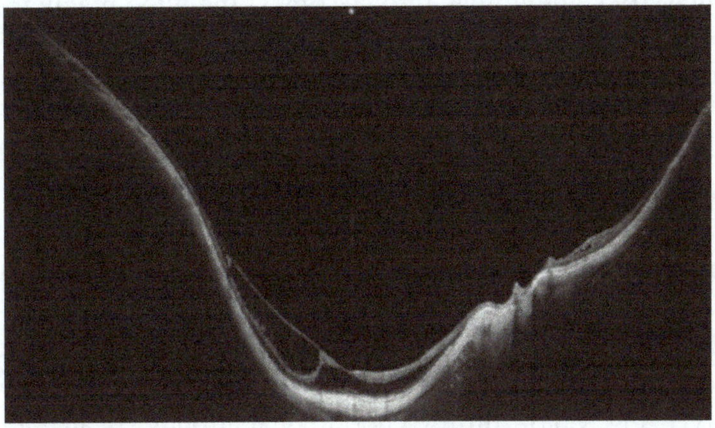

Fig. 9.4 Spatial relationship between myopic macular retinoschisis and posterior staphyloma. In this swept-source wide-field optical coherence tomographic image, the outer and inner retinoschisis is restricted to the area of the posterior staphyloma. It may suggest that the inner retinal structures as compared to the outer retinal structures were not flexible enough to follow the elongated circumference of Bruch's membrane and sclera

An additional advantage of the swept-source WF-OCT technology was the relatively large depth of focus so that structures from the posterior vitreous to the sclera could be imaged in the same image. It allowed the analysis of relationships between vitreoretinal abnormalities and other lesions in the inner retinal layers, such as myopic macular retinoschisis and posterior staphylomas as reported by Shinohara et al. [19] (Fig. 9.4).

9.3.3 Classification (Ohno-Matsui's Modified Classification, Fig. 9.3)

Based upon and modifying Curtin's [20] classical categorization of posterior staphylomas, with Types I–V as primary staphylomas and Types VI–X as compound staphylomas, Ohno-Matsui [17] used 3D-MRI and wide-field fundus

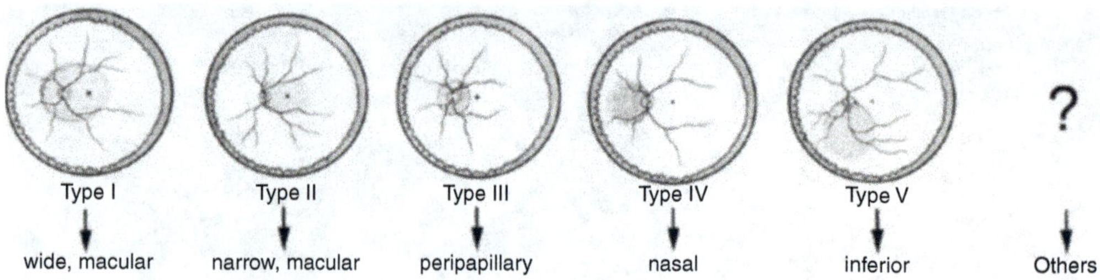

Fig. 9.5 Classification staphyloma (cited from [17] with permission). New classification of posterior staphyloma according to its location and extent. The staphyloma type is renamed according to its location and distribution. Type I → wide, macular staphyloma, Type II → narrow, macular staphyloma, Type III → peripapillary staphyloma, Type IV → nasal staphyloma, Type V → inferior staphyloma, others → staphylomas other than Types I–V

imaging to reclassify staphylomas into six types: the wide macular type, the narrow macular type, the peripapillary type, the nasal type, the inferior type, and others (Fig. 9.5).

9.4 Fundus Complications of Pathologic Myopia

9.4.1 Myopic Chorioretinal Atrophy (META-PM Study, Table 9.1)

In the META-PM classification [7], myopic maculopathy lesions have been categorized into five categories from "no myopic retinal lesions" (Category 0), "tessellated fundus only" (Category 1; Fig. 9.6a), "diffuse chorioretinal atrophy" (Category 2; Fig. 9.6b), "patchy chorioretinal atrophy" (Category 3; Fig. 9.6c), to "macular atrophy" (Category 4; Fig. 9.6d). These categories were defined based on long-term clinical observations that showed the progression patterns and associated factors of the development of myopic choroidal neovascularization (CNV) for each stage. Three additional features were added to these categories and were included as "plus signs": (1) lacquer cracks (Fig. 9.6e) and (2) myopic CNV (Fig. 9.6f) (Table 9.1). Since a Fuchs' spot represented a scarred form of myopic CNV, Fuchs' spots were categorized under the term of myopic CNV. The reason for separately listing the "plus signs" was that all three lesions have been shown to be strongly associated with central vision loss; however, they did not fit into any particular category and might develop from, or coexist, in eyes with any

Table 9.1 Myopic Chorioretinal Atrophy Classification (META-PM Study)

		Plus lesions
Category 0	Normal fundus	Myopic CNV lacquer cracks
Category 1	Tesselated fundus	
Category 2	Diffuse chorioretinal atrophy	
Category 3	Patchy chorioretinal atrophy	
Category 4	Macular atrophy	

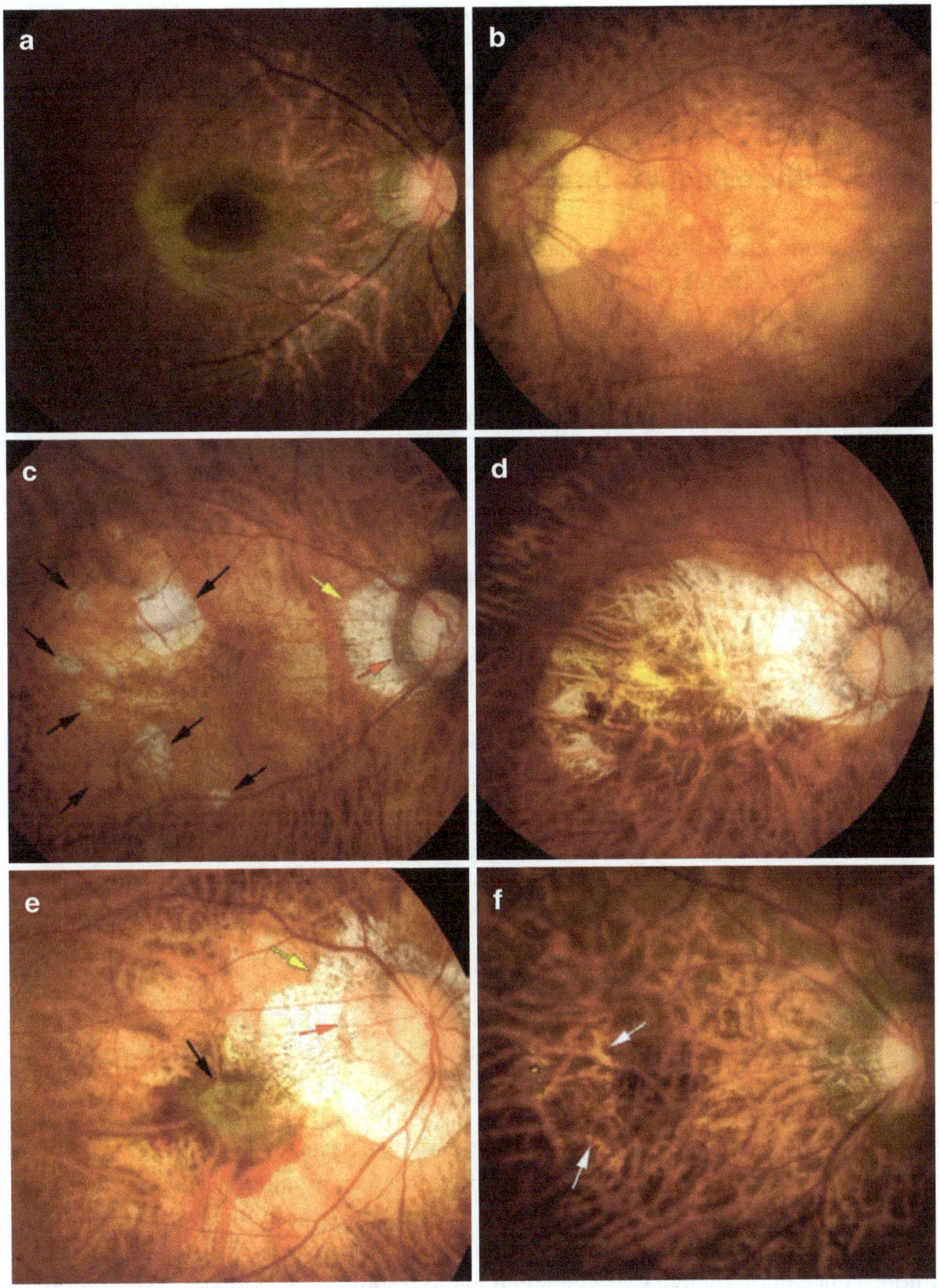

Fig. 9.6 Myopic maculopathy. (**a**) Fundus tessellation temporal to the optic disc. (**b**) Diffuse chorioretinal atrophy. Ill-defined, yellowish atrophy is seen in the posterior fundus. (**c**) Patchy chorioretinal atrophy. Within the area of diffuse atrophy, multiple areas of well-defined, whitish atrophic lesions are seen (arrows); yellow arrows: parapapillary gamma zone; red arrow: parapapillary delta zone. (**d**) Macular atrophy, several years after the formation of myopic choroidal neovascularization (CNV), a well-defined atrophic lesion is seen in the macular area. (**e**) Myopic CNV. Subretinal hemorrhage is seen around the CNV (arrow); yellow arrows: parapapillary gamma zone; red arrow: parapapillary delta zone. (**f**) Lacquer cracks. Multiple yellowish linear lesions are seen (arrows)

of the myopic maculopathy categories described above. Based on this classification, pathologic myopia has now been defined as myopic maculopathy Category 2 or above, or the presence of "plus" sign or posterior staphyloma [7, 21].

9.4.2 Diffuse Chorioretinal Atrophy (Category 2)

Diffuse chorioretinal atrophy is characterized by a yellowish white appearance of the posterior pole. The region of the diffuse atrophy may extend from a restricted area around the optic disc and a part of the macula to the entire posterior pole. The atrophy generally first appears around the optic disc, often increases with age, and finally covers the entire area within a staphyloma if a staphyloma is present. Both older age and longer axial length have been described as risk factors for the development of diffuse atrophy [9]. Marked thinning of the choroidal layer in the area of diffuse atrophy can be detected upon OCT, with occasional large choroidal vessels remaining.

9.4.3 Patchy Chorioretinal Atrophy (Category 3)

Patchy chorioretinal atrophy appears as well-defined, grayish white lesion(s) in the macular area or around the optic disc. Upon OCT, the area of patchy atrophy is characterized by the absence of the entire choroid and the RPE as well as of the outer retina. Hyper-transmission through the underlying sclera can be seen upon OCT. Using swept-source OCT, Ohno-Matsui et al. [22] showed that patchy atrophy was not simply a chorioretinal atrophy but was combined with a defect in Bruch's membrane (BM).

9.4.4 Lacquer Cracks (Plus Sign)

Lacquer cracks appear as yellowish linear lesions in the macula. Lacquer cracks have been considered to represent breaks in BM [9, 23–25]. Progression patterns of lacquer cracks include an increased number, elongation, and progression to patchy atrophy [8, 26].

Detection of lacquer cracks can sometimes be difficult especially in eyes with diffuse atrophy. Assessments of hyper-fluorescence by fluorescein angiography and hypo-fluorescence upon indocyanine green angiography have been useful for the diagnosis. Other linear lesions due to pathologic myopia with a similar hypo-fluorescence upon by indocyanine green angiography, such as myopic stretch lines, have to be differentiated [27].

Due to their small width, linear defects in BM as the base of lacquer cracks are difficult to be directly detected. Instead, hyper-reflective lines of the choroidal and scleral tissue layers on the OCT images indirectly indicate the linear BM defect by an optical window effect (Fig. 9.7). The recently developed imaging technique of OCT angiography may be useful for detecting a rupture of the choriocapillaris in

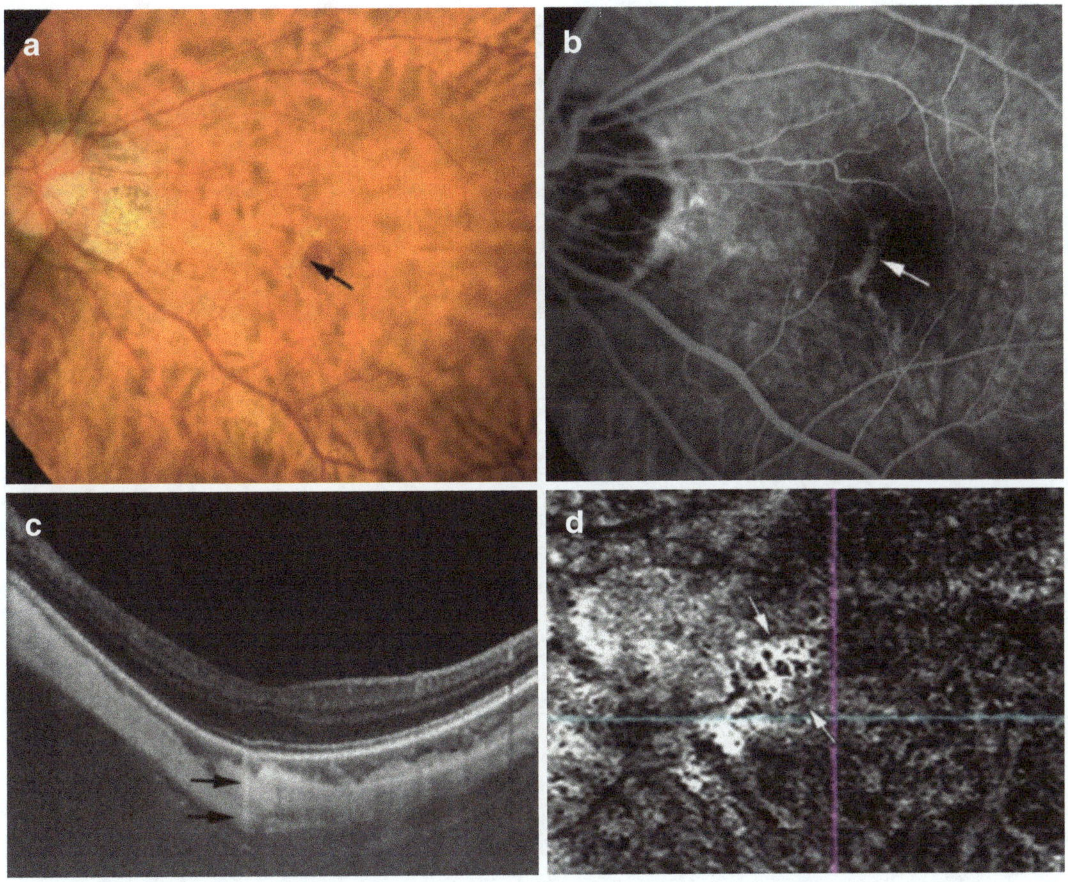

Fig. 9.7 Multimodal imaging of lacquer cracks. (**a**) Left fundus shows lacquer crack as yellowish linear lesion (arrow). (**b**) Fluorescein angiogram shows linear hyper-fluorescence at the site of lacquer crack (arrow). (**c**) Optical coherent tomographic image shows deep penetration of light (arrows) at the site of lacquer cracks. (**d**) OCT angiography shows a defect of choriocapillaris (arrows)

the area of lacquer cracks, again indirectly indicating a defect in BM [28]. Since a subretinal bleeding can often be observed at the onset of the development of lacquer cracks [29–31] (Fig. 9.8), it is important to exclude the presence of a myopic CNV in cases of subretinal bleeding in the region of lacquer cracks.

9.4.5 Myopic CNV and CNV-Related Macular Atrophy

Myopic CNV is a major sight threatening complication of pathologic myopia. It is the most common cause of CNV in individuals younger than 50 years, and it is the second most common cause of CNV overall [25, 32]. Myopic CNV is a Type II CNV and shows a clear hyper-fluorescence by fluorescein angiography. Anti-VEGF therapy is the first-line treatment for myopic CNV, as shown by the RADIANCE study [33] and the MYRROR study [34].

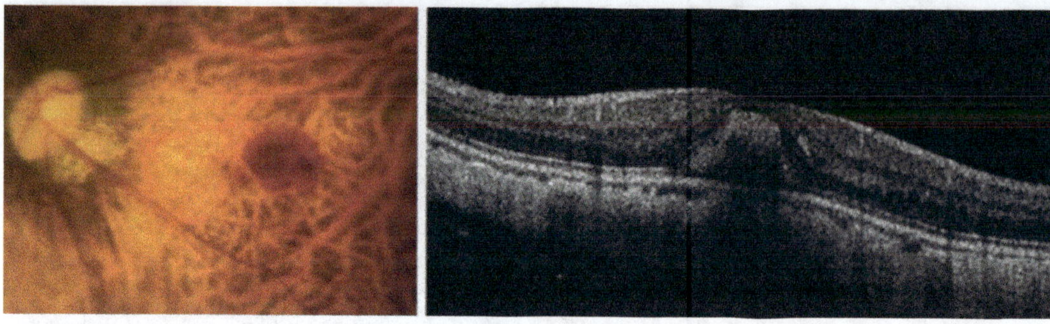

Fig. 9.8 Subretinal bleeding due to new lacquer crack formation. Left fundus shows subretinal bleeding. There are some projections along the temporal border of the hemorrhage. Optical coherent tomographic image shows subretinal hemorrhage. Serous retinal detachment or macular edema is not seen

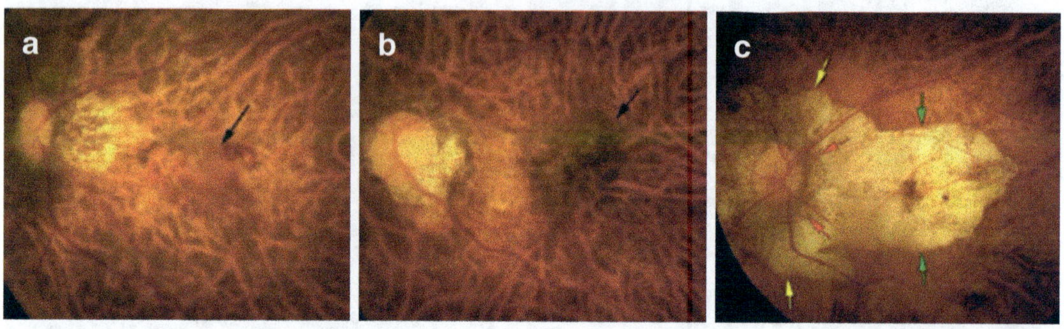

Fig. 9.9 Fundus photographs showing various phases of myopic CNV in different eyes. (**a**) Active phase. Subretinal bleeding is observed around the grayish CNV (black arrow). (**b**) Scar phase with pigmented scarred CNV (black arrow). (**c**) Atrophic phase at about 10 years after the first occurrence of a CNV; a well-defined macular atrophy (green arrows) appears as a macular Bruch's membrane defect, merging with a large parapapillary gamma zone (yellow arrows) around a parapapillary delta zone (red arrows)

In the long-term, both in treated eyes and in eyes exposed to the natural course of the disorder, macular atrophy develops around the scarred CNV and impairs central vision (Fig. 9.9). Swept-source OCT showed that CNV-related macular atrophy was not simply a chorioretinal atrophy but was BM hole [35], like patchy chorioretinal atrophy.

As shown upon OCT-angiography, the CNV maintains its blood flow even when the CNV transforms into the scar phase, including the area of CNV-related macular atrophy (Fig. 9.10). Louzada et al. [36] and Giuffre et al. [37] reported that blood vessels originating from the sclera were found at the site of myopic CNVs. Recently Ishida et al. [38] reported that the blood vessels of myopic CNVs were continuous to scleral branches of short posterior ciliary arteries (Fig. 9.11).

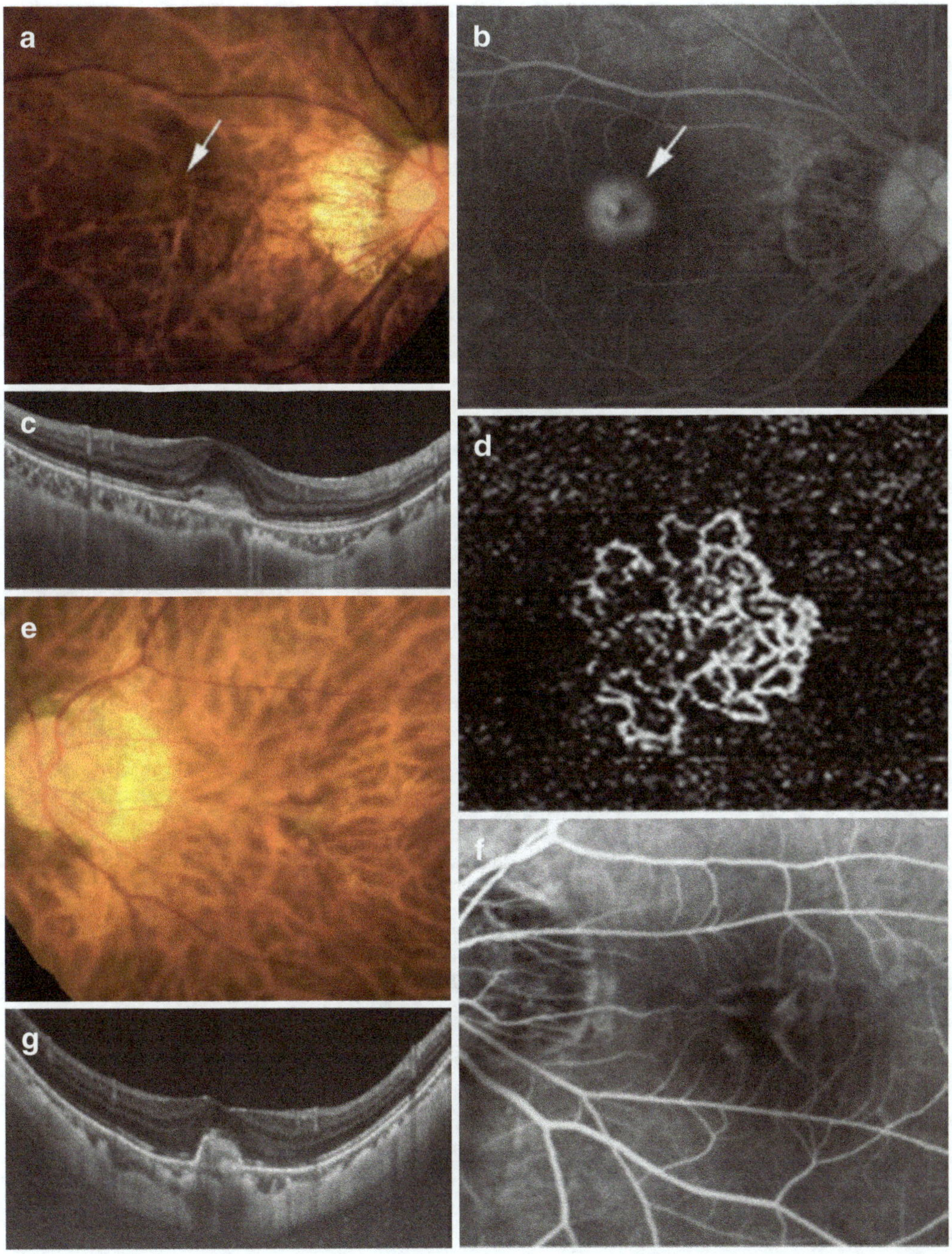

Fig. 9.10 Detection of choroidal neovascularization (CNV) with blood flow in all of the three phases of myopic CNV by optical coherent tomographic angiography (OCTA) [38]. (**a–d**) Active phase. Right fundus shows a grayish CNV (arrow in **a**). Fluorescein angiography (FA) shows hyper-fluorescence at the CNV (arrow in **b**). (**c**) Type II CNV is observed as subretinal tissue with fuzzy border by OCT. (**d**) OCTA shows newly formed vessels. (**e–h**) Scar phase. (**e**) Left fundus shows irregular shape of CNV. (**f**) FA shows tissue staining of irregular shape of CNV. (**g**) OCT shows subretinal CNV with sharp margins. (**h**) OCTA shows spiky shaped CNV. (**i–l**) Atrophic phase. CNV-related macular atrophy (margined by arrowheads) is seen around the remnants of a CNV (arrow in **i**). Fundus autofluorescence shows clear hypo-fluorescence in the area of the macular atrophy around the CNV (arrow in **j**). OCT shows subretinal CNV (arrow in **k**) surrounded by a large defect of Bruch's membrane. The inner retina directly sits on the sclera in the area of macular atrophy. The choroid is barely seen in the area of the macular atrophy. (**l**) OCTA shows CNV with blood flow. Large blood vessels appear to be connected to the CNV

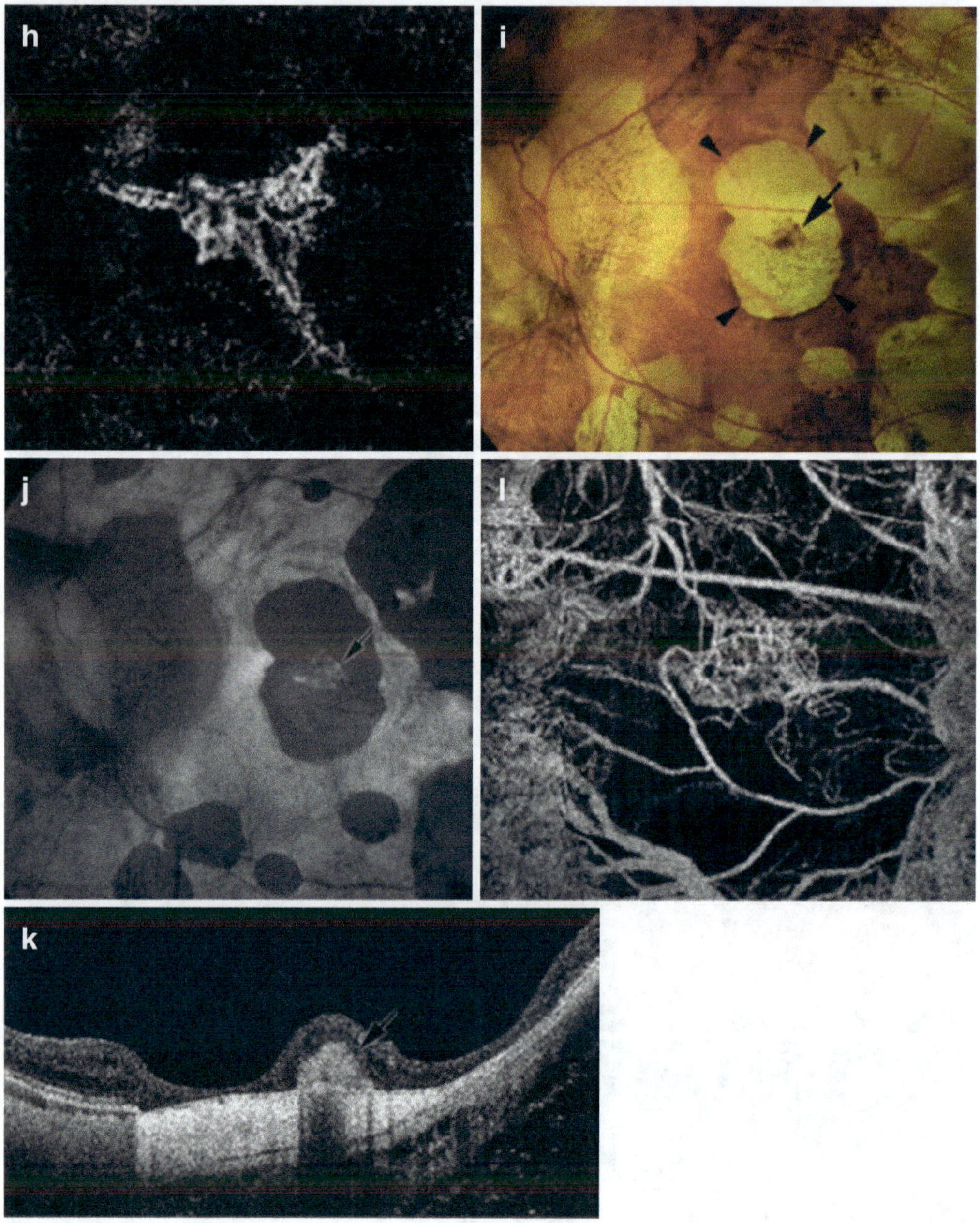

Fig. 9.10 (continued)

9.5 Myopic Macular Retinoschisis

Using optical coherence tomography, Takano and Kishi first demonstrated a foveal retinal detachment and retinoschisis in severely myopic eyes with posterior staphylomas [39]. Panozzo and Mercanti proposed the term "myopic traction maculopathy (MTM)" to encompass various findings characterized by a traction as visualized by OCT in highly myopic eyes [40]. Myopic traction maculopathy,

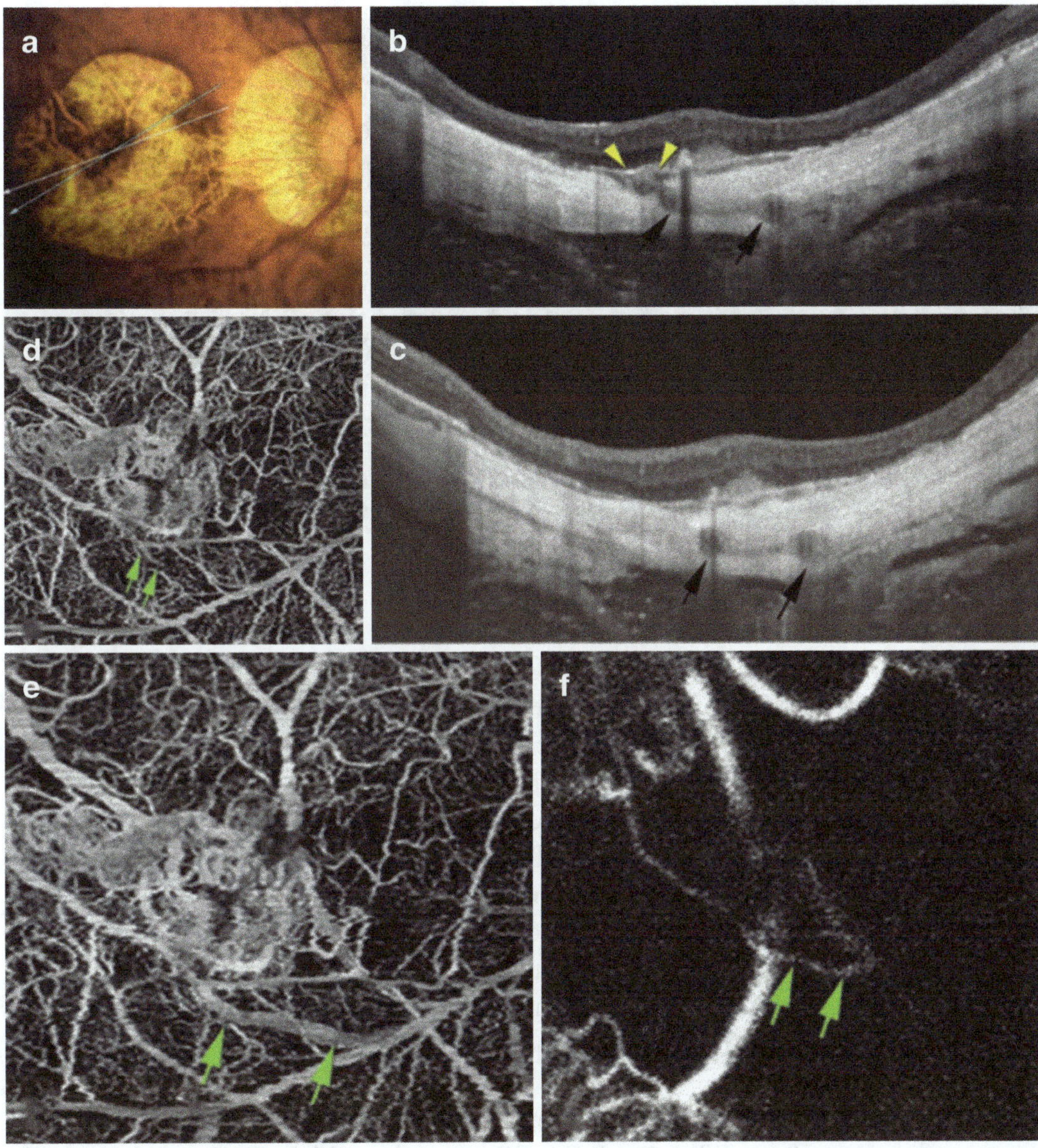

Fig. 9.11 Continuity between scleral perforating vessels and myopic choroidal neovascularization (CNV) in the atrophic phase [38]. (**a**) Fundus photograph of the right eye shows a sharp-margined macular atrophy around a CNV (arrow). Arrows indicate scanned line by OCT. (**b**, **c**) Swept-source OCT images show subretinal CNV. Cross sections of blood vessels coursing within the sclera can be seen (arrows in **c**) in a section scanned by swept-source OCT (blue arrow in **a**). In a serial OCT section (**b**, in a section scanned at white arrow in **a**), this vessel (arrows) is observed to be continuous with the CNV through a defect of Bruch's membrane (between arrowheads). (**d**, **e**) OCT angiogram shows the intrascleral vessel in Fig. 9.4b begins to be seen at the depth just posterior to the CNV (arrows, **d**). At a deeper slab **e**, the longer course of this vessel is seen (arrow, **e**). (**f**, **g**) Arterial phase of ICG angiogram (6 s after dye injection in **f**, and 8 s after dye injection in **g**) shows that the intrascleral vessel shown in OCT angiogram and OCT **b** scans was already filled with dye in the arterial phase (arrows). (**h**) Arterial phase of fluorescein angiogram (10 s after dye injection) shows that the intrascleral vessel observed in **f** and **g** is fairly seen (arrows)

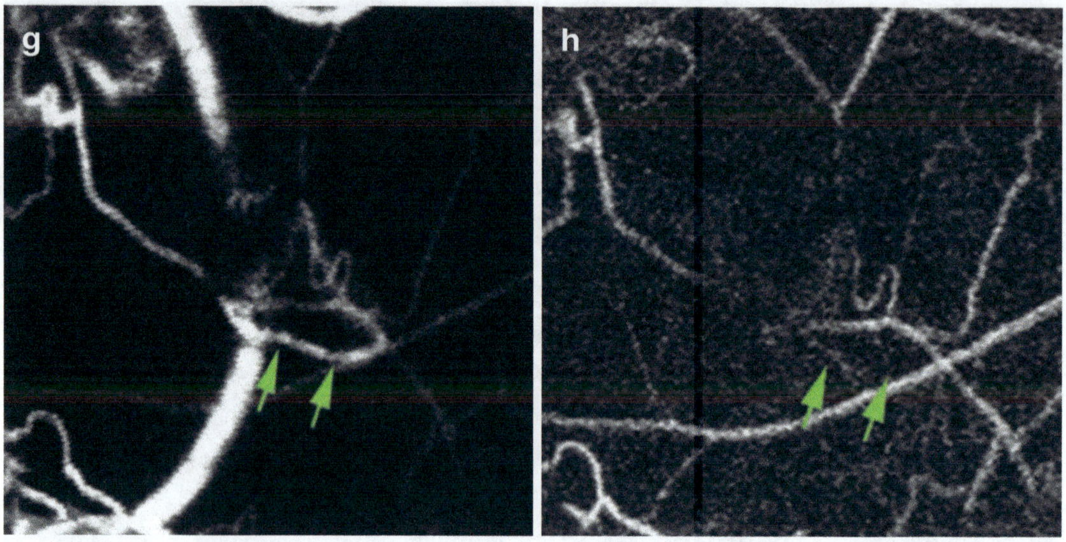

Fig. 9.11 (continued)

also called foveal retinoschisis [39], macular retinoschisis [41], or myopic foveoschisis [42], includes the features of schisis-like inner retinal fluid, schisis-like outer retina fluid, foveal detachment, lamellar or full-thickness macular hole, and/or macular detachment [43]. These features can best be detected by OCT as an indispensable tool to diagnose MTM. Additional examination techniques are a retro-mode imaging which uses an infrared laser in the confocal scanning laser ophthalmoscope and which can produce a pseudo-three-dimensional image showing the details of deep retinal structures (Fig. 9.12). Applying retro-mode imaging, a characteristic fingerprint and firework pattern at the corresponding area of a macular retinoschisis have been detected in the region of a macula retinoschisis [44, 45].

Shimada et al. have classified myopic traction maculopathy according to its location and extent from S0 through S4: S0: no retinoschisis; S1: extrafoveal; S2: foveal; S3: both foveal and extrafoveal but not the entire macula; and S4: entire macula [46].

9.6 Dome-Shaped Macula (DSM)

A dome-shaped macula (DSM) is an inward protrusion of the macula as visualized by OCT (Fig. 9.13) [47–49]. Imamura et al. reported that a DSM was associated with, and caused by, a local thickening of the subfoveal sclera [50]. It was postulated that the local thickening of the subfoveal sclera was an adaptive or

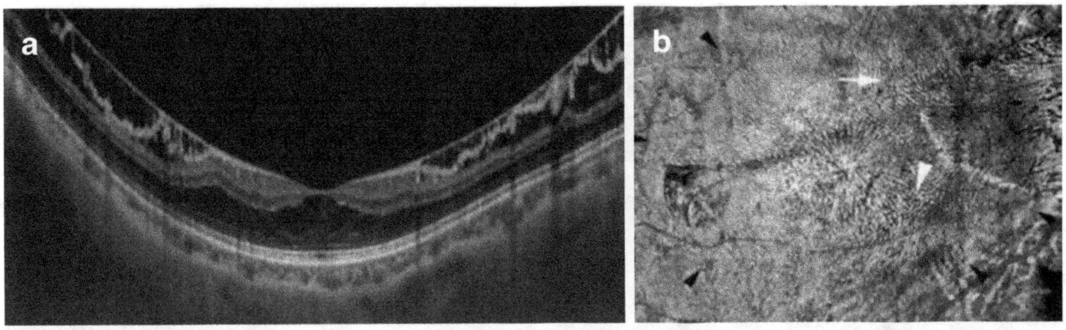

Fig. 9.12 Myopic macular retinoschisis. (**a**) OCT image shows outer and inner retinoschisis. (**b**) Columnar structures are seen within the area of outer retinoschisis (cited from [44]). Retro-mode image by F10 (Nidek, Aichi, Japan) showing a fingerprint pattern (black arrowheads) consisting of central radiating retinal striae and surrounding multiple dots (arrowhead) and lines (arrow). Many lines appear in parallel or in a whorled pattern. The inner lamellar hole appears as a circular defect at the central fovea

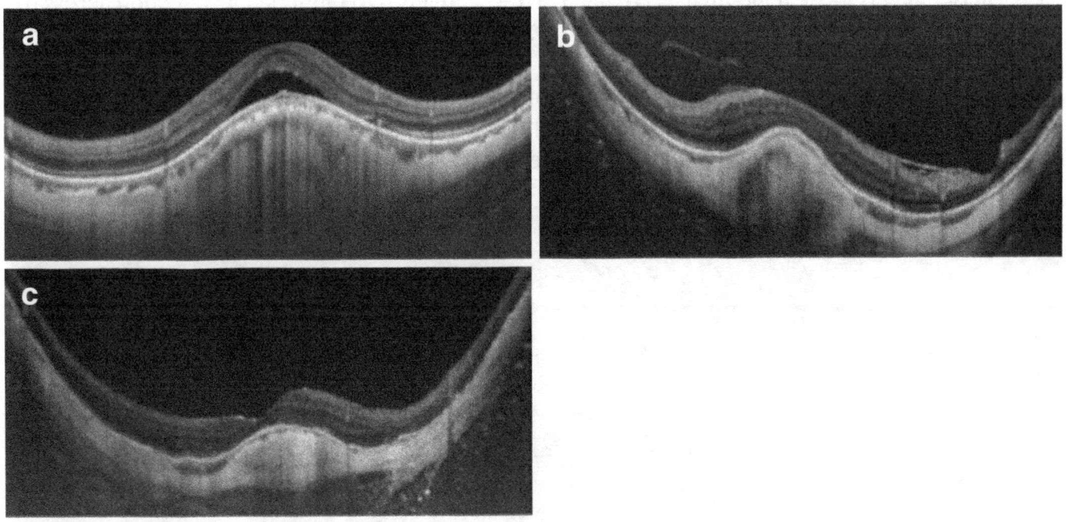

Fig. 9.13 Various types of Dome-shaped macula (DSM). (**a**) Serous retinal detachment is seen on the top of the dome. The sclera is too thick to allow the visualization of its outer surface. (**b**) The subfoveal sclera is thick; however, the scleral outer surface is visible in the surrounding area. (**c**) The subfoveal sclera is thick; however, the scleral outer surface is visible in all regions

compensatory response to the defocus of the image on the fovea in highly myopic eyes. Fang et al. [51] found the high prevalence of macular BM defects around the dome (Figs. 9.14 and 9.15). Ohno-Matsui et al. reported a similar finding [52] as peri-dome choroidal deepening. The morphology of the DSM in association with macular BM defects may be associated with a focal relaxation of the posterior sclera, no longer pushed outward by an expanding BM but allowed to partially bulge inward, leading to the formation of a DSM.

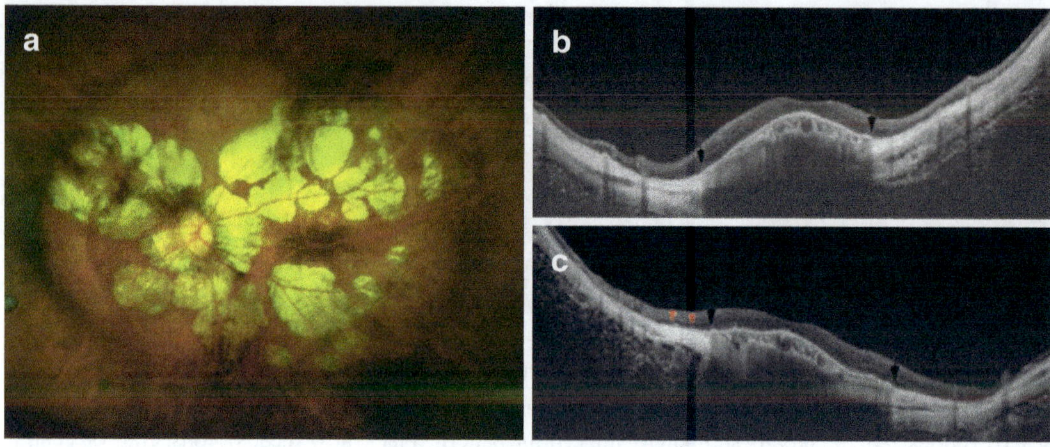

Fig. 9.14 Dome-shaped macula (DSM) coexisting with the macular Bruch's membrane defects (MBMD) associated with patchy atrophy [51]. (**a**) Left fundus of a 65-year-old woman with an axial length of 33.2 mm shows multiple patches of whitish, well-defined patchy atrophy in the regions superior and inferior to the fovea. Two long arrows show scanned lines examined by optical coherence tomography (OCT) in the images (**b**) and (**c**), respectively. (**b**) Oblique OCT section across the fovea demonstrates an inward protrusion due to DSM. Bruch's membrane is present at the center of the macula, but is interrupted abruptly (arrow) on both sides of the dome. (**c**) Oblique OCT section across the fovea shows the inward protrusion of macula due to DSM. Bruch's membrane is present at the center of macula, but is abruptly interrupted (arrow) on both sides of the dome. The remnants of Bruch's membrane are seen near the edge of the macular Bruch's membrane defect (arrowheads)

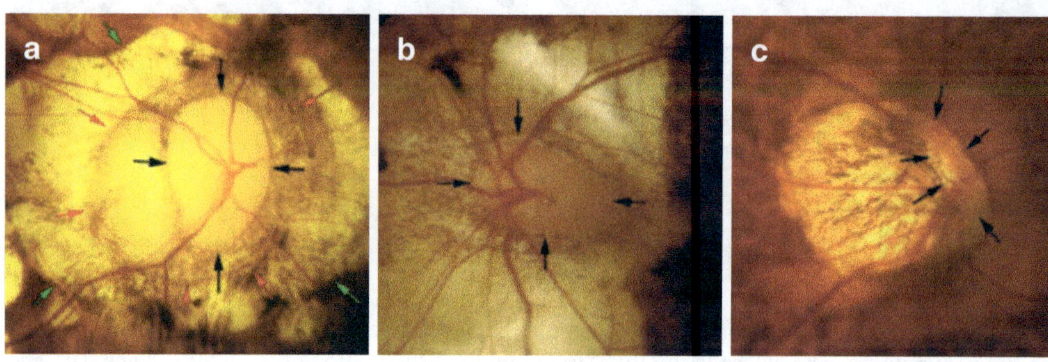

Fig. 9.15 Severe deformity of the optic disc due to pathologic myopia. (**a**) Acquired megalodisc. The optic disc shows irregular shape. (**b**) Horizontally stretched optic disc. (**c**) Extreme tilting of the optic disc. Black arrows: peripapillary rim; red arrows: parapapillary delta zone; green arrows: parapapillary gamma zone

References

1. Iwase A, Araie M, Tomidokoro A, et al. Prevalence and causes of low vision and blindness in a Japanese adult population: the Tajimi Study. Ophthalmology. 2006;113:1354–62.
2. Xu L, Wang Y, Li Y, et al. Causes of blindness and visual impairment in urban and rural areas in Beijing: the Beijing Eye Study. Ophthalmology. 2006;113:1134.e1.

3. You QS, Xu L, Yang H, et al. Five-year incidence of visual impairment and blindness in adult Chinese the Beijing Eye Study. Ophthalmology. 2011;118:1069–75.
4. Yamada M, Hiratsuka Y, Roberts CB, et al. Prevalence of visual impairment in the adult Japanese population by cause and severity and future projections. Ophthalmic Epidemiol. 2010;17:50–7.
5. Hsu WM, Cheng CY, Liu JH, et al. Prevalence and causes of visual impairment in an elderly Chinese population in Taiwan: the Shihpai Eye Study. Ophthalmology. 2004;111:62–9.
6. Ohno-Matsui K, Lai TYY, Cheung CMG, Lai CC. Updates of pathologic myopia. Prog Retin Eye Res. 2016;52:156–87.
7. Ohno-Matsui K, Kawasaki R, Jonas JB, et al. International photographic classification and grading system for myopic maculopathy. Am J Ophthalmol. 2015;159:877–83.
8. Fang Y, Yokoi T, Nagaoka N, et al. Progression of myopic maculopathy during 18-year follow-up. Ophthalmology. 2018;125(6):863–77.
9. Hayashi K, Ohno-Matsui K, Shimada N, et al. Long-term pattern of progression of myopic maculopathy: a natural history study. Ophthalmology. 2010;117:1595–611.
10. Yan YN, Wang YX, Yang Y, et al. Ten-year progression of myopic maculopathy: The Beijing Eye Study 2001-2011. Ophthalmology. 2018;125(8):1253–63.
11. Vongphanit J, Mitchell P, Wang JJ. Prevalence and progression of myopic retinopathy in an older population. Ophthalmology. 2002;109:704–11.
12. Xu L, Wang Y, Wang S, Jonas JB. High myopia and glaucoma susceptibility the Beijing Eye Study. Ophthalmology. 2007;114:216–20.
13. Nagaoka N, Jonas JB, Morohoshi K, et al. Glaucomatous-type optic discs in high myopia. PLoS One. 2015;10:e0138825.
14. Spaide RF. Staphyloma: part 1. New York: Springer; 2014. p. 167–76.
15. Moriyama M, Ohno-Matsui K, Hayashi K, et al. Topographical analyses of shape of eyes with pathologic myopia by high-resolution three dimensional magnetic resonance imaging. Ophthalmology. 2011;118:1626–37.
16. Moriyama M, Ohno-Matsui K, Modegi T, et al. Quantitative analyses of high-resolution 3D MR images of highly myopic eyes to determine their shapes. Invest Ophthalmol Vis Sci. 2012;53:4510–8.
17. Ohno-Matsui K. Proposed classification of posterior staphylomas based on analyses of eye shape by three-dimensional magnetic resonance imaging. Ophthalmology. 2014;121:1798–809.
18. Shinohara K, Shimada N, Moriyama M, et al. Posterior staphylomas in pathologic myopia imaged by widefield optical coherence tomography. Invest Ophthalmol Vis Sci. 2017;58:3750–8.
19. Shinohara K, Tanaka N, Jonas JB, et al. Ultra-widefield optical coherence tomography to investigate relationships between myopic macular retinoschisis and posterior staphyloma. Ophthalmology. 2018;125(10):1575–86.
20. Curtin BJ. The posterior staphyloma of pathologic myopia. Trans Am Ophthalmol Soc. 1977;75:67–86.
21. Verkicharla PK, Ohno-Matsui K, Saw SM. Current and predicted demographics of high myopia and an update of its associated pathological changes. Ophthalmic Physiol Opt. 2015;35:465–75.
22. Ohno-Matsui K, Jonas JB, Spaide RF. Macular Bruch membrane holes in highly myopic patchy chorioretinal atrophy. Am J Ophthalmol. 2016;166:22–8.
23. Gao LQ, Liu W, Liang YB, et al. Prevalence and characteristics of myopic retinopathy in a rural Chinese adult population: the Handan Eye Study. Arch Ophthalmol. 2011;129:1199–204.
24. Zheng Y, Lavanya R, Wu R, et al. Prevalence and causes of visual impairment and blindness in an urban Indian population: the Singapore Indian Eye Study. Ophthalmology. 2011;118:1798–804.
25. Neelam K, Cheung CM, Ohno-Matsui K, et al. Choroidal neovascularization in pathological myopia. Prog Retin Eye Res. 2012;31:495–525.

26. Xu X, Fang Y, Uramoto K, et al. Clinical features of lacquer cracks in eyes with pathologic myopia. Retina. 2018. https://doi.org/10.1097/IAE.0000000000002168.
27. Shinohara K, Moriyama M, Shimada N, et al. Myopic stretch lines: linear lesions in fundus of eyes with pathologic myopia that differ from lacquer cracks. Retina. 2014;34:461–9.
28. Sayanagi K, Ikuno Y, Uematsu S, Nishida K. Features of the choriocapillaris in myopic maculopathy identified by optical coherence tomography angiography. Br J Ophthalmol. 2017;101:1524–9.
29. Ohno-Matsui K, Ito M, Tokoro T. Subretinal bleeding without choroidal neovascularization in pathologic myopia. A sign of new lacquer crack formation. Retina. 1996;16:196–202.
30. Shapiro M, Chandra SR. Evolution of lacquer cracks in high myopia. Ann Ophthalmol. 1985;17:231–5.
31. Klein RM, Green S. The development of lacquer cracks in pathologic myopia. Am J Ophthalmol. 1988;106:282–5.
32. Ohno-Matsui K, Yoshida T, Futagami S, et al. Patchy atrophy and lacquer cracks predispose to the development of choroidal neovascularisation in pathological myopia. Br J Ophthalmol. 2003;87:570–3.
33. Wolf S, Balciuniene VJ, Laganovska G, et al. RADIANCE: a randomized controlled study of ranibizumab in patients with choroidal neovascularization secondary to pathologic myopia. Ophthalmology. 2014;121:682–92.
34. Ikuno Y, Ohno-Matsui K, Wong TY, et al. Intravitreal aflibercept injection in patients with myopic choroidal neovascularization: The MYRROR Study. Ophthalmology. 2015;122:1220–7.
35. Ohno-Matsui K, Jonas JB, Spaide RF. Macular Bruch's membrane holes in choroidal neovascularization-related myopic macular atrophy by swept-source optical coherence tomography. Am J Ophthalmol. 2015;162:133–9.
36. Louzada RN, Ferrara D, Novais EA, et al. Analysis of scleral feeder vessel in myopic choroidal neovascularization using optical coherence tomography angiography. Ophthalmic Surg Lasers Imaging Retina. 2016;47:960–4.
37. Giuffre C, Querques L, Carnevali A, et al. Choroidal neovascularization and coincident perforating scleral vessels in pathologic myopia. Eur J Ophthalmol. 2017;27:e39–45.
38. Ishida T, Watanabe T, Yokoi T, et al. Possible connection of short posterior ciliary arteries to choroidal neovascularisations in eyes with pathologic myopia. Br J Ophthalmol. 2018;103(4):457–62.
39. Takano M, Kishi S. Foveal retinoschisis and retinal detachment in severely myopic eyes with posterior staphyloma. Am J Ophthalmol. 1999;128:472–6.
40. Panozzo G, Mercanti A. Optical coherence tomography findings in myopic traction maculopathy. Arch Ophthalmol. 2004;122:1455–60.
41. Benhamou N, Massin P, Haouchine B, et al. Macular retinoschisis in highly myopic eyes. Am J Ophthalmol. 2002;133:794–800.
42. Ikuno Y, Sayanagi K, Ohji M, et al. Vitrectomy and internal limiting membrane peeling for myopic foveoschisis. Am J Ophthalmol. 2004;137:719–24.
43. Johnson MW. Myopic traction maculopathy: pathogenic mechanisms and surgical treatment. Retina. 2012;32(Suppl 2):S205–10.
44. Tanaka Y, Shimada N, Ohno-Matsui K, et al. Retromode retinal imaging of macular retinoschisis in highly myopic eyes. Am J Ophthalmol. 2010;149:635–40.e1.
45. Su Y, Zhang X, Wu K, et al. The noninvasive retro-mode imaging of confocal scanning laser ophthalmoscopy in myopic maculopathy: a prospective observational study. Eye. 2014;28:998–1003.
46. Shimada N, Tanaka Y, Tokoro T, Ohno-Matsui K. Natural course of myopic traction maculopathy and factors associated with progression or resolution. Am J Ophthalmol. 2013;156:948–57.
47. Gaucher D, Erginay A, Lecleire-Collet A, et al. Dome-shaped macula in eyes with myopic posterior staphyloma. Am J Ophthalmol. 2008;145:909–14.
48. Caillaux V, Gaucher D, Gualino V, et al. Morphologic characterization of dome-shaped macula in myopic eyes with serous macular detachment. Am J Ophthalmol. 2013;156:958–67.

49. Ellabban AA, Tsujikawa A, Matsumoto A, et al. Three-dimensional tomographic features of dome-shaped macula by swept-source optical coherence tomography. Am J Ophthalmol. 2012;3:578.
50. Imamura Y, Iida T, Maruko I, et al. Enhanced depth imaging optical coherence tomography of the sclera in dome-shaped macula. Am J Ophthalmol. 2011;151:297–302.
51. Fang Y, Jonas JB, Yokoi T, et al. Macular Bruch's membrane defect and dome-shaped macula in high myopia. PLoS One. 2017;12:e0178998.
52. Ohno-Matsui K, Fang Y, Uramoto K, et al. Peri-dome choroidal deepening in highly myopic eyes with dome-shaped maculas. Am J Ophthalmol. 2017;183:134–40.

Imaging in Myopia

10

Quan V. Hoang, Jacqueline Chua, Marcus Ang,
and Leopold Schmetterer

Q. V. Hoang
Singapore Eye Research Institute, Singapore, Singapore

Singapore National Eye Centre, Singapore, Singapore

Eye Academic Clinical Program, Duke-NUS Medical School, Singapore, Singapore

Department of Ophthalmology, Harkness Eye Institute, Columbia University Medical Center, New York, NY, USA

J. Chua
Singapore Eye Research Institute, Singapore, Singapore

Singapore National Eye Centre, Singapore, Singapore

Eye Academic Clinical Program, Duke-NUS Medical School, Singapore, Singapore

M. Ang
Singapore Eye Research Institute, Singapore, Singapore

Singapore National Eye Centre, Singapore, Singapore

Eye Academic Clinical Program, Duke-NUS Medical School, Singapore, Singapore

Myopia Centre, Cornea and Refractive Service, Singapore National Eye Centre, Singapore, Singapore

L. Schmetterer (✉)
Singapore Eye Research Institute, Singapore, Singapore

Singapore National Eye Centre, Singapore, Singapore

Eye Academic Clinical Program, Duke-NUS Medical School, Singapore, Singapore

Department of Ophthalmology, Lee Kong Chian School of Medicine, Nanyang Technological University, Singapore, Singapore

School of Chemical and Biomedical Engineering, Nanyang Technological University, Singapore, Singapore

Department of Clinical Pharmacology, Medical University of Vienna, Vienna, Austria

Center for Medical Physics and Biomedical Engineering, Medical University of Vienna, Vienna, Austria
e-mail: leopold.schmetterer@seri.com.sg

M. Ang, T. Y. Wong (eds.), *Updates on Myopia*,
https://doi.org/10.1007/978-981-13-8491-2_10

Key Points

- Advances in ocular imaging devices including optical coherence tomography, ultrasound, and magnetic resonance imaging have enabled the visualization of pathologic changes due to myopia, identifying microscopic changes ranging from the posterior segment (sclera, choroid, retina, and/or the optic nerve) to the anterior segment.
- Imaging-derived measures (imaging biomarkers) are potentially useful in assessing degenerative changes occurring in the myopic fundus, in evaluating the early changes preceding myopic macular degeneration, and in providing objective measures of ocular structures to aid in detecting staphyloma formation and progression, myopic macular degeneration-tilted disc syndrome, and glaucoma in highly myopic eyes.
- Imaging the highly myopic eye is not straightforward and is associated with challenges such as optics-related aberrations, focusing ability of current devices, and morphological alterations of the myopic fundus and optic nerve.
- An understanding of the imaging of microstructural changes associated with pathological myopia, challenges associated with imaging devices, and potential usefulness and limitations of imaging devices will better inform clinicians of its future potential in the diagnosis and management of vision-threatening complications associated with pathological myopia.

10.1 Introduction

In evaluating the myopic eye, imaging has been proven vital in assessing disease complications [1] and prognostication for future management. Early identification of these changes would help predict the development of future complications, which include retinal tears and retinal detachments [2]. Additionally, the possibility of identifying subtle changes in the macula (such as macular schisis or early macular holes; Fig. 10.1) via high-resolution images of the macula could perchance aid clinicians in predicting the development of complications such as macular holes and retinal detachments [3].

Furthermore, imaging may help detect, prognosticate, and guide management of other myopia-related eye diseases. This includes the early detection of atrophy and defects in the basement membrane, located between retinal pigment epithelium (RPE) and Bruch's membrane (BM), which would help predict the risk of developing choroidal neovascularization (CNV) [4]—a leading cause of low vision and blindness in 5–17% of eyes in patients with pathological myopia (PM) [5]. In addition, imaging is vital for monitoring progression of posterior staphylomas and geographic atrophy, both of which can cause visual impairment in older age groups of patients [6].

Optic disc imaging can also be used to predict the development of glaucoma, where visualization of myopic tilting of the optic disc with peripapillary atrophy and pitting of the optic disc [7], is a possible predisposing factor [8, 9]. Serial imaging investigative measures can therefore be utilized for monitoring the development

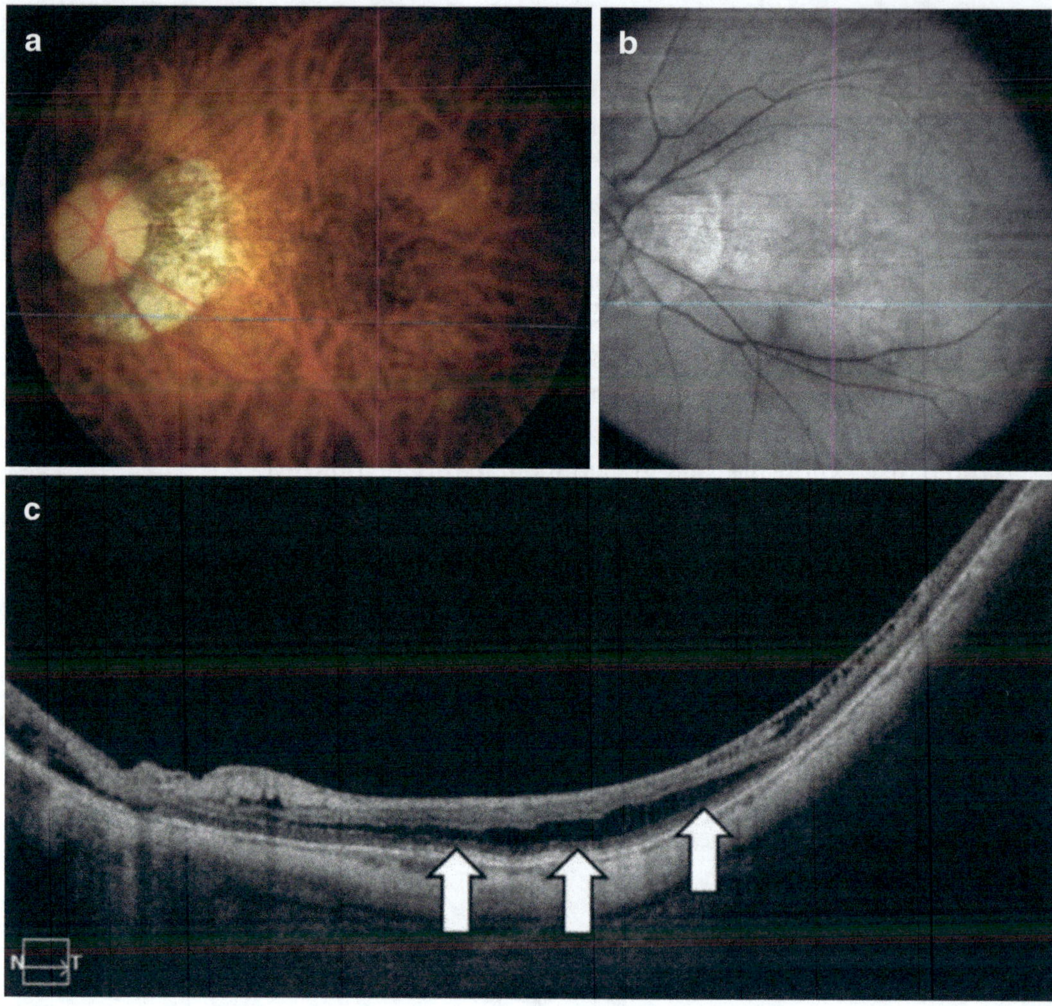

Fig. 10.1 Optical coherence tomography (OCT) imaging findings of a patient with myopic macular degeneration, showing the benefits of using the OCT over color fundus photograph in detecting retinoschisis. (**a**) Color fundus photograph showing tilted disc with large temporal peripapillary atrophy. (**b**, 12 × 12 mm; PLEX Elite, Zeiss) OCT of the fundus showing slight elevation of the retina where the crosshair is positioned. (**c**) OCT B-scan showing distinct retinoschisis (white arrows)

of open-angle, normal-tension glaucoma [10]. With the hope of exploring novel developments and prospective future clinical applications in the field of imaging in myopia, this chapter thus outlines the significance and challenges of imaging myopic eyes (from the anterior and posterior segments and optic nerve).

10.2 Disease Characteristics of Myopia

To best understand how one should approach imaging eyes with myopia, one needs to gear imaging modalities based on the pathophysiology of the disease, which has already been outlined in previous chapters. For example, not only does the sclera of these extremely elongated eyes show marked scleral thinning [12, 13], some eyes thin to the extent that local outpouchings or staphylomas form (Figs. 10.2 and 10.3). Staphylomas are often recognized as the harbinger of PM, reported in up to 90% of

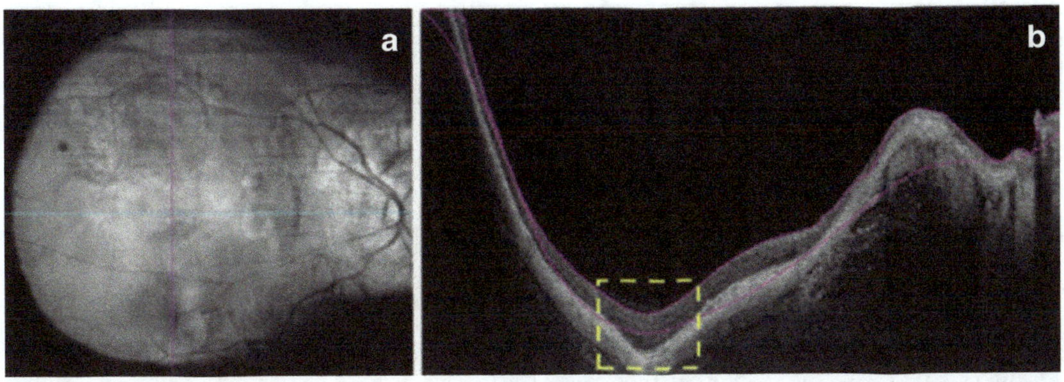

Fig. 10.2 Optical coherence tomography (OCT) imaging findings of a highly myopic patient, showing the benefits of using the OCT over fundus photograph to detect posterior staphyloma. (**a**, 12 × 12 mm; PLEX Elite, Zeiss) OCT fundus photograph showing tilted disc with large temporal peripapillary atrophy. (**b**) OCT B-scan showing distinct posterior staphyloma (yellow dotted box)

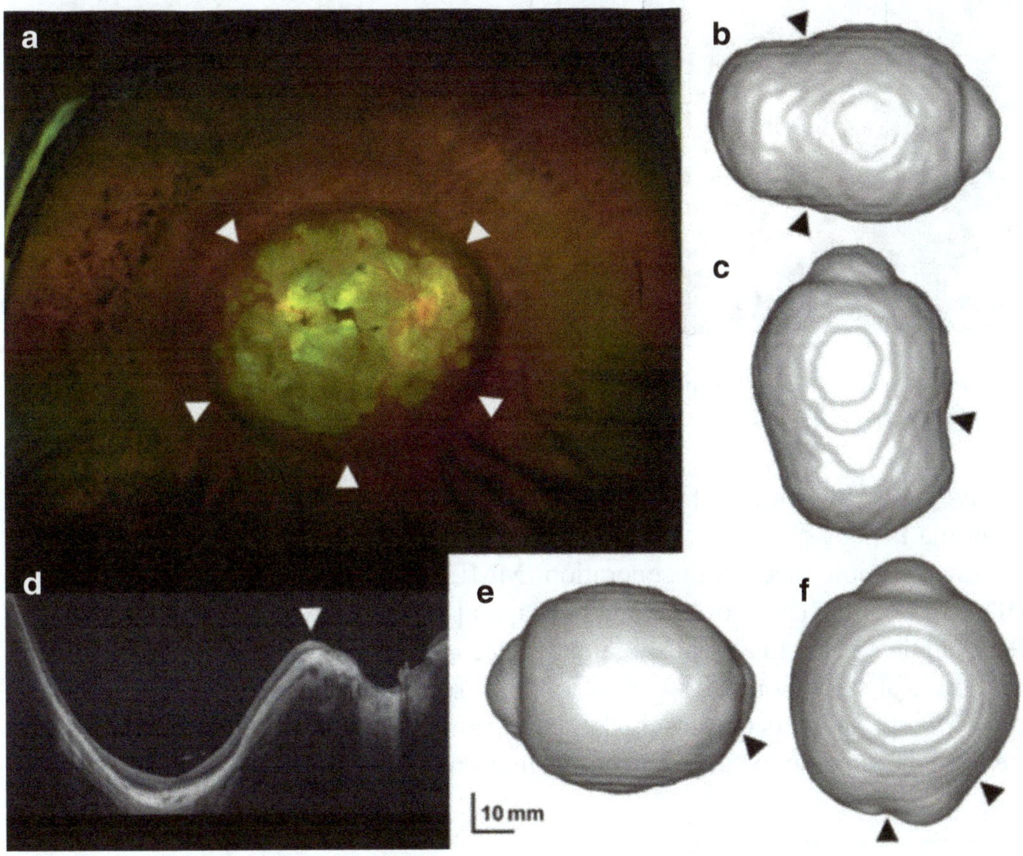

Fig. 10.3 Fundus photography, swept source optical coherence tomography (SSOCT), and 3-dimensional magnetic resonance imaging (MRI) of patients with posterior staphyloma. Patient 1 (**a**, **b**, **c**) was a 58-year-old woman with an axial length of 35.4 mm in the right eye (OD). The right fundus shows a deep, circular-shaped posterior staphyloma, with an abrupt change in scleral curvature (arrowheads) apparent on fundus photography (A) and OD MRI volume renderings (B- temporal view, C- inferior view). Patient 2 (**d**, **e**, **f**) was a 61-year-old woman with an OD axial length of 33.8 mm. A posterior staphyloma was present, with an abrupt change in scleral curvature (arrowheads) apparent on OD SSOCT (D) and OD MRI volume renderings (E- nasal view, F- superior view)

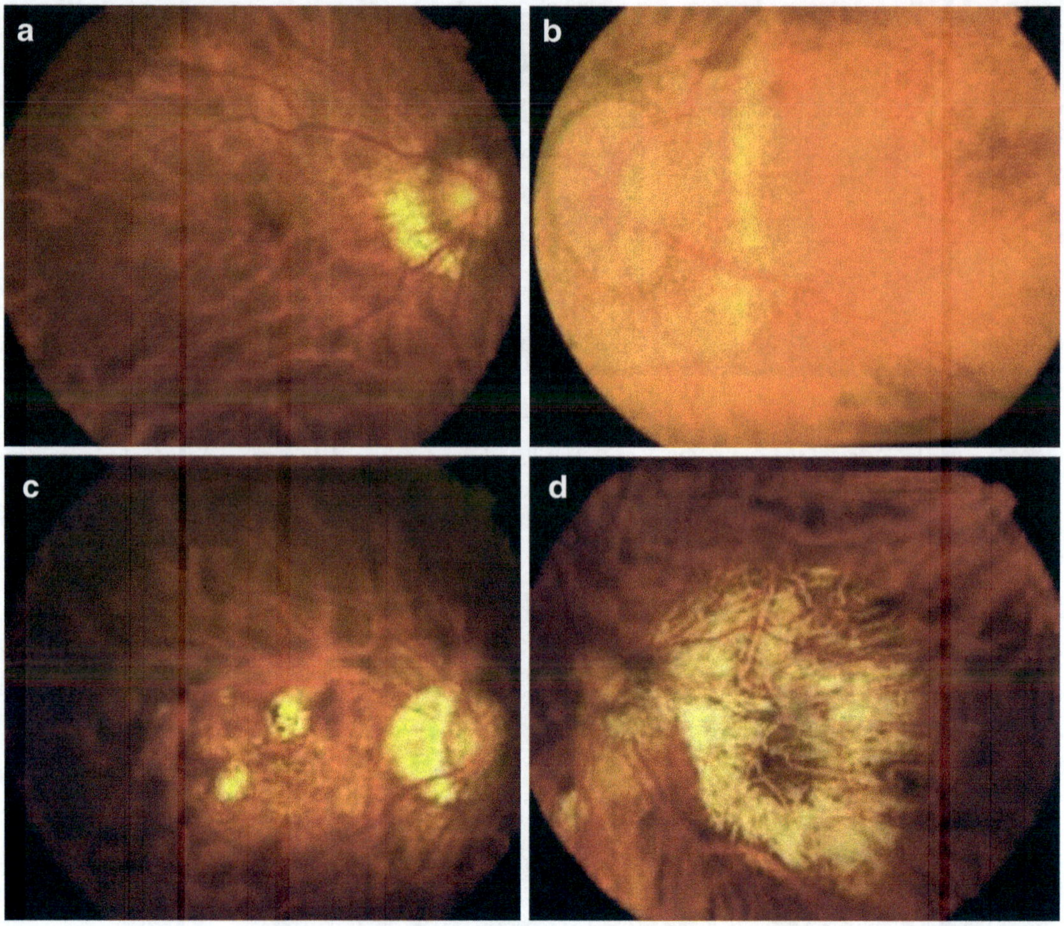

Fig. 10.4 Color fundus photographs showing the worsening levels of myopic macular degeneration; (**a**) Category 1, (**b**) Category 2, (**c**) Category 3 (**c**), and (**d**) Category 4

high myopia (HM) patients [14, 15]. More recent reports noted a severe grade of staphyloma being associated with further eye elongation [16] and more severe and progressive myopic macular degeneration (MMD; Fig. 10.4) [14, 17, 18]. Given that MMD is the leading cause of blindness in Japan [19], and the second leading cause in Chinese adults [20], it highlights the importance of closely monitoring patients with a severe grade of staphyloma. Risk of vision loss from myopic maculopathy (e.g., from splitting of retinal layers (foveoschisis), hole formation, atrophy, and CNV) may correlate with the specific location and conformation [11] of staphylomas [21].

10.3 Key Structures Altered in Myopia and Pathological Myopia

10.3.1 Sclera and Collagen

Changes in sclera and collagen structures may underlie axial elongation and staphyloma formation and progression. The anatomical changes underlying global eye elongation and local staphyloma formation likely occur in the component collagen fibers of the sclera. In mammalian models, there is scleral thinning and tissue loss during myopia development [11, 22] with a net decrease in scleral collagen (with decreased collagen synthesis and increased degradation) evidenced by reduced dry weight and hydroxyproline content [23, 24]. Decreased collagen fiber diameter and decreased collagen crosslinking (CXL) are seen in both mammalian models and HM patients [13, 25]. Specifically, in the guinea pig myopia model, there is scleral remodeling, possibly from greater slippage [26] between collagen fibrils and/or collagen fiber bundles due to fibroblast deactivation, with decreased expression of type I collagen, and α_2 and α_1 integrin [27, 28]. In the tree shrew mammalian myopia model, blockage of collagen crosslinking with β-aminopropionitrile resulted in an increased degree of myopia-induced vitreous elongation and scleral thinning at the posterior pole [29]. Moreover, the development of high myopia and pathologic myopia may be driven by genes such as the scleral remodeling gene LAMA2, leading to scleral thinning and staphyloma formation [30].

10.3.2 Choroidal Changes

Choroidal changes in myopia may contribute to atrophy and myopic macular degeneration. Morphological change such as the thinning of the choroidal vascular layer is closely associated with increasing levels of myopia and MMD (either immediately preceding, concurrent with or immediately following the development of MMD) [31–33]. Specifically, Wei et al. reported that subfoveal choroidal thickness in their Beijing-based cohort decreased by 15 μm per diopter of increased myopia [31]. There are various lesions comprising myopic maculopathy [3, 11, 18, 34, 35] that all involve the choroid, namely, diffuse chorioretinal atrophy, patchy chorioretinal atrophy, macular atrophy (bare sclera), lacquer cracks, and myopic choroidal neovascularization. Diffuse atrophy is a yellowish, ill-defined lesion [34], and is characterized by a marked thinning of the choroid as seen on optical coherence tomography (OCT), but with relatively preserved outer retina and retinal pigment epithelium, allowing for relatively good vision. Patchy chorioretinal atrophy is whitish, well-defined atrophy [34] with complete localized loss of the choroid with only the large choroidal vessels sporadically remaining within the atrophic area. Loss of the choroid is soon followed by loss of outer retina and retinal pigment epithelium. Macular atrophy is similar to patchy atrophy but tends to be centered at the fovea.

10.3.3 Bruch's Membrane and Retinal Pigment Epithelium Changes

The hallmark anatomical changes that occur alongside the development and progression of MMD are changes in BM and RPE as reflected in increasing degrees of atrophy [36]. Moreover, BM changes have been postulated to be the main driver of axial elongation overall [37]. Recently, Ohno-Matsui et al. reported the use of swept-source OCT (SS-OCT) to demonstrate that patchy atrophy was not simply chorioretinal atrophy, but also included a hole in Bruch's membrane [38]. Angiographically observed vessels within the area of patchy atrophy may include large choroidal vessels, intrascleral vessels, and retrobulbar vessels. Lacquer cracks are observed as yellowish linear lesions [34, 39, 40], and represent the mechanical rupture of BM [41]. Jonas et al. have reported an increase in disc–fovea distance due to an increase in the peripapillary gamma zone. Since BM thickness was found to be independent of axial length [42], even in the much larger surface area in an axially elongated eye in a human histomorphometric study, Jonas et al. inferred that the volume of BM increased with longer axial length and BM is actively produced during axial length elongation [37]. They postulated that BM was a primary driver of axial elongation that led to choroidal thinning through "compression." If this was indeed the mechanism, then the RPE is an ideal target for medical intervention in both eyes that are already severely elongated, as well as those undergoing progression, but still only minimally elongated.

10.4 Existing Imaging Modalities to Evaluate the Myopic Eye

10.4.1 Optical Coherence Tomography

Ophthalmic OCT systems can image the anterior segment as well as the posterior segment of the eye such as the retina, BM, RPE, and choroid. Spectral-domain OCT (SD-OCT, Spectralis, Heidelberg Eng., Carlsbad, CA) provides an axial resolution of 4 μm and a lateral resolution of 14 μm, but only about 1 mm of penetration into the retina. The extremely fine resolution of OCT allows better assessment of retinal layers such as photoreceptors, the ganglion cells, plexiform, and nuclear layers [43] and vitreous membranes in proximity to the retina. In contrast to the SD-OCT, SS-OCT uses a tunable laser with a longer wavelength of 1050 nm, which achieves greater penetration of tissue with less signal roll-off, allowing better visualization of choroidal anatomy [38, 44, 45] and has specifically been employed to correlate defects in BM with the atrophy of MMD [38]. In addition to utilizing choroidal thickness as biomarker for myopia progression [31–33], recent developments provide further insight into the function of the choroid, including the calculation of choroidal vascular index (CVI, the vessel-area-to-stromal-area ratio using a validated automated algorithm) [46] and OCTA using the SS-OCT (SS-OCTA, a noninvasive method of imaging choroidal vasculature, and specifically the foveal avascular zone (FAZ) without the administration of intravenous dye) [47, 48]. Newer UWF-OCT systems allow for even wider (100°) scans. Wider scans are likely crucial to accurately depicting staphyloma shape [49].

10.4.2 Ultrasound

Ophthalmic ultrasound can image the entire eye dynamically. Since their introduction in 1958, mechanically scanned, single element 10 MHz transducers have largely been the norm for imaging of the eye [50]. UBM systems (Escalon-Sonomed, Quantel, Ophthalmic Technologies, among others) have been used for diagnostic imaging and biometric characterization [51, 52]. Systems operating at 20 MHz were introduced (Quantel Medical, Bozeman, MT) for examination of the posterior segment of the eye and the vitreoretinal interface [51, 53]. With an axial resolution of about 75 μm, these systems provide superior resolution compared to conventional 10 MHz systems as well as the ability to image the retina. They also provide far deeper penetration than optical modalities (10 mm vs. 1 mm for OCT). Commercial single-element systems are designed such that during a contact examination, the geometric focus of the transducer falls just anterior to the retina. However, the anterior vitreous and anterior-segment structures (cornea, iris, ciliary body, and lens) are poorly visualized because they fall within the unfocused near field of the transducer which makes current ophthalmic systems unsuitable for imaging the entire vitreous. Recent advancements in annular-array imaging technology overcome these technical limits [54].

10.4.3 Magnetic Resonance Imaging

MRI allows for imaging of the whole eye (Fig. 10.3). The standard ophthalmology imaging modalities of ultrasound and optical coherence tomography are limited by a relatively narrow field of view. MRI does allow for imaging of the entire eye globe, but visualizing eye wall distortions at standard MR resolutions minimizes effect sizes and induces aliasing artifacts that obfuscate distortions. Super-resolution is an established MR approach that provides a means of detecting extremely small distortions by increasing signal to noise (with isotropic resolutions down to 50–100 μm), reducing scan time (which would allow patients to more readily maintain fixation, thereby reducing eye movement artifacts), and minimizing aliasing artifacts that can bias estimates [55, 56].

10.5 Challenges in Imaging of the Myopic Eye

10.5.1 Interaction Between Low- and High-Order Aberrations

Given the presence of two positive lenses (the cornea and the crystalline lens) in the eye, any imaging of intraocular structures is contingent on their properties. This makes direct visualization and imaging structures in the posterior segment, secondary to optical imperfections through the cornea and lens, the main challenge in imaging a myopic eye. Examples of such would include light diffraction in the pupil, intraocular scattering, and optical aberrations. As a result of these imperfections, imaging of patients with high myopia using any modality (such as fundus photography) would have a poorer image quality due to an imbalance of low- and high-order aberrations [57, 58]. Other causes to consider include the limitations of focusing lenses used by the imaging device. For example, the device may not be able to compensate (diopter compensation) sufficiently in patients with very high myopia (more than −12.0 D). Pathological myopia is also associated with varying structural changes within the eye (due to the abnormal eye elongation, scleral and corneal curvature irregularities, cataracts leading to poor clarity, or retinal thinning causing abnormal projections of the final image [58, 59]). Such structural changes are demonstrated in altered optic nerve head morphology.

Taking into considerations the challenges faced when imaging the myopic eye, current standards of practice for investigations include fundus photography, dye-based angiography, ultrasound (including biomicroscopy), and magnetic resonance imaging (MRI). The OCT has also become an often-used tool for the characterization of ocular tissue structural changes arising from myopia [60]. Swept source (SS)-OCT has a higher wavelength of 1050 nm and is hence able to penetrate into deeper layers. It is also capable of wide-angle scans, given its speed of capture and software engineering. More recently, OCT angiography (OCTA) has enabled visualization of the vasculature of the eye [61–63]. Nonetheless, there still exists room for improvement and various constraints. In the case of wide-field OCT (WF-OCT), problems with segmentation in the periphery may arise due to inadequate depth range to image the complete anterior–posterior extent of the posterior pole. Further considerations arise regarding the normative databases of OCT systems, where reference and patient cohorts should ideally be derived from the same population to reflect similar comorbidities [64]. Stratifications normally employed for covariates that affect measurements (such as age, ethnicity, and refractive error) are challenging to derive in myopic eyes—a result of large regional variation in refractive error prevalence [65]. In regions with a high prevalence of myopia and pathological myopia, this results in normative databases being poor representations of the existing patient population.

10.5.2 Challenges in Imaging the Anterior Segment

In high myopia, while most refractive errors in myopic eyes arise from an axial length, alterations in the anterior segment lead to significant optical and high-order aberrations [66]. Furthermore, the association between myopia and biomechanical changes in the cornea has implications in the assessment of intraocular pressure and may have a role in the pathogenesis of myopia [67]. Indeed, existing studies report inconsistent results—attributable to different imaging and measurement techniques, and the technological limitations in measuring biomechanical changes in the cornea associated with increasing myopia [68]. Preoperative clinical evaluation of patients with high myopia still necessitates imaging of the cornea and anterior segment, given their increasing risk of developing ectasia proportionate to the amount of corneal tissue removed in laser refractive surgeries [69]. Furthermore, as high myopes are more likely to require phakic lens implantation [70], accurate anterior segment imaging is necessary to ensure adequate safety measures prior to implantation and accurate intraocular lens (IOL) implantation. Especially in high myopes, accurate formulae, anterior segment imaging, and corneal topography are all necessary to prevent refractive surprises [71] and complications postoperatively. Significant improvements in IOL calculations and refractive prediction in high myopes [71] have fortunately been accomplished with new developments in biometry incorporating anterior segment OCT technology [72], coupled with next-generation formulae.

10.5.3 Challenges in Imaging the Retina

Prior to the discovery of modern imaging techniques, there were three main challenges faced in retinal imaging. First, the diagnosis of myopic foveoschisis was challenging based on clinical examination and fundus photography due to the lack of contrast between the retinal tissues and underlying choroid. Second, posterior staphylomas, a hallmark of pathological myopia [73], could not be identified from standalone two-dimensional fundus photography with ease. Finally, it is also challenging to capture lattice degeneration and retinal breaks in the peripheries on traditional 50° fundus photographs.

With the OCT, the way clinicians diagnosed and managed retinal complications of pathological myopia was transformed—with the ability to examine retinal layers *in vivo* and at high resolution. The ability to view distinct retinal layers has enhanced visualization of myopic traction maculopathy (MTM), for which splitting of the retinal layers can be well visualized on cross-sectional OCT scans of the retina. This can be taken a step further using retromode fundus imaging [74]. Examples of features that can be seen include inner or outer retinal schisis, foveal detachment, lamellar, or full thickness macular hole and/or macular detachment [75, 76].

Another aspect in which OCT has advanced the diagnosis and management of myopia-related eye diseases is in the characterization of posterior staphylomas, which are one of the hallmarks of pathological myopia. Nonstereoscopic fundus photographs are inadequate for detailed studies of posterior staphylomas as the change in contour at the staphyloma edge is not always discernible. The OCT overcomes this limitation because of its excellent depth resolution [21, 77]. Comparing their capability in visualizing posterior staphylomas, Shinohara et al. showed no significant differences between using WF-OCT and three-dimensional (3D) MRI imaging. It is noted, however, that ultrawide-field OCT (UWF-OCT) had the advantage in visualizing the spatial relationship of the staphylomas with the optic nerve and macula [78, 79].

Comparing the use of conventional fundus photography to UWF retinal imaging, the former has been shown capable of imaging up to 50° of the retina, while the latter covers a wider field of the retina at 200°. Given the high prevalence of lattice degeneration and retinal breaks in the peripheral retina in patients with highly myopic eyes, the advantages of UWF retinal imaging can be appreciated.

A potentially blinding complication of high myopia, myopic choroidal neovascularization (mCNV) is not easily diagnosed and monitored solely with clinical examinations. Multimodal imaging thus has a pertinent place in assessing mCNV. Verifying the diagnosis of mCNV requires the use of a fundus fluorescein angiography (FFA)—where leakage is seen as increasing size and intensity of hyperfluorescence with time [80]. A feature of pathological myopia, retinal avascularity in the 360° of the periphery, can also be revealed using wide-field FFA [81]. Distinguishing the myriad causes of subretinal exudation in high myopes (i.e., simple lacquer crack hemorrhage, inflammatory lesions, and mCNV [82, 83]) can be achieved with OCTA, which has the ability to identify neovascular membranes noninvasively. However, FFA remains the gold standard for mCNV diagnosis, given OCTA's comparatively lower sensitivity [84]. Furthermore, FFA is still necessary for monitoring disease activity, as OCTA lacks the ability to discern disease activity—where the flow signal may persist in an inactive mCNA [83–85]. Still, OCTA can assist with distinguishing the stages of mCNV via identification of signs of activity. These include ill-defined margins [86], disruption of the external limiting membrane [87], and variable amounts of intraretinal and subretinal fluids. These hyper-reflective lesions coalesce and develop a distinct border with appropriate treatment. Previous studies using the OCTA have suggested that rupture of the Bruch's membranes may be the cause of macular atrophy developing after mCNV [88]. However, the combination of OCTA and SS-OCT in multimodal imaging has given promising results—suggesting that mCNV is directly supplied by the short posterior ciliary artery instead of the choroidal vasculature as previously postulated [89].

10.5.4 Challenges in Imaging the Choroid and Sclera

Lying between the sclera and the RPE, the choroid's anatomical location makes imaging a challenge without the use of methods such as indocyanine green (ICG) angiography, ultrasonography (US), and OCT. Moreover, the choroid in pathological myopia is often extremely thin and thus difficult to measure. The addition of other, varied factors that interfere with choroid imaging in the myopic eye further complicate the process.

Typical fluorescein angiography has limited use in choroidal visualization since melanin impedes most of the spectra emitted from the agent. Imaging is also made near impossible with light absorption and scattering produced by the RPE pigment and choroidal blood. On the other hand, angiography via ICG has better use for the evaluation of various choroidal vasculopathy and inflammatory diseases [90]. This can be attributed to ICG's emitted spectrum being within the near-infrared wavelength—which is not disrupted by the RPE pigment or choroidal blood [91]. Nonetheless, other modalities such as OCT and autofluorescence imaging are still more feasible in the clinical setting and are thus still more often used than ICG angiography. Other modes of imaging include OCTA for assessing choroidal vasculature and its structures [46–48], as well as B-scan ultrasound to image the choroid with better penetration. However, B-scan images provide poorer resolution than those of OCTA—which is subsequently worsened by the thinning of the choroid in PM [53]. Yet, despite its flaws, the ultrasound remains useful in detecting staphylomas and globe contours.

With regard to OCT, we find that spectral domain OCT (SD-OCT) instruments with enhanced depth imaging can visualize the choroid more readily [92]. Inadequacies still exist in OCT images of the choroid, where deeper tissues imaged result in poorer sensitivity. The signals obtained in the choroid are also usually weak due to the high attenuation coefficient of the RPE. Nonetheless, ironically due to thinner choroids and relative depigmentation, full thickness imaging of the choroid is still attainable in high myopes. Yet, OCT image quality may still be compromised by distortions caused by the likely presence of staphylomas and abnormal eyewall contours in these same patients with high myopia. On the other hand, the extent of decreased sensitivities with increased tissue depth is comparatively lower in SS-OCT [93]. Clearly, notwithstanding the technique used, many challenges and limitations still exist in OCT imaging of high myopia—arising from the extreme axial length of highly myopic eyes, curvature deformity exaggeration on OCT, and the production of imaging artifacts [49].

The inability of OCT to readily distinguish the posterior scleral boundary makes scleral imaging a greater challenge than choroid imaging—where the choroid itself (unless extremely thin) reduces scleral image quality by disrupting signals. With the use of "Reflectivity" software, scleral boundaries may be augmented via adaptive compensation based on direct application of pixel intensity exponentiation. This would improve the precision of scleral thickness assessment [94, 95]. In retrospect, we conclude that the use of 3D MRI and ultrasound have more favorable results in visualizing scleral contours and characterizing staphylomas. Using animal experimentations on guinea pigs *ex vivo* and humans *in vivo*, we were able to demonstrate that quantitative ultrasound and super-resolution 3D MRI can be used to localize areas of scleral weakness and elasticity. These modalities could potentially detect scleral weakness preceding staphyloma formation; thereby discerning and even predicting which highly myopic eye is destined to develop staphylomas and MMD. This is critical in research studies targeted toward scleral reinforcement—such as macular buckling [96] or scleral collagen crosslinking [97, 98].

10.5.5 Challenges in Imaging the Optic Nerve

Features such as optic disc tilt (Fig. 10.5), peripapillary atrophy (PPA), and abnormally large or small optic discs are the earliest known structural alterations that potentially predict the development of pathological myopia, and can be observed even in young highly myopic adults. Unfortunately, these features (some also with associations to glaucoma) also interfere with the visualization of optic disc margins [99, 100], and are also not easy to discern in highly myopic eyes [101]. There is also added difficulty in eyes with myopic maculopathy, where visual field defects result in further interference [102]. As such, the answer to these challenges may lie in imaging deep optic nerve head structures (such as parapapillary sclera, scleral wall, and lamina cribrosa) [103] in highly myopic eyes for more precise diagnoses of glaucoma.

Glaucomatous optic nerve damage may be worsened by obstructed axoplasmic flow within the optic nerve head—possibly caused by a disrupted lamina cribrosa (LC) arising from optic disc tilt [104]. Imaging performed to evaluate the integrity of the lamina cribrosa may, therefore, aid in prognosticating risk for eventual glaucoma development. Indeed, Sawada et al. have shown via enhanced depth OCT imaging that LC defects in myopic eyes (with and without primary open-angle glaucoma) are associated with optic disc tilt angle, which can also explain the location and severity of glaucomatous visual field defects [104].

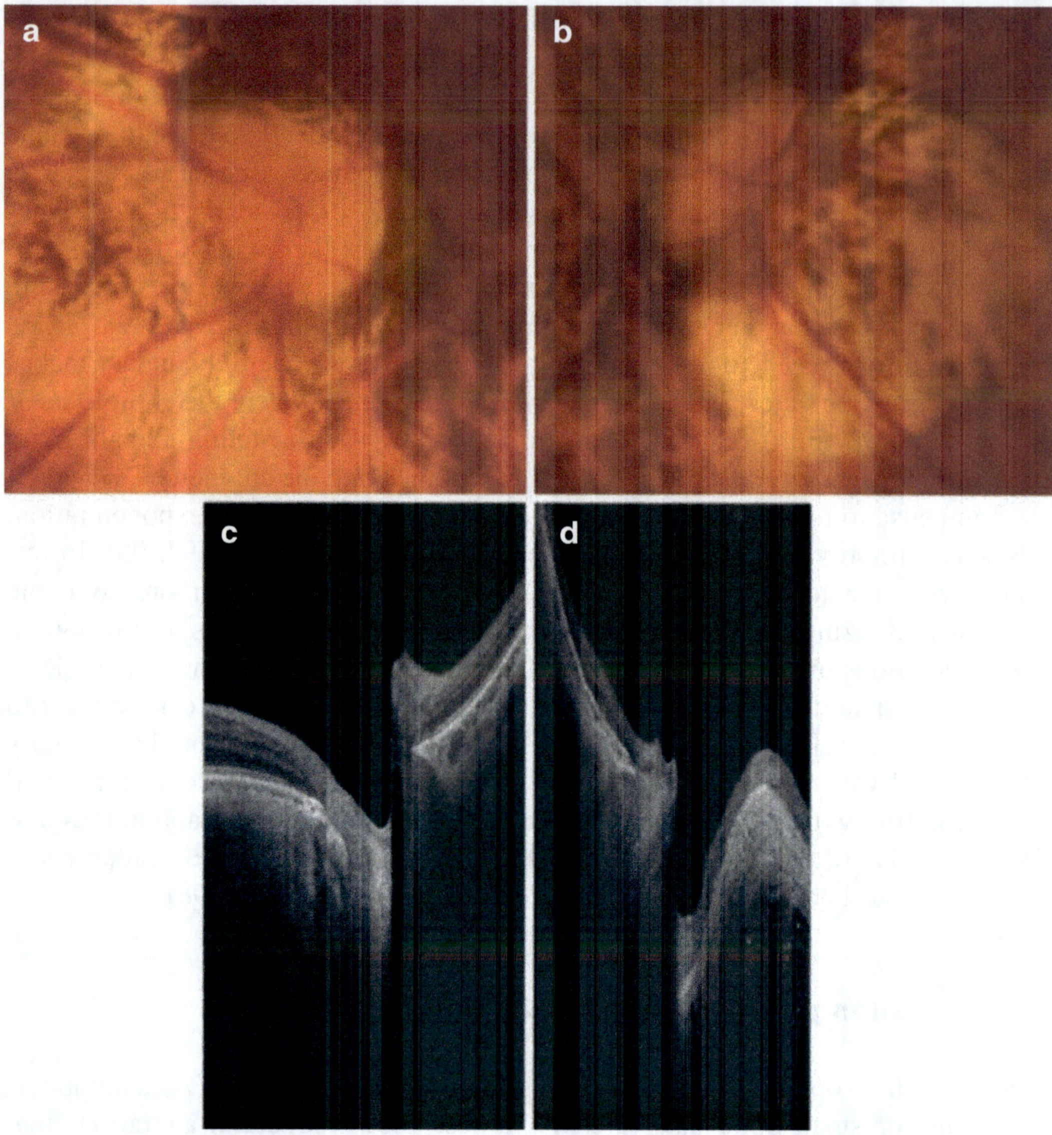

Fig. 10.5 Color photographs (top panels) and optical coherence tomography (bottom panels) of myopic tilted optic nerve discs showing moderately-tilted discs (left panels) and a severely tilted discs (right panels)

The optic nerve exits the eye at the Bruch's membrane opening (BMO), which can be easily discerned on OCT imaging. Using conventional disc margin-based measurements as a standard for comparison, Malik et al. investigated the utility of the BMO as a possible landmark for neuroretinal rim measurements, and has shown the BMO minimum rim width (BMO-MRW) to be markedly more sensitive (71% against 30%) than disc margin rim area (DM-RA) in diagnosing glaucoma [105].

Meanwhile, Enders et al. further demonstrated that a two-dimensional neuroretinal rim parameter based on BMO—namely, the BMO minimum rim area (BMO-MRA), outclassed all other measures (such as BMO-RMW, retinal nerve fiber layer thickness, and DM-RA) in diagnosing glaucoma [106]. Unfortunately, the diagnostic performance of this parameter has yet to be validated in myopic eyes.

Another deep optic nerve head structure that can be imaged on the enhanced depth OCT is the border tissue of Elschnig—a cuff of collagenous tissue arising from the sclera and joining the Bruch's membrane at the optic disc margin [104]. Having reviewed the externally oblique border tissue length (EOBT), optic nerve head tilt angle and optic canal obliqueness, Han et al. have concluded that temporally located maximal values for these parameters were both independently associated with the presence of myopic normal tension glaucoma and consistent with the location of retinal nerve fiber layer defects [103].

Macular ganglion cell complex (GCC) thickness has been reported to have comparable diagnostic power to circumpapillary retinal nerve fiber layer (cp-RNFL) thickness [107–110]—which on its own is strongly suggestive of glaucoma in non-myopic eyes, but faces limitations in interpretation in high myopes with PPA. Zhang et al. have indeed demonstrated that macular GCC parameters are superior to cp-RNFL parameters in diagnosing high myopes with glaucoma—with focal loss volume (FLV) on RTVue-OCT and minimum ganglion cell-inner plexiform layer (GCIPL) on the Cirrus HD OCT having the best diagnostic power among these macular parameters [111]. Yet, two obstacles persist in limiting the use of macular GCC measurements for the diagnosis of glaucoma in high myopes. Namely, these are the lack of a normative database in highly myopic eyes, as well as inaccurate measurements attributable to choroidal atrophy in myopic maculopathy. New developments regarding the use of OCTA on the optic nerve have suggested that it is a prospective adjunctive tool for evaluating the myopic disc for glaucomatous changes. Suwan et al. measured the perfused capillary density (PCD) via a 4.5 × 4.5 mm OCTA scan centered on the optic nerve head and has showed that eyes with myopia and open angle glaucoma had the lowest PCD compared to eyes with glaucoma alone and control eyes [112].

10.6 Future Developments

The primary aim of imaging in myopia would be to study the tissues involved with the pathological elongation of the eye, namely, the sclera as well as the choroid that is the regulator of scleral extracellular matrix remodeling [113], and its biomechanical properties [114]. As the RPE is highly scattering, it makes imaging of the myopic eye highly challenging. To make matters worse, the choroid is highly vascularized and perfused with a high concentration of red blood cells, this also causes a significant amount of light scattering making imaging more complicated [115]. One way to circumvent this problem would be to use OCT systems with wavelengths around 1060 nm to image the choroid [116]; however, the results obtained from this mode are less than satisfactory due to its relatively poor resolution capacity and inability to visualize the microvasculature and cellular structure of the choroid. Due to the complexity of this issue, there is no sensible nomenclature available to classify choroidal layers and boundaries, nor a definition of the choroidal–scleral interface [116]. As such, to facilitate comparisons and meta-analysis of existing data, there is a desperate need for a standardization for choroidal segmentation and OCT-based definition of the choroidal layers.

The OCT itself has its shortcomings: the sclera cannot be visualized using the OCT, higher wavelengths (around 1300 nm range) used for anterior segment OCT would not be able to be used to image the posterior pole either due to the high absorption coefficient of water contained in the vitreous [72]. These limitations also extend to the use of OCTA. There is currently no standard protocol for segmentation, the outcome parameters for OCTA have not been clearly defined either. Although some authors have tried to use analysis of flow voids or signal voids in the choriocapillaris to quantify the area taken up by the microvasculature [117, 118], the data pertaining to myopic patients are but insufficient [119]. Moreover, different authors have used different image analysis methods to quantify signal voids, as such, there is no clear common protocol in place to address the underlying issue. Looking into the future, there is however incipient research suggesting that the comprehension of blood supply and changes in vasculature from the anterior to the posterior segment of the myopic eye is crucial to the understanding of the disease [120–123].

Photoacoustic imaging has shown promise recently to fill the gaps between OCT and ultrasound in terms of penetration depth. Ultrasound biomicroscopy (higher ultrasound frequencies used) of the anterior segment simply does not have enough penetrative depth to image the posterior pole of the eye [124]. Photoacoustic imaging detects the waves generated by the absorption of pulsed laser light in tissues [125]; meanwhile, other modalities use contrast solely based on absorption. This modality has been used before to image the posterior pole of the eye in vitro and in animal models *in vivo*. This can also be used in concurrence with angiography, measuring oxygen saturation and pigment imaging [126]. However, there are some limitation pertaining to this modality notwithstanding moderate depth resolution, pure optical absorption sensing, need for contact detection with ultrasound sensor, and a relatively long acquisition time. In view of these limitations, we have yet to receive tangible results from photoacoustic imaging for posterior pole imaging in humans.

Recently, there has been a shift to elastography approaches to study the biochemical properties of ocular tissues with either OCT [127] or with ultrasound [128], the visualization of biochemical properties of the eye coats *in vivo* would otherwise be incredibly challenging This perspective is propelled by several studies proposing the measurement of ocular rigidity using noninvasive measures instead [129, 130]. However, none of these studies have addressed or included patients with myopia. The crux of this technique pertains to using an internal or external force to induce movement of tissue that is subsequently picked up using imaging devices, most *in vivo* work would be aimed at biochemical properties of the cornea [131, 132]. *In vivo* imaging using an ocular pulse with an internal excitation source is not yet able to produce results of biochemical parameters [133, 134]. Meanwhile, some *in vivo* work has been pursued involving the use of acoustic radiation force optical coherence elastography [135].

References

1. Chen L, et al. Rhegmatogenous retinal detachment due to paravascular linear retinal breaks over patchy chorioretinal atrophy in pathologic myopia. Arch Ophthalmol. 2010;128(12):1551–4.
2. Mitry D, et al. The epidemiology of rhegmatogenous retinal detachment: geographical variation and clinical associations. Br J Ophthalmol. 2010;94(6):678–84.
3. Hayashi K, et al. Long-term pattern of progression of myopic maculopathy: a natural history study. Ophthalmology. 2010;117(8):1595–611.
4. Yoshida T, et al. Myopic choroidal neovascularization: a 10-year follow-up. Ophthalmology. 2003;110(7):1297–305.
5. Ikuno Y, et al. Ocular risk factors for choroidal neovascularization in pathologic myopia. Invest Ophthalmol Vis Sci. 2010;51(7):3721–5.
6. Ohno-Matsui K, et al. Intrachoroidal cavitation in macular area of eyes with pathologic myopia. Am J Ophthalmol. 2012;154(2):382–93.
7. Samarawickrama C, et al. Myopia-related optic disc and retinal changes in adolescent children from singapore. Ophthalmology. 2011;118(10):2050–7.
8. Jonas JB, et al. Histology of the parapapillary region in high myopia. Am J Ophthalmol. 2011;152(6):1021–9.
9. Park HY, Lee K, Park CK. Optic disc torsion direction predicts the location of glaucomatous damage in normal-tension glaucoma patients with myopia. Ophthalmology. 2012;119(9):1844–51.
10. Marcus MW, et al. Myopia as a risk factor for open-angle glaucoma: a systematic review and meta-analysis. Ophthalmology. 2011;118(10):1989–1994.e2.
11. Curtin BJ. The myopias: basic science and clinical management. Philadelphia: Harper and Row; 1985.
12. Curtin BJ, Teng CC. Scleral changes in pathological myopia. Trans Am Acad Ophthalmol Otolaryngol. 1958;62(6):777–88.
13. Avetisov ES, et al. A study of biochemical and biomechanical qualities of normal and myopic eye sclera in humans of different age groups. Metab Pediatr Syst Ophthalmol. 1983;7(4):183–8.
14. Hsiang HW, et al. Clinical characteristics of posterior staphyloma in eyes with pathologic myopia. Am J Ophthalmol. 2008;146(1):102–10.
15. Curtin BJ, Karlin DB. Axial length measurements and fundus changes of the myopic eye. I. The posterior fundus. Trans Am Ophthalmol Soc. 1970;68:312–34.
16. Saka N, et al. Changes of axial length measured by IOL master during 2 years in eyes of adults with pathologic myopia. Graefes Arch Clin Exp Ophthalmol. 2013;251(2):495–9.
17. Lin LL, et al. Epidemiologic study of the prevalence and severity of myopia among schoolchildren in Taiwan in 2000. J Formos Med Assoc. 2001;100(10):684–91.
18. Steidl SM, Pruett RC. Macular complications associated with posterior staphyloma. Am J Ophthalmol. 1997;123(2):181–7.
19. Iwase A, et al. Prevalence and causes of low vision and blindness in a Japanese adult population: the Tajimi Study. Ophthalmology. 2006;113(8):1354–62.
20. Saka N, et al. Long-term changes in axial length in adult eyes with pathologic myopia. Am J Ophthalmol. 2010;150(4):562–568.e1.
21. Ohno-Matsui K, et al. Association between shape of sclera and myopic retinochoroidal lesions in patients with pathologic myopia. Invest Ophthalmol Vis Sci. 2012;53(10):6046–61.
22. McBrien NA, Cornell LM, Gentle A. Structural and ultrastructural changes to the sclera in a mammalian model of high myopia. Invest Ophthalmol Vis Sci. 2001;42(10):2179–87.
23. McBrien NA, Lawlor P, Gentle A. Scleral remodeling during the development of and recovery from axial myopia in the tree shrew. Invest Ophthalmol Vis Sci. 2000;41(12):3713–9.
24. Norton TT, Rada JA. Reduced extracellular matrix in mammalian sclera with induced myopia. Vis Res. 1995;35(9):1271–81.
25. Wollensak G, Iomdina E. Crosslinking of scleral collagen in the rabbit using glyceraldehyde. J Cataract Refract Surg. 2008;34(4):651–6.

26. McBrien NA, Jobling AI, Gentle A. Biomechanics of the sclera in myopia: extracellular and cellular factors. Optom Vis Sci. 2009;86(1):E23–30.
27. Wang Q, et al. Form-deprivation myopia induces decreased expression of bone morphogenetic protein-2, 5 in guinea pig sclera. Int J Ophthalmol. 2015;8(1):39–45.
28. Tian XD, et al. Expressions of type I collagen, alpha2 integrin and beta1 integrin in sclera of guinea pig with defocus myopia and inhibitory effects of bFGF on the formation of myopia. Int J Ophthalmol. 2013;6(1):54–8.
29. McBrien NA, Norton TT. Prevention of collagen crosslinking increases form-deprivation myopia in tree shrew. Exp Eye Res. 1994;59(4):475–86.
30. Li YT, Xie MK, Wu J. Association between Ocular axial length-related genes and high myopia in a Han Chinese population. Ophthalmologica. 2016;235(1):57–60.
31. Wei WB, et al. Subfoveal choroidal thickness: the Beijing Eye Study. Ophthalmology. 2013;120(1):175–80.
32. Wang NK, et al. Choroidal thickness and biometric markers for the screening of lacquer cracks in patients with high myopia. PLoS One. 2013;8(1):e53660.
33. Wang S, et al. Choroidal thickness and high myopia: a cross-sectional study and meta-analysis. BMC Ophthalmol. 2015;15:70.
34. Tokoro T. Types of fundus changes in the posterior pole. In: Atlas of posterior fundus changes in pathologic myopia. Tokyo: Springer; 1998. p. 5–22.
35. Ohno-Matsui K. Myopic chorioretinal atrophy. In: Spaide RF, Ohno-Matsui K, Yannuzzi LA, editors. Pathologic myopia. New York: Springer; 2014. p. 187–209.
36. Ohno-Matsui K, et al. International photographic classification and grading system for myopic maculopathy. Am J Ophthalmol. 2015;159(5):877–83.e7.
37. Jonas JB, et al. Bruch membrane and the mechanism of myopization: a new theory. Retina. 2017;37(8):1428–40.
38. Ohno-Matsui K, Jonas JB, Spaide RF. Macular bruch membrane holes in highly myopic patchy chorioretinal atrophy. Am J Ophthalmol. 2016;166:22–8.
39. Ohno-Matsui K, Tokoro T. The progression of lacquer cracks in pathologic myopia. Retina. 1996;16(1):29–37.
40. Pruett RC, Weiter JJ, Goldstein RB. Myopic cracks, angioid streaks, and traumatic tears in Bruch's membrane. Am J Ophthalmol. 1987;103(4):537–43.
41. Grossniklaus HE, Green WR. Pathologic findings in pathologic myopia. Retina. 1992;12(2):127–33.
42. Bai HX, et al. Bruch's membrane thickness in relationship to axial length. PLoS One. 2017;12(8):e0182080.
43. Puliafito CA, et al. Imaging of macular diseases with optical coherence tomography. Ophthalmology. 1995;102(2):217–29.
44. Tan CS, Ngo WK, Cheong KX. Comparison of choroidal thicknesses using swept source and spectral domain optical coherence tomography in diseased and normal eyes. Br J Ophthalmol. 2015;99(3):354–8.
45. Tan CS, et al. Comparison of retinal thicknesses measured using swept-source and spectral-domain optical coherence tomography devices. Ophthalmic Surg Lasers Imaging Retina. 2015;46(2):172–9.
46. Alshareef RA, et al. Subfoveal choroidal vascularity in myopia: evidence from spectral-domain optical coherence tomography. Ophthalmic Surg Lasers Imaging Retina. 2017;48(3):202–7.
47. Takase N, et al. Enlargement of foveal avascular zone in diabetic eyes evaluated by en face optical coherence tomography angiography. Retina. 2015;35(11):2377–83.
48. Tan CS, et al. Optical coherence tomography angiography evaluation of the parafoveal vasculature and its relationship with ocular factors. Invest Ophthalmol Vis Sci. 2016;57(9):224–34.
49. Shinohara K, et al. Ultrawide-field OCT to investigate relationships between myopic macular retinoschisis and posterior staphyloma. Ophthalmology. 2018;125:1575–86.
50. Baum G, Greenwood I. The application of ultrasonic locating techniques to ophthalmology. II. Ultrasonic slit lamp in the ultrasonic visualization of soft tissues. AMA Arch Ophthalmol. 1958;60(2):263–79.

51. Coleman DJ, et al. High-resolution ultrasonic imaging of the posterior segment. Ophthalmology. 2004;111(7):1344–51.
52. Reinstein DZ, Silverman RH, Coleman DJ. High-frequency ultrasound measurement of the thickness of the corneal epithelium. Refract Corneal Surg. 1993;9(5):385–7.
53. Hewick SA, et al. A comparison of 10 MHz and 20 MHz ultrasound probes in imaging the eye and orbit. Br J Ophthalmol. 2004;88(4):551–5.
54. Silverman RH, et al. Pulse-encoded ultrasound imaging of the vitreous with an annular array. Ophthalmic Surg Lasers Imaging. 2012;43(1):82–6.
55. Van Reeth E, et al. Isotropic reconstruction of a 4-D MRI thoracic sequence using super-resolution. Magn Reson Med. 2015;73(2):784–93.
56. Milanfar P. Super-resolution imaging. Boca Raton: CRC Press; 2010.
57. Collins MJ, Buehren T, Iskander DR. Retinal image quality, reading and myopia. Vis Res. 2006;46(1-2):196–215.
58. Pope JM, et al. Three-dimensional MRI study of the relationship between eye dimensions, retinal shape and myopia. Biomed Opt Express. 2017;8(5):2386–95.
59. Kuo AN, et al. Posterior eye shape measurement with retinal OCT compared to MRI. Invest Ophthalmol Vis Sci. 2016;57(9):196–203.
60. Ng DS, et al. Advances of optical coherence tomography in myopia and pathologic myopia. Eye. 2016;30(7):901–16.
61. Ang M, et al. Optical coherence tomography angiography: a review of current and future clinical applications. Graefes Arch Clin Exp Ophthalmol. 2018;256(2):237–45.
62. Tan ACS, et al. An overview of the clinical applications of optical coherence tomography angiography. Eye. 2018;32(2):262–86.
63. Ang M, et al. Optical coherence tomography angiography and indocyanine green angiography for corneal vascularisation. Br J Ophthalmol. 2016;100(11):1557–63.
64. Realini T, et al. Normative databases for imaging instrumentation. J Glaucoma. 2015;24(6):480–3.
65. Hashemi H, et al. Global and regional estimates of prevalence of refractive errors: systematic review and meta-analysis. J Curr Ophthalmol. 2018;30(1):3–22.
66. Kasahara K, et al. Characteristics of higher-order aberrations and anterior segment tomography in patients with pathologic myopia. Int Ophthalmol. 2017;37(6):1279–88.
67. Chansangpetch S, et al. Impact of myopia on corneal biomechanics in glaucoma and nonglaucoma patients. Invest Ophthalmol Vis Sci. 2017;58(12):4990–6.
68. Schehlein EM, Novack G, Robin AL. New pharmacotherapy for the treatment of glaucoma. Expert Opin Pharmacother. 2017;18(18):1939–46.
69. Chan C, et al. Validation of an objective scoring system for forme fruste keratoconus detection and post-LASIK Ectasia Risk Assessment in Asian eyes. Cornea. 2015;34(9):996–1004.
70. Lu Y, et al. Four-year follow-up of the changes in anterior segment after phakic collamer lens implantation. Am J Ophthalmol. 2017;178:140–9.
71. Chong EW, Mehta JS. High myopia and cataract surgery. Curr Opin Ophthalmol. 2016;27(1):45–50.
72. Ang M, et al. Anterior segment optical coherence tomography. Prog Retin Eye Res. 2018;66(9):132–56.
73. Ohno-Matsui K. What is the fundamental nature of pathologic myopia? Retina. 2017;37(6):1043–8.
74. Tanaka Y, et al. Retromode retinal imaging of macular retinoschisis in highly myopic eyes. Am J Ophthalmol. 2010;149(4):635–640.e1.
75. Johnson MW. Myopic traction maculopathy: pathogenic mechanisms and surgical treatment. Retina. 2012;32(Suppl 2):S205–10.
76. Wong CW, et al. Is choroidal or scleral thickness related to myopic macular degeneration? Invest Ophthalmol Vis Sci. 2017;58(2):907–13.
77. Shinohara K, et al. Characteristics of peripapillary staphylomas associated with high myopia determined by swept-source optical coherence tomography. Am J Ophthalmol. 2016;169:138–44.

78. Shinohara K, et al. Posterior staphylomas in pathologic myopia imaged by widefield optical coherence tomography. Invest Ophthalmol Vis Sci. 2017;58(9):3750–8.
79. Ohno-Matsui K, et al. Features of posterior staphylomas analyzed in wide-field fundus images in patients with unilateral and bilateral pathologic myopia. Retina. 2017;37(3):477–86.
80. Iacono P, et al. Fluorescein angiography and spectral-domain optical coherence tomography for monitoring anti-VEGF therapy in myopic choroidal neovascularization. Ophthalmic Res. 2014;52(1):25–31.
81. Kaneko Y, et al. Areas of nonperfusion in peripheral retina of eyes with pathologic myopia detected by ultra-widefield fluorescein angiography. Invest Ophthalmol Vis Sci. 2014;55(3):1432–9.
82. Miyata M, et al. Detection of myopic choroidal neovascularization using optical coherence tomography angiography. Am J Ophthalmol. 2016;165:108–14.
83. Bruyere E, et al. Neovascularization secondary to high myopia imaged by optical coherence tomography angiography. Retina. 2017;37(11):2095–101.
84. Querques G, et al. Optical coherence tomography angiography of choroidal neovascularization secondary to pathologic myopia. Dev Ophthalmol. 2016;56:101–6.
85. Querques L, et al. Optical coherence tomography angiography of myopic choroidal neovascularisation. Br J Ophthalmol. 2017;101(5):609–15.
86. Ohno-Matsui K, et al. Updates of pathologic myopia. Prog Retin Eye Res. 2016;52:156–87.
87. Battaglia Parodi M, Iacono P, Bandello F. Correspondence of leakage on fluorescein angiography and optical coherence tomography parameters in diagnosis and monitoring of myopic choroidal neovascularization treated with bevacizumab. Retina. 2016;36(1):104–9.
88. Ohno-Matsui K, Jonas JB, Spaide RF. Macular bruch membrane holes in choroidal neovascularization-related myopic macular atrophy by swept-source optical coherence tomography. Am J Ophthalmol. 2016;162:133–139.e1.
89. Ishida T, et al. Possible connection of short posterior ciliary arteries to choroidal neovascularisations in eyes with pathologic myopia. Br J Ophthalmol. 2018;103(4):457–62.
90. Hayashi K, et al. Value of indocyanine green angiography in the diagnosis of occult choroidal neovascular membrane. Jpn J Ophthalmol. 1988;42:827–9.
91. Geeraets WJ, Berry ER. Ocular spectral characteristics as related to hazards from lasers and other light sources. Am J Ophthalmol. 1968;66(1):15–20.
92. Spaide RF, Koizumi H, Pozonni MC. Enhanced depth imaging spectral-domain optical coherence tomography. Am J Ophthalmol. 2008;146(4):496–500.
93. Choma MA, et al. Sensitivity advantage of swept source and Fourier domain optical coherence tomography. Opt Express. 2003;11(18):2183–9.
94. Chung CW, et al. Enhancement of corneal visibility in optical coherence tomography images with corneal opacification. Transl Vis Sci Technol. 2016;5(5):3.
95. Girard MJ, et al. Enhancement of corneal visibility in optical coherence tomography images using corneal adaptive compensation. Transl Vis Sci Technol. 2015;4(3):3.
96. Alkabes M, Mateo C. Macular buckle technique in myopic traction maculopathy: a 16-year review of the literature and a comparison with vitreous surgery. Graefes Arch Clin Exp Ophthalmol. 2018;256(5):863–77.
97. Wollensak G, Iomdina E. Long-term biomechanical properties of rabbit sclera after collagen crosslinking using riboflavin and ultraviolet A (UVA). Acta Ophthalmol. 2009;87(2):193–8.
98. Kim M, et al. Pharmacologic alternatives to riboflavin photochemical corneal cross-linking: a comparison study of cell toxicity thresholds. Invest Ophthalmol Vis Sci. 2014;55(5):3247–57.
99. Chang RT, Singh K. Myopia and glaucoma: diagnostic and therapeutic challenges. Curr Opin Ophthalmol. 2013;24(2):96–101.
100. Jonas JB, Gusek GC, Naumann GO. Optic disk morphometry in high myopia. Graefes Arch Clin Exp Ophthalmol. 1988;226(6):587–90.
101. Jonas JB, et al. Intraocular pressure and glaucomatous optic neuropathy in high myopia. Invest Ophthalmol Vis Sci. 2017;58(13):5897–906.
102. Ohno-Matsui K, et al. Long-term development of significant visual field defects in highly myopic eyes. Am J Ophthalmol. 2011;152(2):256–265.e1.

103. Han JC, et al. The characteristics of deep optic nerve head morphology in myopic normal tension glaucoma. Invest Ophthalmol Vis Sci. 2017;58(5):2695–704.
104. Sawada Y, et al. Multiple temporal lamina cribrosa defects in myopic eyes with glaucoma and their association with visual field defects. Ophthalmology. 2017;124(11):1600–11.
105. Malik R, et al. Diagnostic accuracy of optical coherence tomography and scanning laser tomography for identifying glaucoma in myopic eyes. Ophthalmology. 2016;123(6):1181–9.
106. Enders P, et al. Novel Bruch's membrane opening minimum rim area equalizes disc size dependency and offers high diagnostic power for glaucoma. Invest Ophthalmol Vis Sci. 2016;57(15):6596–603.
107. Nakanishi H, et al. Sensitivity and specificity for detecting early glaucoma in eyes with high myopia from normative database of macular ganglion cell complex thickness obtained from normal non-myopic or highly myopic Asian eyes. Graefes Arch Clin Exp Ophthalmol. 2015;253(7):1143–52.
108. Hung KC, et al. Macular diagnostic ability in OCT for assessing glaucoma in high myopia. Optom Vis Sci. 2016;93(2):126–35.
109. Akashi A, et al. The ability of macular parameters and circumpapillary retinal nerve fiber layer by three SD-OCT instruments to diagnose highly myopic glaucoma. Invest Ophthalmol Vis Sci. 2013;54(9):6025–32.
110. Mwanza JC, et al. Diagnostic performance of optical coherence tomography ganglion cell--inner plexiform layer thickness measurements in early glaucoma. Ophthalmology. 2014;121(4):849–54.
111. Zhang Y, Wen W, Sun X. Comparison of several parameters in two optical coherence tomography systems for detecting glaucomatous defects in high myopia. Invest Ophthalmol Vis Sci. 2016;57(11):4910–5.
112. Suwan Y, et al. Association of myopia with peripapillary perfused capillary density in patients with glaucoma: an optical coherence tomography angiography study. JAMA Ophthalmol. 2018;136(5):507–13.
113. Summers JA. The choroid as a sclera growth regulator. Exp Eye Res. 2013;114:120–7.
114. Campbell IC, Coudrillier B, Ross Ethier C. Biomechanics of the posterior eye: a critical role in health and disease. J Biomech Eng. 2014;136(2):021005.
115. Kiss B, et al. Ocular hemodynamics during isometric exercise. Microvasc Res. 2001;61(1):1–13.
116. Ferrara D, Waheed NK, Duker JS. Investigating the choriocapillaris and choroidal vasculature with new optical coherence tomography technologies. Prog Retin Eye Res. 2016;52:130–55.
117. Spaide RF. Choriocapillaris flow features follow a power law distribution: implications for characterization and mechanisms of disease progression. Am J Ophthalmol. 2016;170:58–67.
118. Zhang Q, et al. A novel strategy for quantifying choriocapillaris flow voids using swept-source OCT angiography. Invest Ophthalmol Vis Sci. 2018;59(1):203–11.
119. Al-Sheikh M, et al. Quantitative OCT angiography of the retinal microvasculature and the choriocapillaris in myopic eyes. Invest Ophthalmol Vis Sci. 2017;58(4):2063–9.
120. Ang M, et al. Comparison of anterior segment optical coherence tomography angiography systems for corneal vascularisation. Br J Ophthalmol. 2018;102(7):873–7.
121. Cai Y, et al. Serial optical coherence tomography angiography for corneal vascularization. Graefes Arch Clin Exp Ophthalmol. 2017;255(1):135–9.
122. Ang M, et al. En face optical coherence tomography angiography for corneal neovascularisation. Br J Ophthalmol. 2016;100(5):616–21.
123. Grudzi E, et al. Modern diagnostic techniques for the assessment of ocular blood flow in myopia: current state of knowledge. J Ophthalmol. 2018;2018:8.
124. Silverman RH, et al. 75 MHz ultrasound biomicroscopy of anterior segment of eye. Ultrason Imaging. 2006;28(3):179–88.
125. Liu W, Zhang HF. Photoacoustic imaging of the eye: a mini review. Photoacoustics. 2016;4(3):112–23.
126. Xie D, et al. In vivo blind-deconvolution photoacoustic ophthalmoscopy with total variation regularization. J Biophotonics. 2018;11(9):e201700360.

127. Larin KV, Sampson DD. Optical coherence elastography - OCT at work in tissue biomechanics. Biomed Opt Express. 2017;8(2):1172–202.
128. Li G-Y, Cao Y. Mechanics of ultrasound elastography. Proc Math Phys Eng Sci. 2017;473(2199):20160841.
129. Karyotakis NG, et al. Manometric measurement of the outflow facility in the living human eye and its dependence on intraocular pressure. Acta Ophthalmol. 2015;93(5):e343–8.
130. Beaton L, et al. Non-invasive measurement of choroidal volume change and ocular rigidity through automated segmentation of high-speed OCT imaging. Biomed Opt Express. 2015;6(5):1694–706.
131. Sit AJ, et al. In vivo noninvasive measurement of young's modulus of elasticity in human eyes: a feasibility study. J Glaucoma. 2017;26(11):967–73.
132. Zaitsev VY, et al. Optical coherence elastography for strain dynamics measurements in laser correction of cornea shape. J Biophotonics. 2017;10(11):1450–63.
133. O'Hara KE, et al. Measuring pulse-induced natural relative motions within human ocular tissue in vivo using phase-sensitive optical coherence tomography. J Biomed Opt. 2013;18(12):121506.
134. Dragostinoff N, et al. Time course and topographic distribution of ocular fundus pulsation measured by low-coherence tissue interferometry. J Biomed Opt. 2013;18(12):121502.
135. Qu Y, et al. In vivo elasticity mapping of posterior ocular layers using acoustic radiation force optical coherence elastography. Invest Ophthalmol Vis Sci. 2018;59(1):455–61.

11 Glaucoma in High Myopia

Jost B. Jonas, Songhomitra Panda-Jonas, and Kyoko Ohno-Matsui

Key Points

- In all highly myopic eyes, glaucomatous optic neuropathy may specifically be ruled out, in attempt not to miss the diagnosis
- High axial myopia is a major risk factor for glaucomatous or glaucoma-like optic neuropathy, even at a normal intraocular pressure.
- Morphological risk factors for glaucoma in high myopia may be an enlarged optic disc and enlarged parapapillary delta zone.
- Histological hallmarks of the highly myopic optic nerve head are an elongated and thinned lamina cribrosa, steepened trans-lamina cribrosa pressure gradient, enlarged optic disc, elongated peripapillary scleral flange (as equivalent of parapapillary delta zone), and a shallowing of the physiological optic cup.

11.1 Introduction

Axial myopization leads to marked changes in the morphology of the posterior ocular segment including the anatomy of the optic nerve head. The changes of the optic nerve head include an enlargement of all three layers of the optic disc (i.e., optic disc Bruch's membrane opening, optic disc choroidal opening, and optic disc scleral

J. B. Jonas (✉) · S. Panda-Jonas
Department of Ophthalmology, Medical Faculty Mannheim, Ruprecht-Karls-University Heidelberg, Mannheim, Germany
e-mail: jost.jonas@medma.uni-heidelberg.de

K. Ohno-Matsui
Department of Ophthalmology and Visual Science, Tokyo Medical and Dental University, Tokyo, Japan

M. Ang, T. Y. Wong (eds.), *Updates on Myopia*,
https://doi.org/10.1007/978-981-13-8491-2_11

opening) with the development of a secondary macrodisc, and an enlargement and shallowing of the cup. Further morphological changes are an elongation and thinning of the lamina cribrosa with a secondary reduction in the distance between the intraocular space with the intraocular pressure (IOP) and the retro-lamina compartment with the orbital cerebrospinal fluid pressure, and a direct exposure of the peripheral posterior lamina cribrosa surface to the orbital cerebrospinal fluid space. In the parapapillary region, an elongation and thinning of the peripapillary scleral flange with development and enlargement of the parapapillary gamma zone (defined as the parapapillary Bruch's membrane free region) and delta zone (defined as the region between the optic disc border and the merging line of the optic nerve dura mater with the posterior sclera) occurs, in addition to an elongation and thinning of the peripapillary border tissue of the choroid (Jacoby). The optic rotates around the vertical axis, and less often and to a minor degree around the horizontal axis und the sagittal axis. These changes make it more difficult to differentiate between myopic changes and (additional) glaucoma-associated changes such as a loss of neuroretinal rim and thinning of the retinal nerve fiber layer, and these changes may make the optic nerve head more vulnerable potentially explaining the increased prevalence of glaucomatous optic neuropathy in highly myopic eyes.

11.2 Anatomy of the Optic Nerve Head in High Myopia

The anatomy of the optic nerve head in primary high myopia is markedly influenced by the axial elongation. This process of sagittal enlargement of the myopic globe takes place predominantly in the posterior hemisphere of the eye, and the changes are more pronounced the closer to the posterior pole [1–5]. Histological studies have shown that with longer axial length, the axial elongation-associated thinning of the sclera was most pronounced close to the posterior pole, while the scleral thickness in the pars plana region did not vary significantly between eyes of various axial length. In a similar manner, the thinning of the choroid was more marked the closer to the macula [6].

It has been postulated that the main driver for the scleral and choroidal thinning in the process of axial elongation may be a new production and elongation of Bruch's membrane in the equatorial and retroequatorial region of the eye [7]. Findings leading to this hypothesis were the following:

- the volume of the scleral and choroid did not markedly increase after the end of the second year of life and that both parameters were independent of axial length [3, 5];
- the thickness of Bruch's membrane was not associated with axial length so that its volume increased in the process of axial myopization [8];
- the main determinant of the process of emmetropization (and myopization) is the length of the optical axis which ends at the photoreceptor outer segments and not at the scleral posterior surface;
- the structure with a minimum of biomechanical strength and being located closest to the photoreceptor outer segments is Bruch's membrane;
- a biomechanical study revealed that the stiffness of Bruch's membrane was comparable or higher than those of other ocular tissues and that it could sustain a relatively high pressure of 80 mmHg or higher before rupture [9];

- the density of the retinal pigment epithelium cells and the retinal thickness decreased in the midperiphery with increasing axial length, while both parameters, measured in the macular region, were independent of axial length [10, 11]; and
- the optic disc-fovea distance increased with longer axial length by the development and enlargement of parapapillary gamma zone while the length of Bruch's membrane in the macular region was independent of axial length [12–14].

These anatomical findings and the postulated mechanism of Bruch's membrane enlargement in the midperiphery as the driver for the cylindrical-like sagittal enlargement of the globe are associated with typical myopic changes in the anatomy of the optic nerve head. These include the following: an enlargement of the optic nerve head with the development of a secondary or acquired macrodisc [15, 16]; enlargement and shallowing of the optic cup, so that the spatial contrast between the height of the neuroretinal rim and the depth of the optic cup is decreased; elongation and thinning of the lamina cribrosa [17, 18]; development and enlargement of parapapillary gamma zone and delta zone [19, 20]; and rotation of the optic disc mostly around the vertical axis [21, 22].

The enlargement of the optic disc (as defined by the peripapillary ring) affects all three optic disc layers: Bruch's membrane opening; the choroidal opening, in which the choroid is separated from the intrapapillary compartment by the peripapillary border tissue of the choroid (Jacoby); and the scleral opening which is spanned by the lamina cribrosa. The (passive) enlargement of all three optic disc layers may be due to the finding that the myopic axial elongation additionally includes a widening of the eye in the horizontal and vertical directions [23]. For each millimeter increase in axial length, both the horizontal globe diameter and the vertical globe diameter increase by approximately 0.2 mm [23]. Since the primary and active enlargement of Bruch's membrane may occur in the equatorial region, an increased tension within Bruch's membrane and within the choroid and the sclera may develop at the posterior pole. It would lead to a stretching of the openings of all three optic disc layers. It has been discussed that if the increased tension within Bruch's membrane is not sufficiently released by the enlargement of the physiological Bruch's membrane opening in the optic disc, secondary defects in Bruch's membrane may develop starting with the formation of lacquer cracks and ending the formation of macular Bruch's membrane defects [24–27]. If the enlargement of the optic disc Bruch's membrane opening is more marked than the enlargement of the optic disc choroidal opening, a part of the parapapillary region will no longer be covered by Bruch's membrane, so that parapapillary gamma zone as Bruch's membrane-free region develops [19, 20]. The uneven enlargement of the opening of the various layers of the optic disc may thus be one of the reasons for the development of parapapillary gamma zone.

The enlargement of the optic disc in axially elongating eyes leads secondarily to an enlargement of the optic cup, while the shape of the neuroretinal rim may still follow the so-called ISNT (inferior–superior–nasal–temporal) rule, with the small rim part being located usually in the temporal horizontal disc region [28]. Due to the stretching and enlargement of the optic disc and cup, the spatial contrast between the height of the neuroretinal rim and the depth of the optic cup appears to diminish, so that it becomes clinically more difficult to delineate the optic cup form the neuroretinal rim.

The enlargement of the opening in the scleral layer of the optic disc is associated with a stretching and thinning of the lamina cribrosa [17, 18]. Since the diameter of the retrobulbar optic nerve is not directly affected by the process of axial elongation, the myopic enlargement of the posterior surface of the lamina cribrosa has as consequence that a peripheral annular-like region of the lamina is no longer covered or buffered by the solid optic nerve but is directly facing the orbital cerebrospinal fluid space.

Outside of the optic disc border, parapapillary gamma zone and delta zone develop during axial elongation (Fig. 11.1) [19–21, 24, 29–35]. Gamma zone has been defined as the Bruch's membrane-free zone at the optic disc border. It is usually larger on the temporal side than on the nasal side. Prevalence and size of gamma zone is strongly associated with myopic axial elongation and the amount of the optic disc rotation around the vertical axis [21]. Two mechanisms may lead to the development of gamma zone. As pointed out above, gamma zone may develop if the enlargement of the optic disc Burch's membrane opening is more marked than the enlargement of the optic disc choroidal opening. A second mechanism may be connected with a shift of the three optic disc layers during axial elongation. One may assume that at birth all three optic disc layers are aligned to each other. If in the process of axial elongation Bruch's membrane is newly formed and enlarged in the equatorial region, the optic disc Bruch's membrane opening may shift in direction to the macula. If this movement is less marked for the optic disc choroidal layer and scleral layer than it is for the Bruch's membrane opening, a misalignment of the layers will occur, with the Bruch's membrane opening being located most to the macular side and the scleral opening being located most to the nasal side. This

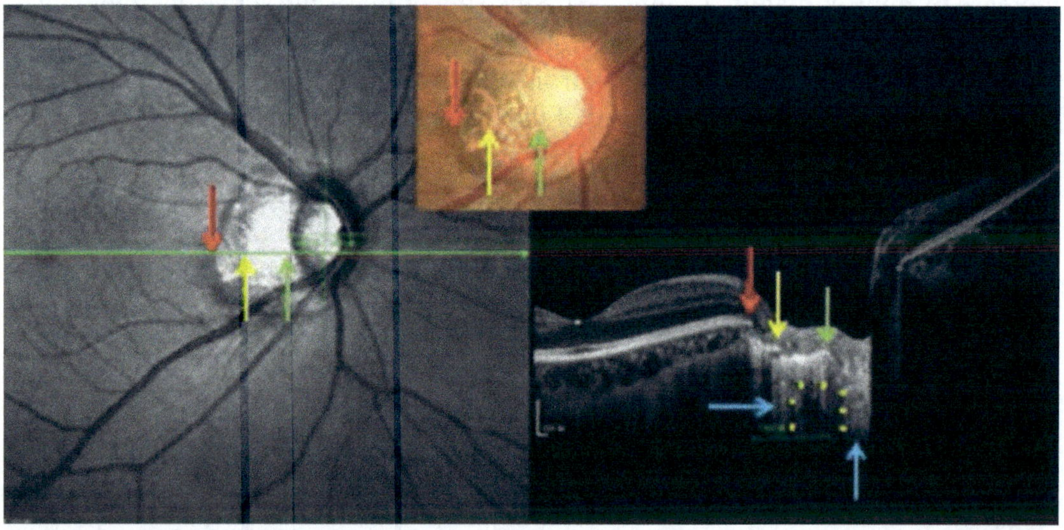

Fig. 11.1 Optical coherence tomographic image of the optic nerve head, showing parapapillary gamma zone (between red arrow and yellow arrow) with Bruch's membrane being absent, and parapapillary delta zone (between yellow arrow and green arrow (optic disc border)) showing an elongated peripapillary scleral flange as anterior border of the orbital cerebrospinal fluid space (yellow stars) between the optic nerve dura mater (horizontal blue arrow) and the optic nerve with its surrounding pia mater (vertical blue arrow)

phenomenon would explain the overhanging of Bruch's membrane on the nasal side of the optic disc in moderately myopic eyes, and it could be a second mechanism for the development of parapapillary gamma zone [36]. It would also explain the paradoxical course of the optic nerve through the optic nerve head channel with the optic nerve entering the canal from nasal anteriorly and reaching the vitreous compartment temporal posteriorly, although the optic nerve arrives at the eye globe coming from the posterior part of the orbit.

Parapapillary delta zone is located at the optic disc border within gamma zone and has been defined as the region of the elongated and thinned peripapillary scleral flange [19, 20]. The peripapillary scleral flange is the continuation of the inner half of the posterior sclera and continues into the lamina cribrosa, separated from the latter by the peripapillary scleral border tissue of Elschnig [37, 38]. It forms the anterior end of the orbital cerebrospinal fluid space. In axially elongated eyes, in particular beyond an axial length of 26.5 mm, the peripapillary scleral flange gets markedly elongated and thinned [37, 39]. It may change its dimensions from a normal thickness and length of about 0.5 mm to a length of 5 mm and a thickness of less than 100 μm. The ophthalmoscopical delineation between gamma zone and delta zone can be facilitated by searching for the peripapillary arterial circle of Zinn-Haller which is usually located at the merging line of the optic nerve dura mater with the sclera, i.e., at the peripheral end of delta zone [40, 41].

The optic disc shape as perceived upon ophthalmoscopy is normally slightly oval [42, 43]. It has to be taken into account that the ophthalmoscopically determined optic disc shape is different from the true optic disc shape, since the location of the optic disc close to the nasal side leads to perspective distortion, usually resulting in a perspective shortening of the horizontal disc diameter [44]. In addition, the optic disc undergoes rotational changes in the process of myopic axial elongation [22]. These are mainly an optic disc rotation around the vertical axis, and to a minor degree a rotation around the horizontal axis and the sagittal axis. A rotation round the vertical axis leads to a perspective shortening of the horizontal disc diameter, a rotation round the horizontal axis leads to a perspective shortening of the vertical disc diameter, a rotation round the sagittal axis does not change the perspective appearance of the disc diameters [44]. The rotation around the vertical axis is associated with the development and enlargement of gamma zone at the temporal side, and a rotation around the horizontal axis is associated with the development and enlargement of gamma zone at the inferior border of the optic disc. These optic disc rotations explain the ophthalmoscopical appearance of the markedly vertically oval shape of optic discs in highly myopic eyes [15, 16]. The difference between the two-dimensional ophthalmoscopical optic disc shape and the optic disc shape as determined three-dimensionally by optical coherence tomography increases with longer axial length, due to the progressing disc rotation around the vertical axis [44]. It has remained elusive which forces lead to the disc rotation around the vertical axis in progressive axial myopia. One reason could be, as outlined above, the increasing misalignment of the three optic disc openings, with the Bruch's membrane opening moving in temporally and the scleral opening staying partially behind. The resulting overhanging of Bruch's membrane into the nasal part of the optic disc channel leads to a shortening of the effective horizontal disc diameter. A second mechanism could be a backward strain or pull of the optic nerve dura mater on the peripapillary region [45, 46]. In a recent study, Demer and colleagues proposed that the backward pull of the optic nerve on the optic nerve head in markedly axially elongated eyes could lead to a novel mechanical load on the globe at the optic nerve head in ocular adduction [45]. Since the optic nerve originates in the nasal superior region of the orbit and inserts in the posterior nasal region of the eye, adduction of the globe would lead in axially elongated eyes to a backward pull of the optic nerve on the temporal and temporal inferior side of the optic nerve head. Such a mechanism could explain the marked rotation of the optic nerve head mainly around its vertical axis (and a slight rotation around its horizontal axis with a backward movement of the inferior optic disc pole) in highly elongated eyes. Since the optic nerve dura mater as compared to the pia mater or the neural tissue of the optic nerve may be biomechanically the strongest element, one may assume that the traction is forwarded by the optic nerve dura mater to its insertion on the globe, i.e., the merging line of the dura mater with the posterior sclera or the peripheral end of the peripapillary scleral flange. Traction on the merging line could also lead to an elongation of the peripapillary scleral flange and indirectly to the development and enlargement of parapapillary gamma zone. The study by Demer has been confirmed and extended by investigations conducted by Wang and colleagues who found that that the optic nerve head strains due to the pull by the optic nerve dura mater on the peripapillary sclera during a lateral eye movement of 13° were as high as, or higher than, those resulting from an IOP of 50 mmHg [46]. Fitting with the notion of a biomechanical role the optic nerve may play for the anatomy and physiology of the optic nerve head is the finding of peripapillary suprachoroidal cavitations which are located mostly in the inferior peripapillary region in about 17% of highly myopic eyes [47–50]. Their development may also be explained by a backward pull of the optic nerve dura mater on the temporal and inferior peripapillary sclera. Correspondingly, peripapillary suprachoroidal cavitations are associated with an optic disc rotation around the vertical disc axis and high axial myopia [50].

The cutoff for the differentiation between moderate myopia and high myopia at which the axial elongation associated enlargement of the optic nerve head starts has not concisely been assessed so far. According to hospital-based investigations and population-based studies, the optic disc and parapapillary gamma zone start to increase at about a value of approximately −8.00 diopters or an axial length of about 26.5 mm [51, 52]. At the same cutoff values, the prevalence of myopic retinopathy increases [53–55].

11.3 Increased Prevalence of Glaucoma in High Myopia and Associated Factors

Population-based investigations and hospital-based studies have shown that the prevalence of glaucomatous optic neuropathy (GON) was higher in highly myopic eyes than in emmetropic eyes [53, 56–69]. To cite an example, in the Beijing

Eye Study the prevalence of GON was significantly higher in eyes with a myopic refractive error exceeding −6 diopters than in the remaining eyes, while between the hyperopic eyes, the emmetropic eyes and the eyes with low to moderate myopia (myopic refractive up to −6 diopters or less), the frequency of glaucoma did not vary significantly [53]. Since the IOP pressure did not differ significantly between the highly myopic eyes and the remaining eyes, it suggested a higher glaucoma susceptibility in the highly myopic eyes. In the Blue Mountains Eye Study, the glaucoma prevalence was higher in moderate to high myopes (4.4%) than in emmetropes (1.5%) [63]. In the Barbados Eye Study, myopia increased the odds of having glaucoma while hyperopia reduced it [61]. In the Malmö eye survey on more than 30,000 individuals, the glaucoma prevalence increased with increasing myopia, and the association between myopia and glaucoma was strong at lower IOP levels, and weakened gradually with increasing IOP [64, 67]. The reason for a discrepancy between studies on an association between myopia and glaucoma may be that not all studies differentiated between moderate myopia, which may not be associated with an increased glaucoma prevalence, and high myopia with an increased frequency of GON [65]. Accordingly, in the Beijing Eye Study the low to moderate myopic group, the emmetropic group and the hyperopic group did not vary significantly in the prevalence of glaucoma in the present study [53]. By the same token, in non-highly myopic individuals, inter-eye differences in refractive error were not significantly correlated with inter-eye differences in neuroretinal rim area and mean visual field defect nor were the neuroretinal rim area, the horizontal and vertical cup/disk diameter ratios and the mean visual field loss correlated with refractive error in an interindividual statistical analysis [65].

A previous study revealed that at a given IOP in patients with chronic open-angle glaucoma, the amount of optic nerve damage was more marked in highly myopic eyes with large optic discs than in non-highly myopic eyes [68]. This observation was supported by a hospital-based study in which Nagaoka and colleagues examined 172 patients with a mean axial length of 30.1 ± 2.3 mm (range: 24.7–39.1 mm) and in which the prevalence of GON (overall: 28%) was 3.2 times higher ($P < 0.001$) in large optic discs (>3.79 mm^2) than in normal-sized discs or small discs (<1.51 mm^2) after adjusting for older age. Interestingly, axial length was not significantly ($P = 0.38$) associated with glaucoma prevalence in that model [70]. It suggested that the axial elongation-associated enlargement of the optic disc as compared to the axial elongation itself was one of the main factors for the increased glaucoma susceptibility in the highly myopic eyes. In a following study, it was additionally detected that an enlarged parapapillary delta zone, together with an enlarged optic disc, was associated with the increased glaucoma prevalence in highly myopic eyes, while in the multivariate analysis, parapapillary gamma zone was not related with the glaucoma prevalence [71]. In that study on 519 eyes with a mean axial length of 29.5 ± 2.2 mm, prevalence of GON increased from 12.2% in the group with an axial length of <26.5 mm to 28.5% (24.4, 32.5) in the group with an axial length of ≥26.5 mm, to 32.6% in the group with an axial length of ≥28 mm, to 36.0% in the group with an axial length of ≥29 mm, and to 42.1% in eyes with an axial length of ≥30 mm.

11.4 Potential Reasons for the Association Between Glaucoma and High Myopia

The main factors associated with the increased prevalence of GON in the highly myopic eyes were the size of the optic disc and the prevalence and size of parapapillary delta zone. Histomorphometric studies have revealed that the axial elongation-associated enlargement of the optic disc is associated with an elongation and thinning of the lamina cribrosa. Since the lamina cribrosa is the functional border tissue between the intraocular compartment with the IOP and the retrobulbar compartment with the orbital cerebrospinal fluid pressure, a thinning of the lamina cribrosa leads to a decreased distance between both compartments and to a steepening of the trans-lamina cribrosa pressure gradient between both compartments [17, 18]. An elevated the trans-lamina cribrosa pressure difference or a steepening of the trans-lamina cribrosa pressure gradient have been discussed to be associated with the glaucomatous damage to the retinal ganglion cell axons when passing through the lamina cribrosa [72–76]. The thinning of the lamina cribrosa may thus be one of the reasons for the association between an enlargement of the optic disc size and a higher prevalence of GON. Additional potential reasons for the increased glaucoma susceptibility in highly myopic optic disc may be a rearrangement of the lamina cribrosa pores and the whole lamina cribrosa architecture by the axial elongation-associated stretching of the lamina cribrosa. Theoretically, it may have a similar effect as the scarring of the lamina cribrosa due to the glaucomatous process itself, what may also lead to increased glaucoma susceptibility at a given IOP [77].

Histological studies have additionally shown that the myopic enlargement of the posterior surface of the lamina cribrosa leads to an exposure of a peripheral annular-like region of the lamina directly to the orbital cerebrospinal fluid space [18]. Since the cerebrospinal fluid in contrast to the solid optic nerve tissue cannot resist a local backward bowing of the lamina cribrosa, the exposure of the posterior lamina cribrosa surface to the cerebrospinal fluid space may allow the development of acquired pits of the optic nerve head which are typically located at the optic disc border.

The peripapillary scleral flange is the biomechanical anchor of the lamina cribrosa to the posterior sclera, with both tissues being partially separated from each other by the peripapillary border tissue of Elschnig the scleral flange [38]. In the process of axial elongation, the length of the peripapillary scleral flange can increase by a factor of 10×, and its thickness can get reduced to 10% of its original value [19, 78]. These marked anatomical changes may have an effect on the biomechanical properties of the flange as the anchor of the lamina cribrosa and may be one of the reasons for the increased glaucoma susceptibility in high myopia. This notion fits with the observation that the size of parapapillary gamma zone, after adjusting for axial length was not significantly associated with the glaucoma prevalence. Gamma is the zone free of Bruch's membrane, and Bruch's membrane, connected with the lamina cribrosa by the thin peripapillary choroidal border tissue of Jacoby may not directly be involved in the biomechanics of the lamina cribrosa in glaucoma.

The lamina cribrosa is nourished by vessels originating from the peripapillary arterial circle of Zinn-Haller, which is located approximately at the merging point of the posterior sclera with the dura mater of the optic nerve [40, 41, 79]. The longer the peripapillary scleral flange, the larger is the distance between the arterial circle and the optic nerve head. The axial elongation-associated elongation of the peripapillary scleral flange may thus potentially have importance for the blood supply of the lamina cribrosa and be another factor for an increased susceptibility of a highly myopic disc for optic nerve damage.

It has remained unclear whether the axial elongation-associated enlargement of the optic disc is an independent risk factor for an increased GON susceptibility in high myopia. In non-highly myopic eyes, the optic disc size was not associated with the prevalence and amount of GON [77, 80, 81]. Since the elongation and thinning of the lamina cribrosa and of the peripapillary scleral flange are strongly associated with the optic disc enlargement, one may assume that the disc enlargement is secondarily, and not causally, associated with the increased prevalence of GON in high myopia. It has also remained elusive whether the axial elongation-associated thinning of the peripapillary choroid has an influence on the GON susceptibility [82].

11.5 Intraocular Pressure and Glaucoma in High Myopia

In a recent pilot study on 517 eyes with a mean axial length of 29.5 ± 2.2 mm, the IOP did not differ significantly ($P = 0.53$) between the glaucoma group ($n = 141$ (27.3%) eyes) and the non-glaucomatous group ($n = 376$ (72.7%)) (14.5 ± 3.3 mmHg versus 14.7 ± 2.5 mmHg) [83]. Only in the eyes with an axial length of equal to or less than 27.4 mm, the prevalence of GON was correlated with higher IOP ($P = 0.037$; odds ratio (OR): 1.35; 95% confidence interval (CI):1.02, 1.80), while in the eyes with a longer axial length, the prevalence of GON was not significantly ($P = 0.97$) associated with IOP in a multivariate analysis adjusting for age, axial length, shorter vertical diameter of the temporal arterial arcade and longer minimal optic disc diameter. There were major limitations of the study as follows: the diagnosis of GON was based on the ophthalmoscopic appearance of the optic nerve head, without taking into account results of visual field examinations or findings obtained by optical coherence tomography; and the glaucomatous group as compared to the non-glaucomatous group had a significantly higher prevalence of anti-glaucomatous therapy. It could suggest that the lack of a difference in IOP between both groups was due to the higher prevalence of IOP-lowering therapy in the glaucomatous group. In the multivariate analysis with adjustment for the prevalence of anti-glaucomatous treatment however, the IOP was not significantly associated with the glaucomatous versus non-glaucoma group.

If the results of the study are valid, it may not indicate that there is no association between IOP and glaucoma in high myopia, but that highly myopic glaucomatous eyes as compared with non-highly myopic glaucomatous eyes may have a markedly lower IOP threshold to develop optic nerve damage. It could indicate that an IOP of perhaps lower than 10 mmHg might be necessary to prevent the development of GON in these highly myopic eyes, and that in highly myopic eyes with axial elongation associated enlargement and stretching of the optic disc and parapapillary region as the main risk factors for GON in high myopia a normal IOP may be sufficient to lead to GON.

11.6 Therapy of Glaucoma in High Myopia

Although it has not yet been firmly proven that GON in high myopia is dependent on IOP, and although a randomized trial on the effect of lowering of IOP as therapy of glaucoma in highly myopic eyes has not been performed yet, most researchers recommend lowering IOP in highly myopic patients with glaucoma. Based on the morphological findings described above, the target pressure in highly myopic glaucoma may be lower than in non-highly myopic glaucoma. A factor markedly complicating the clinical situation is the difficulty in detecting the presence of GON and, in particular, in detecting the progression of optic nerve damage in highly myopic glaucoma. Due to the peculiar anatomy of the optic nerve head in highly myopic eyes, most diagnostic procedures fail in precisely assessing the status of the optic nerve in highly myopic eyes with glaucoma. It includes factors such as:

- a decreased spatial and color contrast between the neuroretinal rim and the optic cup making a delineation of both structures more difficult;
- a peripapillary retinoschisis leading to an incorrect segmentation of the retinal nerve fiber layer upon optical coherence tomography;
- a large gamma zone (and delta zone) which makes using the end of Bruch's membrane as reference point for the measurement of the neuroretinal rim useless;
- a large gamma zone also markedly further reduces the anyway relatively low value of parapapillary beta zone as indicator for GON; and
- macular Bruch's membrane defects and other reasons for non-glaucomatous visual field defects which reduces the diagnostic precision of perimetry for the detection of presence and progression of GON.

The mode of therapy of lowering IOP in highly myopic glaucoma is similar to the therapy of open-angle glaucoma in non-highly myopic eyes and includes topically applied drugs reducing the production of aqueous humor and/or increasing the outflow of aqueous humor, laser procedures aimed at the trabecular meshwork to increase aqueous humor outflow, and surgical procedures for increase of aqueous humor outflow or reduction of aqueous humor production. If fistulating procedures, such as trabeculectomy, are performed, one may have to take into account a potentially increased risk of postoperative choroidal swelling and detachment and even expulsive hemorrhage. Potential reasons might be the marked thinning (compression) of the choroid in highly myopic eyes and an oblique course of the short posterior ciliary arteries (and potentially vortex veins) through the sclera in highly myopic eyes, while in emmetropic eyes the short posterior ciliary arteries run almost perpendicularly through the sclera (Fig. 11.2).

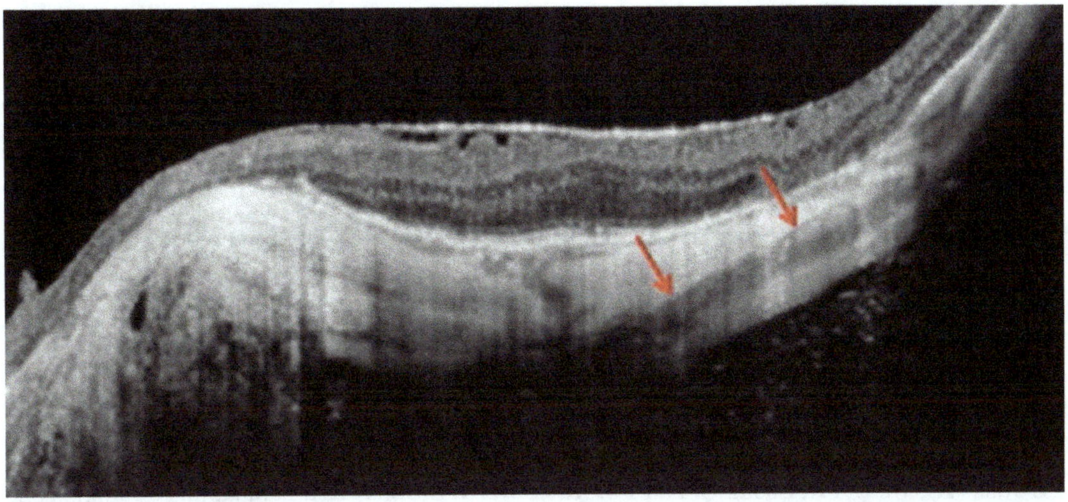

Fig. 11.2 Optical coherence tomographic image of the posterior sclera in a highly myopic eye showing the oblique course of a short posterior ciliary artery (red arrows) through the sclera

References

1. Heine L. Beiträge zur Anatomie des myopischen Auges. Arch Augenheilk. 1899;38:277–90.
2. Vurgese S, Panda-Jonas S, Jonas JB. Sclera thickness in human globes and its relations to age, axial length and glaucoma. PLoS One. 2012;7:e29692.
3. Jonas JB, Holbach L, Panda-Jonas S. Scleral cross section area and volume and axial length. PLoS One. 2014;9:e93551.
4. Shen L, Xu X, You QS, Gao F, Zhang Z, Li B, Jonas JB. Scleral thickness in Chinese eyes. Invest Ophthalmol Vis Sci. 2015;56:2720–7.
5. Shen L, You QS, Xu X, Gao F, Zhang Z, Li B, Jonas JB. Scleral and choroidal volume in relation to axial length in infants with retinoblastoma versus adults with malignant melanomas or end-stage glaucoma. Graefes Arch Clin Exp Ophthalmol. 2016;254:1779–86.
6. Wei WB, Xu L, Jonas JB, Shao L, Du KF, Wang S, Chen CX, Xu J, Wang YX, Zhou JQ, You QS. Subfoveal choroidal thickness: the Beijing Eye Study. Ophthalmology. 2013;120:175–80.
7. Jonas JB, Ohno-Matsui K, Jiang WJ, Panda-Jonas S. Bruch membrane and the mechanism of myopization. A new theory. Retina. 2017;37:1428–40.
8. Jonas JB, Holbach L, Panda-Jonas S. Bruch's membrane thickness in high myopia. Acta Ophthalmol. 2014;92:e470–4.
9. Wang X, Teoh CKG, Chan ASY, Thangarajoo S, Jonas JB, Girard MJA. Biomechanical properties of Bruch's membrane-choroid complex and their influence on optic nerve head biomechanics. Invest Ophthalmol Vis Sci. 2018;59:2808–17.
10. Jonas JB, Ohno-Matsui K, Holbach L, Panda-Jonas S. Retinal pigment epithelium cell density in relationship to axial length in human eyes. Acta Ophthalmol. 2017;95:e22–8.
11. Jonas JB, Xu L, Wei WB, Pan Z, Yang H, Holbach L, Panda-Jonas S, Wang YX. Retinal thickness and axial length. Invest Ophthalmol Vis Sci. 2016;57:1791–7.
12. Jonas RA, Wang YX, Yang H, Li JJ, Xu L, Panda-Jonas S, Jonas JB. Optic disc - fovea distance, axial length and parapapillary zones. The Beijing Eye Study 2011. PLoS One. 2015;10:e0138701.
13. Guo Y, Liu LJ, Tang P, Feng Y, Wu M, Lv YY, Xu L, Jonas JB. Optic disc-fovea distance and myopia progression in school children: the Beijing Children Eye Study. Acta Ophthalmol. 2018. https://doi.org/10.1111/aos.13728.

14. Jonas JB, Wang YX, Zhang Q, Liu Y, Xu L, Wei WB. Macular Bruch's membrane length and axial length. The Beijing Eye Study. PLoS ONE. 2015;10:e0136833.
15. Jonas JB, Dichtl A. Optic disc morphology in myopic primary open-angle glaucoma. Graefes Arch Clin Exp Ophthalmol. 1997;235:627–33.
16. Xu L, Li Y, Wang S, et al. Characteristics of highly myopic eyes. The Beijing Eye Study. Ophthalmology. 2007;114:121–6.
17. Jonas JB, Berenshtein E, Holbach L. Lamina cribrosa thickness and spatial relationships between intraocular space and cerebrospinal fluid space in highly myopic eyes. Invest Ophthalmol Vis Sci. 2004;45:2660–5.
18. Jonas JB, Berenshtein E, Holbach L. Anatomic relationship between lamina cribrosa, intraocular space, and cerebrospinal fluid space. Invest Ophthalmol Vis Sci. 2003;44:5189–95.
19. Jonas JB, Jonas SB, Jonas RA, Holbach L, Dai Y, Sun X, Panda-Jonas S. Parapapillary atrophy: histological gamma zone and delta zone. PLoS One. 2012;7(10):e47237.
20. Dai Y, Jonas JB, Huang H, et al. Microstructure of parapapillary atrophy: beta zone and gamma zone. Invest Ophthalmol Vis Sci. 2013;54:2013–8.
21. Jonas JB, Wang YX, Zhang Q, Fan YY, Xu L, Wei WB, Jonas RA. Parapapillary gamma zone and axial elongation-associated optic disc rotation: The Beijing Eye Study. Invest Ophthalmol Vis Sci. 2016;57:396–402.
22. Fan YY, Jonas JB, Wang YX, Chen CX, Wei WB. Horizontal and vertical optic disc rotation. The Beijing Eye Study. PLoS One. 2017;12:e0175749.
23. Jonas JB, Ohno-Matsui K, Holbach L, Panda-Jonas S. Association between axial length and horizontal and vertical globe diameters. Graefes Arch Clin Exp Ophthalmol. 2017;255:237–42.
24. Jonas JB, Ohno-Matsui K, Spaide RF, et al. Macular Bruch's membrane holes in high myopia: associated with gamma zone and delta zone of parapapillary region. Invest Ophthalmol Vis Sci. 2013;54:1295–30.
25. You QS, Peng XY, Xu L, Chen CX, Wei WB, Wang YX, Jonas JB. Macular Bruch's membrane defects in highly myopic eyes. The Beijing Eye Study. Retina. 2016;36:517–23.
26. Ohno-Matsui K, Jonas JB, Spaide RF. Macular Bruch's membrane holes in choroidal neovascularization-related myopic macular atrophy by swept-source optical coherence tomography. Am J Ophthalmol. 2015;162:133–9.
27. Shinohara K, Tanaka N, Jonas JB, Shimada N, Moriyama M, Yoshida T, Ohno-Matsui K. Ultrawide-field OCT to investigate relationships between myopic macular retinoschisis and posterior staphyloma. Ophthalmology. 2018. https://doi.org/10.1016/j.ophtha.2018.03.053.
28. Jonas JB, Gusek GC, Naumann GO. Optic disc, cup and neuroretinal rim size, configuration and correlations in normal eyes. Invest Ophthalmol Vis Sci. 1988;29:1151–8.
29. Na JH, Moon BG, Sung KR, Lee Y, Kook MS. Characterization of peripapillary atrophy using spectral domain optical coherence tomography. Korean J Ophthalmol. 2010;24:353–9.
30. Lee KY, Tomidokoro A, Sakata R, Konno S, Mayama C, Saito H, Hayashi K, Iwase A, Araie M. Cross-sectional anatomic configurations of peripapillary atrophy evaluated with spectral domain-optical coherence tomography. Invest Ophthalmol Vis Sci. 2010;51:666–71.
31. Park SC, De Moraes CG, Tello C, Liebmann JM, Ritch R. In-vivo microstructural anatomy of beta-zone parapapillary atrophy in glaucoma. Invest Ophthalmol Vis Sci. 2010;51:6408–13.
32. Manjunath V, Shah H, Fujimoto JG, Duker JS. Analysis of peripapillary atrophy using spectral domain optical coherence tomography. Ophthalmology. 2011;118:531–6.
33. Nonaka A, Hangai M, Akagi T, Mori S, Nukada M, Nakano N, Yoshimura N. Biometric features of peripapillary atrophy beta in eyes with high myopia. Invest Ophthalmol Vis Sci. 2011;52:6706–13.
34. Park SC, De Moraes CG, Teng CC, Tello C, Liebmann JM, Ritch R. Enhanced depth imaging optical coherence tomography of deep optic nerve complex structures in glaucoma. Ophthalmology. 2012;119:3–9.
35. Hayashi K, Tomidokoro A, Lee KY, Konno S, Saito H, Mayama C, Aihara M, Iwase A, Araie M. Spectral-domain optical coherence tomography of β-zone peripapillary atrophy: influence of myopia and glaucoma. Invest Ophthalmol Vis Sci. 2012;53:1499–505.

36. Reis AS, Sharpe GP, Yang H, Nicolela MT, Burgoyne CF, Chauhan BC. Optic disc margin anatomy in patients with glaucoma and normal controls with spectral domain optical coherence tomography. Ophthalmology. 2012;119:738–47.
37. Jonas JB, Jonas SB, Jonas RA, Holbach L, Panda-Jonas S. Histology of the parapapillary region in high myopia. Am J Ophthalmol. 2011;152:1021–9.
38. Jonas JB, Holbach L, Panda-Jonas S. Peripapillary ring: histology and correlations. Acta Ophthalmol. 2014;92:e273–9.
39. Jonas JB, Jonas RA, Jonas SB, Panda-Jonas S. Lamina cribrosa thickness correlated with peripapillary sclera thickness. Acta Ophthalmol. 2012;90:e248–50.
40. Jonas JB, Jonas SB. Histomorphometry of the circular arterial ring of Zinn-Haller in normal and glaucomatous eyes. Acta Ophthalmol. 2010;88:e317–22.
41. Jonas JB, Holbach L, Panda-Jonas S. Peripapillary arterial circle of Zinn-Haller: location and spatial relationships. PLoS One. 2013;8:e78867.
42. Jonas JB, Papastathopoulos KI. Optic disc shape in glaucoma. Graefes Arch Clin Exp Ophthalmol. 1996;234:S167–73.
43. Guo Y, Liu LJ, Xu L, Lv YY, Tang P, Feng Y, Zhou JQ, Meng M, Jonas JB. Optic disc ovality in primary school children in Beijing. Invest Ophthalmol Vis Sci. 2015;56:4547–53.
44. Dai Y, Jonas JB, Ling Z, Sun X. Ophthalmoscopic-perspectively distorted optic disc diameters and real disc diameters. Invest Ophthalmol Vis Sci. 2015;56:7076–83.
45. Demer JL. Optic nerve sheath as a novel mechanical load on the globe in ocular ductionoptic nerve sheath constrains duction. Invest Ophthalmol Vis Sci. 2016;57:1826–38.
46. Wang X, Rumpel H, Lim WE, Baskaran M, Perera SA, Nongpiur ME, Aung T, Milea D, Girard MJ. Finite element analysis predicts large optic nerve head strains during horizontal eye movements. Invest Ophthalmol Vis Sci. 2016;57:2452–62.
47. Jonas JB, Dai Y, Panda-Jonas S. Peripapillary suprachoroidal cavitation, parapapillary gamma zone and optic disc rotation due to the biomechanics of the optic nerve dura mater. Invest Ophthalmol Vis Sci. 2016;57:4373.
48. Wang X, Rumpel H, Lim WE, Baskaran M, Perera SA, Nongpiur ME, Aung T, Milea D, Girard MJ. Author Response: Peripapillary suprachoroidal cavitation, parapapillary gamma zone and optic disc rotation due to the biomechanics of the optic nerve dura mater. Invest Ophthalmol Vis Sci. 2016;57:4374–5.
49. Ohno-Matsui K, Shimada N, Akiba M, Moriyama M, Ishibashi T, Tokoro T. Characteristics of intrachoroidal cavitation located temporal to optic disc in highly myopic eyes. Eye. 2013;27:630–8.
50. Dai Y, Jonas JB, Ling Z, Wang X, Sun X. Unilateral peripapillary intrachoroidal cavitation and optic disc rotation. Retina. 2015;35:655–9.
51. Jonas JB. Optic disc size correlated with refractive error. Am J Ophthalmol. 2005;139:346–8.
52. Xu L, Wang YX, Wang S, Jonas JB. Definition of high myopia by parapapillary atrophy. The Beijing Eye Study. Acta Ohthalmol. 2010;88:e350–1.
53. Xu L, Wang Y, Wang S, Wang Y, Jonas JB. High myopia and glaucoma susceptibility. The Beijing Eye Study. Ophthalmology. 2007;114:216–20.
54. Liu HH, Xu L, Wang YX, Wang S, You QS, Jonas JB. Prevalence and progression of myopic retinopathy in Chinese adults: The Beijing Eye Study. Ophthalmology. 2010;117:1763–8.
55. Nakazawa M, Kurotaki J, Ruike H. Longterm findings in peripapillary crescent formation in eyes with mild or moderate myopia. Acta Ophthalmol. 2008;86:626–9.
56. Podos S, Becker B, Mortion W. High myopia and primary open-angle glaucoma. Am J Ophthalmol. 1966;62:1039–43.
57. Greve EL, Furuno F. Myopia and glaucoma. Graefes Arch Clin Exp Ophthalmol. 1980;213:33–41.
58. Daubs JG, Crick RP. Effect of refractive error on the risk of ocular hypertension and open angle glaucoma. Trans Ophthalmol Soc Aust. 1981;101:121–6.
59. Phelps CD. Effect of myopia on prognosis in treated primary open-angle glaucoma. Am J Ophthalmol. 1982;93:622–8.

60. Perkins ES, Phelps CD. Open angle glaucoma, ocular hypertension, low-tension glaucoma, and refraction. Arch Ophthalmol. 1982;100:1464–7.
61. Leske MC, Connell AM, Wu SY, Hyman LG, Schachat AP. Risk factors for open-angle glaucoma. The Barbados Eye Study. Arch Ophthalmol. 1995;113:918–24.
62. Chihara E, Liu X, Dong J, Takashima Y, Akimoto M, Hangai M, Kuriyama S, Tanihara H, Hosoda M, Tsukahara S. Severe myopia as a risk factor for progressive visual field loss in primary open-angle glaucoma. Ophthalmologica. 1997;211:66–71.
63. Mitchell P, Hourihan F, Sandbach J, Wang JJ. The relationship between glaucoma and myopia: the Blue Mountains Eye Study. Ophthalmology. 1999;106:2010–5.
64. Grodum K, Heijl A, Bengtsson B. Refractive error and glaucoma. Acta Ophthalmol Scand. 2001;79:560–6.
65. Jonas JB, Martus P, Budde WM. Anisometropia and degree of optic nerve damage in chronic open-angle glaucoma. Am J Ophthalmol. 2002;134:547–51.
66. Wong TY, Klein BE, Klein R, Knudtson M, Lee KE. Refractive errors, intraocular pressure, and glaucoma in a white population. Ophthalmology. 2003;110:211–7.
67. Leske MC, Heijl A, Hussein M, Bengtsson B, Hyman L, Komaroff E, Early Manifest Glaucoma Trial Group. Factors for glaucoma progression and the effect of treatment: the early manifest glaucoma trial. Arch Ophthalmol. 2003;121:48–56.
68. Jonas JB, Budde WM. Optic nerve damage in highly myopic eyes with chronic open-angle glaucoma. Eur J Ophthalmol. 2005;15:41–7.
69. Kuzin AA, Varma R, Reddy HS, Torres M, Azen SP, Los Angeles Latino Eye Study Group. Ocular biometry and open-angle glaucoma: the Los Angeles Latino Eye Study. Ophthalmology. 2010;117:1713–9.
70. Nagaoka N, Jonas JB, Morohoshi K, Moriyama M, Shimada N, Yoshida T, Ohno-Matsui K. Glaucomatous-type optic discs in high myopia. PLoS One. 2015;10:e0138825.
71. Jonas JB, Weber P, Nagaoka N, Ohno-Matsui K. Glaucoma in high myopia and parapapillary delta zone. PLoS One. 2017;12:e0175120.
72. Balaratnasingam C, Morgan WH, Johnstone V, et al. Histomorphometric measurements in human and dog optic nerve and an estimation of optic nerve pressure gradients in human. Exp Eye Res. 2009;89:618–28.
73. Morgan WH, Yu DY, Balaratnasingam CX. The role of cerebrospinal fluid pressure in glaucoma pathophysiology: the dark side of the optic disc. J Glaucoma. 1998;17:408–13.
74. Berdahl JP, Allingham RR, Johnson DH. Cerebrospinal fluid pressure is decreased in primary open-angle glaucoma. Ophthalmology. 2008;115:763–8.
75. Ren R, Jonas JB, Tian G, Zhen Y, Ma K, Li S, Wang H, Li B, Zhang X, Wang N. Cerebrospinal fluid pressure in glaucoma. A prospective study. Ophthalmology. 2010;117:259–66.
76. Jonas JB, Wang N, Yang D, Ritch R, Panda-Jonas S. Facts and myths of cerebrospinal fluid pressure for the physiology of the eye. Prog Retin Eye Res. 2015;46:67–83.
77. Burgoyne CF, Morrison JC. The anatomy and pathophysiology of the optic nerve head in glaucoma. J Glaucoma. 2001;10:S16–8.
78. Dichtl A, Jonas JB, Naumann GO. Histomorphometry of the optic disc in highly myopic eyes with absolute secondary angle closure glaucoma. Br J Ophthalmol. 1998;82:286–9.
79. Hayreh SS. Blood supply of the optic nerve head and its role in optic atrophy, glaucoma, and oedema of the optic nerve. Br J Ophthalmol. 1969;53:721–48.
80. Jonas JB, Xu L, Zhang L, Wang Y, Wang Y. Optic disk size in chronic glaucoma. The Beijing Eye Study. Am J Ophthalmol. 2006;142:168–70.
81. Wang YX, Hu LN, Yang H, Jonas JB, Xu L. Frequency and associated factors of structural progression of open-angle glaucoma in the Beijing Eye Study. Br J Ophthalmol. 2012;96:811–5.
82. Jiang R, Wang YX, Wei WB, Xu L, Jonas JB. Peripapillary choroidal thickness in adult Chinese: The Beijing Eye Study. Invest Ophthalmol Vis Sci. 2015;56:4045–52.
83. Jonas JB, Nagaoka N, Fang YX, Weber P, Ohno-Matsui K. Intraocular pressure and glaucomatous optic neuropathy in high myopia. Invest Ophthalmol Vis Sci. 2017;58:5897–906.

Clinical Management of Myopia in Adults: Treatment of Retinal Complications

12

Jerry K. H. Lok, Raymond L. M. Wong, Lawrence P. L. Iu, and Ian Y. H. Wong

Key Points

- MTM is an important treatable cause of visual loss among individuals with high myopia.
- A certain proportion of cases of MTM do not progress. Treatment should be offered to patients with more advanced disease with progressive visual loss.
- Fovea-sparing instead of complete peeling of the ILM and avoidance of gas tamponade could prevent the formation of secondary macular hole in MTM.
- Surgical adjuncts should be considered for macular hole especially in high-risk cases (persistent macular hole despite initial surgery, large and chronic macular hole, atrophic macula, etc.)

J. K. H. Lok
Department of Ophthalmology, Hong Kong Eye Hospital, Kowloon, Hong Kong

R. L. M. Wong
Department of Ophthalmology, Hong Kong Eye Hospital, Kowloon, Hong Kong

Department of Ophthalmology, LKS Faculty of Medicine, University of Hong Kong, Pok Fu Lam, Hong Kong

L. P. L. Iu
Department of Ophthalmology, LKS Faculty of Medicine, University of Hong Kong, Pok Fu Lam, Hong Kong

Department of Ophthalmology, Prince of Wales Hospital, Sha Tin, Hong Kong

I. Y. H. Wong (✉)
Department of Ophthalmology, LKS Faculty of Medicine, University of Hong Kong, Pok Fu Lam, Hong Kong

Department of Ophthalmology, Hong Kong Sanatorium and Hospital, Happy Valley, Hong Kong

M. Ang, T. Y. Wong (eds.), *Updates on Myopia*,
https://doi.org/10.1007/978-981-13-8491-2_12

12.1 Introduction

As described in the previous chapter, myopic foveal retinoschisis was first described in 1958 [1], then by Takano and Kishi in 1999 through the advent of optical coherence tomography (OCT) [2]. Subsequently, the various pathological effects of traction on the macula in patients with high myopia were collectively termed *myopic traction maculopathy* (MTM) by Panozzo and Mercanti in 2004 [3]. It was estimated to occur in approximately 8–34% in individuals with high myopia [4–6]. The term MTM originally encompassed retinal thickening, macular retinoschisis, foveal detachment, and lamellar macular hole with or without epiretinal membrane and/or vitreomacular traction [3]. The spectrum was extended to include full-thickness macular hole (HM) with or without retinal detachment.

Central to the pathogenesis of MTM is traction, which was postulated to arise from one or more of the following mechanisms [7]: vitreomacular traction associated with perifoveal posterior vitreous detachment (PVD) [8–10]; relative incompliance of inner retinal structures (e.g., internal limiting membrane [ILM] [11–15], epiretinal membrane [ERM] [6, 8, 16–18], and cortical vitreous remnant after PVD [19]) to the outer retina which conforms to the shape of the posterior staphyloma; and traction exerted by retinal arterioles [14, 20, 21].

Not all patients with MTM require interventions [10, 22, 23]. A study on the natural history of MTM with 207 eyes found that while 12% of cases progressed during a mean follow-up period of 36 months, the majority (84%) remained stable and a small proportion (4%) even had improvement or complete resolution of the disease [24]. The extent of macular retinoschisis was identified as a predictor of progression, with stage 4 disease (i.e., involving the entire macula) having the higher chance of progression than any other stages [24]. It is generally accepted that eyes with complications such as foveal detachment or full-thickness MH with or without retinal detachment, or eyes with significant progression in the extent of macular retinoschisis on OCT should undergo intervention early. On the other hand, an early macular retinoschisis involving only a limited area of the macula with preserved vision should be monitored with OCT for any progression.

There are numerous reported interventions for MTM. The principles of the treatment are: (1) to relieve traction, mainly achieved through pars plana vitrectomy (PPV) with or without ILM peeling; (2) to minimize surgical damage to the weakened macula through technique modifications in order to prevent the formation of postoperative MH; and (3) in the presence of full-thickness MH to maximize the chance of hole closure through the use of various surgical adjuncts.

12.2 Surgical Procedures

12.2.1 Pars Plana Vitrectomy

PPV serves several purposes in the treatment of MTM. It allows removal of all premacular tractional forces, including posterior vitreous cortex and ERM. It also creates a potential space in the posterior segment for gas tamponade to be performed.

12.2.1.1 Microincision Vitrectomy Surgery

With the advent of microincision vitrectomy system, PPV can be performed with small sclerotomy wounds and instruments in the size of 23 gauge, 25 gauge, or 27 gauge. Small sclerotomy wounds tend to be self-sealing and do not require sutures. It has the advantages of reduced ocular trauma, reduced inflammation, less conjunctival scarring, shorter operation time, better patient comfort, and faster postoperative recovery [25]. The design of closer opening near the tip of vitreous cutter probe also facilitates engagement and induction of PVD.

12.2.1.2 Induction of Posterior Vitreous Detachment

Since the pathogenesis of MTM involves abnormal vitreoretinal traction at the macula, induction of PVD is crucial to a successful operation. After core vitrectomy, induction of PVD is performed by using an aspiration port, usually the vitreous cutter probe, to engage the posterior hyaloid just anterior to optic disc. Once the posterior hyaloid is engaged by applying aspiration, the port is lifted upward to detach the posterior hyaloid from the retinal surface.

Induction of PVD can be difficult in MTM due to tight vitreoretinal adhesion and presence of vitreoschisis. Vitreoschisis refers to splitting of posterior vitreous cortex which occurs when there is vitreous gel liquefaction but without dehiscence at the vitreoretinal interface [26]. Vitreoschisis is common in MTM and is present in around half of the patients with MH [27]. To facilitate induction of PVD, triamcinolone acetonide [28] or trypan blue can be injected to stain the posterior hyaloid to improve visualization. If PVD cannot be induced by aspiration, intraocular forceps or diamond-dusted membrane scraper can be used to lift and assist detachment of the posterior hyaloid [29, 30].

12.2.1.3 Epiretinal Membrane Peeling

It is necessary to remove all ERM if any present on the macula. Removal of ERM allows removal of tractional forces on the macula, and allows access and identification of the underlying ILM with vital dyes.

Trypan blue is useful to stain the ERM to enhance visualization [31, 32]. Trypan blue is often injected after fluid-air exchange [33], or it can be mixed with 10% glucose isovolumetrically to create a heavy dye denser than balanced salt solution so that it will fall onto the macula with less dispersion in vitreous cavity [34]. There are also products combining trypan blue, brilliant blue, and polyethylene glycol with increased molecular weight so that the dye falls onto the macula to enhance tissue staining.

12.2.1.4 Internal Limiting Membrane Peeling

ILM is the innermost layer of a normal retina. It has significant contribution to retinal rigidity [35]. ILM peeling therefore improves retinal compliance and allows the retina to restore its normal anatomy [35]. The potential complications of ILM peeling include iatrogenic damage to retinal nerve fiber layer, retinal hemorrhage, and retinal defect formation, especially at sites of ILM flap creation and grasping points [35]. Due to the thinner retina and longer distance required to reach the posterior pole, ILM peeling is more technically challenging in highly myopic eyes than normal eyes and complications may be more common.

ILM is barely visible and requires staining with vital dyes for identification. Triamcinolone acetonide and trypan blue do not stain ILM well. The better dyes for ILM staining are brilliant blue and indocyanine green (ICG) [31, 32]. ICG adheres well to the extracellular matrix of ILM such as collagen type 4 and laminin and allows good visualization of ILM [31]. However, there are concerns of potential retinal toxicity, especially when ICG is in direct contact with the photoreceptors and retinal pigment epithelium through a MH [31]. ICG retinal toxicity has been shown with electrophysiology and histological studies in animal models [36, 37]. The risk increases with endoillumination light exposure [32]. In comparison, brilliant blue is a much safer alternative. A recent meta-analysis showed that postoperative visual acuity was better with brilliant blue than ICG in MH surgeries [38].

After ILM staining, an ILM flap can be created at the extrafoveal region using intraocular forceps by direct pinch method [35]. Alternatively, a pick, diamond-dusted membrane scraper or flexible nitinol loop can be used to create an ILM flap by scrapping [11]. The ILM flap is then lifted with intraocular forceps and moved in a circular fashion so that the whole ILM is peeled off from the macula.

Full-Thickness Macular Hole

In full-thickness MH, ILM peeling helps to reduce retinal rigidity and improve retinal compliance and thus the chance of MH closure [35]. It also helps to reduce postoperative ERM formation and risk of MH reopening [35]. A meta-analysis of four randomized controlled trials showed that ILM peeling for stages 2, 3, and 4 full-thickness MH has a significantly higher closure rate than without ILM peeling [39]. Another meta-analysis showed that MH reopening rate reduced from 7 to 1% when ILM peeling was performed.

Concerning the extent of ILM peeling, there is no consensus on the optimal size required [35]. Extended ILM peeling up to arcade is often performed for large MH to ensure traction has been sufficiently removed. Extended ILM peeling, however, is performed at the expense of longer operation time and higher risk of iatrogenic retinal trauma due to repeated ILM grasping [35]. Dissociated optic nerve fiber layer (DONFL) and swelling of arcuate retinal nerve fiber layer (SANFL), which can be shown on imaging modalities such as OCT scan and infrared fundus photographs, are two known structural changes secondary to ILM peeling [40, 41]. ILM flap initiation techniques might affect the chance of these structural complications, with pinch technique shown to be less damaging than diamond dust membrane scraping [40].

Myopic Foveoschisis

For myopic foveoschisis, ILM peeling helps to ensure that all tractional forces from premacular glial cells and vitreous cortex are completely removed [42]. It increases retinal compliance and allows the retina to better conform to the posterior staphyloma [42].

Favorable anatomical and visual outcomes have been reported for combined PPV, ILM peeling, and gas tamponade. However, development of postoperative full-thickness MH is not uncommon and occurs in around 13–28% of patients [43].

Shimada et al. [44] and Ho et al. [45] introduced the technique of *fovea-sparing ILM peel* in 2012. Instead of complete ILM removal, this technique involves removal of the perifoveal ILM only and leaving the ILM over the central foveola intact. It is believed that preservation of foveolar ILM would preserve foveolar Muller cells integrity and therefore reduce the risk of postoperative MH development [46]. Although studies suggested this technique might be useful to reduce the risk of MH development and foveolar thinning [46], leaving ILM on the fovea could result in late ILM contraction and retinal thickening [44]. This technique is also more technically demanding and requires more tissue manipulation than conventional complete ILM peeling.

In view of the risk of secondary macular hole development in foveoschisis patients undergone ILM peeling, conservative treatment can be considered in foveoschisis patients without foveal detachment.

12.2.1.5 Gas Tamponade

The commonly used gases for tamponade include air, sulfur hexafluoride (SF_6), and perfluoropropane (C_3F_8). Gas tamponade is commonly performed for MTM, particularly in cases with FTMH. For myopic foveoschisis without FTMH, it is still controversial whether gas tamponade is necessary. Gas tamponade may help the retina to adhere better to the posterior staphyloma and tamponade against unnoticeable macular holes [47]. In the presence of outer retinal detachment, the subretinal fluid (SRF) could be displaced toward areas with healthier retinal pigment epithelial (RPE) cells, which can facilitate SRF absorption [48–50]. More rapid resolution of foveoschisis was also reported by a study [51]. However, the study showed that the chance of successful resolution was similar between the group with gas tamponade and that without gas tamponade [51]. Indeed, a meta-analysis showed that for eyes undergoing vitrectomy for myopic foveoschisis, gas tamponade did not have significant impact on visual acuity or the rate of resolution of foveoschisis, yet it was associated with more complications [42]. Several studies also reported the paradoxical occurrence of FTHM from the use of gas tamponade, which could squeeze SRF within the limited space through the weak point of fovea [52–54]. The use of gas tamponade as an adjunct for FTMH would be discussed below.

12.2.2 Additional Measures (Adjuncts) to Improve Outcome of Macular Hole Surgery

12.2.2.1 Endotamponade

PPV with endotamponade agents is the most commonly employed technique for the management of myopic macular hole with or without retinal detachment. Gas tamponade with long-acting gases, commonly SF_6 and C_3F_8, has the advantages of high surface tension and buoyancy compared to silicone oil. A study comparing C_3F_8 and silicone oil as a tamponade agent for myopic MH retinal detachment (MHRD) showed higher initial success rate for C_3F_8 than silicone oil [55]. Due to lower buoyancy, silicone oil is less conforming to posterior staphyloma, rendering it less effective for MHRD. However, silicone oil still has advantages over gases for longer duration of tamponade, shorter duration of face down posturing, earlier visual recovery as well as allowing immediate air travel.

12.2.2.2 Inverted Internal Limiting Membrane Flap

Even with extended ILM peeling, a proportion of large chronic MH remains open after operation. Michalewska et al. introduced the *inverted ILM flap technique* in 2009 and reported closure rate of large MH reached 98% [56]. Instead of complete ILM removal, this technique involves leaving a hinge of ILM flap at the edge of MH during ILM peeling. This ILM flap is then inverted upside-down to cover or fill the MH. Some surgeons would inject an ophthalmic viscosurgical device on the inverted ILM flap in order to keep it in place. It is postulated that this technique facilitates MH closure by (1) providing a flap which contains Muller cell fragments to induce glial cells proliferation, and (2) providing a scaffold for retinal tissue to approximate [56]. Despite an apparently promising closure rate for large or persistent MH, it has been reported that the visual recovery and recovery of retinal microstructures such as external limiting membrane and the ellipsoid zone are worse among cases managed with inverted ILM flap when compared to conventional complete ILM peeling [57]. This can possibly be due to mechanical obstruction of functional recovery of retinal layers by the presence of an ILM plug in the MH.

12.2.2.3 Autologous Internal Limiting Membrane Transplantation

Although the inverted ILM flap technique proposed by Michalewska and associates seems to be a good surgical adjunct for anatomical closure of large MH, this method cannot be applied to patients who suffer from persistent macular hole after vitrectomy and conventional ILM peeling, since ILM surrounding MH has already been removed in the previous procedure. In view of this limitation, Morizane et al. introduced a new method of ILM flap, which is the autologous ILM transplantation (free ILM flap) [58]. Brilliant Blue G solution is used to stain the remaining ILM in those refractory MH cases. Subsequently appropriately sized ILM is peeled off, which is supposed to match the size of the macular hole, and is placed as a free flap onto the persistent MH. Infusion should be turned off during the procedure in order to avoid accidental loss of the ILM flap. In order to stabilize the flap, an ophthalmic viscosurgical device is injected on the top of the flap before fluid-air exchange is performed. It has been demonstrated that with this method of autologous ILM transplantation, up to 90% of refractory MH (with previous vitrectomy and ILM peeled) could achieve MH closure [58, 59].

12.2.2.4 Autologous Blood

In order to prevent subretinal migration of dye and the resultant retinal toxicity associated with vital stains, it was proposed to use autologous blood to cover the MH before injection of brilliant blue dye. Ghosh et al. collected autologous heparinized whole blood from patients' antecubital vein and injected to MH before injection of brilliant blue dye assisted ILM peeling. It has been demonstrated that compared to conventional method, the use of prestaining autologous blood led to better visual acuity outcomes and continuity of ellipsoid zone at all postoperative time points; and the outer retinal layer is thicker as well [60].

Apart from being used in the prevention of subretinal migration of dye, the therapeutic effect of autologous blood in persistent and refractory MH has also been investigated. It has been shown that injection of autologous blood or platelet concentrate into MH after ILM peeling can improve closure rate of macular hole and visual recovery [61–63]; and the efficacy of autologous platelet concentrate might even be better than whole blood. In one study in which 75 subjects were included, MH closure rate after revitrectomy plus autologous platelet concentrate was 85.2% versus 7.1% in the group using autologous whole blood instead [64].

12.2.2.5 Lens Capsular Flap Transplantation

Due to the possible lack of residual accessible ILM in reoperative cases of persistent MH, transplantation of lens capsules to MH have been proposed to increase the surgical success rate. In patients with cataract, phacoemulsification would be performed in the same setting and capsular flap would be harvested during continuous curvilinear capsulorhexis and stained with indocyanine green solution or brilliant blue solution for better visualization. In aphakic or pseudophakic patients with insufficient anterior capsule, capsular flap can be harvested from their fellow eyes requiring cataract operations. Alternatively, posterior capsular flap can be used instead. Since capsular flaps are more rigid than ILM flap, it is easier to manipulate during the operation. Moreover, due to the higher specific gravity of capsular flap, it will sink in balanced salt solution, therefore shall fall nicely onto the preretinal surface, unlike ILM flap that is tended to float inside the vitreous cavity. Chen et al. demonstrated a 100% MH closure rate with anterior capsular transplantation among patients with refractory MH, whereas the complete closure rate of MH after posterior capsular transplantation was only 50% and with another 30% enjoyed partial MH closure [65]. Similarly, Peng et al. reported a 90% MH closure rate after transplantation of anterior capsule to refractory MH [66].

12.2.2.6 Macular Buckle

One of the major etiological factors of MTM is the elongation of axial length of the globe leading to tension and traction on retinal layers. The aim of vitrectomy is to remove vitreous traction and ILM peeling to reduce the rigidity and improve the compliance of retina. Nevertheless, none of these procedures tackle the primary pathology, which is the long axial length in high myopes.

Macula buckles have been used to shorten the axial length of myopic eyeballs in conditions such as MHRD, myopic foveoschisis with or without foveal detachment and MH with foveoschisis. There are many types of macular buckle, including scleral sponge, T-shaped or L-shaped buckle, Ando Plombe, wire-strengthened sponge exoplant, and even donor sclera and suprachoroidal injectable long-acting hyaluronic acid. Chandelier light is attached to the indenting head of macular buckle when necessary for better localization and positioning of the buckle. The purpose of all the aforementioned macular buckles is to shape the globe back to normal length along the visual axis, thereby reducing the anteroposterior traction on retina and the tension within retinal layers [67].

Studies have been carried out to compare the efficacy of vitrectomy and macular buckle in inducing retinal reattachment and MH closure in patients suffering from MHRD. Fifty to seventy-nine percent of patients with previous vitrectomy had their retina successfully reattached whereas 93.3–100% of the patients managed with macular buckles enjoyed flattening of the retina [68–70]. The differences in MH closure rates between the two treatment modalities are even higher. Similarly, comparing to less than 50% MH closure rate by vitrectomy, macular buckle surgeries achieved a 100% closure rate in patients with MH and concomitant foveoschisis, and more than 80% of these patients had improvement in final visual acuity [67]. In patients with very poor MTM, combined vitrectomy and macular buckle surgeries can be considered.

Despite the high success rate in the latest macular buckle surgeries, these procedures are technically demanding and are not without risks. Complications of macular buckles include globe perforation, problems with extraocular movement, squint, choroidal effusion, changes in retinal pigment epithelium and the need for removal of buckle.

12.2.2.7 Autologous Neurosensory Retinal Transplantation

In 2016, Grewal and Mahmoud reported the technique of autologous neurosensory retinal free flap transplantation for the closure of refractory macular hole after initial PPV with peeling of ILM [71].

The technique involves bimanually harvesting a free flap of neurosensory retina superior to the superotemporal arcade, with the harvest site first secured by endolaser barricade and endodiathermy. The free flap was translocated in its correct orientation over the macular hole and perfluoro-*n*-octane heavy liquid (PFC) was instilled over it, followed by direct PFC-silicone oil exchange.

In order to prevent flap dislocation intraoperatively and postoperatively, the intraocular pressure should be lowered to reduce fluid turbulence [72]. The edge of the flap could be tucked underneath the edge of MH [72]. A technique combining autologous blood and autologous retinal free flap transplantation was described to secure the flap with blood clot [72].

There were small case series using similar techniques with good results, in terms of both anatomical closure rate and visual recovery [73–75]. The recovery of vision was postulated to be in part due to integration of the free flap to the surrounding retinal tissue with partial recovery of the ellipsoid zone and external limiting membrane, as observed postoperatively using OCT. It was hypothesized that the flap served more than a scaffold, providing glial cells and growth factors for structural and functional restoration. The implications of this observation to other macular diseases are yet to be determined.

12.3 Conclusion

The pathological changes associated with high myopia lead to a range of retinal complications, including MTM. An understanding of the pathogenesis and natural history of the disease sheds light on its management. Advances in surgical instruments and skills have shown promises in the management of this challenging condition.

References

1. Philips C. Retinal detachment at the posterior pole. Br J Ophthalmol. 1958;42(12):749–53.
2. Takano M, Kishi S. Foveal retinoschisis and retinal detachment in severely myopic eyes with posterior staphyloma. Am J Ophthalmol. 1999;128(4):472–6. https://doi.org/10.1016/S0002-9394(99)00186-5.
3. Panozzo G, Mercanti A. Optical coherence tomography findings in myopic traction maculopathy. Arch Ophthalmol. 2004;122(10):1455–60. https://doi.org/10.1001/archopht.122.10.1455.
4. Wu PC, Chen YJ, Chen YH, et al. Factors associated with foveoschisis and foveal detachment without macular hole in high myopia. Eye. 2009;23(2):356–61. https://doi.org/10.1038/sj.eye.6703038.
5. Baba T, Ohno-Matsui K, Futagami S, et al. Prevalence and characteristics of foveal retinal detachment without macular hole in high myopia. Am J Ophthalmol. 2003;135(3):338–42. https://doi.org/10.1016/S0002-9394(02)01937-2.
6. Fang X, Weng Y, Xu S, et al. Optical coherence tomographic characteristics and surgical outcome of eyes with myopic foveoschisis. Eye. 2009;23(6):1336–42. https://doi.org/10.1038/eye.2008.291.
7. Vanderbeek BL, Johnson MW. The diversity of traction mechanisms in myopic traction maculopathy. Am J Ophthalmol. 2012;153(1):93–102. https://doi.org/10.1016/j.ajo.2011.06.016.
8. Yeh S-I, Chang W-C, Chen L-J. Vitrectomy without internal limiting membrane peeling for macular retinoschisis and foveal detachment in highly myopic eyes. Acta Ophthalmol. 2008;86(2):219–24. https://doi.org/10.1111/j.1600-0420.2007.00974.x.
9. Smiddy WE, Kim SS, Lujan BJ, Gregori G. Myopic traction maculopathy: spectral domain optical coherence tomographic imaging and a hypothesized mechanism. Ophthalmic Surg Lasers Imaging. 2009;40(2):169–73. https://doi.org/10.3928/15428877-20090301-21.
10. Gaucher D, Haouchine B, Tadayoni R, et al. Long-term follow-up of high myopic foveoschisis: natural course and surgical outcome. Am J Ophthalmol. 2007;143(3):455–62. https://doi.org/10.1016/j.ajo.2006.10.053.
11. Ikuno Y, Sayanagi K, Soga K, Oshima Y, Ohji M, Tano Y. Foveal anatomical status and surgical results in vitrectomy for myopic foveoschisis. Jpn J Ophthalmol. 2008;52(4):269–76. https://doi.org/10.1007/s10384-008-0544-8.
12. Ikuno Y, Sayanagi K, Ohji M, et al. Vitrectomy and internal limiting membrane peeling for myopic foveoschisis. Am J Ophthalmol. 2004;137(4):719–24. https://doi.org/10.1016/j.ajo.2003.10.019.
13. Kuhn F. Internal limiting membrane removal for macular detachment in highly myopic eyes. Am J Ophthalmol. 2003;135(4):547–9. https://doi.org/10.1016/S0002-9394(02)02057-3.
14. Panozzo G, Mercanti A. Vitrectomy for myopic traction maculopathy. Arch Ophthalmol. 2007;125(6):767–72. https://doi.org/10.1001/archopht.125.6.767.
15. Kumagai K, Furukawa M, Ogino N, Larson E. Factors correlated with postoperative visual acuity after vitrectomy and internal limiting membrane peeling for myopic foveoschisis. Retina. 2010. https://doi.org/10.1097/IAE.0b013e3181c703fc.
16. Kwok AKH, Lai TYY, Yip WWK. Vitrectomy and gas tamponade without internal limiting membrane peeling for myopic foveoschisis. Br J Ophthalmol. 2005. https://doi.org/10.1136/bjo.2005.069427.
17. Tang J, Rivers MB, Moshfeghi AA, Flynn HW, Chan C-C. Pathology of macular foveoschisis associated with degenerative myopia. J Ophthalmol. 2010. https://doi.org/10.1155/2010/175613.
18. Sayanagi K, Morimoto Y, Ikuno Y, Tano Y. Spectral-domain optical coherence tomographic findings in myopic foveoschisis. Retina. 2010. https://doi.org/10.1097/IAE.0b013e3181ca4e7c.
19. Spaide RF, Fisher Y. Removal of adherent cortical vitreous plaques without removing the internal limiting membrane in the repair of macular detachments in highly myopic eyes. Retina. 2005. https://doi.org/10.1097/00006982-200504000-00007.

20. Sayanagi K, Ikuno Y, Gomi F, Tano Y. Retinal vascular microfolds in highly myopic eyes. Am J Ophthalmol. 2005. https://doi.org/10.1016/j.ajo.2004.11.025.
21. Ikuno Y, Gomi F, Tano Y. Potent retinal arteriolar traction as a possible cause of myopic foveoschisis. Am J Ophthalmol. 2005. https://doi.org/10.1016/j.ajo.2004.09.078.
22. Ripandelli G, Rossi T, Scarinci F, Scassa C, Parisi V, Stirpe M. Macular vitreoretinal interface abnormalities in highly myopic eyes with posterior staphyloma: 5-year follow-up. Retina. 2012. https://doi.org/10.1097/IAE.0b013e318255062c.
23. Benhamou N, Massin P, Haouchine B, Erginay A, Gaudric A. Macular retinoschisis in highly myopic eyes. Am J Ophthalmol. 2002. https://doi.org/10.1016/S0002-9394(02)01394-6.
24. Shimada N, Tanaka Y, Tokoro T, Ohno-Matsui K. Natural course of myopic traction maculopathy and factors associated with progression or resolution. Am J Ophthalmol. 2013. https://doi.org/10.1016/j.ajo.2013.06.031.
25. Mohamed S, Claes C, Tsang CW. Review of Small Gauge Vitrectomy: Progress and Innovations. J Ophthalmol. 2017. https://doi.org/10.1155/2017/6285869.
26. Sebag J. Vitreoschisis. Graefe's Arch Clin Exp Ophthalmol. 2008. https://doi.org/10.1007/s00417-007-0743-x.
27. Gupta P, Yee KMP, Garcia P, et al. Vitreoschisis in macular diseases. Br J Ophthalmol. 2011. https://doi.org/10.1136/bjo.2009.175109.
28. Peyman GA, Cheema R, Conway MD, Fang T. Triamcinolone acetonide as an aid to visualization of the vitreous and the posterior hyaloid during pars plana vitrectomy. Retina. 2000. https://doi.org/10.1097/00006982-200005000-00024.
29. Takeuchi M, Takayama K, Sato T, Ishikawa S, Fujii S, Sakurai Y. Non-aspiration technique to induce posterior vitreous detachment in minimum incision vitrectomy system. Br J Ophthalmol. 2012. https://doi.org/10.1136/bjophthalmol-2012-301628.
30. Gómez-Resa M, Burés-Jelstrup A, Mateo C. Myopic traction maculopathy. Dev Ophthalmol. 2014. https://doi.org/10.1159/000360468.
31. Rodrigues EB, Costa EF, Penha FM, et al. The use of vital dyes in ocular surgery. Surv Ophthalmol. 2009. https://doi.org/10.1016/j.survophthal.2009.04.011.
32. Farah M, Maia M, Rodrigues E. Dyes in ocular surgery: principles for use in chromovitrectomy. Am J Ophthalmol. 2009;148(3):332–40.
33. Badaro E, Novais EA, Penha FM, Maia M, Farah ME, Rodrigues EB. Vital dyes in ophthalmology: a chemical perspective. Curr Eye Res. 2014. https://doi.org/10.3109/02713683.2013.865759.
34. Lesnik Oberstein SY, De Smet MD. Use of heavy trypan blue in macular hole surgery. Eye. 2010. https://doi.org/10.1038/eye.2010.3.
35. Chatziralli I, Theodossiadis P, Steel D. Internal limiting membrane peeling in macular hole surgery; why, when and how? Retina. 2018;38(5):870–82.
36. Enaida H, Sakamoto T, Hisatomi T, Goto Y, Ishibashi T. Morphological and functional damage of the retina caused by intravitreous indocyanine green in rat eyes. Graefe's Arch Clin Exp Ophthalmol. 2002. https://doi.org/10.1007/s00417-002-0433-7.
37. Penha FM, Maia M, Farah ME, et al. Effects of subretinal injections of indocyanine green, trypan blue, and glucose in rabbit eyes. Ophthalmology. 2007. https://doi.org/10.1016/j.ophtha.2006.09.028.
38. Azuma K, Noda Y, Hirasawa K, Ueta T. Brilliant blue G-assisted internal limiting membrane peeling for macular hole: a systematic review of literature and meta-analysis. Retina. 2016. https://doi.org/10.1097/IAE.0000000000000968.
39. Spiteri Cornish K, Lois N, Scott N, et al. Vitrectomy with internal limiting membrane (ILM) peeling versus vitrectomy with no peeling for idiopathic full-thickness macular hole (FTMH). Cochrane Database Syst Rev. 2013. https://doi.org/10.1002/14651858.CD009306.pub2.
40. Steel DHW, Dinah C, Habib M, White K. ILM peeling technique influences the degree of a dissociated optic nerve fibre layer appearance after macular hole surgery. Graefe's Arch Clin Exp Ophthalmol. 2015. https://doi.org/10.1007/s00417-014-2734-z.

41. A S, G G, E A, et al. Arcuate nerve fiber layer changes after internal limiting membrane peeling in idiopathic epiretinal membrane. Retina. 2018;38(9):1777–85.
42. Meng B, Zhao L, Yin Y, et al. Internal limiting membrane peeling and gas tamponade for myopic foveoschisis: a systematic review and meta-analysis. BMC Ophthalmol. 2017. https://doi.org/10.1186/s12886-017-0562-8.
43. Lee C, Wu W, Chen K, Chiu L, Wu K, Chang Y. Modified internal limiting membrane peeling technique (maculorrhexis) for myopic foveoschisis surgery. Acta Ophthalmol. 2017;95(2):e128–31.
44. Shimada N, Sugamoto Y, Ogawa M, Takase H, Ohno-Matsui K. Fovea-sparing internal limiting membrane peeling for myopic traction maculopathy. Am J Ophthalmol. 2012. https://doi.org/10.1016/j.ajo.2012.04.013.
45. Ho TC, Chen MS, Huang JS, Shih YF, Ho H, Huang YH. Foveola nonpeeling technique in internal limiting membrane peeling of myopic foveoschisis surgery. Retina. 2012. https://doi.org/10.1097/IAE.0B013E31824D0A4B.
46. Ho TC, Yang CM, Huang JS, et al. Long-term outcome of foveolar internal limiting membrane nonpeeling for myopic traction maculopathy. Retina. 2014. https://doi.org/10.1097/IAE.0000000000000149.
47. Rizzo S, Giansanti F, Finocchio L, et al. Vitrectomy with internal limiting membrane peeling and air tamponade for myopic foveoschisis. Retina. 2018. https://doi.org/10.1097/IAE.0000000000002265.
48. Wu TY, Yang CH, Yang CM. Gas tamponade for myopic foveoschisis with foveal detachment. Graefe's Arch Clin Exp Ophthalmol. 2013. https://doi.org/10.1007/s00417-012-2192-4.
49. Li X, Wang W, Tang S, Zhao J. Gas injection versus vitrectomy with gas for treating retinal detachment owing to macular hole in high myopes. Ophthalmology. 2009. https://doi.org/10.1016/j.ophtha.2009.01.003.
50. Chen FT, Yeh PT, Lin CP, Chen MS, Yang CH, Yang CM. Intravitreal gas injection for macular hole with localized retinal detachment in highly myopic patients. Acta Ophthalmol. 2011. https://doi.org/10.1111/j.1755-3768.2009.01649.x.
51. Kim K, Lee S, Lee W. Vitrectomy and internal limiting membrane peeling with and without gas tamponade for myopic foveoschisis. Am J Ophthalmol. 2012;153(2):320–6.
52. Hirakata A, Hida T. Vitrectomy for myopic posterior retinoschisis or foveal detachment. Jpn J Ophthalmol. 2006. https://doi.org/10.1007/s10384-005-0270-4.
53. Zheng B, Chen Y, Zhao Z, et al. Vitrectomy and internal limiting membrane peeling with perfluoropropane tamponade or balanced saline solution for myopic foveoschisis. Retina. 2011. https://doi.org/10.1097/IAE.0b013e3181f84fc1.
54. Lim SJ, Kwon YH, Kim SH, You YS, Kwon OW. Vitrectomy and internal limiting membrane peeling without gas tamponade for myopic foveoschisis. Graefe's Arch Clin Exp Ophthalmol. 2012. https://doi.org/10.1007/s00417-012-1983-y.
55. Mancino R, Ciuffoletti E, Martucci A, et al. Anatomical and functional results of macular hole retinal detachment surgery in patients with high myopia and posterior staphyloma treated with perfluoropropane gas or silicone oil. Retina. 2013. https://doi.org/10.1097/IAE.0b013e3182670fd7.
56. Michalewska Z, Michalewski J, Adelman RA, Nawrocki J. Inverted internal limiting membrane flap technique for large macular holes. Ophthalmology. 2010. https://doi.org/10.1016/j.ophtha.2010.02.011.
57. Iwasaki M, Kinoshita T, Miyamoto H, Imaizumi H. Influence of inverted internal limiting membrane flap technique on the outer retinal layer structures after a large macular hole surgery. Retina. 2018. https://doi.org/10.1097/IAE.0000000000002209.
58. Morizane Y, Shiraga F, Kimura S, et al. Autologous transplantation of the internal limiting membrane for refractory macular holes. Am J Ophthalmol. 2014. https://doi.org/10.1016/j.ajo.2013.12.028.

59. Leisser C, Hirnschall N, Döller B, et al. Internal limiting membrane flap transposition for surgical repair of macular holes in primary surgery and in persistent macular holes. Eur J Ophthalmol. 2018. https://doi.org/10.5301/ejo.5001037.
60. Ghosh B, Arora S, Goel N, et al. Comparative evaluation of sequential intraoperative use of whole blood followed by brilliant blue versus conventional brilliant blue staining of internal limiting membrane in macular hole surgery. Retina. 2016. https://doi.org/10.1097/IAE.0000000000000948.
61. Lyu W-J, Ji L-B, Xiao Y, Fan Y-B, Cai X-H. Treatment of refractory giant macular hole by vitrectomy with internal limiting membrane transplantation and autologous blood. Int J Ophthalmol. 2018;11(5):818–22.
62. Dimopoulos S, William A, Voykov B, Ziemssen F, Bartz-Schmidt KU, Spitzer MS. Anatomical and visual outcomes of autologous thrombocyte serum concentrate in the treatment of persistent full-thickness idiopathic macular hole after ILM peeling with brilliant blue G and membrane blue dual. Acta Ophthalmol. 2017. https://doi.org/10.1111/aos.12971.
63. Figueroa MS, Govetto A, De Arriba-Palomero P. Short-term results of platelet-rich plasma as adjuvant to 23-G vitrectomy in the treatment of high myopic macular holes. Eur J Ophthalmol. 2015. https://doi.org/10.5301/ejo.5000729.
64. Purtskhvanidze K, Frühsorger B, Bartsch S, Hedderich J, Roider J, Treumer F. Persistent full-thickness idiopathic macular hole: anatomical and functional outcome of revitrectomy with autologous platelet concentrate or autologous whole blood. Ophthalmologica. 2017. https://doi.org/10.1159/000481268.
65. Chen SN, Yang CM. Lens capsular flap transplantation in the management of refractory macular hole from multiple etiologies. Retina. 2016. https://doi.org/10.1097/IAE.0000000000000674.
66. Peng J, Chen C, Jin H, Zhang H, Zhao P. Autologous lens capsular flap transplantation combined with autologous blood application in the management of refractory macular hole. Retina. 2017;38(11):2177–83. https://doi.org/10.1097/IAE.0000000000001830.
67. Alkabes M, Mateo C. Macular buckle technique in myopic traction maculopathy: a 16-year review of the literature and a comparison with vitreous surgery. Graefes Arch Clin Exp Ophthalmol. 2018;256(5):863–77. https://doi.org/10.1007/s00417-018-3947-3.
68. Ripandelli G, Coppe AM. Evaluation of Primary Surgical Procedures for Retinal Detachment with Macular Hole in highly myopic eyes. Ophthalmology. 2001;108(12):2258–64.
69. Ando F, Ohba N, Touura K, Hirose H. Anatomical and visual outcomes after episcleral macular buckling compared with those after pars plana vitrectomy for retinal detachment caused by macular hole in highly myopic eyes. Retina. 2007;27(1):37–44. https://doi.org/10.1097/01.iae.0000256660.48993.9e.
70. Qi Y, Duan AL, You QS, Jonas JB, Wang N. Posterior scleral reinforcement and vitrectomy for myopic foveoschisis in extreme myopia. Retina. 2015;35(2):351–7. https://doi.org/10.1097/IAE.0000000000000313.
71. Grewal DS, Mahmoud TH. Autologous neurosensory retinal free flap for closure of refractory myopic macular holes. JAMA Ophthalmol. 2016;134(2):229–30. https://doi.org/10.1001/jamaophthalmol.2015.5237.
72. Wu A-L, Chuang L-H, Wang N-K, et al. Refractory macular hole repaired by autologous retinal graft and blood clot. BMC Ophthalmol. 2018;18:213.
73. Thomas AS, Mahmoud TH. Subretinal transplantation of an autologous retinal free flap for chronic retinal detachment with proliferative vitreoretinopathy with and without macular hole. Retina. 2017;38(Suppl 1):S121–4. https://doi.org/10.1097/IAE.0000000000002026.
74. Ding C, Li S, Zeng J. Autologous neurosensory retinal transplantation for unclosed and large macular holes. Ophthalmic Res. 2018;61(2):88–93.
75. de Giacinto C, D'Aloisio R, Cirigliano G, Pastore MR, Tognetto D. Autologous neurosensory retinal free patch transplantation for persistent full-thickness macular hole. Int Ophthalmol. 2018;39(5):1147–50.

Clinical Management of Myopia in Adults: Treatment of Myopic CNV

13

Shaun Sim, Chee Wai Wong, and Gemmy C. M. Cheung

Key Points

- The prevalence of myopic choroidal neovascularization (CNV) was between 5.2% and 11.3% in individuals with pathological myopia and was more common in females.
- Fundus fluorescein angiography (FFA) and optical coherence tomography are the imaging modalities of choice to diagnose myopic CNV and assess activity.
- Current evidence supports the use of intravitreal anti-vascular endothelial growth factor as the gold standard of treatment for myopic CNV, following a pro re nata (PRN) treatment regimen without a loading phase.
- Long-term visual outcomes remain less favorable, largely due to the development of chorioretinal atrophy around the regressed CNV.

13.1 Disease Overview

Myopic choroidal neovascularization (myopic CNV), a subtype of CNV associated with pathological myopia, is the second most common cause of CNV after age-related macular degeneration (AMD) [1, 2]. Compared to CNV secondary to AMD, key differences include occurrence in a younger age group, less prominent exudative and hemorrhagic changes, generally smaller choroidal

S. Sim · C. W. Wong · G. C. M. Cheung (✉)
Singapore National Eye Centre, Singapore, Singapore

Singapore Eye Research Institute, Singapore, Singapore
e-mail: gemmy.cheung.c.m@singhealth.com.sg

M. Ang, T. Y. Wong (eds.), *Updates on Myopia*,
https://doi.org/10.1007/978-981-13-8491-2_13

neovascular membranes, excellent response to anti-vascular endothelial growth factor treatment and better long-term visual prognosis [3–5]. It is one of the most sight-threatening complications of pathological myopia [6, 7], with individuals typically reporting acute loss of central vision. Estimated to develop in 5–10% of eyes with pathological myopia, myopic CNV is the most common cause of CNV in people aged 50 years or younger [1], with significant social and economic burden.

13.2 Incidence and Prevalence

Owing to a lack of uniform diagnostic criteria, the reported incidence and the prevalence of myopic CNV have varied widely and may be well underestimated. A recent systematic review reported that the prevalence of myopic CNV was between 5.2% and 11.3% in individuals with pathological myopia [8], with female preponderance seen in most studies [1, 2, 6, 9]. Myopic CNV was also bilateral in approximately 15% of individuals [1, 9]. Table 13.1 shows the prevalence as reported in population-based studies and in individuals with pathological myopia.

Table 13.1 Prevalence of myopic CNV

Reference	Definition of PM	Definition of CNV-type lesion	Age	Subjects (eyes)	Prevalence of CNV
Pathological myopia studies					
Curtin et al. (1970) [9]	AL >26.5 mm	Fuchs' spot	All ages	(538)	5.2%, bilateral in 16.7%
Grossniklaus et al. (1992) [10]	AL 25.5–26.5 mm, refractive error −5.0 to −7.5 D	Subretinal neovascularization, Fuchs' spot	All ages	202 (308)	5.2%—subretinal neovascularization 3.2%—Fuchs' spot
Hayashi et al. (2010) [11]	AL ≥26.5 mm or refractive error ≥−8 D	CNV	All ages	429 (806)	11.3%
General population studies					
The Blue Mountains Eye Study	"Myopic retinopathy"	CNV or Fuchs' spot	≥49 years	44 (67)	6.0%—CNV 1.5%—Fuchs' spot
The Beijing Eye Study	"Myopic retinopathy"	Fuchs' spot	≥40 years	132 (198)	1.5%

PM pathological myopia, *AL* axial length, *CNV* choroidal neovascularization

13.3 Natural History

The long-term outcome of CNV is poor if left untreated. In a 10-year follow-up study of 25 patients with myopic CNV, visual acuity deteriorated to 20/200 or worse in 89% and 96% of eyes in 5 and 10 years respectively [2]. Approximately 35% of individuals with myopic CNV in one eye developed CNV in the fellow eye, with a mean period of 8 years between eyes [12].

In the late twentieth century, Tokoro et al. classified myopic CNV into three stages; active, scar, and atrophic stages [13]. Several other authors subsequently examined longitudinally the natural course of CNV and the three stages associated with visual loss [14, 15]. In the active phase, myopic CNV is characterized by hemorrhage with or without serous retinal detachment. In the scar phase, there is absorption of hemorrhage with development of fibrotic scars, some of which can become hyperpigmented, known classically as Fuchs' spots. Finally, in the atrophic phase, as the myopic CNV regresses, the development of macular chorioretinal atrophy ensues. Recent studies using swept source optical coherence tomography have revealed the presence of macular Bruch's membrane defect associated with myopic CNV. The expansion of these defects was found to be related to the enlargement of chorioretinal atrophy surrounding a regressed CNV [16]. In a small proportion of patients, poor visual outcome might be due to formation of myopic macular hole, particularly in eyes where chorioretinal atrophy is greater than one disc area [17].

13.4 Risk Factors

Compared to systemic risk factors, ocular risk factors have a much stronger influence on the development of myopic CNV. A prospective study found that eyes with myopic CNV had higher grade myopic maculopathy (with patchy retinal atrophy or worse) than eyes without myopic CNV. In the same series, eyes with higher grade myopic maculopathy were also 3.55 times more likely to develop myopic CNV than those with lower grade myopic maculopathy [18]. Higher grade lacquer cracks defined as crisscrossing lacquer cracks with or without linear cracks were also found in a significantly higher proportion of eyes with myopic CNV as compared to the fellow uninvolved eye [19, 20]. Choroidal thinning, in particular the subfoveal and inferior choroid, was found to be significantly thinner in eyes with myopic CNV than in the fellow uninvolved eyes [19, 21]. Furthermore, in patients with newly diagnosed myopic CNV, it was reported that the incidence of myopic CNV development in the fellow eye was 34.8% compared to 6.1% in those with no previous CNV [12]. Other studies have also established an association between highly myopic eyes with higher aqueous humor levels of the inflammatory cytokines interleukin 6 and 8 [22, 23]. Systemic risk factors implicated in the development of myopic CNV include higher levels of C-reactive protein and complement factors C3 and CH50 [24]. Older age (>40 years), subfoveal CNV location, larger baseline lesion size

(>400 μm), and lower best corrected visual acuity (BCVA) at baseline have been identified as factors leading to poorer visual outcomes [8, 25].

13.5 Pathogenesis

The pathogenesis of myopic CNV has not been clarified although several theories have been proposed. The mechanical theory postulates that progressive elongation of the anteroposterior axis leads to breaks in the retinal pigment epithelium (RPE)–Bruch's membrane–choriocapillaris complex with formation of lacquer cracks, which in turn facilitates neovascularization from choriocapillaris [26–28]. Lacquer cracks have been more frequently observed in fellow eyes of patients with unilateral myopic CNV, hence the suggestion that breaks in Bruch's membrane as the predisposing factor for development of CNV in pathological myopia [12]. It has also been reported that in vitro, progressive elongation of the posterior pole results in mechanical stress of the RPE cell layer, thus upregulating the expression and secretion of angiogenic factors [29]. The increased expression of vascular endothelial growth factor (VEGF) in aqueous humor of eyes with myopic CNV compared to cataract controls has also been reported in a comparative study [22]. Notably, VEGF levels in myopic CNV were lower than those in CNV secondary to AMD and can be explained by the smaller size of CNV membranes in myopic CNV. It is the imbalance between pro-angiogenic and anti-angiogenic factors that results in the development of myopic CNV.

The heredo-degenerative theory has been supported by genetic factors associated with myopic CNV based on twin and familial aggregation studies of pathologic myopia [30]. In a recent study that analyzed 15 genes associated with age-related macular degeneration, it was found that a single nucleotide polymorphism in the complement factor I (*CFI*) gene was significantly associated with myopic CNV [31]. Complement factor I is a regulatory protein involved in three complement pathways and is expressed by macrophages, lymphocytes, and fibroblasts, suggesting that inflammation via the complement pathway may be involved in the development of myopic CNV.

The hemodynamic theory suggests that alterations in choroidal perfusion of myopic eyes with choroidal filling delay may result in choroidal ischemia [32]. This leads to subsequent upregulation of angiogenic factors and the subsequent development of myopic CNV [7]. Doppler ultrasound imaging of the retrobulbar vessels revealed significantly higher vascular flow resistance in the posterior ciliary artery in eyes with myopic CNV as compared to the fellow eye, thus further implicating dysfunction of choroidal circulation in the development of myopic CNV [33].

13.6 Diagnosis and Monitoring

On slit-lamp biomicroscopy, myopic CNV manifests as a small, flat, grayish subretinal lesion adjacent to or beneath the fovea [2, 6, 34, 35]. There may be associated macular hemorrhage with or without exudation or subretinal fluid. Spectral

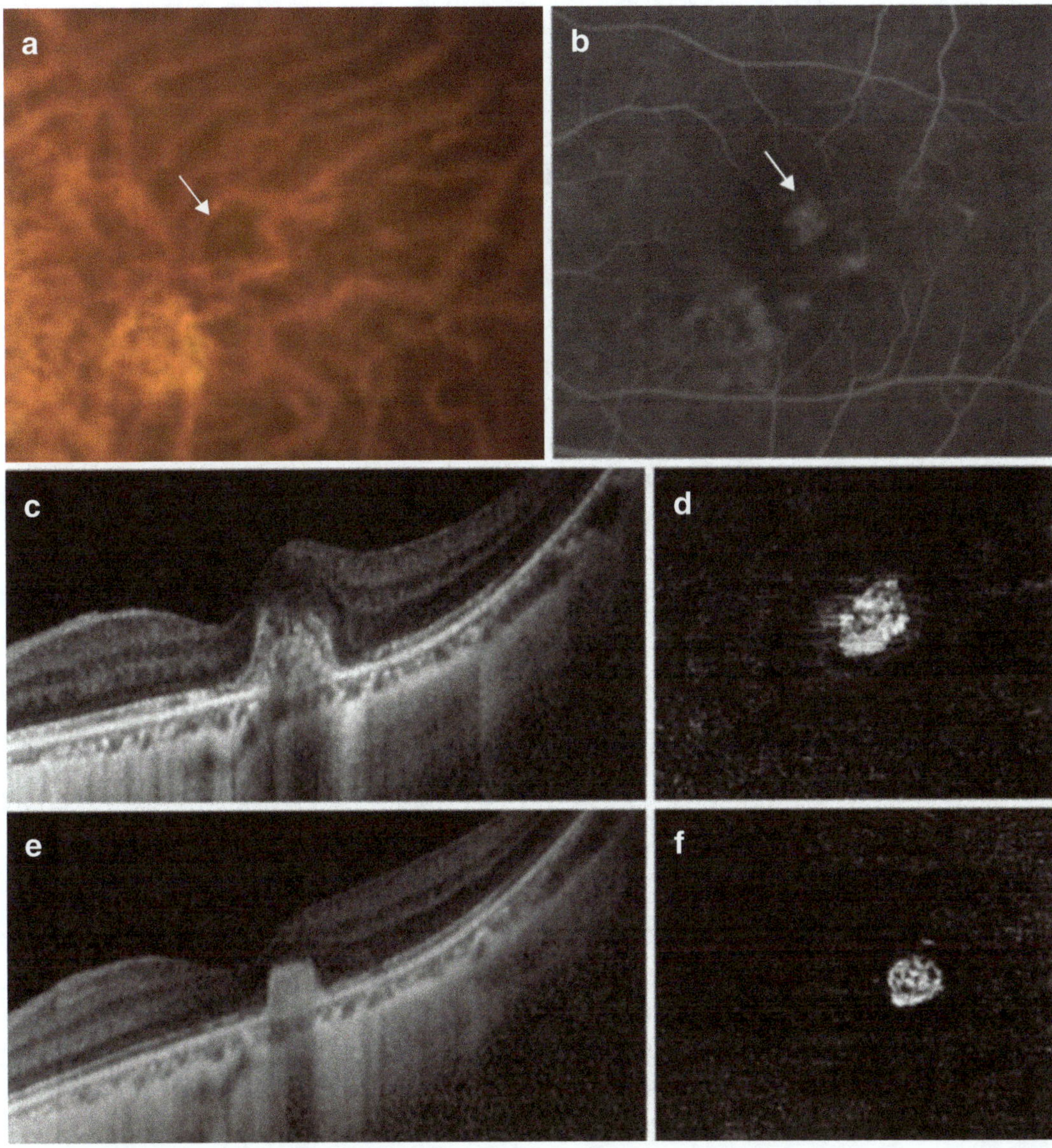

Fig. 13.1 Myopic CNV in a 57-year-old female. (**a**) Fundus photo shows a spot of subretinal hemorrhage (white arrow). (**b**) Fundus fluorescein angiogram shows early hyperfluorescence (white arrow) with a halo of hypofluoresence. (**c**) Optical coherence tomography (OCT) B scan shows a subretinal hyper-reflective lesion with indistinct margins, representing a type 2 CNV. (**d**) OCT angiography shows flow signals representing the choroidal neovascular membrane in the outer retina slab. (**e**) OCT B scan after treatment with a single intravitreal injection of anti-vascular endothelial growth factor. The subretinal hyper-reflective lesion is now inactive and has acquired well-demarcated margins. (**f**) OCT angiography shows persistence of flow signals despite inactivity

domain optical coherence tomography (SD-OCT) is a useful non-invasive screening tool that can be performed rapidly. On SD-OCT, myopic CNV presents as a hyper-reflective material above the RPE band (type 2 CNV), with a variable amount of subretinal fluid (Fig. 13.1). OCT appearance is helpful to assess the activity of mCNV: signs of activity include ill-defined margins and disruption of the external limiting membrane, with a variable amount of intraretinal or subretinal fluid. As the lesion becomes inactive, it consolidates and acquires a distinct border.

Clinical diagnosis is confirmed by fundus fluorescein angiography (FFA). Most myopic CNVs are type 2 neovascularization and present with a "classic" pattern on fluorescein angiography (FA). The amount of leakage may vary, depending on the level of the activity, the size of the lesion and the health of the RPE. FA has been shown to have higher sensitivity for detecting the activity than OCT. In some eyes, subtle late leakage on FA may be the only sign of myopic CNV activity [35]. Myopic CNV with dense macular hemorrhage may result in masking of both early hyperfluorescence and late leakage. Indocyanine green angiography (ICGA) is useful in these cases to detect CNV. In addition, imaging also provides important prognostic indications. The size and location of the lesion can be better evaluated on FFA, while lacquer cracks and chorio-retinal atrophy are best seen with ICGA [3]. ICGA also aids in exclusion of polypoidal choroidal vasculopathy (PCV) in those with macular hemorrhage, particularly important amongst Asian patients with the higher prevalence of PCV [36].

OCT angiography (OCTA) allows non-invasive imaging of the retinal and choroidal microvasculature. It is able to detect type 2 CNV with high sensitivity and specificity when compared against FFA and ICGA [37]. OCTA is able to detect flow within myopic CNV vascular complexes and hence delineates vascular networks in these myopic neovascular membranes that lie above the RPE where flow signals are spared from attenuation [38]. On OCTA, CNV shape could be described as circular or irregular, margins could be well defined or poorly defined and appearance could be interlacing or tangled/disorganized vascular loops. In eyes with active myopic CNV lesions, the OCTA appearance is primarily interlacing, while inactive CNV neovascular networks appear primarily tangled [39–41]. OCTA is also able to clearly visualize the choriocapillaris in myopic eyes, with varying loss of choriocapillaris depending on the extent of myopic maculopathy and the presence of lacquer cracks [42, 43]. Although sensitivity and specificity compared to FFA as gold standard have not been fully evaluated for the diagnosis of myopic CNV, it is felt that OCTA may reduce the need for FFA if CNV is clearly visualized on OCTA at the commencement of anti-VEGF therapy. However, there remain limitations concerning OCTA: It is currently still unable to provide information on the disease activity as flow signals can persist in an inactive myopic CNV [39–41]. Therefore, activity assessment should be evaluated with clinical examination and multi-modal imaging, including structural OCT with or without FA. Motion or image artifacts and segmentation errors may further complicate its interpretation. Therefore, it is still recommended to complement SD-OCT and FFA to increase diagnostic accuracy and monitoring of the disease activity.

The imaging features of various stages of myopic CNV are summarized in Table 13.2.

Table 13.2 Imaging characteristics of the different phases of myopic choroidal neovascularization

Phase	Fundus appearance	Fluorescein angiography	Indocyanine green angiography	Optical coherence tomography
Active	Small grayish subretinal lesion at or near the fovea, with or without hemorrhage	Early hyperfluorescence increasing in size and intensity with time	Late hyperfluorescence	Ill-defined subretinal hyper-reflective lesion with or without subretinal fluid
Scar	Grayish white, sometimes pigmented spot. Absence of hemorrhage	Early hyperfluorescence decreasing in intensity with time, indicating fluorescein staining of subretinal scar	Hypofluorescence	Subretinal hyper-reflective lesion with well-demarcated margins
Atrophic	Well-demarcated whitish lesion centered on fovea. Absence of hemorrhage	Hypofluorescence	Hypofluorescence	Absence of RPE–Bruch's membrane–choriocapillaris complex with hypertransmission of signal into the underlying sclera and retro-orbital fat

13.7 Differential Diagnosis

There are several differential diagnoses that must be excluded from myopic CNV.

13.7.1 Macular Hemorrhage Secondary to Lacquer Cracks (Fig. 13.2)

In individuals with macular hemorrhage, it is critical to differentiate eyes with myopic CNV from those with simple hemorrhage associated with lacquer cracks (Fuch's hemorrhage). Eyes with Fuch's hemorrhage secondary to lacquer cracks tend to have better prognosis than myopic CNV and do not require anti-VEGF therapy [44]. In cases with thick blood, the myopic CNV may not be visible even in FA or OCTA due to masking. In these cases, late phases of ICGA will be able to visualize the myopic CNV if it is present [20].

13.7.2 Inflammatory CNV

Punctate inner choroidopathy (PIC) with or without secondary CNV may present with OCT appearance similar to that of myopic CNV. The clinical manifestation

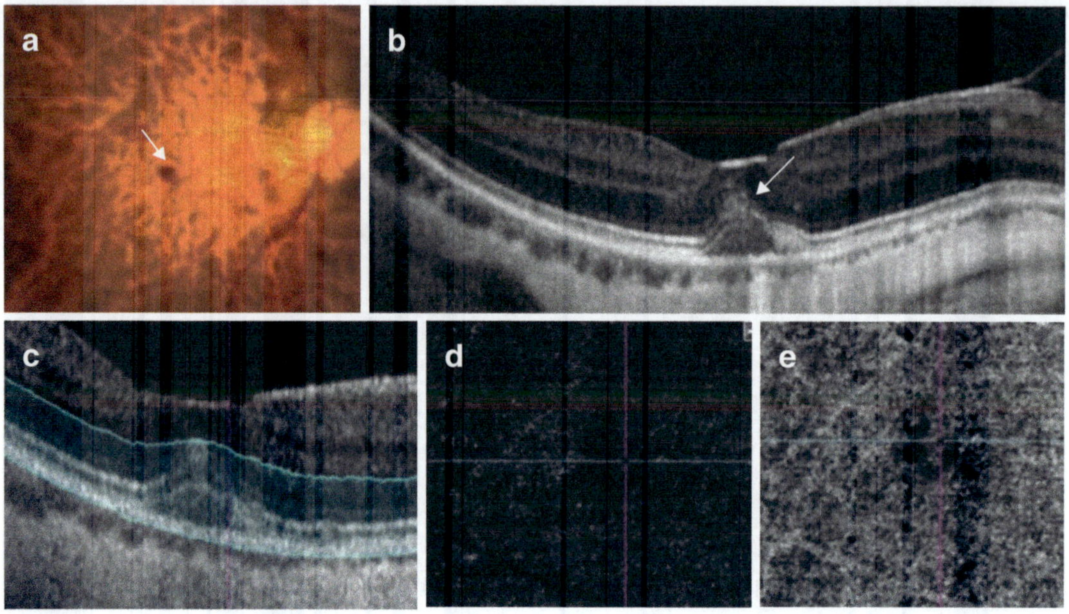

Fig. 13.2 A 51-year-old highly myopic male with lacquer crack hemorrhage. (**a**) Fundus photo shows a red spot suggestive of subretinal hemorrhage (white arrow). (**b**) Optical coherence tomographic scan shows a separation between the RPE and the underlying Bruch's membrane in the subfoveal position (white arrow head), with hyper-reflectivity in the subretinal space (white arrow) corresponding to the area of subretinal hemorrhage. Optical coherence tomographic angiography of the region of interest (**c**) shows no flow signals suggestive of choroidal neovascularization in the outer retinal slab (**d**) or the choriocapillaris slab (**e**)

of punctate inner choroidopathy differs from myopic CNV, with characteristic creamy yellow-white lesions located at the RPE and inner choroid. A prospective series revealed that PIC lesions go through a five-stage evolution process with differing SD-OCT findings at each stage: choroidal infiltration (stage I: mostly normal but can present with hyper-reflective fine spots within the outer nuclear layer), formation of sub-RPE nodules (stage II: focal elevation of RPE with corresponding ellipsoid zone disruption), chorioretinal nodules (stage III: nodule that breaks through the RPE and progresses towards and replaces the photoreceptor layer that eventually domes the outer plexiform layer (OPL)), regression (stage IV: noted to begin from the apex towards the choroid and with herniation of the OPL and inner retina through the RPE break) and retinal herniation (stage V: sagging of the OPL and inner retina with loss of photoreceptor layer and RPE proliferation that relieves the retinal hernia) [45]. Of these various stages, only stage III may ostensibly be misdiagnosed as myopic CNV. The use of OCTA and its ability to identify vascular network can be particularly useful in this instance to distinguish myopic CNV from PIC as inflammatory lesions do not manifest vascular flow signals [46]. Unlike myopic CNV, the late phases of ICGA would reveal multiple areas of hypercyanescence in punctate inner choroidopathy [47].

13.7.3 Dome-Shaped Maculopathy with Serous Detachment

Dome-shaped maculopathy (DSM) is characterized by an inward bulge within the chorioretinal posterior concavity of the eye in the macular area [48, 49]. Serous foveal detachment is a complication of DSM that has been postulated to be related to the abnormal curvature of the macula [50]. On FFA, DSM with serous retinal detachment can be distinguished from myopic CNV where it may be associated with pinpoint leakage. On ICGA, it presents as punctate hypercyanescent spots [51]. The absence of macular hemorrhage, with the characteristic dome-shaped profile of the macula visualized on OCT, and the leakage of dye in later frames help differentiate this entity from myopic CNV.

13.8 Management

13.8.1 Anti-Vascular Endothelial Growth Factor Drugs

Prior to the advent of anti-VEGF therapy, the main treatment options for myopic CNV were limited to thermal laser photocoagulation [52] and photodynamic therapy with verteporfin (vPDT) [53, 54]. These treatments had limited efficacy in improving vision significantly and have now largely been relegated to the annals of history by the anti-vascular endothelial growth factor (anti-VEGF) therapy [55].

13.9 Ranibizumab

Ranibizumab is a Fab fragment of humanized monoclonal antibody against all isoforms of VEGF-A, and it was the first anti-VEGF agent to be FDA approved for the treatment of myopic CNV. The strongest evidence of anti-VEGF use for myopic CNV comes from two large multi-centered, double-masked, randomized, controlled clinical trials [56, 57]. The RADIANCE study ($n = 277$) was a 12-month, phase III, randomized, double-masked, multicenter study comparing the efficacy and safety of intravitreal ranibizumab 0.5 mg versus vPDT in patients with myopic CNV [56]. This trial demonstrated the superiority of ranibizumab 0.5 mg, with a mean visual acuity gain of 10.5–10.6 letters compared to 2.2 letters with vPDT at 3 months and maintained through 12 months. The study further compared two retreatment protocols and showed that the disease activity guided retreatment based on OCT could achieve similar visual outcomes with a lower median number of injections (2.0) compared to retreatment according to visual acuity stabilization (4.0 injections). The RADIANCE study confirmed the results of the REPAIR trial, a phase II prospective, open-label, multicenter study of intravitreal ranibizumab 0.5 mg in myopic CNV in 65 eyes. In this study, a mean visual gain of 13.8 letters was achieved with a mean of 3.6 ranibizumab injections over 12 months in a cohort of treatment-naïve patients with myopic CNV [58]. These trials were performed in predominantly Caucasian populations. To support the use of ranibizumab for Asian patients with myopic CNV, the BRILLIANCE study was conducted with a design similar to the RADIANCE study. This was a 12-month, double-masked trial in which study participants with myopic CNV were randomized into one of three treatment groups: ranibizumab guided by visual acuity stabilization criteria (group 1, $n = 182$), ranibizumab guided by disease activity (group 2, $n = 184$) and vPDT followed by ranibizumab/vPDT/both treatments at month 3, guided by the disease activity (group 3, $n = 91$) [55]. Findings from the BRILLIANCE study corroborated with those from the RADIANCE study. Both ranibizumab arms experienced significantly better visual acuity gains at 3 months compared to the vPDT arm (Group I/II: +9.5/+9.8 letters vs. Group III: +4.5 letters; both $P < 0.001$), and ranibizumab treatment guided by disease activity was noninferior to treatment guided by visual acuity stabilization, achieving similar visual acuity outcomes with a median of three and four injections over 12 months, respectively. These results confirmed the efficacy of ranibizumab for the treatment of myopic CNV in Asian patients.

In a large post-marketing surveillance study of ranibizumab for the treatment of Japanese patients with myopic CNV ($n = 318$) over a 12-month observation period, ranibizumab was found to be safe (incidence of 0.6% and 0.3% of adverse drug reactions and serious adverse events, respectively) and effective with a low number of injections needed for the therapeutic effect (median injection number of 1 and 52.2% requiring only 1 injection) [59].

13.10 Aflibercept

Aflibercept is a recombinant human fusion protein that acts as a soluble decoy receptor for VEGF family members VEGF-A, VEGF-B and placental growth factor, preventing these ligands from binding to, and activating, their receptors. The MYRROR trial was a 48-week, phase III, multicenter, randomized, double-masked, sham-controlled study investigating the efficacy and safety of intravitreal aflibercept 2 mg for the treatment of myopic CNV [57]. Patients treated with intravitreal aflibercept ($n = 91$) achieved a mean visual gain of 12 letters compared to a 2-letter loss in the sham group ($n = 31$). The mean number of injections was low in this study (4.2 injections over 48 weeks). Significant improvement in the quality of life (National Eye Institute Visual Function Questionnaire 25 and EuroQol-5 Dimension score) was also demonstrated in patients treated with aflibercept.

13.11 Bevacizumab

Bevacizumab was the first angiogenesis inhibitor to be approved for clinical use, initially for the treatment of metastatic colorectal cancer. Since then, it has been used as an open-label drug and a lower cost option for the treatment of choroidal neovascularization, including myopic CNV. There is a lack of randomized controlled trials assessing the efficacy of bevacizumab in the treatment of myopic CNV, but many clinical case series have reported significant visual gains ranging from 5 to 20 letters with the open-label use of bevacizumab [60–64]. Long-term studies have also demonstrated maintenance of visual gains for up to 4 years after the initial treatment [52, 65].

13.12 Conbercept

Conbercept is a recombinant fusion protein containing the second Ig-like domain of VEGFR-1, the third and fourth Ig-like domains of VEGFR-2 and a human IgG Fc fragment, with binding affinity to VEGF and placental growth factor (PIGF) [66]. There are no prospective interventional trials on the use of conbercept for myopic CNV. Yan et al. performed a retrospective analysis of 42 consecutive eyes with myopic CNV treated with three loading doses of conbercept at monthly intervals, followed by as-needed injections based on monthly follow-up visits till month 12. BCVA improved from 0.67 logMAR at baseline to 0.32 at 12 months, with 71.4% achieving three lines or more improvement at final follow-up with a mean of 3.76 injections [67].

13.13 Factors Related to Treatment Outcomes

As previously mentioned, older age, subfoveal location of CNV, larger lesion size and poorer presenting visual acuity are poor prognostic factors for myopic CNV [8, 25, 68]. In addition, subretinal hemorrhage, duration of CNV and previous photodynamic therapy were found to confer a poorer prognosis after treatment [68]. Similarly, older age, larger CNV size and greater central macular thickness were factors associated with the need for retreatment [69–71]. Thinner choroid and lacquer cracks were also found to be associated with the need for a higher number of intravitreal injections [71].

The presence of vitreomacular abnormalities, in particular epiretinal membrane (ERM), is common in high myopes. ERM often coexists with myopic CNV. The presence of ERM has been shown to hamper visual gains after treatment of myopic CNV with ranibizumab compared to eyes without ERM (visual stabilization from a baseline of 0.3–0.4 compared to improvement from 0.3 to 0.1, $p = 0.008$). The coexistence of ERM with myopic CNV neither influenced the median number of injections (3) nor the reduction in central foveal thickness [72]. As regards the myopic macular retinoschisis (MRS), a post hoc analysis of the RADIANCE trial showed that eyes with MRS received more injections (5.8 ± 2.1 vs 4.0 ± 2.9; $P = 0.0001$), had slower visual gain at 3 months (+2.8 letters vs +12.3 letters) and poorer visual outcomes at 12 months (+7.1 letters vs +14.4 letters) than eyes without MRS [73]. Post hoc analysis further evaluated whether baseline myopic macular degeneration (MMD) influenced the treatment outcomes in 115 eyes. Change in BCVA from baseline to week 48 was not significantly different between eyes with mild MMD

(META-PM category 1–2) and eyes with severe MMD (META-PM category 1–2) (+13.5 letters vs +12.4 letters, $p = 0.83$), and were achieved with a similar number of injections (3.9 vs 5.4, $p = 0.23$) [74].

13.14 Recurrence

The recurrence rate of myopic CNV is generally low, with most recurrences occurring during the first year. Yang et al. reported a recurrence rate of 23.3% in a retrospective series of 103 eyes of 89 consecutive patients with subfoveal myopic CNV, followed over 2 years. 72.7% of recurrences occurred in the first year of treatment. Baseline CNV size was found to be a significant prognostic factor for recurrence on multivariate analysis [71]. In the post-RADIANCE observation study (12–48 months), only 10% of eyes experienced a recurrence [75]. These findings reinforce the importance of monitoring for recurrences in the first year of treatment.

13.15 Treatment Regimen and Follow-Up

Once active myopic CNV is diagnosed, prompt treatment with intravitreal anti-VEGF therapy should be administered as soon as possible [56, 58]. Current evidence suggests that a pro re nata (PRN) regimen without a loading phase can be considered in most patients. Patients should be monitored monthly with OCT and treatment administered until cessation of the disease activity on OCT or visual stabilization. FA may be performed to confirm inactive disease before stopping treatment, especially if there are uncertainties regarding activity based on OCT. Thereafter, review can be progressively lengthened on an individualized basis if no further activity is observed in the first year to monitor for recurrence or development of myopic CNV in the fellow eye. After the first year of treatment, patients without recurrence can have their visit interval prolonged to 6 months. Patients should be advised to return if vision drops or metamorphopsia recurs [3].

13.16 Long-Term Outcomes

Although anti-VEGF therapy for myopic CNV has demonstrated remarkable short- and mid-term efficacy, longer term visual outcomes are generally less favorable, with most studies reporting a gradual decline back to baseline visual acuity [60, 61, 75–79]. Onishi et al. reported the 5-year outcomes of 51 patients who received treatment with ranibizumab for myopic CNV. Mean baseline BCVA (0.38 logMAR) was significantly improved at 1 year (0.27 logMAR) but not in the subsequent years (0.31, 0.35 and 0.32 logMAR at 2, 4 and 5 years, respectively). Sarao et al. reported similar findings in a prospective interventional study with mean BCVA improvement of −0.13 at 24 months in 101 eyes with myopic CNV treated with bevacizumab and an increase in the area of chorioretinal atrophy in the same period [61]. In contrast, the long-term visual outcomes of 41 patients who had completed the RADIANCE trial were shown to be sustained up to 48 months post initiation of treatment. Mean visual gain from baseline (56.5 ± 12.1 letters) was significant up to 48 months (+16.3 ± 18.7, $n = 16$, $p = 0.0034$). Of the 16 patients who completed 48 months of follow-up, 63% gained ≥10 letters and 13% lost ≥10 letters. Over the post-RADIANCE observation period (months 12–48), 83% of patients required no further treatment and 10% experienced recurrences [75].

Similar results were reported in Caucasian patients with myopic CNV ($n = 40$) treated with intravitreal ranibizumab: baseline visual acuity improved from 55.4 letters to 63.4 letters at 3 years ($p = 0.039$) and 35% gained 15 letters or more at the final follow-up, achieved with a mean of 4.1 injections in the first year, 2.4 in the second year and 1.1 in the third year [76]. A longer term follow-up study in Caucasian eyes treated with bevacizumab or ranibizumab found that visual gains could be maintained at 3 (+9.0 letters, $n = 52$), 4 (+9.0 letters, $n = 28$) and 5 years (+9.8 letters, $n = 13$) [77]. A 5-year outcome study by the PAN-American Collaborative Retina Study Group with intravitreal bevacizumab ($n = 33$) reported a significant decline in visual acuity from 0.65 ± 0.33 logMAR at baseline to 0.73 ± 0.50 logMAR units at final follow-up ($p = 0.003$) [80].

In the longest follow-up study to date, Pastore et al. reported on the visual outcomes of 17 eyes with myopic CNV, treated with ranibizumab according to a strict pro re nata regimen over 9 years. Mean visual acuity was significantly improved from baseline (56.2 ± 13.5 letters) at 1 (69.7 ± 12.2 letters) and 2 years (69.9 ± 12.8 letters) post treatment initiation, but gradually receded towards baseline at 9 years (57.4 ± 17.7 letters). Only 11.8% of eyes lost 3 lines or more, while 17.7% maintained 3 lines or more gain in vision at 9 years, achieved with a mean of 1.24 ± 1.70 injections per year (range 2–25) [78]. Despite a loss of visual gains, these results demonstrate a considerably superior visual prognosis for patients with myopic CNV than patients with CNV secondary to age-related macular degeneration over the long term [81, 82].

Myopic CNV-related chorioretinal atrophy (CRA) is the major culprit for the loss of visual gain over the long term. Ohno Matsui et al. found that the macular atrophy developing after myopic CNV may be related to rupture of Bruch's membrane. This defect in Bruch's membrane may continue to expand in spite of adequate treatment of myopic CNV, leading to macular atrophy and loss of vision [16]. This point was demonstrated in a 5-year outcome study of eyes with myopic CNV treated with intravitreal ranibizumab ($n = 51$), in which visual stability was achieved (baseline best corrected visual acuity 20/49 compared to 20/42) at 5 years, where good visual outcome was shown to be significantly associated with a lack of enlargement of CNV-related macular atrophy, in addition to better baseline visual acuity and a lower number of injections [79]. These outcomes were achieved with a mean of 1.6 injections over 5 years, and two-thirds received only 1 injection. Another study by Ohno Matsui's group observed similar findings in patients treated with bevacizumab ($n = 36$). Visual acuity improved significantly from a baseline of 0.5 logMAR to 0.31 and 0.39 at years 2 and 4, respectively, but not at 6 years (0.45), achieved with a mean of 1.78 injections. Again, visual outcomes at 6 years were correlated with the size of CNV-related macular atrophy, as well as baseline visual acuity and CNV size. Further, in a long-term (mean follow-up 80.6 ± 28.0 months) retrospective review of 54 eyes with myopic CNV treated with photodynamic therapy and/or intravitreal ranibizumab and eyes with myopic maculopathy alone, the progression of macular atrophy was significantly greater in myopic CNV eyes compared to the eyes with only myopic maculopathy. The risk of progression was related to age, degree of myopia and presence of staphyloma, but not the type of treatment [83].

13.17 Conclusions

Myopic CNV is a sight-threatening complication of pathologic myopia that, fortunately, has an effective treatment in the form of anti-VEGF injections. Early detection, accurate diagnosis with multimodal imaging, early initiation of treatment, and careful post-treatment monitoring are key to achieving good treatment outcomes. Although FFA and OCT remain the gold standard for diagnosis, OCTA is emerging as a good adjunct imaging modality to screen for the presence of neovascular networks in patients with suspected myopic CNV. Anti-VEGF therapy has been shown to be efficacious and safe with a low treatment burden. Finally, long-term visual outcomes remain less favorable, largely due to the development of chorioretinal atrophy around the regressed CNV. Therapeutic strategies to prevent the enlargement of CNV-related atrophy should form the focus of future research for the treatment of myopic CNV.

References

1. Cohen SY, Laroche A, Leguen Y, Soubrane G, Coscas GJ. Etiology of choroidal neovascularization in young patients. Ophthalmology. 1996;103(8):1241–4.
2. Yoshida T, Ohno-Matsui K, Yasuzumi K, et al. Myopic choroidal neovascularization: a 10-year follow-up. Ophthalmology. 2003;110(7):1297–305.
3. Ohno-Matsui K, Ikuno Y, Lai TYY, Gemmy Cheung CM. Diagnosis and treatment guideline for myopic choroidal neovascularization due to pathologic myopia. Prog Retin Eye Res. 2018;63:92–106.
4. Cheung CMG, Arnold JJ, Holz FG, et al. Myopic choroidal neovascularization: review, guidance, and consensus statement on management. Ophthalmology. 2017;124(11):1690–711.
5. Ohno-Matsui K, Lai TY, Lai CC, Cheung CM. Updates of pathologic myopia. Prog Retin Eye Res. 2016;52:156–87.
6. Avila MP, Weiter JJ, Jalkh AE, Trempe CL, Pruett RC, Schepens CL. Natural history of choroidal neovascularization in degenerative myopia. Ophthalmology. 1984;91(12):1573–81.
7. Neelam K, Cheung CM, Ohno-Matsui K, Lai TY, Wong TY. Choroidal neovascularization in pathological myopia. Prog Retin Eye Res. 2012;31(5):495–525.
8. Wong TY, Ferreira A, Hughes R, Carter G, Mitchell P. Epidemiology and disease burden of pathologic myopia and myopic choroidal neovascularization: an evidence-based systematic review. Am J Ophthalmol. 2014;157(1):9–25.e12.
9. Curtin BJ, Karlin DB. Axial length measurements and fundus changes of the myopic eye. I. The posterior fundus. Trans Am Ophthalmol Soc. 1970;68:312–34.

10. Grossniklaus HE, Green WR. Pathologic findings in pathologic myopia. Retina. 1992;12(2):127–33.
11. Hayashi K, Ohno-Matsui K, Shimada N, Moriyama M, Kojima A, Hayashi W, Yasuzumi K, Nagaoka N, Saka N, Yoshida T, Tokoro T, Mochizuki M. Long-term pattern of progression of myopic maculopathy: a natural history study. Ophthalmology. 2010;117(8):1595–611. 1611.e1–4.
12. Ohno-Matsui K, Yoshida T, Futagami S, et al. Patchy atrophy and lacquer cracks predispose to the development of choroidal neovascularisation in pathological myopia. Br J Ophthalmol. 2003;87(5):570–3.
13. Tokoro T. Atlas of posterior fundus changes in pathologic myopia. Tokyo: Springer; 1998.
14. Ohno-Matsui K. What is the fundamental nature of pathologic myopia? Retina. 2017;37(6):1043–8.
15. Ohno-Matsui K, Yoshida T. Myopic choroidal neovascularization: natural course and treatment. Curr Opin Ophthalmol. 2004;15(3):197–202.
16. Ohno-Matsui K, Jonas JB, Spaide RF. Macular Bruch membrane holes in choroidal neovascularization-related myopic macular atrophy by swept-source optical coherence tomography. Am J Ophthalmol. 2016;162:133–139.e131.
17. Shimada N, Ohno-Matsui K, Yoshida T, Futagami S, Tokoro T, Mochizuki M. Development of macular hole and macular retinoschisis in eyes with myopic choroidal neovascularization. Am J Ophthalmol. 2008;145(1):155–61.
18. Cheung CM, Loh BK, Li X, et al. Choroidal thickness and risk characteristics of eyes with myopic choroidal neovascularization. Acta Ophthalmol. 2013;91(7):e580–1.
19. Ikuno Y, Jo Y, Hamasaki T, Tano Y. Ocular risk factors for choroidal neovascularization in pathologic myopia. Invest Ophthalmol Vis Sci. 2010;51(7):3721–5.
20. Kim YM, Yoon JU, Koh HJ. The analysis of lacquer crack in the assessment of myopic choroidal neovascularization. Eye. 2011;25(7):937–46.
21. Ng WY, Ting DS, Agrawal R, et al. Choroidal structural changes in myopic choroidal neovascularization after treatment with antivascular endothelial growth factor over 1 year. Invest Ophthalmol Vis Sci. 2016;57(11):4933–9.
22. Tong JP, Chan WM, Liu DT, et al. Aqueous humor levels of vascular endothelial growth factor and pigment epithelium-derived factor in polypoidal choroidal vasculopathy and choroidal neovascularization. Am J Ophthalmol. 2006;141(3):456–62.
23. Yamamoto Y, Miyazaki D, Sasaki S, et al. Associations of inflammatory cytokines with choroidal neovascularization in highly myopic eyes. Retina. 2015;35(2):344–50.
24. Long Q, Ye J, Li Y, Wang S, Jiang Y. C-reactive protein and complement components in patients with pathological myopia. Optom Vis Sci. 2013;90(5):501–6.
25. Wong TY, Ohno-Matsui K, Leveziel N, et al. Myopic choroidal neovascularisation: current concepts and update on clinical management. Br J Ophthalmol. 2015;99(3):289–96.
26. Curtin BJ, Karlin DB. Axial length measurements and fundus changes of the myopic eye. Am J Ophthalmol. 1971;71(1 Pt 1):42–53.
27. Noble KG, Carr RE. Pathologic myopia. Ophthalmology. 1982;89(9):1099–100.
28. Lloyd RI. Clinical studies of the myopic macula. Trans Am Ophthalmol Soc. 1953;51:273–84.
29. Seko Y, Fujikura H, Pang J, Tokoro T, Shimokawa H. Induction of vascular endothelial growth factor after application of mechanical stress to retinal pigment epithelium of the rat in vitro. Invest Ophthalmol Vis Sci. 1999;40(13):3287–91.
30. Young TL. Dissecting the genetics of human high myopia: a molecular biologic approach. Trans Am Ophthalmol Soc. 2004;102:423–45.
31. Leveziel N, Yu Y, Reynolds R, et al. Genetic factors for choroidal neovascularization associated with high myopia. Invest Ophthalmol Vis Sci. 2012;53(8):5004–9.
32. Wakabayashi T, Ikuno Y. Choroidal filling delay in choroidal neovascularisation due to pathological myopia. Br J Ophthalmol. 2010;94(5):611–5.
33. Dimitrova G, Tamaki Y, Kato S, Nagahara M. Retrobulbar circulation in myopic patients with or without myopic choroidal neovascularisation. Br J Ophthalmol. 2002;86(7):771–3.
34. Ohno-Matsui K, Kawasaki R, Jonas JB, et al. International photographic classification and grading system for myopic maculopathy. Am J Ophthalmol. 2015;159(5):877–883.e877.
35. Lai TY, Cheung CM. Myopic choroidal neovascularization: diagnosis and treatment. Retina. 2016;36(9):1614–21.

36. Cheung CMG, Lai TYY, Ruamviboonsuk P, et al. Polypoidal choroidal vasculopathy: definition, pathogenesis, diagnosis, and management. Ophthalmology. 2018;125(5):708–24.
37. Soomro T, Talks J, Medscape. The use of optical coherence tomography angiography for detecting choroidal neovascularization, compared to standard multimodal imaging. Eye. 2018;32(4):661–72.
38. Jia Y, Bailey ST, Wilson DJ, et al. Quantitative optical coherence tomography angiography of choroidal neovascularization in age-related macular degeneration. Ophthalmology. 2014;121(7):1435–44.
39. Bruyere E, Miere A, Cohen SY, et al. Neovascularization secondary to high myopia imaged by optical coherence tomography angiography. Retina. 2017;37(11):2095–101.
40. Miyata M, Ooto S, Hata M, et al. Detection of myopic choroidal neovascularization using optical coherence tomography angiography. Am J Ophthalmol. 2016;165:108–14.
41. Querques L, Giuffre C, Corvi F, et al. Optical coherence tomography angiography of myopic choroidal neovascularisation. Br J Ophthalmol. 2017;101(5):609–15.
42. Sayanagi K, Ikuno Y, Uematsu S, Nishida K. Features of the choriocapillaris in myopic maculopathy identified by optical coherence tomography angiography. Br J Ophthalmol. 2017;101(11):1524–9.
43. Wong CW, Teo YCK, Tsai STA, et al. Characterization of the choroidal vasculature in myopic maculopathy with optical coherence tomographic angiography. Retina. 2018. https://doi.org/10.1097/IAE.0000000000002233.
44. Moriyama M, Ohno-Matsui K, Shimada N, et al. Correlation between visual prognosis and fundus autofluorescence and optical coherence tomographic findings in highly myopic eyes with submacular hemorrhage and without choroidal neovascularization. Retina. 2011;31(1):74–80.
45. Zhang X, Zuo C, Li M, Chen H, Huang S, Wen F. Spectral-domain optical coherence tomographic findings at each stage of punctate inner choroidopathy. Ophthalmology. 2013;120(12):2678–83.
46. Tan ACS, Tan GS, Denniston AK, et al. An overview of the clinical applications of optical coherence tomography angiography. Eye. 2018;32(2):262–86.
47. Spaide RF, Goldberg N, Freund KB. Redefining multifocal choroiditis and panuveitis and punctate inner choroidopathy through multimodal imaging. Retina. 2013;33(7):1315–24.
48. Gaucher D, Erginay A, Lecleire-Collet A, et al. Dome-shaped macula in eyes with myopic posterior staphyloma. Am J Ophthalmol. 2008;145(5):909–14.
49. Caillaux V, Gaucher D, Gualino V, Massin P, Tadayoni R, Gaudric A. Morphologic characterization of dome-shaped macula in myopic eyes with serous macular detachment. Am J Ophthalmol. 2013;156(5):958–967.e951.
50. Ellabban AA, Tsujikawa A, Matsumoto A, et al. Three-dimensional tomographic features of dome-shaped macula by swept-source optical coherence tomography. Am J Ophthalmol. 2013;155(2):320–328.e322.
51. Viola F, Dell'Arti L, Benatti E, et al. Choroidal findings in dome-shaped macula in highly myopic eyes: a longitudinal study. Am J Ophthalmol. 2015;159(1):44–52.
52. Virgili G, Menchini F. Laser photocoagulation for choroidal neovascularisation in pathologic myopia. Cochrane Database Syst Rev. 2005;4:CD004765.
53. Blinder KJ, Blumenkranz MS, Bressler NM, et al. Verteporfin therapy of subfoveal choroidal neovascularization in pathologic myopia: 2-year results of a randomized clinical trial--VIP report no. 3. Ophthalmology. 2003;110(4):667–73.
54. Verteporfin in Photodynamic Therapy Study G. Photodynamic therapy of subfoveal choroidal neovascularization in pathologic myopia with verteporfin. 1-year results of a randomized clinical trial--VIP report no. 1. Ophthalmology. 2001;108(5):841–52.
55. Chen Y, Sharma T, Li X, et al. Ranibizumab versus verteporfin photodynamic therapy in asian patients with myopic choroidal neovascularization: brilliance, a 12-month, randomized, double-masked study. Retina. 2018. https://doi.org/10.1097/IAE.0000000000002292.
56. Wolf S, Balciuniene VJ, Laganovska G, et al. RADIANCE: a randomized controlled study of ranibizumab in patients with choroidal neovascularization secondary to pathologic myopia. Ophthalmology. 2014;121(3):682–692.e682.

57. Ikuno Y, Ohno-Matsui K, Wong TY, et al. Intravitreal aflibercept injection in patients with myopic choroidal neovascularization: the MYRROR study. Ophthalmology. 2015;122(6):1220–7.
58. Tufail A, Narendran N, Patel PJ, et al. Ranibizumab in myopic choroidal neovascularization: the 12-month results from the REPAIR study. Ophthalmology. 2013;120(9):1944–1945.e1941.
59. Ohno-Matsui K, Suzaki M, Teshima R, Okami N. Real-world data on ranibizumab for myopic choroidal neovascularization due to pathologic myopia: results from a post-marketing surveillance in Japan. Eye. 2018;32(12):1871–8.
60. Kasahara K, Moriyama M, Morohoshi K, et al. Six-year outcomes of intravitreal bevacizumab for choroidal neovascularization in patients with pathologic myopia. Retina. 2017;37(6):1055–64.
61. Sarao V, Veritti D, Macor S, Lanzetta P. Intravitreal bevacizumab for choroidal neovascularization due to pathologic myopia: long-term outcomes. Graefes Arch Clin Exp Ophthalmol. 2016;254(3):445–54.
62. Baba T, Kubota-Taniai M, Kitahashi M, Okada K, Mitamura Y, Yamamoto S. Two-year comparison of photodynamic therapy and intravitreal bevacizumab for treatment of myopic choroidal neovascularisation. Br J Ophthalmol. 2010;94(7):864–70.
63. Ikuno Y, Nagai Y, Matsuda S, et al. Two-year visual results for older Asian women treated with photodynamic therapy or bevacizumab for myopic choroidal neovascularization. Am J Ophthalmol. 2010;149(1):140–6.
64. Gharbiya M, Cruciani F, Parisi F, Cuozzo G, Altimari S, Abdolrahimzadeh S. Long-term results of intravitreal bevacizumab for choroidal neovascularisation in pathological myopia. Br J Ophthalmol. 2012;96(8):1068–72.
65. Peiretti E, Vinci M, Fossarello M. Intravitreal bevacizumab as a treatment for choroidal neovascularisation secondary to myopia: 4-year study results. Can J Ophthalmol. 2012; 47(1):28–33.
66. Wu Z, Zhou P, Li X, et al. Structural characterization of a recombinant fusion protein by instrumental analysis and molecular modeling. PLoS One. 2013;8(3):e57642.
67. Yan M, Huang Z, Lian HY, Song YP, Chen X. Conbercept for treatment of choroidal neovascularization secondary to pathologic myopia. Acta Ophthalmol. 2018. https://doi.org/10.1111/aos.13632.
68. Wang J, Kang Z. Summary of prognostic factors for choroidal neovascularization due to pathological myopia treated by intravitreal bevacizumab injection. Graefes Arch Clin Exp Ophthalmol. 2012;250(12):1717–23.
69. Iacono P, Battaglia Parodi M, Selvi F, et al. Factors influencing visual acuity in patients receiving anti-vascular endothelial growth factor for myopic choroidal neovascularization. Retina. 2017;37(10):1931–41.
70. Ng DS, Kwok AK, Tong JM, Chan CW, Li WW. Factors influencing need for retreatment and long-term visual outcome after intravitreal bevacizumab for myopic choroidal neovascularization. Retina. 2015;35(12):2457–68.
71. Yang HS, Kim JG, Kim JT, Joe SG. Prognostic factors of eyes with naive subfoveal myopic choroidal neovascularization after intravitreal bevacizumab. Am J Ophthalmol. 2013;156(6):1201–1210.e1202.
72. Iacono P, Battaglia Parodi M, Iuliano L, Bandello F. How vitreomacular interface modifies the efficacy of anti-Vegf therapy for myopic choroidal neovascularization. Retina. 2018;38(1):84–90.
73. Ceklic L, Munk MR, Wolf-Schnurrbusch U, Gekkieva M, Wolf S. Visual acuity outcomes of ranibizumab treatment in pathologic myopic eyes with macular retinoschisis and choroidal neovascularization. Retina. 2017;37(4):687–93.
74. Gemmy Chui Ming Cheung KO-M, Tien Yin Wong, Tummy Li, Friedrich Asmus, Sergio L, et al. Influence of myopic macular degeneration (MMD) severity on treatment outcomes of myopic choroidal neovascularization (mCNV) in the MYRROR Study. In: Presented at the American Academy of Ophthalmology (AAO) Congress Chicago, IL 2016.

75. Tan NW, Ohno-Matsui K, Koh HJ, et al. Long-term outcomes of ranibizumab treatment of myopic choroidal neovascularization in East-Asian patients from the radiance study. Retina. 2017;38(11):2228–38.
76. Franqueira N, Cachulo ML, Pires I, et al. Long-term follow-up of myopic choroidal neovascularization treated with ranibizumab. Ophthalmologica. 2012;227(1):39–44.
77. Freitas-da-Costa P, Pinheiro-Costa J, Carvalho B, et al. Anti-VEGF therapy in myopic choroidal neovascularization: long-term results. Ophthalmologica. 2014;232(1):57–63.
78. Pastore MR, Capuano V, Bruyere E, et al. Nine-year outcome of ranibizumab monotherapy for choroidal neovascularization secondary to pathologic myopia. Ophthalmologica. 2018;239(2-3):133–42.
79. Onishi Y, Yokoi T, Kasahara K, et al. Five-year outcomes of intravitreal ranibizumab for choroidal neovascularization in patients with pathologic myopia. Retina. 2018. https://doi.org/10.1097/IAE.0000000000002164.
80. Chhablani J, Paulose RM, Lasave AF, et al. Intravitreal bevacizumab monotherapy in myopic choroidal neovascularisation: 5-year outcomes for the PAN-American Collaborative Retina Study Group. Br J Ophthalmol. 2018;102(4):455–9.
81. Rofagha S, Bhisitkul RB, Boyer DS, Sadda SR, Zhang K, Group S-US. Seven-year outcomes in ranibizumab-treated patients in anchor, marina, and horizon: a multicenter cohort study (SEVEN-UP). Ophthalmology. 2013;120(11):2292–9.
82. Maguire MG, Martin DF, Comparison of Age-related Macular Degeneration Treatments Trials Research G, et al. Five-year outcomes with anti-vascular endothelial growth factor treatment of neovascular age-related macular degeneration: the comparison of age-related macular degeneration treatments trials. Ophthalmology. 2016;123(8):1751–61.
83. Farinha CL, Baltar AS, Nunes SG, et al. Progression of myopic maculopathy after treatment of choroidal neovascularization. Ophthalmologica. 2014;231(4):211–20.

Optical Interventions for Myopia Control 14

Wing Chun Tang, Myra Leung, Angel C. K. Wong,
Chi-ho To, and Carly S. Y. Lam

Key Points

- Optical intervention for myopia control can slow down myopia progression by 50–60%.
- Simultaneous myopic defocus and refractive error correction have been proved to be effective in myopia control.
- Different myopia control methods and their pros and cons aid clinicians to select the best treatment for patients.

14.1 Introduction

A variety of clinical methods are currently utilized for retarding myopia progression. However, none of the methods have been proven to cease the development or progression of myopia completely and they may not work for some individuals. As described in previous chapters, the main clinical interventions for myopia control currently include optical lenses, pharmaceutical agents and outdoor activities. This chapter provides an overview of the various types of optical interventions for slowing down myopia progression. The findings of the clinical trials of these methods are summarized and the relative effectiveness of these methods in myopia control is compared. In general, the optical methods for myopia control in children can be summarized into two categories: spectacle lenses and contact lenses.

The original version of this chapter was revised. A correction to this chapter can be found at https://doi.org/10.1007/978-981-13-8491-2_15.

W. C. Tang · M. Leung · A. C. K. Wong · C.-h. To · C. S. Y. Lam (✉)
Centre for Myopia Research, School of Optometry, The Hong Kong Polytechnic University, Kowloon, Hong Kong
e-mail: Carly.lam@polyu.edu.hk

M. Ang, T. Y. Wong (eds.), *Updates on Myopia*,
https://doi.org/10.1007/978-981-13-8491-2_14

14.2 Spectacle Lenses

14.2.1 Under-Correction of Myopia

Studies using animals, such as chicks and mammals, have shown that the use of optical lenses to impose myopic defocus inhibits myopic eye growth in developing eyes [1–5]. These studies have led to the hypothesis that under-correction of myopia, that is, prescribing spectacles for distance vision that does not fully correct the myopic refraction, may be a viable method for slowing myopia progression in humans. As near work and accommodation were proposed as key factors for the development and progression of myopia, in theory, under-correction could reduce accommodative demand during near viewing, thereby halting the myopia progression of myopia.

Contrary to the animal studies, two clinical trial studies showed that under-correction actually accelerates myopia development and progression in myopic humans [6, 7]. In a randomized study by Chung et al. [6], children in the experimental group were assigned to wear spectacle lenses that were under corrected by 0.50–0.75 D to achieve distance visual acuity of 6/12, while children in the control group were prescribed their full correction. After 2 years, the under-correction group had greater myopia progression of −1.00 D as compared to the control group who progressed by −0.77 D. A retrospective study investigating clinical data from a private optometric practice also found that under-correction resulted in greater myopia progression compared to full correction [7].

One recent study in Beijing reported that children with no spectacle correction had slower myopia progression and less axial elongation than those given a full spectacle correction over 2 years [8]. In this study, myopia progression decreased significantly with an increasing amount of under-correction, but the effect on slowing myopia progression was slowed by only 0.27 D over 2 years, which is not clinically meaningful. In view of these conflicting results, there is no convincing evidence to indicate that under-correction should be used for slowing myopia progression in children.

14.2.2 Bifocal or Multifocal Spectacles

Over the past decades, numerous studies have assessed the effect of bifocal, multifocal, and progressive addition lens (PALs) spectacles on myopia progression. Table 14.1 summarizes the clinical trials of using the different spectacle lens types. Bifocals and PALs allow the wearers to clearly see objects in the distance through the upper part of the glasses by providing correction of distance refractive error. The bottom part of the lens consists of an addition power that may retard myopia progression by reducing accommodative effort and lag at near in a similar way as under-correction.

The majority of these studies have shown that PALs have an insignificant effect on slowing myopia progression rate (less than 0.2 D per year) overall (Table 14.1)

Table 14.1 Myopia control studies using PALs, bifocal and multifocal spectacles

Authors and years	Study duration (years)	Design	Age (years), ethnicity	Subject Rx range, diopters (D)	Interventions and sample size (*n*)	Treatment effect in slowing myopia progression during study period, D (%)
Fulk et al. (2000) [15]	2.5	Randomized, masked	6–13	−0.50 to −6.00 (under 9 years old) or −8.00 (9 years old or older)	SV, $n = 40$ Bifocals with 1.50 D add, $n = 42$	0.25 (20%)
Edward et al. (2002) [9]	2	Randomized, double masked	7–10.5, Chinese	−1.25 to −4.50	SV, $n = 132$ PAL (1.5 D add), $n = 121$	0.14 (11%)
Gwiazda et al. (2003) [10]	3	Randomized, masked	6–11, diverse ethnicity	−1.25 to −4.50	SV, $n = 233$ PAL (2 D add), $n = 229$	0.20 (14%)
Yang et al. (2009) [11]	2	Randomized, masked	7–13, Chinese	−0.50 to −3.00	SV, $n = 75$ PAL (1.5 D add), $n = 74$	0.26 (17%)
COMET2 (2011) [12]	3	Randomized, masked, multicenter	8–12, diverse ethnicity	−0.75 to −2.50	SV, $n = 58$ PAL (2 D add), $n = 52$	0.28 (24%)
Sankaridurg et al. (2011) [17]	1	Randomized	6–16, Chinese	−0.75 to −3.50	Type I, III lenses, SV, $n = 50$ each group Type II, $n = 60$	Type III lens: 0.29 (30% only in a subgroup of children with myopic parents)
Berntsen et al. (2012) [13]	1	Randomized, masked, all subjects worn SV in 2nd year	6–11	−0.75 to −4.50	SV, $n = 42$ PAL (2 D add), $n = 41$	0.18 (35%)
Hasbe et al. (2014) [14]	1.5	Randomized, masked, cross-over	6–12, Japanese	−1.25 to −6.00	SV, $n = 44$ PAL (1.5 D add), $n = 42$	1st period: 0.31 (18%) 2nd period: 0.02 (2%)
Cheng et al. (2014) [16]	3	Randomized, masked	8–13, Chinese	−1 to −5.50	SV, $n = 41$ BF (1.5 D add), $n = 48$ PBF (1.5 D add, 3ΔBI), $n = 46$	BF: 0.81 (39%) PBF: 1.05 (51%)
Lam et al. (2019) [19]	2	Randomized, masked	8–13, Chinese	−1.00 to −5.00	SV = 90 DIMS = 93	0.44 (52%)

COMET2 and PEDIG Correction of Myopia Evaluation Trial 2 Study Group and the Paediatric Eye Disease Investigator Group, *SV* single vision spectacle lens, *PAL* progressive addition lens, *BF* bifocal spectacle lens, *PBF* prismatic bifocal lens, *DIMS* defocus incorporated multiple segments spectacle lens

[9–14]. Some myopic children with esophoria and accommodative lag may benefit from PALs, but the retardation effect is not clinically significant.

For bifocal spectacles, an early randomized trial performed by Fulk et al. [15] found that bifocals with +1.5 D add slowed myopia progression by 20% in the children with esophoria. The clinical trial by Cheng et al. [16] found that both executive top bifocals with and without 3Δ base-in prism have shown a more meaningful myopia control effect in a selected group of fast progressing myopic children when compared with single vision spectacles. The myopia progression rate was reduced by approximately 40–50% over 3 years, with the effect being more prominent among those with low accommodative lag. The inclusion of base-in prism in the experimental lenses was an attempt to reduce fusional vergence demand to enhance the treatment effects of the bifocals. A positive effect of myopia control was exhibited as changes in spherical equivalent refraction in the study. Axial length changes were similar between those with and without base-in prism in their bifocals; it is rather unclear whether there is a benefit in having base-in prism in the bifocal lens. This option may also not be preferable for some children having anisometropia, and it results in poor cosmesis.

Another hypothesis is that the correction or reduction of relative peripheral hyperopia may have an effect on myopia progression [17, 18]. Sankaridurg et al. [17] performed a clinical trial to test this hypothesis by using three custom-designed spectacle lenses that reduced peripheral hyperopic defocus while maintaining clear central vision. After 12 months of lens wear, no significant reduction in myopia progression was found between the treatment groups and the control group. Only one type of the treatment lenses showed 30% reduction of myopia progression in a subgroup of the children whose parents were myopes. A similar clinical trial in soft contact lens [18], based on the same hypothesis, exhibited meaningful effects and will be discussed later in the section on soft multifocal contact lenses.

More recently, a specially designed bifocal spectacle lens, called Defocus Incorporated Multiple Segments (DIMS) spectacle lens (also known as multisegment of myopic defocus (MSMD) spectacle lens), has been used for myopia control in a randomized trial by Lam et al. [19]. DIMS lens design is based on the principle of simultaneous vision with myopia defocus for myopia control where it comprises a central optical zone for correcting refractive error and multiple segments of constant myopic defocus (+3.50 D) surrounding the central zone. This enables the lens to provide clear vision and myopic defocus simultaneously for wearers regardless of whether they are looking at distance, intermediate or near objects. The results from the clinical trial showed that the children wearing DIMS lenses had 52% less myopia progression and 62% less axial elongation when compared with children wearing single vision spectacle lenses over 2 years. Moreover, about 20% of the DIMS lens wearers had no myopia progression during the study period. Further studies in other study populations are required to validate these promising results.

Figure 14.1 presents a comparison of the percentage myopia progression that slowed down from PALs, bifocals, and prismatic bifocals use as well as other types of multiple spectacle lenses [9–16].

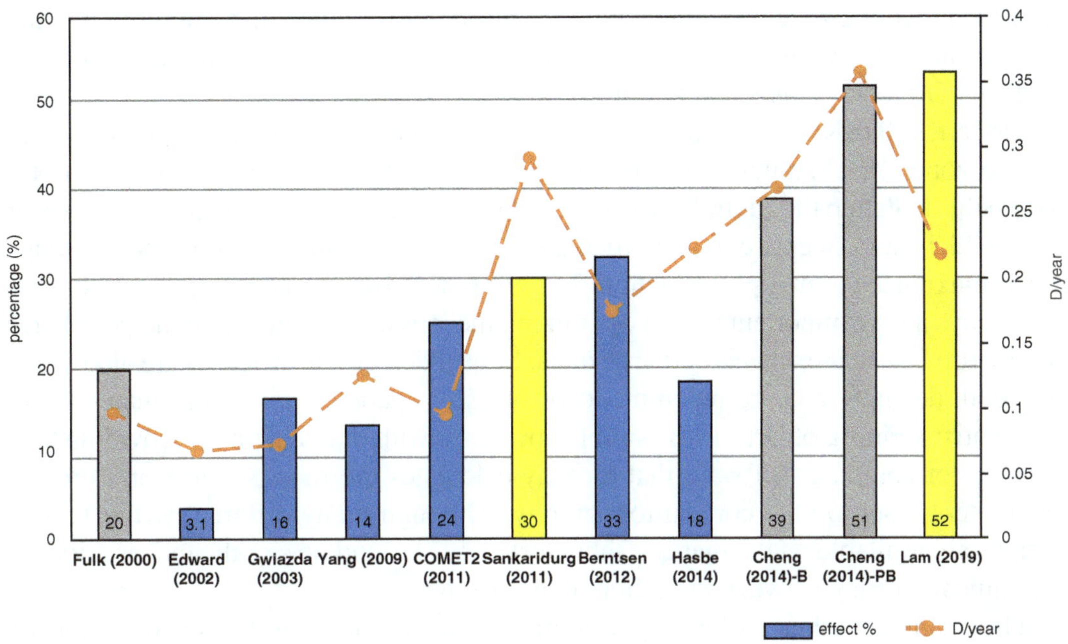

Fig. 14.1 The effect on slowing of myopia progression, in terms of percentage within the study period (effect %) and diopter per year (D/year), reported by various controlled clinical studies using bifocal or multifocal spectacles. The bars represent effect % using bifocals (gray), progressive addition lenses (blue) and other types of multifocal spectacle lenses (yellow). The value of effect % is indicated in the bar. The dotted line represents treatment effect in D/year (*B* bifocals, *PB* prismatic bifocals)

14.3 Contact Lenses

14.3.1 Rigid Gas Permeable Contact Lenses

Several studies in the later part of the twentieth century investigated whether daytime wear of rigid gas permeable (RGP) contact lenses slowed myopia progression, but all those studies had various limitations in their study designs, such as subject criteria outside the expected age of progression, lack of randomization, and unequal loss to follow-up [20–22]. Two randomized clinical trials [23, 24] showed that RGP contact lenses did not retard axial eye growth. However, Walline et al. [23] reported significant slower myopia progression in the group of RGP lenses compared with soft contact lenses. Despite that no differences were found in axial elongation between the groups. The proposed reason for a treatment effect on the refractions may be due to the changes in corneal curvature. As wear of RGP contact lenses is likely to induce only temporary changes in corneal curvature, the retardation of myopia progression may be transient. Therefore, the authors concluded that RGP lens wear does not slow myopia progression.

14.3.2 Orthokeratology

Orthokeratology (Ortho-K) lenses are specially designed RGP contact lenses that are worn overnight to reshape the cornea and thereby temporarily correct low to moderate myopia. It has become a popular modality for controlling myopia in children in the last few decades. In addition to the enhancement of unaided vision at daytime, Ortho-K is also able to control myopia progression.

Modern Ortho-K lens designs include four zones, namely the central optic zone, the reverse zone, the alignment zone and the peripheral zone [25, 26]. The central optic zone helps to flatten the central cornea and is used for refractive correction. The reverse zone, which has a steeper curvature than the central zone, enhances the corneal reshaping to maximize the myopic reduction. The alignment zone, usually aspherical or tangent, plays a very important role in optimizing the lens centration, while the peripheral curve promotes tear exchange. Apart from spherical designs, toric lenses are also available commercially and are recommended for use in patients with more than 1.50 D astigmatism. Fitting of Ortho-K is simple nowadays with manufacturers providing trial lens sets or computer software that directly calculates the most suitable and precise parameters based on the corneal topography. Although many different Ortho-K lens designs are available on the market, Tahhan et al. [27] found no significant variation on the clinical efficacy between the different lens designs.

The main hypothesis of myopia control using Ortho-K is the introduction of myopic defocus on the peripheral retina [27]. It is proposed that after Ortho-K treatment, the corneal shape changes to an oblate shape, which results in a peripheral refraction that has less hyperopic defocus [28]. Another hypothesis of the mechanism behind the myopia control effect of Ortho-K is that the changes in lag of accommodation may be due to increasing positive spherical aberration and changes in choroidal thickness [29, 30]. It seems that further investigation is required in order to determine the actual mechanism for the efficacy of Ortho-K.

Various clinical studies have demonstrated the effectiveness of inhibiting myopic progression with Ortho-K. Table 14.2 summarizes recent clinical trials using Ortho-K for myopia control in children. The effect of slowing axial length elongation ranges from 32% to 63% [31–38]. The overall treatment effect is around 50%. Figure 14.2 shows a comparison of the effect on retarding axial elongation using Ortho-K among different studies [31–37].

A recent study by Swabrick et al. [39] used a contralateral eye cross-over study design to investigate the effects of Ortho-K on axial length growth over 1 year. The results revealed that there were no changes in axial length at each 6-month phase of Ortho-K wear, while significant increases in axial length were found in the control group who wore daytime gas permeable lenses.

To the best of our knowledge, there is no research investigating the maximum power of myopia reduction with overnight Ortho-K, and most studies use −4.00 D as the exclusion criteria. Charm et al. investigated the myopic control effect of Ortho-K by partial reduction to the power of −4.00 D as the target in children with high myopia (spherical equivalent refraction at least −5.75 D and myopia ≥−5.00 D). The remaining refractive error was corrected by single vision spectacles. The myopia control effect was comparable to other studies of Ortho-K in low–moderate myopic subjects over 2 years [37]. As the risk of having corneal staining and lens decentration increases with the amount of myopia correction [39], partial reduction of myopia might be a better option in high myopes instead of the full correction.

Table 14.2 Myopia control studies using Ortho-K lenses

Authors and years	Study design	Study duration (years)	Control group	Mean change in AL (mm)		Treatment effect in retarding axial length elongation, mean difference in mm (%)
				Ortho-K	Control	
Cho et al. (2005) [31]	Self-selected prospective	2	SV	0.29	0.54	0.25 (46)
Walline et al. (2009) [32]	Prospective, historical controls	2	SVCL	0.25	0.57	0.32 (56)
Kakita et al. (2011) [33]	Self-selected retrospective	2	SV	0.39	0.61	0.22 (36)
Cho and Cheung (2012) [34]	Randomized, single-masked	2	SV	0.36	0.63	0.27 (43)
Hiraoka et al. (2012) [35]	Self-selected retrospective	5	SV	0.99	1.41	0.42 (30)
Santodomingo-Rubido et al. (2012) [36]	Self-selected prospective	2	SV	0.47	0.69	0.22 (32)
Charm and Cho (2013) [37]	Randomized, single-masked	2	SV	0.19	0.51	0.32 (63)
Chen et al. (2013) [38]	Self-selected prospective	2	SV	0.31	0.64	0.33 (52)

SV single vision spectacle lens, *SVCL* single vision soft contact lens

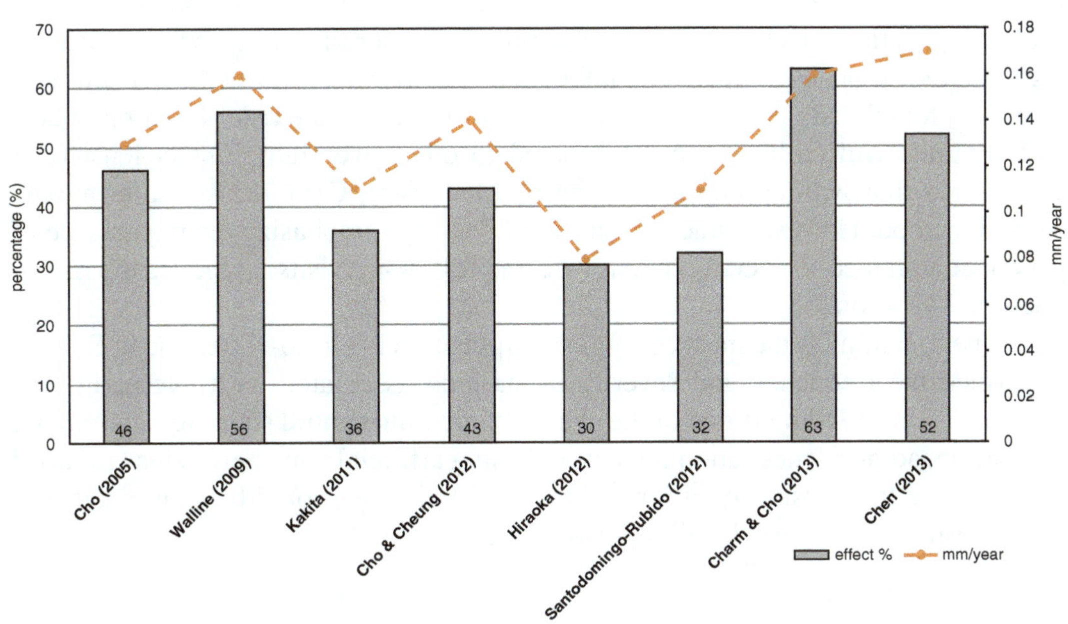

Fig. 14.2 Effect on slowing axial elongation reported by various studies using orthokeratology. The bar represents the treatment effect within the study period in terms of percentage (%) as compared to controls. The dotted line represents reduction in changes of axial length per year (mm/year)

Although Ortho-K is useful for myopic control in numerous studies, all the results were reported as an average value. Lipson et al [26] evaluated the axial length change over 3 years in children receiving Ortho-K treatment. Around 65% of the children had 0.5 mm or less axial elongation, while axial eye growth of more than 1.0 mm was seen in 15% of the children. Hence, the myopic control effect of Ortho-K lenses shows a large variation among individuals. Some researchers believed that the age at which Ortho-K is started, baseline myopia, cornea profile, and pupil size may be possible factors affecting the effectiveness of myopic control among Ortho-K wearers [26, 31, 34, 35, 40].

Interestingly, a recent study in Japan [41] showed that the combination of Ortho-K and low-concentration atropine (0.01%) eye drops was more effective in slowing axial elongation over 12 months than Ortho-K treatment alone in myopic children. More research is needed to show if this effect can be sustained in the longer term.

Although hypoxic reactions are rarely seen with Ortho-K wear due to the use of highly oxygen permeable materials, the need to wear contact lenses overnight may remain a concern for clinicians, as this type of lens wear pattern is associated with a higher risk of infectious keratitis [42–44]. A review of 50 cases of microbial keratitis done by Watt and Swarbrick [44] revealed that the majority of microbial keratitis cases are related to contamination of lenses due to patient non-compliance, such as improper lens handling or cleaning. A detailed systematic review on the safety of Ortho-K wear by Liu and Xie [45] also suggested that the training of practitioners and wearers, appropriate fitting procedures, compliance to lens care regimens and follow-up schedule are all factors affecting the incidence of microbial keratitis. A recent retrospective study compared the adverse events in Ortho-K wearers versus soft contact lens wearers over a 10-year period. The number of corneal complications such as keratitis and infiltrates were found to be significantly higher in the Ortho-K group, but no infectious keratitis was reported [46]. Bullimore et al. [47] found that there was no significant difference in the risk of getting microbial keratitis with Ortho-K wear compared to other overnight contact lens wear. This shows that with appropriate fitting and lens care, Ortho-K is a safe myopic control method. However, practitioners should always emphasize the importance of patient compliance, especially in lens care and follow-up visits, to reduce the risk of microbial keratitis [45].

Corneal staining is the most common complication in Ortho-K treatment. Studies confirmed the frequency and severity of staining associated with overnight lens wear [44]. Lens binding is one of the causes of creating central staining. Optimizing lens fitting, adding fenestration on lens and using artificial tears before lens removal could reduce the possibility of lens adhesion. Clinicians should be cautious if persistent or recurrent corneal staining is observed.

14.3.3 Soft Bifocal and Multifocal Contact Lenses

Soft contact lenses in the form of bifocal and multifocal have been designed to slow myopia progression in children, and there has been a rising interest in this area over the recent decade. These lenses are worn during the daytime. Compared to spectacles, contact lenses are more cosmetically acceptable and are more convenient for daily activities of some children, especially during sports activities [48, 49]. Also, they are generally able to be competently handled and worn by children [48]. For most of eye care practitioners, the fitting procedures of soft bifocal contact lenses are relatively simpler than those of Ortho-K.

Table 14.3 and Fig. 14.3 summarize recent clinical trials using soft bifocal contact lenses for myopia control [18, 50–56]. Generally, two main approaches are employed for the design of soft contact lenses for myopia control. Both lens designs incorporate a central distance zone to correct myopia. One design manipulates the peripheral lens curvature in order to lower peripheral hyperopic defocus. The other design uses concentric rings of alternating myopia defocus using addition (plus) powers and myopia correction powers in the periphery. This design is sometimes called 'dual power or dual focus' contact lenses in the literature. Both approaches allow the lens wearers to have good vision in their daily life and receive therapeutic optical defocus at the same time.

Several lens types, with a design to reduce peripheral hyperopia, have been reported to be promising in retarding myopia progression. Examples include a lens type used in a study by Sankaridurg et al. [18] and a multifocal contact lens used in a study by Walline et al. [50]. The former was reported to retard myopia progression by 34% over 1 year and the latter by 50% over 2 years. Paune et al. [51] carried out a study using 'soft radial refractive gradient' (SRRG) contact lens, which corrects the central refraction while producing peripheral myopic defocus that increases gradually from the central optical axis towards the periphery. After 2 years, children wearing the SRRG contact lens had retardation in myopia progression by 43%. Cheng et al. [52] developed a soft contact lens for myopia control that included a positive spherical aberration (+SA) in the optical design to shift retinal hyperopic defocus in the opposite direction, resulting in the reduction of relative peripheral hyperopia. The greatest effect of myopia control (56%) was observed during the first 6 months, and it decreased greatly to 20% by 12 months. The overall treatment effects of these contact lenses were better than ophthalmic lenses that used a similar approach [17]. This may be due to the soft contact lenses moving with the eye, and hence the optical correction remains centered for all viewing gazes.

Anstice and Phillips [53] investigated the use of a concentric bifocal power (also called dual-focus or dual power) soft contact lens with 2D of myopic defocus in retarding myopia progression in children. Children participating in their study were randomly assigned to wear the treatment lens in one eye and an ordinary single vision contact lens in the fellow eye for 10 months. The lens types were then switched between the eyes and the lenses were worn for another 10 months. On average, the eyes with the bifocal contact lenses showed about 45% less myopia progression than the eyes with single vision contact lenses. Several randomized clinical trials showed that concentric bifocal contact lenses exhibited meaningful effects on myopia control. Lam et al. [54] reported that the use of Defocus Incorporated Soft Contact (DISC) lens for at least 7 hours a day resulted in more effective myopia control, reaching nearly 60% reduction in myopia progression and

Table 14.3 Myopia control studies using soft bifocal and multifocal contact lenses

Authors and years	Study duration (months)	Study design	Age (years old), ethnicity	Subject Rx range (D)	Interventions and sample size (*n*)	Effect in slowing myopia progression in study period, D (%)
Anstice and Phillips (2011) [53]	20	Randomized, paired eye control, cross-over	11–14, diverse ethnicity	−1.25 to −4.50	DF (2 D add), $n = 40$ SVCL, $n = 40$	1st 10-month: 0.25 (37%) 2nd 10-month: 0.2 (54%)
Sankaridurg et al. (2011) [18]	12	Randomized	7–14, Chinese	−0.75 to −3.50	RPH CL, $n = 45$ SV, $n = 40$	0.29 (34%)
Walline et al. (2013) [50]	24	Matched study	8–11, diverse ethnicity	−1.00 to −6.00	Proclear multifocal D (2 D add), $n = 40$ Matched SVCL, $n = 40$	0.52 (50%)
Lam et al. (2014) [54]	24	Randomized, double-masked	8–13, Chinese	−1.00 to −5.00	DISC (2.5 D add), $n = 65$ SVCL, $n = 63$	0.21 (25%) 0.44 (50%) > 6 h 0.54 (58%) > 7 h 0.53 (60%) > 8 h
Paune et al. (2014) [51]	24	Prospective, nonrandomized	9–16, Caucasian	−0.75 to −7.00	SRRG, $n = 30$ OK, $n = 29$ SV, $n = 41$	0.42 (43%)
Aller et al. (2016) [57]	12	Randomized, masked	8–18,	−0.50 to −6.00	BFSCL, $n = 39$ SVCL, $n = -40$	0.57 (72% in children with eso fixation disparities)
Cheng et al. (2016) [52]	24 (only 12-month data)	Randomized, double-masked	8–11	−0.75 to −4.00	+SA, $n = 64$ SVCL, $n = 63$	6-month: 0.21 (56%) 12-month: 0.12 (20%)
Chamberlain et al. (2018) [55]	36	Randomized, double-masked	8–12	−0.75 to −4.00	DF (2 D add), $n = 70$ SVCL, $n = 74$	0.73 (59%)
Ruiz-Pomeda et al. (2018) [56]	24	Randomized, double-masked, multicenter	8–12	−0.75 to −4.00	DF (2 D add), $n = 46$ SVCL, $n = 33$	0.29 (39%)

DF dual focus contact lens, *SVCL* single vision contact lens, *RPH CL* contact lens designed to reduce relative peripheral hyperopia, *SV* single vision spectacle lens, *DISC* Defocus Incorporated Soft Contact lens, *SRRG* soft radial refractive gradient contact lens, *OK* Ortho-K, *BFSCL* bifocal soft contact lens, *+SA* soft contact lens with positive special aberration

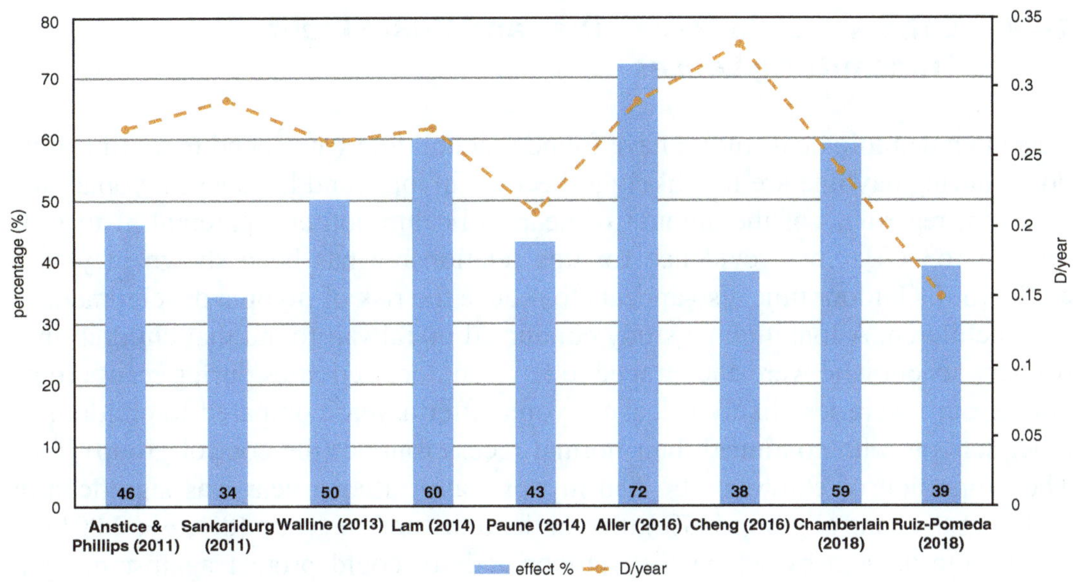

Fig. 14.3 Comparison of the treatment effect on slowing myopia progression among the studies using soft bifocal and multifocal contact lenses. The bar represents treatment effect within the study period in terms of percentage as compared with controls. The dotted line represents reduction of myopia progression per year (D/year)

axial length growth. The amount of myopic defocus used in the DISC lens was 2.50 D. Two more recent studies have indicated that a Dual-Focus 1-Day soft contact lens using 2D of myopic defocus also slows myopia progression in children. The multicenter study by Chamberlain et al. [55] has shown that the Dual-Focus 1-Day soft contact lens slows myopic progression and axial elongation in children by 59% and 52%, respectively, over 3 years. However, another study in Spain showed less myopia control effect, 39% and 36% in terms of refractive changes and axial growth, respectively [56]. A study by Aller et al. [57] reported the most promising effect of 70% with another type of bifocal soft contact lenses, but this was seen only for the children with eso fixation disparities at near.

Among the optical interventions for myopia control, Ortho-K lenses (45%), soft bifocal contact lenses (50%), prismatic bifocals (50%) and the very recent DIMS spectacle lenses (52%) have shown clinically significant treatment effects. However, the treatment effect of these methods is still inferior to that of pharmaceutical eye drops. The average reduction in myopia progression using regular dose (1%) of atropine is approximately 70% or above [58, 59]. Yet, the associated side effects, such as blurring of near vision, light sensitivity and possible allergic reactions and post-treatment rebound effects [58, 59], will be obstacles for the widespread application of atropine 1% in clinical practice. Lower doses of atropine (such as 0.5%, 0.02%, 0.01%) have been found to have minimal side effects, but long-term safety is unclear [60–62]. Atropine 0.01% has been found to have the least side effects with good myopia control and least rebound effects [61, 62]. However, optical treatment regimens are less invasive than those by pharmacological treatment and have been found to be more popular.

14.4 Others: Outdoor Activities and Violet Light Transmitting Lenses

Recent epidemiological studies have found that children who spend more time outdoors during daytime are less likely to become myopic and have less myopia progression, regardless of the amount of near work duration and parental history of myopia [63–65]. Some evidence for this relationship has been shown in young adults [63]. Outdoor time also appears to reduce the risk of myopia development in schoolchildren. A longitudinal study conducted in Taiwan found that children in a primary school who were encouraged to have outdoor activities during recess (outdoor group) were less likely to have myopia after a year compared to children in other schools who continued their normal recess routine (the control group) [64]. The proportion of children who had myopia onset after a year was significantly higher in the control group (18%) than in the intervention group (8%, $p < 0.001$).

The mechanism by which the outdoor activity could protect against myopia development is still unknown. However, there are a number of theories, such as relaxed accommodation for viewing distance receiving more myopic defocus in outdoor environments and higher light intensity in outdoor environments [65, 66]. The spectral composition of sunlight may also play a role in myopia control. Sunlight has a large portion of short-wavelength visible and non-visible light, such as blue light and ultraviolet light [67]. Animal studies have demonstrated that blue light has a suppressive effect against myopia [68, 69]. Recently, Torri et al. [70] proposed that violet light (VL) (which has a shorter wavelength than blue light), which is a missing light component in indoor environments, may play a role in the inhibition of myopia development and progression. They demonstrated that exposure to VL inhibited myopic shift and axial elongation in chicks. On the basis of the animal findings, they conducted a clinical trial in which myopic children were assigned to wear VL blocking eyeglasses, partially VL blocking contact lenses or VL transmitting contact lenses [70]. The results showed that children who wore VL transmitting contact lenses had significantly less axial length elongation compared to those wearing the other types of lenses over 1 year. These data provide evidence that VL may contribute to the protective effect against myopia progression. Further investigation is needed to determine whether VL transmitting lenses could slow myopia progression or prevent myopia in children.

14.5 Comparison of the Effectiveness on Myopia Control by Different Optical Interventions

Several studies have reviewed and compared the outcomes of the effect on myopia control using various treatments and methodologies [71–74]. In a review of nine randomized controlled trials that compared the effects of multifocal and single vision spectacle lenses, multifocals with add power ranging from +1.50 to +2.00 D were associated with a statistically significant decrease in myopia progression in school-age children compared with single vision lenses [74]. The effect was more prominent in children with a higher degree of myopia at baseline and could be sustained for a period of 24 months or more. Asian children were found to have greater benefit from the interventions than Caucasian children. A study comparing the treatment effect of atropine, soft bifocal and Ortho-K contact lens indicated that both atropine and Ortho-K showed treatment effects reaching over 75%, while soft bifocals had effects up to 48% [71].

In another study, a meta-analysis was performed to determine and compare 16 interventions for myopia control in children using pharmaceuticals or optical methods [73]. Among the optical methods, spectacle lens, contact lenses and Ortho-K were included. They concluded that atropine, pirenzepine, Ortho-K, soft contact lenses with myopia control features and progressive addition spectacle lenses are effective at reducing myopia progression in terms of refraction or axial length. For the pharmaceutical treatment, the average treatment effects reported in the literature are around 50%. For spectacle treatments, the effects range from minimal in the PAL trials to moderately effective in a study on executive bifocals. The investigators also compare different interventions with single vision spectacle lenses/placebo [73]. Atropine was found to be the most effective as it can retard myopia progression by around 0.50–0.60 D per year.

14.6 Conclusions

In summary, under-correction of myopia is not recommended for myopia control as it is likely to speed up myopia progression instead. Among spectacles, PALs and multifocal lenses do not yield clinically meaningful effects on slowing myopia progression in children. One single center study using prismatic bifocals in children with rapid progressing myopia showed a moderate treatment effect. Ortho-K, soft bifocal contact lenses and the very recent DIMS spectacle lenses have all shown clinically significant treatment effects ranging from 45% to 60% reduction in myopia progression. These methods demonstrated that myopic defocus as natural optical signals can inhibit refractive eye growth and control myopia progression through different optical designs. Although the effectiveness of myopia control with atropine is relatively better than those of optical methods, the associated side effects, such as sensitivity to light and near blur, hinder its widespread clinical application. Optical interventions are less invasive, which will make it likely to become more popular compared to pharmaceutical treatments.

Although there are a number of clinical methods currently available for myopia control for children, none of them have been proven to definitely halt the development or progression of myopia. The treatment effect also varies among individuals. Each therapy has its advantages and limitations. The suitable choice of treatment for each patient can vary and should be determined by the eye care professionals based on age, parental history, myopic progression rate, corneal health and lifestyle of the children. More research is needed to enhance the treatment effects of myopia control, particularly to prevent myopia before its onset through improved designs of optical lenses or pharmaceuticals. Several clinical trials are also testing the possibility of better myopia control with combined treatments, for example, optical lenses (soft bifocals, Ortho-K or DIMS spectacle lenses) with ophthalmic pharmaceutical (low-concentration atropine) or with other non-optical modalities (outdoor activities, intense bright light for near work). Also, there is still room for research on new myopia control methods, such as VL transmitting contact lenses or spectacles. When there is more evidence in the treatment effect, there is hope to reduce the prevalence of myopia and high myopia and its related ocular complications.

References

1. Siegwart JT, Norton TT. Binocular lens treatment in tree shrews: effect of age and comparison of plus lens wear with recovery from minus lens-induced myopia. Exp Eye Res. 2010;91:660–9. https://doi.org/10.1016/j.exer.2010.08.010.
2. Howlett MHC, McFadden SA. Spectacle lens compensation in the pigmented guinea pig. Vis Res. 2009;49:219–27. https://doi.org/10.1016/j.visres.2008.10.008.
3. Whatham AR, Judge SJ. Compensatory changes in eye growth and refraction induced by daily wear of soft contact lenses in young marmosets. Vis Res. 2001;41:267–73.
4. Smith EL, Hung L-F, Arumugam B. Visual regulation of refractive development: insights from animal studies. Eye (Lond). 2014;28:180–8. https://doi.org/10.1038/eye.2013.277.
5. Schaeffel F, Glasser A, Howland HC. Accommodation, refractive error and eye growth in chickens. Vis Res. 1988;28:639–57.
6. Chung K, Mohidin N, O'Leary DJ. Undercorrection of myopia enhances rather than inhibits myopia progression. Vis Res. 2002;42:2555–9.
7. Adler D, Millodot M. The possible effect of under correction on myopic progression in children. Clin Exp Optom. 2006;89:315–21. https://doi.org/10.1111/j.1444-0938.2006.00055.x.
8. Sun Y-Y, Li S-M, Li S-Y, et al. Effect of uncorrection versus full correction on myopia progression in 12-year-old children. Graefes Arch Clin Exp Ophthalmol. 2017;255:189–95. https://doi.org/10.1007/s00417-016-3529-1.
9. Edwards MH, Li RW-H, Lam CS-Y, et al. The Hong Kong progressive lens myopia control study: study design and main findings. Invest Ophthalmol Vis Sci. 2002;43:2852–8.
10. Gwiazda J, Hyman L, Hussein M, et al. A randomized clinical trial of progressive addition lenses versus single vision lenses on the progression of myopia in children. Invest Ophthalmol Vis Sci. 2003;44:1492–500.
11. Yang Z, Lan W, Ge J, et al. The effectiveness of progressive addition lenses on the progression of myopia in Chinese children. Ophthalmic Physiol Opt. 2009;29:41–8. https://doi.org/10.1111/j.1475-1313.2008.00608.x.
12. Correction of Myopia Evaluation Trial 2 Study Group for the Pediatric Eye Disease Investigator Group. Progressive-addition lenses versus single-vision lenses for slowing progression of myopia in children with high accommodative lag and near esophoria. Invest Ophthalmol Vis Sci. 2011;52:2749–57. https://doi.org/10.1167/iovs.10-6631.
13. Berntsen DA, Sinnott LT, Mutti DO, Zadnik K. A randomized trial using progressive addition lenses to evaluate theories of myopia progression in children with a high lag of accommodation. Invest Ophthalmol Vis Sci. 2012;53:640–9. https://doi.org/10.1167/iovs.11-7769.
14. Hasebe S, Jun J, Varnas SR. Myopia control with positively aspherized progressive addition lenses: a 2-year, multicenter, randomized, controlled trial. Invest Ophthalmol Vis Sci. 2014;55:7177–88. https://doi.org/10.1167/iovs.12-11462.
15. Fulk GW, Cyert LA, Parker DE. A randomized trial of the effect of single-vision vs. bifocal lenses on myopia progression in children with esophoria. Optom Vis Sci. 2000;77:395–401.
16. Cheng D, Woo GC, Drobe B, Schmid KL. Effect of bifocal and prismatic bifocal spectacles on myopia progression in children: three-year results of a randomized clinical trial. JAMA Ophthalmol. 2014;132:258–64. https://doi.org/10.1001/jamaophthalmol.2013.7623.
17. Sankaridurg P, Donovan L, Varnas S, et al. Spectacle lenses designed to reduce progression of myopia: 12-month results. Optom Vis Sci. 2010;87:631–41. https://doi.org/10.1097/OPX.0b013e3181ea19c7.

18. Sankaridurg P, Holden B, Smith E, et al. Decrease in rate of myopia progression with a contact lens designed to reduce relative peripheral hyperopia: one-year results. Invest Ophthalmol Vis Sci. 2011;52:9362–7. https://doi.org/10.1167/iovs.11-7260.
19. Lam CSY, Tang WC, Tse DY, et al. Defocus Incorporated Multiple Segments (DIMS) spectacle lenses slow myopia progression: a 2-year randomised clinical trial. Br J Ophthalmol. 2019 May 29. http://dx.doi.org/10.1136/bjophthalmol-2018-313739.
20. Khoo CY, Chong J, Rajan U. A 3-year study on the effect of RGP contact lenses on myopic children. Singap Med J. 1999;40:230–7.
21. Perrigin J, Perrigin D, Quintero S, Grosvenor T. Silicone-acrylate contact lenses for myopia control: 3-year results. Optom Vis Sci. 1990;67:764–9.
22. Stone J. The possible influence of contact lenses on myopia. Br J Physiol Opt. 1976;31:89–114.
23. Walline JJ, Jones LA, Mutti DO, Zadnik K. A randomized trial of the effects of rigid contact lenses on myopia progression. Arch Ophthalmol. 2004;122:1760–6. https://doi.org/10.1001/archopht.122.12.1760.
24. Katz J, Schein OD, Levy B, et al. A randomized trial of rigid gas permeable contact lenses to reduce progression of children's myopia. Am J Ophthalmol. 2003;136:82–90.
25. Swarbrick HA. Orthokeratology review and update. Clin Exp Optom. 2006;89:124–43. https://doi.org/10.1111/j.1444-0938.2006.00044.x.
26. Lipson MJ, Brooks MM, Koffler BH. The role of orthokeratology in myopia control: a review. Eye Contact Lens. 2018;44:224–30. https://doi.org/10.1097/ICL.0000000000000520.
27. Tahhan N, Du Toit R, Papas E, et al. Comparison of reverse-geometry lens designs for overnight orthokeratology. Optom Vis Sci. 2003;80:796–804.
28. Kang P, Swarbrick H. Peripheral refraction in myopic children wearing orthokeratology and gas-permeable lenses. Optom Vis Sci. 2011;88:476–82. https://doi.org/10.1097/OPX.0b013e31820f16fb.
29. Han X, Xu D, Ge W, et al. A comparison of the effects of orthokeratology lens, medcall lens, and ordinary frame glasses on the accommodative response in myopic children. Eye Contact Lens. 2018;44:268–71. https://doi.org/10.1097/ICL.0000000000000390.
30. Chen Z, Xue F, Zhou J, et al. Effects of orthokeratology on choroidal thickness and axial length. Optom Vis Sci. 2016;93:1064–71. https://doi.org/10.1097/OPX.0000000000000894.
31. Cho P, Cheung SW, Edwards M. The longitudinal orthokeratology research in children (LORIC) in Hong Kong: a pilot study on refractive changes and myopic control. Curr Eye Res. 2005;30:71–80.
32. Walline JJ, Jones LA, Sinnott LT. Corneal reshaping and myopia progression. Br J Ophthalmol. 2009;93:1181–5. https://doi.org/10.1136/bjo.2008.151365.
33. Kakita T, Hiraoka T, Oshika T. Influence of overnight orthokeratology on axial elongation in childhood myopia. Invest Ophthalmol Vis Sci. 2011;52:2170–4. https://doi.org/10.1167/iovs.10-5485.
34. Cho P, Cheung S-W. Retardation of myopia in Orthokeratology (ROMIO) study: a 2-year randomized clinical trial. Invest Ophthalmol Vis Sci. 2012;53:7077–85. https://doi.org/10.1167/iovs.12-10565.
35. Hiraoka T, Kakita T, Okamoto F, et al. Long-term effect of overnight orthokeratology on axial length elongation in childhood myopia: a 5-year follow-up study. Invest Ophthalmol Vis Sci. 2012;53:3913–9. https://doi.org/10.1167/iovs.11-8453.
36. Santodomingo-Rubido J, Villa-Collar C, Gilmartin B, Gutiérrez-Ortega R. Myopia control with orthokeratology contact lenses in Spain: refractive and biometric changes. Invest Ophthalmol Vis Sci. 2012;53:5060–5. https://doi.org/10.1167/iovs.11-8005.
37. Charm J, Cho P. High myopia-partial reduction ortho-k: a 2-year randomized study. Optom Vis Sci. 2013;90:530–9. https://doi.org/10.1097/OPX.0b013e318293657d.
38. Chen C, Cheung SW, Cho P. Myopia control using toric orthokeratology (TO-SEE study). Invest Ophthalmol Vis Sci. 2013;54:6510–7. https://doi.org/10.1167/iovs.13-12527.
39. Swarbrick HA, Alharbi A, Watt K, et al. Myopia control during orthokeratology lens wear in children using a novel study design. Ophthalmology. 2015;122:620–30. https://doi.org/10.1016/j.ophtha.2014.09.028.

40. Santodomingo-Rubido J, Villa-Collar C, Gilmartin B, Gutiérrez-Ortega R. Factors preventing myopia progression with orthokeratology correction. Optom Vis Sci. 2013;90:1225–36. https://doi.org/10.1097/OPX.0000000000000034.
41. Kinoshita N, Konno Y, Hamada N, et al. Additive effects of orthokeratology and atropine 0.01% ophthalmic solution in slowing axial elongation in children with myopia: first year results. Jpn J Ophthalmol. 2018;62:544–53. https://doi.org/10.1007/s10384-018-0608-3.
42. Dart JK, Stapleton F, Minassian D. Contact lenses and other risk factors in microbial keratitis. Lancet. 1991;338:650–3.
43. Cheng KH, Leung SL, Hoekman HW, et al. Incidence of contact-lens-associated microbial keratitis and its related morbidity. Lancet. 1999;354:181–5. https://doi.org/10.1016/S0140-6736(98)09385-4.
44. Watt K, Swarbrick HA. Microbial keratitis in overnight orthokeratology: review of the first 50 cases. Eye Contact Lens. 2005;31:201–8.
45. Liu YM, Xie P. The safety of orthokeratology--a systematic review. Eye Contact Lens. 2016;42:35–42. https://doi.org/10.1097/ICL.0000000000000219.
46. Hiraoka T, Sekine Y, Okamoto F, et al. Safety and efficacy following 10-years of overnight orthokeratology for myopia control. Ophthalmic Physiol Opt. 2018;38:281–9. https://doi.org/10.1111/opo.12460.
47. Bullimore MA, Sinnott LT, Jones-Jordan LA. The risk of microbial keratitis with overnight corneal reshaping lenses. Optom Vis Sci. 2013;90:937–44. https://doi.org/10.1097/OPX.0b013e31829cac92.
48. Walline JJ, Gaume A, Jones LA, et al. Benefits of contact lens wear for children and teens. Eye Contact Lens. 2007;33:317–21. https://doi.org/10.1097/ICL.0b013e31804f80fb.
49. Rah MJ, Walline JJ, Jones-Jordan LA, et al. Vision specific quality of life of pediatric contact lens wearers. Optom Vis Sci. 2010;87:560–6. https://doi.org/10.1097/OPX.0b013e3181e6a1c8.
50. Walline JJ, Greiner KL, McVey ME, Jones-Jordan LA. Multifocal contact lens myopia control. Optom Vis Sci. 2013;90:1207–14. https://doi.org/10.1097/OPX.0000000000000036.
51. Pauné J, Queiros A, Quevedo L, et al. Peripheral myopization and visual performance with experimental rigid gas permeable and soft contact lens design. Cont Lens Anterior Eye. 2014;37:455–60. https://doi.org/10.1016/j.clae.2014.08.001.
52. Cheng X, Xu J, Chehab K, et al. Soft contact lenses with positive spherical aberration for myopia control. Optom Vis Sci. 2016;93:353–66. https://doi.org/10.1097/OPX.0000000000000773.
53. Anstice NS, Phillips JR. Effect of dual-focus soft contact lens wear on axial myopia progression in children. Ophthalmology. 2011;118:1152–61. https://doi.org/10.1016/j.ophtha.2010.10.035.
54. Lam CSY, Tang WC, DY-Y T, et al. Defocus incorporated soft contact (DISC) lens slows myopia progression in Hong Kong Chinese schoolchildren: a 2-year randomised clinical trial. Br J Ophthalmol. 2014;98:40–5. https://doi.org/10.1136/bjophthalmol-2013-303914.
55. Chamberlain P, Back A, Lazon P, et al. 3 year effectiveness of a dual-focus 1 day soft contact lens for myopia control. Cont Lens Anterior Eye. 2018;41:S71–2. https://doi.org/10.1016/j.clae.2018.03.097.
56. Ruiz-Pomeda A, Pérez-Sánchez B, Valls I, et al. MiSight Assessment Study Spain (MASS). A 2-year randomized clinical trial. Graefes Arch Clin Exp Ophthalmol. 2018;256:1011–21. https://doi.org/10.1007/s00417-018-3906-z.
57. Aller TA, Liu M, Wildsoet CF. Myopia control with bifocal contact lenses: a randomized clinical trial. Optom Vis Sci. 2016;93:344–52. https://doi.org/10.1097/OPX.0000000000000808.
58. Chua W-H, Balakrishnan V, Chan Y-H, et al. Atropine for the treatment of childhood myopia. Ophthalmology. 2006;113:2285–91. https://doi.org/10.1016/j.ophtha.2006.05.062.
59. Tong L, Huang XL, Koh ALT, et al. Atropine for the treatment of childhood myopia: effect on myopia progression after cessation of atropine. Ophthalmology. 2009;116:572–9. https://doi.org/10.1016/j.ophtha.2008.10.020.
60. Wu P-C, Yang Y-H, Fang P-C. The long-term results of using low-concentration atropine eye drops for controlling myopia progression in schoolchildren. J Ocul Pharmacol Ther. 2011;27:461–6. https://doi.org/10.1089/jop.2011.0027.

61. Chia A, Chua W-H, Cheung Y-B, et al. Atropine for the treatment of childhood myopia: safety and efficacy of 0.5%, 0.1%, and 0.01% doses (atropine for the treatment of myopia 2). Ophthalmology. 2012;119:347–54. https://doi.org/10.1016/j.ophtha.2011.07.031.
62. Clark TY, Clark RA. Atropine 0.01% eyedrops significantly reduce the progression of childhood myopia. J Ocul Pharmacol Ther. 2015;31:541–5. https://doi.org/10.1089/jop.2015.0043.
63. Schmid KL, Leyden K, Chiu Y, et al. Assessment of daily light and ultraviolet exposure in young adults. Optom Vis Sci. 2013;90:148–55. https://doi.org/10.1097/OPX.0b013e31827cda5b.
64. Wu P-C, Tsai C-L, Wu H-L, et al. Outdoor activity during class recess reduces myopia onset and progression in school children. Ophthalmology. 2013;120:1080–5. https://doi.org/10.1016/j.ophtha.2012.11.009.
65. Karouta C, Ashby RS. Correlation between light levels and the development of deprivation myopia. Invest Ophthalmol Vis Sci. 2014;56:299–309. https://doi.org/10.1167/iovs.14-15499.
66. Li W, Lan W, Yang S, et al. The effect of spectral property and intensity of light on natural refractive development and compensation to negative lenses in guinea pigs. Invest Ophthalmol Vis Sci. 2014;55:6324–32. https://doi.org/10.1167/iovs.13-13802.
67. Thorne HC, Jones KH, Peters SP, et al. Daily and seasonal variation in the spectral composition of light exposure in humans. Chronobiol Int. 2009;26:854–66. https://doi.org/10.1080/07420520903044315.
68. Foulds WS, Barathi VA, Luu CD. Progressive myopia or hyperopia can be induced in chicks and reversed by manipulation of the chromaticity of ambient light. Invest Ophthalmol Vis Sci. 2013;54:8004–12. https://doi.org/10.1167/iovs.13-12476.
69. Rucker F, Britton S, Spatcher M, Hanowsky S. Blue light protects against temporal frequency sensitive refractive changes. Invest Ophthalmol Vis Sci. 2015;56:6121–31. https://doi.org/10.1167/iovs.15-17238.
70. Torii H, Kurihara T, Seko Y, et al. Violet light exposure can be a preventive strategy against myopia progression. EBioMedicine. 2017;15:210–9. https://doi.org/10.1016/j.ebiom.2016.12.007.
71. Smith MJ, Walline JJ. Controlling myopia progression in children and adolescents. Adolesc Health Med Ther. 2015;6:133–40. https://doi.org/10.2147/AHMT.S55834.
72. Walline JJ. Myopia control: a review. Eye Contact Lens. 2016;42:3–8. https://doi.org/10.1097/ICL.0000000000000207.
73. Huang J, Wen D, Wang Q, et al. Efficacy comparison of 16 interventions for myopia control in children: a network meta-analysis. Ophthalmology. 2016;123:697–708. https://doi.org/10.1016/j.ophtha.2015.11.010.
74. Li S-M, Ji Y-Z, Wu S-S, et al. Multifocal versus single vision lenses intervention to slow progression of myopia in school-age children: a meta-analysis. Surv Ophthalmol. 2011;56:451–60. https://doi.org/10.1016/j.survophthal.2011.06.002.

Correction to: Optical Interventions for Myopia Control

Wing Chung Tang, Myra Leung, Angel C. K. Wong, Chi-ho To, and Carly S. Y. Lam

Correction to: M. Ang, T. Y. Wong (eds.), *Updates on Myopia*, https://doi.org/10.1007/978-981-13-8491-2_14

In the original version of Chapter 14, the chapter author name was wrongly given as Wing Chung Tang.

The name of the author should be Wing Chun Tang.

The updated online version of this chapter can be found at https://doi.org/10.1007/978-981-13-8491-2_14.

M. Ang, T. Y. Wong (eds.), *Updates on Myopia*,
https://doi.org/10.1007/978-981-13-8491-2_15

www.ingramcontent.com/pod-product-compliance
Lightning Source LLC
LaVergne TN
LVHW082117200926
848484LV00008B/1971
9781013274091

Diet and the Microbiome

At all stages of life, humans are associated with microorganisms and their products. Diet plays a crucial role in shaping the composition of the gut microbiome. Different dietary patterns, such as vegan, vegetarian, and omnivorous diets, result in distinct microbiome profiles. Recent research is rapidly strengthening the appreciation that associated microorganisms make essential contributions to human health and well-being. A low diversity of microorganisms is associated with a plethora of diseases including allergy, diabetes, obesity, arthritis, inflammatory bowel diseases, and even neuropsychiatric disorders. Thus, an interaction of microorganisms with the host immune system is required for a healthy body. The microbiome in humans is also not constant during lifespan but rather changes with age. Culture and location also have a profound impact on the microbiome. Diet is a particularly important factor in determining the microbiota composition of the gut. Thus, vegans, vegetarians, and omnivores have distinct microbiomes.

Sunil Thomas is a Research Professor at the Lankenau Institute for Medical Research in Wynnewood, Pennsylvania, where he leads interdisciplinary work spanning cell biology, microbiology, and translational medicine. His research focuses on next-generation immunotherapies for chronic conditions such as inflammatory bowel disease and Alzheimer's disease, with particular emphasis on how the human microbiome influences disease progression and treatment response.

Over his career, he has contributed to infectious disease research, vaccine development, and viral structural biology, helping advance diagnostics, therapeutics, and preventive strategies. He earned his Ph.D. in Environmental Biotechnology from Cochin University of Science and Technology in India and completed postdoctoral training at the Mount Sinai School of Medicine. He has authored over 70 peer-reviewed publications, contributed to books on vaccines and infectious diseases, and holds multiple patents.

Diet and the Microbiome

Edited by
Sunil Thomas

CRC Press
Taylor & Francis Group
Boca Raton London New York

CRC Press is an imprint of the
Taylor & Francis Group, an **informa** business

Designed cover image: Sunil Thomas

First edition published 2027
by CRC Press
2385 NW Executive Center Drive, Suite 320, Boca Raton FL 33431

and by CRC Press
4 Park Square, Milton Park, Abingdon, Oxon, OX14 4RN

CRC Press is an imprint of Taylor & Francis Group, LLC

ISBN: 978-1-041-06987-4 (hbk)
ISBN: 978-1-041-06988-1 (pbk)
ISBN: 978-1-003-63829-2 (ebk)

DOI: 10.1201/9781003638292

Typeset in Joanna
by Newgen Publishing UK

CONTENTS

PREFACE

Microorganisms represent the earliest and most enduring forms of life on Earth. Long before the emergence of complex multicellular organisms, microbial life shaped the planet's atmosphere, soils, waters, and biogeochemical cycles. Even today, all eukaryotic life—including plants, animals, and humans—remains fundamentally rooted in microbial ancestry. Modern eukaryotic cells themselves are conserved amalgamations of ancient microbial partnerships, a testament to the central role microorganisms have played in the evolution of life.

Higher organisms cannot exist in isolation from microorganisms. From plants drawing nutrients through symbiotic soil microbes to animals relying on gut bacteria for digestion, microorganisms are indispensable partners in survival. The collective community of microorganisms that inhabit a host or environment is known as the microbiome.These microbial communities are not passive inhabitants; rather, they form dynamic, interactive systems that profoundly influence the health, development, and resilience of their hosts.

The microbiome—comprising trillions of bacteria, archaea, fungi, viruses, and protozoa—acts much like a vital organ. In humans and animals, it supports digestion, synthesizes essential vitamins, regulates metabolism, trains the immune system to distinguish friend from foe, and influences inflammation, behavior, mood, and disease susceptibility. In plants, the microbiome enhances nutrient uptake, improves stress tolerance, and protects against pathogens. Microbial diversity is a defining feature of a healthy microbiome, conferring stability and adaptability to changing conditions.

Beneficial microorganisms produce a wide array of secondary metabolites that are critical for maintaining physiological balance and overall well-being. When this balance is disrupted—a condition known as dysbiosis—the consequences can be severe. Dysbiosis has been linked to infections, allergies, autoimmune diseases, metabolic disorders, reduced crop productivity, and even neurological and behavioral conditions. Understanding the mechanisms that govern microbial balance is therefore essential for advancing health, agriculture, and environmental sustainability.

Recent breakthroughs in high-throughput sequencing, metagenomics, and bioinformatics have revolutionized microbiome research. These technologies allow rapid identification and functional analysis of microbial communities associated with different hosts, diets, environments, and lifestyles. What once took decades to uncover can now be achieved in a fraction of the time, opening new frontiers in medicine, nutrition, agriculture, ecology, and biotechnology.

The six interconnected volumes listed below present a comprehensive exploration of microbial life across biological systems and ecosystems:

Volume 1: The Human Microbiome

Volume 2: Diet and the Microbiome

Volume 3: Animal Microbiomes

Volume 4: Plant Microbiomes

Volume 5: Insect Microbiomes

Volume 6: The Environmental Microbiome

Together, these volumes provide an integrated perspective on how microbial communities shape life on Earth.

I extend my sincere and heartfelt gratitude to all the authors who contributed chapters to this book series. Their expertise, dedication, and scholarly insight form the foundation of these volumes. Each contribution reflects a commitment to scientific rigor and a shared passion for advancing knowledge in the rapidly evolving field of microbiome research.

The collective efforts of these authors have enriched the depth, breadth, and quality of this series, transforming it into a comprehensive and authoritative resource. Their willingness to share ideas, collaborate across disciplines, and invest their time and intellect has been invaluable. This work stands as a testament to their contributions, and I am deeply thankful for their role in bringing this series to fruition.

This year marks the 100th anniversary of the Lankenau Institute for Medical Research. The anniversary represents decades of unwavering commitment to scientific inquiry, education, and the advancement of medical knowledge. The Lankenau Institute for Medical Research has played a pivotal role in shaping and supporting my scientific endeavors. Its culture of intellectual rigor, encouragement, and dedication to research excellence has provided an environment in which curiosity could thrive, and ideas could evolve into meaningful scientific contributions.

This six-volume Microbiome book series is presented as a tribute to the Lankenau Institute for Medical Research. It stands as a testament to the Institute's enduring legacy, its profound impact on generations of researchers, and its mission to advance science for the betterment of human health and society. Through this work, I honor its past achievements, acknowledge its present influence, and celebrate its continued inspiration for future scientific discovery.

CONTRIBUTORS

SUGATO BANERJEE
Department of Pharmacology and Toxicology
National Institute of Pharmaceutical Education and Research
Kolkata, West Bengal, India

VALENTINA BIAGIOLI
Department of Neurosciences, Rehabilitation, Ophthalmology, Genetics, Maternal and Child Health
University of Genoa
Genoa, Italy
Microbiota International Clinical Society (MICS)
Turin, Italy

PATRICIA MARTINS BOCK
Department of Physiology and Postgraduate Program in Pharmacology and Therapeutics
Federal University of Rio Grande do Sul (UFRGS)
Santa Cecilia, Porto Alegre-RS, Brazil

TATIANA DIACOVA
UCLA Center for Human Nutrition
University of California
Los Angeles, California, USA

GOPAL KHODVE
Department of Pharmacology and Toxicology
National Institute of Pharmaceutical Education and Research
Kolkata, West Bengal, India

CHARMY R. KOTHARI
Department of Biotechnology
Christ College, Gujarat, India

RAMESH K. KOTHARI
Department of Biosciences
Saurashtra University
Gujarat, India

MAURÍCIO DA SILVA KRAUSE
Department of Physiology
Federal University of Rio Grande do Sul (UFRGS)
Santa Cecilia, Porto Alegre – RS, Brazil

ZHAOPING LI
UCLA Center for Human Nutrition
University of California
Los Angeles, California, USA

LEIDIANE DE MEDEIROS OLIVEIRA LIMA
Postgraduate Program in Pharmacology and Therapeutics
Federal University of Rio Grande do Sul (UFRGS)
Brazil

OLIVIA LUTZ
Lankenau Institute for Medical Research
Wynnewood, Pennsylvania, USA

ALEX MUPPASANI
Lankenau Institute for Medical Research
Wynnewood, Pennsylvania, USA

KINJAL J. PARMAR
Department of Biosciences
Saurashtra University
Gujarat, India

SUPARNA ROY SARKAR
Department of Pharmaceutical Sciences and Technology
Birla Institute of Technology—Mesra
Ranchi, Jharkhand, India

PASQUALE STRIANO
Department of Neurosciences, Rehabilitation, Ophthalmology, Genetics, Maternal and Child Health
University of Genoa
Genoa, Italy
Pediatric Neurology and Muscular Diseases Unit
Genoa, Italy

SUNIL THOMAS
Lankenau Institute for Medical Research
Wynnewood, Pennsylvania, USA

GABRIEL MAYER TOSSI
Postgraduate Program in Physiology
Federal University of Rio Grande do Sul (UFRGS)
Santa Cecilia, Porto Alegre-RS, Brazil

CHAPTER 1

Feeding the Microbiome

HOW DIET SHAPES HUMAN HEALTH

Valentina Biagioli and Pasquale Striano

1.1 FROM BREAST MILK TO ADULT HEALTH: HOW FOOD COMMUNICATES WITH BACTERIA

At birth, we come into contact with a microcosm invisible to the eye, yet one that will accompany us for the rest of our lives: the microbiota. Physiologically, newborns have an immature intestinal mucosa and immune system, allowing them to feed exclusively on breast milk (Dominguez-Bello et al., 2010). Human milk not only serves a purely nutritional function but also represents a veritable treasure trove of bioactive substances that modulate and guide intestinal and immune system maturation (Biagioli, Volpedo, et al., 2024; Xu et al., 2025). Breastfeeding should therefore be exclusive until the infant is 6 months old, after which the first solid foods should be gradually introduced. Early weaning is not recommended, as only from the sixth month onward is the infant able to adequately absorb solid foods, thanks to a progressive reduction in breast milk intake and the gradual introduction of the first solid nutrients (Barends et al., 2013; D'Auria et al., 2018). This slow transition from milk to solid food is a significant event for all the bacteria that colonize the infant's gut, which will undergo the greatest change in their gut microbiota, from the infantile microbial trajectory to the adult stage (Dominguez-Bello et al., 2016; Hickman et al., 2024; Ma et al., 2020). This transition will be complete around age 4 and will then stabilize until adulthood. Complementary feeding, defined by the World Health Organization (WHO), is the administration of any food or beverage in addition to milk when breast milk or formula alone is no longer adequate to meet the infant's nutritional needs. This age group also coincides with a developmental period in which children must learn to accept healthy foods and beverages and establish long-term dietary patterns. This developmental stage is also the one most at risk for stunted growth, delayed psychomotor development, nutritional deficiencies, morbidity, and mortality (Borghi et al., 2024; Calcaterra et al., 2023). The first two years of life are also a critical period for the development of the brain, higher cognitive functions, vision and hearing, and language acquisition. Recent estimates by UNICEF (United Nations Children's Fund), WHO, and the World Bank on child malnutrition indicate that globally, stunting, wasting, and overweight affect 22.3% (148 million), 6.8% (45 million), and 5.6% (37 million) of boys and girls under five years of age, respectively (de Onis & Branca, 2016).

With complementary feeding, there is a gradual increase in the consumption of plant fiber and animal proteins, and a reduction in breast milk consumption. This translates into a progressive reduction in the predominance of bifidogenic species, such as *Lactobacillaceae* and Enterobacteriaceae, and an increase in bacteria typical of the adult gut microbiota, including Ruminococcaceae, *Akkermansia muciniphila*, *Bacteroides*, and Firmicutes

DOI: 10.1201/9781003638292-1

(Ding et al., 2025). These microorganisms are capable of fermenting more complex substrates, introduced with the new solid diet.

As the microbiota matures, bacterial diversity increases significantly: Firmicutes and Bacteroidetes account for approximately 95% of the total, while phyla such as Actinobacteria and Proteobacteria, prevalent during the neonatal period, decline. Stewart et al. (2018), through a longitudinal analysis, highlighted how the introduction of the first solid foods leads to an increase in microbial biodiversity, with positive effects also on immune and metabolic development. These results underscore the importance of offering a varied diet rich in different solid foods from an early age to promote a balanced and resilient microbiota. A diversified diet, in fact, helps maintain the homeostasis of the intestinal microbial consortium. Microbiota-accessible carbohydrates such as resistant starches, fructooligosaccharides (FOS), galactooligosaccharides (GOS), and inulin, present in seasonal fruits and vegetables, stimulate the growth of *Lactobacillus*, *Bacteroides*, and *Bifidobacterium* (Grüber et al., 2015; Okburan & Kızıler, 2023; W. Zhang et al., 2024). These bacteria produce short-chain fatty acids (SCFAs), which are essential for the health of the intestinal mucosa and the maintenance of eubiosis. Protein-rich foods, such as meat, eggs, and dairy products, on the other hand, favor bacteria with proteolytic activity, such as *Clostridium*, *Streptococcus*, and *Hafnia*. The latter, widely used in the dairy industry, is currently a subject of scientific interest for its potential role as a precision probiotic in modulating hunger–satiety mechanisms (Ramos-Vivas, 2020). Dietary variety, therefore, is not only a matter of nutritional balance but also a means of promoting a diverse and functional microbial composition, in which each bacterial phylum contributes specific metabolic and fermentative activities.

The complementary feeding phase is therefore crucial not only for the formation of the microbiota but also for the child's future nutritional education. The development of the senses of taste and smell begins in the fetal period: the olfactory bulbs are functional around the 24th week of gestation. The ingestion of amniotic fluid allows the fetus to perceive the aromas and flavors derived from the mother's diet. The same phenomenon is repeated during breastfeeding, as the aromatic substances ingested with the mother's diet are transferred into the milk, contributing to its "flavoring." This early exposure to flavors influences the food preferences of newborns when solid foods are introduced (Mennella et al., 2001; Mennella & Beauchamp, 1991). Eating habits acquired in early childhood profoundly influence not only the intestinal microbiota, but also long-term metabolic health. Gracner et al. (2024) analyzed, using data from the UK Biobank, the effects of sugar rationing that occurred in the United Kingdom during the Second World War on individuals exposed in utero and in the first thousand days of life. The results indicate that lower sugar intake during this critical growth phase had a protective effect against cardiovascular disease, hypertension, and type 2 diabetes.

In summary, the gut microbiota and the formation of taste preferences are primarily determined perinatally and during the first year of life. This time window represents a crucial moment for microbial, metabolic, and immune development, and for the child's overall long-term health.

1.1.1 The Gut Microbiome as a Key Metabolic Organ

The set of microbial communities colonizing the human gastrointestinal tract can now be considered a fully fledged metabolic system functionally integrated into host homeostasis. Beyond its mere digestive function, the gut microbiome plays an active role in the transformation, modulation, and systemic distribution of metabolic signals, participating in the regulation of key processes such as energy balance, lipid and carbohydrate metabolism, chronic low-grade inflammation, and insulin sensitivity (Kwon et al., 2024; Nohesara et al., 2025; Siddiqui et al., 2025; Zhu et al., 2013).

Biochemically, the microbiota substantially expands the metabolic repertoire of the human body, enabling the transformation of dietary substrates indigestible by host enzymes into a wide range of biologically active metabolites. Among these, SCFAs such as acetate, propionate, and butyrate, microbial bile acid derivatives, indoles, and other products of aromatic amino acid metabolism represent central mediators of communication between the intestinal lumen and peripheral compartments (Macfarlane & Macfarlane, 2003). For this scientific rationale, it is no longer sufficient to focus on what an individual eats, but rather on how the microbiota metabolizes it for them. The study by Shimizu et al. (2025) identified *Streptococcus salivarius* as a commensal bacterium with distinctive anti-obesity properties. The results indicate that *S. salivarius* is able to prevent obesity induced by high sucrose intake in male mice through the exopolysaccharide (EPS)–SCFA–carbohydrate metabolic axis. Specifically, *S. salivarius* strains derived from healthy human donors produced high levels of EPS from sucrose, but not from other sugars. Comparative analysis also showed that the abundance of *S. salivarius* is significantly reduced in obese donors compared to healthy donors, with attenuation of the EPS–SCFA metabolism of carbohydrates. These data highlight a fundamental interaction between host and commensal bacteria in glycometabolism, which regulates energy balance, and suggest that EPS-producing bacteria and their metabolites may represent a promising target for preventing lifestyle-related diseases.

Microbial products (metabolites) not only perform local energy functions but also act as ligands for specific cellular receptors, modulating endocrine, immune, and neurometabolic signaling pathways. In this sense, the microbiome can be conceptualized as a "distributed metabolic organ," lacking a defined anatomical structure but endowed with a regulatory capacity comparable to that of classic endocrine organs. Evidence from germ-free models, microbiota transplant studies, and multi-omic analyses in humans demonstrates that qualitative and quantitative alterations in gut microbial communities are associated with profound changes in dietary energy extraction efficiency, plasma lipid composition, and glycemic regulation (Turnbaugh et al., 2006; Wang et al., 2016; Zeevi et al., 2015a). These observations strengthen the hypothesis that the microbiome contributes causally, rather than merely associatively, to the pathophysiology of obesity, type 2 diabetes, and metabolic syndrome (Fasano, 2025).

1.1.2 Integration of the Gut Microbiome with the Enteroendocrine Signaling Axis

The gut is the largest endocrine organ in the human body, thanks to the presence of a highly specialized population of enteroendocrine cells (EECs) dispersed throughout the intestinal epithelium (Latorre et al., 2016; Sun et al., 2019). These cells, despite constituting a minimal fraction of the total epithelial count, orchestrate a complex hormonal signaling network that connects the luminal environment to the central nervous system and peripheral metabolic organs. EECs act as multimodal chemical sensors, capable of simultaneously detecting nutrients derived from digestion and metabolites produced by the gut microbiome. In response to these stimuli, they secrete a broad spectrum of hormones and neuropeptides, glucagon-like peptide-1 (GLP-1), peptide YY (PYY), glucose-dependent insulinotropic polypeptide (GIP), cholecystokinin (CCK), and serotonin, which modulate insulin secretion, gastrointestinal motility, hunger–satiety sensation, and energy distribution (Amaro et al., 2022; Schneeberger et al., 2015).

A crucial aspect of this regulation lies in the functional interaction between the microbiome and EECs. Microbial metabolites, including SCFAs, activate G protein–coupled receptors, particularly free fatty acid receptor 2 (FFAR2) and free fatty acid receptor 3 (FFAR3), inducing the secretion of incretin and anorectic hormones (O'Riordan et al., 2022). Similarly, the microbial transformation of primary bile acids into secondary forms alters the activation profiles of farnesoid X receptor (FXR) and the G protein–coupled receptor TGR5 (Takeda G protein–coupled receptor 5), influencing glucose and lipid metabolism and energy expenditure (Chiang & Ferrell, 2020).

This signaling system does not operate in isolation but integrates with the gut–brain axis via neural and hormonal pathways, contributing to central regulation of appetite and eating behavior. Peripheral signals generated by the interaction between diet and the microbiome are integrated at the hypothalamic level, where they modulate neuronal circuits sensitive to the body's energy status (Rusch et al., 2023).

Taken together, these interactions delineate a functional continuum from digestion to systemic endocrine regulation, placing the gut microbiome at the center of a communication network that coordinates nutrient sensing, hormonal response, and metabolic adaptation (Qi et al., 2021). Understanding these mechanisms provides a fundamental interpretative key to explaining how dietary and environmental factors can translate into persistent alterations in metabolic homeostasis and the risk of chronic diseases.

1.1.3 How Diet Shapes the Gut Microbiome

Diet can be defined as the set of dietary choices that characterize an individual's food and beverage consumption over time. It represents one of the main environmental factors influencing the composition and function of the gut microbiome. Differences in dietary habits contribute significantly to interindividual variability in microbial communities, with potential health implications (Biagioli et al., 2025; Kolodziejczyk et al., 2019a). To fully understand these relationships, however, it is necessary to move beyond a reductionist approach that considers diet solely in terms of macronutrients (carbohydrates, lipids, and proteins). A truly informative analysis must instead address the quality of these components, such as the type of carbohydrates, lipids, and protein sources, as well as the degree and method of food processing, the frequency of consumption, and the timing of intake (Adhikari et al., 2022; Comerford et al., 2021; Shan et al., 2019). Only by adopting an integrated view, which conceives of diet as a complex and dynamic system, is it possible to fully grasp the interactions between nutrition, gut microbiota, and host health (Figure 1.1). From this perspective, the multilevel analysis of food data, which includes overall dietary patterns, individual foods, and nutritional components, allows us to better understand the complexity of the interactions between diet and the gut microbiome (Troisi et al., 2020).

Analyzing the diet as a whole is particularly relevant because foods are consumed in combination, and their biological effects cannot be interpreted as the simple sum of their individual nutrients. This approach has led to growing interest in the role of dietary patterns in modulating the gut microbiome and, consequently, health.

The gut microbiome is capable of responding to both acute and sustained dietary changes. Intervention studies indicate that short-term dietary changes can induce rapid changes in the composition and function of the microbiome, often observable within a few days or weeks (Wu et al., 2011; Zeevi et al., 2015b). These rapid responses reflect the high plasticity of gut microbial communities. In contrast, prolonged dietary interventions tend to result in more

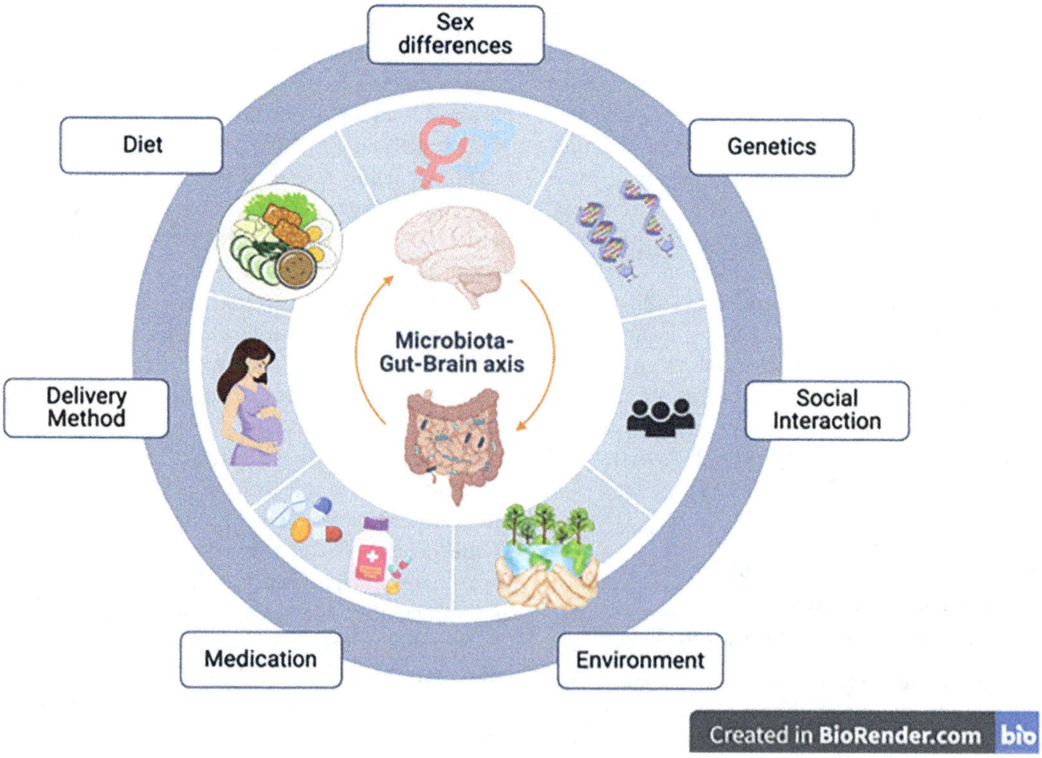

Figure 1.1 The microbiota–gut–brain axis as a dynamic system shaped by diet, host-related, environmental, and social factors within a One Health framework.

modest changes in the overall structure of the microbiome, suggesting the existence of stability and resilience mechanisms. This does not, however, exclude persistent changes in the abundance of specific microorganisms, which can have a significant impact on host metabolism and long-term health. The differences between short- and long-term responses can be explained by the intensity of the initial dietary changes and the difficulty of maintaining high adherence to modified diets over prolonged periods (David et al., 2014; Wu et al., 2011).

An additional element of complexity is the temporal dimension of nutrition. The gut microbiome follows daily oscillations synchronized with the host's circadian rhythms, which regulate fundamental physiological processes such as digestion, metabolism, and immune response. Alterations in sleep–wake rhythms or feeding–fasting cycles can interfere with these oscillations, with potential negative health consequences (Abdollahpour et al., 2025; Bashore et al., 2025).

1.1.4 Dietary Components and Food Groups in Relation to the Gut Microbiome

Alongside the analysis of overall dietary patterns, the study of individual food categories has provided important insights into the relationships between diet and the microbiome. Some observational studies conducted in diverse populations show that regular consumption of fruits, vegetables, and whole grains is generally associated with greater microbial diversity (García-Vega et al., 2020; Wang et al., 2023). Conversely, diets characterized by a high intake of ultra-processed foods (UPFs), sugary drinks, fried foods, and red or processed meats tend to be associated with lower gut microbiome diversity, promoting an "industrial" microbial signature that is far from supporting host health (Khoury et al., 2024; Więckowska-Gacek et al., 2021).

Taken together, these findings reflect the following: diets rich in plant-based, minimally processed foods are associated with greater microbial diversity and better health indicators, while dietary patterns typical of Western diets show the opposite associations. However, further detailed study of the associations between foods and microorganisms remains necessary, considering differences within food categories and specificities at the microbial species, strain, and function levels.

In this context, the international standardization and harmonization of dietary data represent a crucial step to effectively integrate nutritional information into microbiome studies and to translate scientific evidence into increasingly targeted and contextualized nutritional recommendations.

1.1.5 Mediterranean Diet: A Model of Microbial Resilience

The first study of the world's most studied and renowned diet came to light thanks to Ancel Keys, an American physiologist. In the 1950s, through the epidemiological study "Seven Countries Study," he observed that populations in southern Italy, particularly in the Cilento region, had low rates of cardiovascular disease and above-average longevity (KEYS et al., 1986). Keys attributed these results to a diet rich in monounsaturated fats, such as olive oil, and low in saturated fat, along with a moderate consumption of fish, legumes, fruits, and vegetables. This diet, combined with an active lifestyle and strong social bonds, became known as the Mediterranean diet. In 2010, UNESCO provided an expanded definition of the Mediterranean diet, recognizing it as "a set of skills, knowledge, practices, and traditions that extend from field to fork, including cultivation, harvesting, fishing, preservation, preparation, and consumption of food" (Bonaccio et al., 2022). This dietary pattern emphasizes, first and foremost, the consumption of fruits, vegetables, whole grains, legumes, fish, extra virgin olive oil, and nuts. It is low in red meat, UPFs, and refined sugars. It promotes the growth of bacteria such as *Faecalibacterium prausnitzii*, a key producer of butyrate, contributing to the reduction of oxidative stress and chronic inflammation. The high presence of polyphenols, monounsaturated fatty acids (MUFAs), and omega-3s makes this dietary pattern a cornerstone for promoting intestinal and systemic health (Tsigalou et al., 2024).

The PREDIMED study (Estruch et al., 2018), a multicenter trial conducted in Spain among 7447 participants at high cardiovascular risk (aged 55–80, 57% women) but without cardiovascular disease at enrollment, compared three dietary regimens: a Mediterranean diet enriched with extra virgin olive oil, a Mediterranean diet enriched with nuts, and a control diet (low-fat). The primary endpoint was a major cardiovascular event (heart attack, stroke, or cardiovascular death). The results showed a significant reduction in cardiovascular risk with both variants of the Mediterranean diet: HR 0.69 (95% CI, 0.53–0.91) for extra virgin olive oil and HR 0.72 (95% CI, 0.54–0.95) for nuts, compared to the control group. These results confirm the effectiveness of the Mediterranean diet, enriched with extra virgin olive oil or nuts, in the primary prevention of cardiovascular events. Furthermore, the cross-sectional observational study by De Filippis et al. (2016) analyzed the role of diet in modulating the composition of the gut microbiota and the associated metabolomic profile. To this end, daily dietary data were collected, and the gut microbiota and metabolome were analyzed in 153 individuals who consistently followed omnivorous, vegetarian, or vegan diets. Most vegetarians and vegans, as well as approximately 30% of omnivores, had a high adherence to the Mediterranean diet. Participants were stratified both by diet type and degree of adherence to the Mediterranean diet, based on their dietary patterns and associated microbiota characteristics. The analysis highlighted a significant relationship between plant-based diets and increased fecal levels of SCFAs, as well as a greater abundance of *Prevotella* and some Firmicutes involved in the degradation of dietary fiber. Conversely, higher urinary levels of trimethylamine N-oxide (TMAO) were found in subjects with lower adherence to the Mediterranean diet.

Current scientific evidence emphasizes that the benefits of the Mediterranean diet derive from the overall combination of healthy foods rather than the isolated effect of individual nutrients. In other words, adopting the entire dietary pattern produces a greater protective effect than consuming individual foods or nutrients individually.

1.1.6 Western Diet and Loss of Microbial Biodiversity

In recent decades, the diets of industrialized populations have undergone a profound transformation, characterized by the emergence of energy-dense foods low in fresh plant foods. The so-called Western diet is characterized by high caloric intake, an abundance of animal proteins, saturated fats, simple sugars, and industrially processed foods, combined with an insufficient consumption of fiber, fruits, and vegetables. This nutritional structure significantly impacts the composition and function of the gut microbiome, contributing to a reorganization of microbial communities with systemic consequences (Agus et al., 2016; Horner et al., 2025; Więckowska-Gacek et al., 2021).

One of the most consistently observed effects is the reduction in microbial diversity, considered a key indicator of gut ecosystem health. In this context, the microbiome tends to assume a structure dominated by taxa adapted to a high availability of easily assimilated nutrients, such as some species belonging to the genus *Bacteroides*. Alongside these, other bacterial groups are also frequently increased, including *Alistipes*, *Blautia*, and *Bilophila*, whose relative abundance reflects adaptation to an intestinal environment shaped by a diet high in fat and low in fermentable fiber (Heiman & Greenway, 2016; Malesza et al., 2021; Yang et al., 2023).

Dietary fiber deficiency is a key element of this process. Fiber is one of the main sources of substrates for microbial fermentation and the production of SCFAs, molecules essential for maintaining the integrity of the intestinal barrier, modulating immune responses, and regulating energy metabolism. Reduced fiber availability limits these protective functions and promotes a state of chronic, low-grade inflammation (Gibson et al., 2017; Koh et al., 2016a).

UPF foods play a particularly critical role in the Western diet. These products are not only characterized by their high sugar, salt, and fat content, but also, above all, by the presence of ingredients typical of industrial processing, such as emulsifiers, thickeners, preservatives, flavorings, and colorings (Khoury et al., 2024; Lane et al., 2022; Mengist et al., 2025; Rondinella et al., 2025). The European Food Safety Authority (EFSA) has authorized several non-caloric artificial sweeteners (NAS), including acesulfame potassium (E-950), aspartame (E-951), cyclamate (E-952), saccharin (E-954), sucralose (E-955), and neotame (E-961) (Mortensen, 2006). However, a recent systematic review of human and animal studies found that the consumption of these artificial sweeteners, including acesulfame potassium, aspartame, saccharin, sucralose, cyclamate, and neotame, is associated with changes in the composition of the gut microbiota, promoting dysbiosis and a reduction in gut biodiversity (Cao et al., 2020).

Emulsifiers, widely present in industrial products such as sauces, puddings, margarines, and ice cream, and particularly common in the Western diet, are amphiphilic molecules used in the food industry both to facilitate technological processes and to improve the consistency and shelf life of processed foods. Recently, Elmén et al. (2020) analyzed the in vitro effects of different emulsifiers, such as glycerol monoacetate, glycerol monostearate, glycerol monolaurate, propylene glycol monostearate, and sodium stearoyl lactylate, on the fecal microbiota. They found that exposure to sodium stearoyl lactylate (0.025% in aqueous solution) resulted in a reduction in the Clostridiaceae, Lachnospiraceae, and Ruminococcaceae families, accompanied by an increase in the abundance of Bacteroidaceae and Enterobacteriaceae.

These substances are therefore capable of directly or indirectly interfering with the gut microbiome, altering its composition, metabolic function, and interaction with the intestinal epithelium. The widespread distribution of these foods has contributed to the emergence of an "industrialized" microbiome, adapted to a nutritional environment profoundly different from that in which the human species evolved. Overall, habitual consumption of UPF has been linked to an increased risk of obesity, metabolic disorders, cardiovascular disease, and chronic inflammatory conditions, suggesting the involvement of the microbiome as a biological mediator of these effects (Khoury et al., 2024).

Another characteristic of the Western diet is its high intake of red meat and animal products. These foods introduce compounds such as choline and carnitine, which can be metabolized by the gut microbiota into trimethylamine and subsequently converted by the liver into TMAO, a metabolite associated with an increased risk of cardiovascular and metabolic diseases (Budoff et al., 2025; Canyelles et al., 2023). This example highlights how the interaction between specific dietary components and microbial metabolism can generate biologically active molecules with significant systemic effects. However, the potential negative impact of red meat on health is not attributable to its consumption per se, but rather to excessive and inadequately balanced intake within the overall dietary context. In particular, a diet characterized by a high meat intake and a low consumption of plant-based foods, rich in fiber, can promote alterations in the gut microbiota and associated metabolic processes. Conversely, an adequate intake of dietary fiber appears to play a protective role, modulating the effects of meat on the composition and function of the gut microbiota and attenuating the potential adverse effects associated with diets high in animal protein (Rinninella et al., 2023).

Another important factor concerns the preparation and cooking methods of meat. High-temperature cooking methods, such as grilling or frying, are associated with the formation of potentially harmful compounds, such as heterocyclic amines and polycyclic aromatic hydrocarbons, while more controlled cooking techniques at moderate temperatures can reduce the production of these substances while preserving the nutritional quality of the food (Adeyeye et al., 2025).

Finally, meat quality is a key factor in assessing its impact on health. Meat from animals raised in extensive systems and fed primarily on grass (grass-fed) generally has a more favorable lipid profile, with a higher presence of polyunsaturated fatty acids, particularly omega-3, and a higher content of bioactive compounds (Davis et al., 2022). Therefore, the consumption of high-quality meat, included in a balanced, fiber-rich diet, and combined with appropriate cooking methods, should not be considered intrinsically harmful, but rather evaluated within a comprehensive dietary approach (Geiker et al., 2021).

Within this framework, excessive salt consumption also deserves particular attention. In addition to its well-known effects on blood pressure and cardiovascular health, high sodium intake has been associated with changes in the composition of the gut microbiome and a reduction in specific beneficial bacterial groups (Elmén et al., 2020; Hammer et al., 2017). Experimental studies suggest that salt can influence the activity of the intestinal immune system, promoting pro-inflammatory responses and altering the balance between commensal and potentially pathogenic microorganisms. In this sense, salt is not only a direct risk factor but also an indirect modulator of the intestinal ecosystem and systemic inflammation (Miranda et al., 2018; Wang et al., 2024).

Taken together, these elements paint a coherent picture in which the Western diet, through high consumption of UPF, poor-quality red meat, salt, and a lack of fiber and plant-based foods, contributes to a less diverse and functionally altered microbiome. This configuration promotes a state of chronic, low-grade inflammation, which represents a common basis for the development of numerous non-communicable diseases.

In light of the available evidence, it is clear that overall dietary quality, rather than individual nutrients, is a key determinant of gut microbiome health. Nutritional strategies aimed at reducing UPFs, limiting salt intake, and increasing consumption of fiber-rich plant foods can help preserve microbial biodiversity and support a more balanced interaction between the microbiome and the host, with potential long-term benefits for human health.

1.1.7 Plant-Based Diet and Gut Microbiota

Plant-based diets (PBDs) are attracting growing interest for their potential benefits on human health. Numerous studies have analyzed the impact of PBDs on the composition and function of the gut microbiota, highlighting their role in modulating host metabolic and immune processes.

PBDs are predominantly based on the consumption of plant-based foods. A vegan diet completely excludes all animal products and consists exclusively of fiber-rich foods, such as fruits, vegetables, grains, legumes, nuts, and seeds. A vegetarian diet, on the other hand, eliminates meat and meat products but may include, to varying degrees, other animal-based foods such as eggs and dairy products. The high content of dietary fiber, polyphenols, and other bioactive compounds characteristic of PBDs selectively promotes the growth of beneficial gut bacteria, particularly those involved in the production of SCFAs (Tomova et al., 2019; Xiao et al., 2022). Since the human body lacks the enzymes necessary for the fermentation of complex carbohydrates, this function is performed by intestinal microorganisms, which express specific enzymes, such as propionate CoA-transferase and propionaldehyde dehydratase, allowing the conversion of carbohydrates into SCFAs. In the gastrointestinal tract, over 95% of SCFAs are acetate, propionate, and butyrate. Acetate is produced mainly by bacteria belonging to the phylum Bacteroidetes and genera such as *Lactobacillus*, *Bifidobacterium*, *Akkermansia*, *Bacteroides*, *Prevotella*, *Ruminococcus*, and *Streptococcus* (Dalile et al., 2019; Macfarlane & Macfarlane, 2003). Propionate is synthesized by various taxa, including *Phascolarctobacterium*, *Bacteroides*, *Dialister*, *Veillonella*, and *Roseburia*, via the succinate, acrylate, and propanediol pathways (Koh et al., 2016b). Butyrate is produced primarily by bacteria such as *F. prausnitzii*, *Roseburia* spp., *Eubacterium rectale*, and *Anaerostipes caccae*, through the butyryl-CoA and phosphotransbutyrylase/butyrate kinase pathways (Louis et al., 2010; Stoeva et al., 2021).

However, some evidence suggests that inadequately planned PBD may be associated with an increased risk of nutritional deficiencies, particularly of vitamin B12, vitamin D, iron, calcium, zinc, and long-chain omega-3 fatty acids (EPA and DHA) (Chouraqui, 2023). These deficiencies can negatively impact the balance of the gut microbiota and, consequently, the host's overall health through alterations in the metabolome. Furthermore, the consumption of raw or minimally processed plant foods introduces environmental and plant-associated microorganisms into the intestinal tract, which can temporarily or permanently alter the diversity and functionality of the microbiota (Berg et al., 2025). It should also be considered that the use of antibiotics and pesticides in agricultural practices can promote the spread of antibiotic-resistant bacteria, potentially attenuating the beneficial effects of PBDs (Manyi-Loh et al., 2018). In this context, the importance of not only the quantity of plant-based foods consumed, but also their quality, emerges once again, suggesting that the consumption of organic and locally sourced plant-based foods can further contribute to favorably modulating the gut microbiota and metabolic profile, thanks to a lower content of chemical residues and a higher density of bioactive compounds.

A large-scale metagenomic study conducted by Fackelmann et al. (2025) analyzed the association between dietary patterns (omnivorous, vegetarian, and vegan) and gut microbiota composition in a population of 21,561 individuals belonging to five independent multinational cohorts. The results show that red meat consumption is associated with the enrichment of bacterial species such as *Ruminococcus torques*, *Bilophila wadsworthia*, and *Alistipes putredinis*, which were negatively correlated with indicators of host cardiometabolic health. In contrast, vegan diets are characterized by specific microbial signatures associated with more favorable cardiometabolic profiles. The study also highlights a partial overlap between the gut microbiota and the microbiome of consumed foods, particularly with regard to dairy-derived microorganisms (e.g., *Streptococcus thermophilus*) and bacteria typically found in soil, which are more represented in vegan subjects. PBDs can therefore influence the microbiome not only indirectly, through the food substrates provided, but also directly, through the introduction of microbial communities derived from the foods themselves. For this reason, it is important to highlight how the microbiomes of the rhizosphere, endosphere, and phyllosphere are closely interconnected and constitute an essential ecological continuum for the human food chain (Anand et al., 2026). Therefore, the adoption of sustainable agricultural practices, characterized by a reduction in the use of fertilizers and antibiotics, represents a benefit not only for environmental protection but also for the maintenance of human and microbial health.

Overall, these observations underscore the biological continuity between soil, plants, humans, and the microbiota, indicating that the health of soil, ecosystems, and the planet is a fundamental prerequisite for human health and the balance of the human intestinal microbiota.

1.1.8 Special Diets: Metabolic and Microbial Impacts

The very low–carbohydrate ketogenic diet (KD) (VLCKD) is a nutritional approach introduced in the 1920s as a treatment for drug-resistant epilepsy and, in recent years, has attracted growing interest as a therapeutic strategy for obesity and metabolic diseases (De Giorgis et al., 2023). Due to its unique nutritional characteristics, the impact of VLCKD on the composition and function of the intestinal microbiota has become a topic of increasing relevance. VLCKD is characterized by a severe restriction of carbohydrates, equal to 5–10% of total energy intake or less than 50 g/day, to stimulate the endogenous production of ketone bodies (De Giorgis et al., 2023). Recent evidence suggests potential benefits of VLCKD in neurological disorders such as autism spectrum disorder (ASD), Alzheimer's disease, glucose transporter type 1 deficiency syndrome, and autoimmune multiple sclerosis (Pietrzak et al., 2022).

Due to its highly restrictive nature, more flexible variants have been developed, including the modified Atkins diet (MAD) and the low-glycemic index diet (LGID) (Gauthier et al., 2020; Zafar et al., 2019). These approaches show comparable efficacy in controlling epileptic seizures, but with better tolerability and a lower incidence of side effects (De Giorgis et al., 2023). Compared to the MAD, the LGID places greater emphasis on the exclusion of high-glycemic index carbohydrates to maintain stable glucose levels, a condition associated with seizure control (Sharawat et al., 2025). Both regimens allow for greater flexibility in food choice, without the need to rigorously calculate the ketogenic ratio, focusing on adequate fat intake, both qualitatively and quantitatively.

The VLCKD shares several metabolic mechanisms typical of the fasting state. After several days of marked carbohydrate restriction (<20 g/day or approximately 5% of total energy), glucose availability becomes insufficient for both the tricarboxylic acid cycle and the energy needs of the central nervous system, prompting the body to use lipids as the primary energy source (Paoli et al., 2013). Free fatty acids do not cross the blood–brain barrier; therefore, the brain obtains energy from the ketone bodies, β-hydroxybutyrate (3HB), acetoacetate (AcAc), and acetone, produced in the liver via ketogenesis. This process occurs in the hepatic mitochondria, where fatty acids are transported by carnitine palmitoyltransferase, β-oxidized to acetyl-CoA, condensed into acetoacetyl-CoA by thiolase, transformed into 3-hydroxy-3-methylglutaryl-coenzyme A (HMG-CoA) by HMG-CoA synthase, and finally converted to AcAc by HMG-CoA lyase. AcAc can be decarboxylated to acetone or reduced to 3HB by the enzyme 3HB dehydrogenase. Among ketone bodies, 3HB represents the main alternative energy source under conditions of low carbohydrate intake (Paoli et al., 2013).

Preclinical and clinical studies highlight that VLCKD can modulate the gut microbiota with beneficial effects on neurodegenerative and autoimmune diseases. In murine models, a 16-week KD containing MUFA and polyunsaturated fatty acid (PUFA) improved neurovascular parameters, reduced the risk of Alzheimer's disease, and increased beneficial bacteria such as *A. muciniphila* and *Lactobacillus*, producers of SCFA, while reducing pro-inflammatory microbes such as *Desulfovibrio* and *Turicibacter* (Ma et al., 2018). In patients with autoimmune multiple sclerosis, the colonic microbiota was characterized by reduced bacterial concentration and diversity, with marked decreases in *Roseburia*, *Bacteroides*, and *F. prausnitzii*. Ten patients followed a VLCKD for six months, showing biphasic effects: in the short term, bacterial concentration and diversity further decreased, but from week 12 a recovery was observed that exceeded baseline values at the end of the study (Swidsinski et al., 2017). These findings suggest that the KD can normalize gut microbial composition and colonic biofermentative function, indicating a potential therapeutic role for dietary modulation of the microbiota in MS patients.

However, reducing fermentable carbohydrates alters the availability of substrates for gut bacteria, resulting in changes in the composition and functionality of the microbiome. Recent studies indicate that the KD often results in a decrease in beneficial bacteria such as *Bifidobacterium*, which can produce SCFAs essential for intestinal barrier integrity and inflammation modulation. At the same time, some species capable of metabolizing proteins and fats, such as *Alistipes* or *Parabacteroides*, increase in abundance, suggesting a functional adaptation of the microbiome to the new available energy sources (Wang et al., 2025).

In summary, VLKD, KD, MAD, and LGID offer documented metabolic benefits, including weight loss, improved glycemia, and plasma lipid regulation, but also significantly impact the gut microbiome. Dietary choice should therefore balance metabolic efficacy with microbial health, ensuring a personalized and sustainable approach. Monitoring the response of the microbiome, its metabolites, and the balance of macronutrients and micronutrients can help maximize metabolic benefits and minimize potential negative effects on intestinal and systemic function in the long term.

1.1.9 Fermented Foods: Living Foods

According to one of the oldest narratives, the birth of the first fermented foods is that of a shepherd, carrying fresh milk in a bag made from the dried stomach of a ruminant, observed that, after several hours of exposure to heat, the contents had separated into two fractions: a liquid (whey) and a solid, creamy consistency. The milk coagulated due to residual enzymes, particularly renin (or chymosin), naturally present in the gastric mucosa of the bag. Tasting the product revealed a pleasant-tasting food, more stable and long-lasting than fresh milk. This event, which has become an archetype in the oral tradition of many pastoral peoples, is considered the possible mythical origin of the first fermented food, the ancestor of yogurt and fresh cheeses. Variants of the same legend are found in different geographical and cultural contexts: in Mesopotamia and ancient Egypt, where the observation of spontaneously acidified doughs or beverages is said to have led to the invention of leavened bread and beer; in Central Asia, nomadic populations developed similar techniques for fermenting mare's milk (kumis) or camel milk. Although the historical reconstruction of the first fermentations remains undocumented, legend testifies to humanity's progressive ability to observe, understand, and ultimately control natural processes of microbial transformation, converting them into dietary practices and preservation technologies that played a decisive role in the development of agro-pastoral civilizations, which are still ongoing. Current research highlights the role of regular consumption of fermented foods, such as yogurt, kefir, kombucha, kimchi, miso, tempeh, fermented vegetables, legumes, and cheeses, among the most promising strategies for modulating the intestinal microbiota (Leeuwendaal et al., 2022; Stiemsma et al., 2020).These products derive from microbial fermentation, such as lactic, acetic, propionic, or alcoholic, of raw materials such as dairy products, grains, or vegetables. They are characterized by a high concentration of probiotics, as well as bioactive properties, aiding digestion and having a lower glycemic index (Padhi et al., 2025). Fermentation also allows for the production of postbiotics, molecules produced by microorganisms that can have beneficial effects on the microbiota and host health. According to the FAO (Food and Agriculture Organization of the United Nations), fermentation processes improve the availability of proteins and minerals, promote the formation of beneficial fats, and increase the vitamin content of foods (Samtiya et al., 2021). Significant examples of fermented foods rich in live microorganisms include nutrients in Table 1.1.

The quantity and diversity of live microorganisms present at the time of consumption are crucial for the potential positive effect on the gut microbiota. Even foods that normally cause bloating can become more digestible if fermented (Park & Mannaa, 2025; Veiga et al., 2014). Currently, there is no recommended daily allowance for fermented foods in nutritional guidelines, but it is recommended to consume them regularly. This promotes gut microbial diversity and allows the bioactive molecules produced by the microorganisms to be absorbed, helping to promote health and well-being.

1.1.10 The Microbiome Toolkit: Prebiotics, Probiotics, and Postbiotics

1.1.10.1 Probiotics

Probiotics are defined by the FAO, ISAPP (International Scientific Association for Probiotics and Prebiotics), and WHO as live microorganisms that, when administered in adequate quantities, confer a health benefit on the host (Hill

TABLE 1.1

The synergy between fermented foods and live bacteria that lead from the raw matrix to the finished food product

Food	Origin/base	Main microorganisms	Notes on postbiotics/fermentation
Yogurt	Milk	Live lactic acid bacteria (e.g., *Lactobacillus bulgaricus*, *Streptococcus thermophilus*)	Produces lactic acid; postbiotics are limited compared to kefir
Kefir	Milk	Lactic acid bacteria + yeasts	Produces a wider range of postbiotics and bioactive compounds than yogurt
Water kefir	Sweetened water	Lactic acid bacteria + yeasts	Slightly fizzy; postbiotics similar to milk kefir but with a different composition
Kombucha	Sweetened tea	Yeasts + bacteria (SCOBY)	Produces organic acids, enzymes, and antioxidant compounds
Miso	Soybeans	*Aspergillus oryzae* + lactic acid bacteria	Contains enzymes and amino acids derived from fermentation
Tempeh	Legumes (soy)	*Rhizopus oligosporus*	Rich in protein and bioactive compounds from fungal fermentation
Lactic acid–fermented vegetables	Vegetables (cabbage, cucumbers, etc.)	Lactic acid bacteria	Produces lactic acid, vitamins, enzymes, and other beneficial compounds

et al., 2014a). However, even before they achieved global fame, humans consumed them in ancient and unsuspecting times, purely casually, through fermented foods. The difference between spontaneous fermentations and potential probiotics currently on the market lies in the rigorous standards established to ensure product quality and safety. In 2013, ISAPP convened a group of experts, including nutritionists, pediatricians, microbiologists, and gastroenterologists, and, through their combined expertise, reached a consensus on the characteristics required to define a probiotic as such (Hill et al., 2014b). These include the following: the probiotic must be safe for human use; it must consist of live, viable microorganisms in adequate quantities (the minimum amount of microorganisms is 5 billion colony forming units (CFU) for pediatrics and 10 billion CFU for adults); its components must be able to adequately colonize and reach the target site; and they must provide a documented beneficial effect. The choice of probiotics must therefore be aimed at achieving a specific objective based on the patient's clinical profile and the current diagnostic hypothesis (Sanders et al., 2010). Therefore, based on the patient's age, sex, lifestyle, diet, current therapies, and medical history, it will be possible to choose the most appropriate probiotic, the number of CFU, the method of administration, and the timing of administration.

Probiotics have species- and strain-specific mechanisms of action, thanks to their colonization characteristics, production of metabolites and byproducts, and competitive activity. Once they reach their target, probiotics are competitive for space and nutrients and are able to colonize, inhibiting potential pathogens (Tan et al., 2021). This is achieved by producing antimicrobial substances such as hydrogen peroxide, carbon dioxide, SCFA, bacteriocins, and acetaldehyde. These byproducts can alter the pH and the environment in which they are located, rendering them inhospitable to potential pathogens or attacking them, for example, through the action of bacteriocins, a heterogeneous class of bactericidal or bacteriostatic peptides (Premkumar & Pammi, 2025; Szajewska et al., 2016). By altering the permeability of the pathogens' barrier, they inhibit their DNA or RNA synthesis and thus their replication. Furthermore, probiotics, having site-specific trophism, must be chosen based on the desired prophylactic–therapeutic goal. Some strains have a specific trophism for the vaginal niche, others for the oral or intestinal niche. Based on these characteristics, it is possible to choose the best probiotic for the therapeutic needs. Finally, each probiotic is capable of producing hormones, neurotransmitters, participating in the metabolism of vitamins B and K, and cytokines (Baucells et al., 2023; Beghetti et al., 2021; Shaaban et al., 2018). These bioproducts can have local or distal organ effects, thus regulating numerous functions even between anatomically distant systems. It is also important to emphasize that the situation becomes even more complex when considering the complex mechanisms of positive or negative covariance between microbial species, a phenomenon known as cross-feeding (FitzGerald et al., 2022). That is, a probiotic may be the choice not so much for the strain itself, but for its ability to negatively covariate with a strain whose colonization and growth we wish to reduce. Alternatively, we can opt for a bacterial strain that positively covaries with commensal microorganisms whose colonization is of interest in increasing. This is because the supplemented strain may possess the ability to produce metabolites that the commensal microorganism requires for growth. An example is Bifidobacteria, which can positively covary with *Eubacterium hallii* or *F. prausnitzii*, both major butyrate producers (Ryan et al., 2025; Schöpping et al., 2022; Turroni et al., 2018). Therefore, we understand that the choice of probiotics goes well beyond the marketing campaign; it requires a thorough understanding of the microbiological mechanisms underlying each probiotic used in order to maximize its final therapeutic effect.

1.1.10.2 Prebiotics

The term prebiotic has been defined by ISAPP as a substrate selectively utilized by host microorganisms and which provides health benefits to the host (Gibson et al., 2017). The FAO has outlined that prebiotics must be safe for both men and women (Guarino et al., 2020). Furthermore, in addition to their positive effect on the gastrointestinal system, they can provide extraintestinal benefits such as cardiometabolic health, bone metabolism, cognitive function, and brain metabolism (Biagioli et al., 2025; Grüber et al., 2015; Kazemi et al., 2019; Leo et al., 2021). Prebiotics, in addition to being commonly used orally, are currently added to numerous compounds such as cosmetic formulations and detergents. A key characteristic of prebiotics, often misunderstood, is that all prebiotics are fibers, but not all fibers have purely prebiotic effects. It is therefore necessary to refer to the characteristic of selectivity, meaning that a prebiotic is such to the extent that it is selectively utilized as a food substrate by one or a few bacterial species present in or capable of colonizing the host (Gibson et al., 2017). For this reason, cellulose and pectin, despite being substrates fermented by intestinal bacteria and indigestible to us, are not considered prebiotics due to their low specificity. Among the prebiotics most studied in the scientific literature for their interesting health effects on the host are breast milk oligosaccharides (HMOs), GOS, FOS, plant polyphenols, lactulose, resistant starches, guar gum, beta-glucans, and glucomannans (Marzorati et al., 2023; Walsh et al., 2023).

HMOs are one of the most studied classes of prebiotics. They represent a heterogeneous family of over 200 molecules derived from lactose, modified by fucosylation and sialylation, with functions that vary based on genetic factors and maternal health (Dinleyici et al., 2023). These structural differences translate into diverse effects on neural and immune development in the newborn. Biochemically, HMOs are synthesized in the alveolar cells of the mammary gland from five main monosaccharides: fucose, glucose, galactose, N-acetylglucosamine, and sialic acid. The ability to add fucose residues depends on the expression of the Secretor (Se) and Lewis (Le) genes, which encode the FUT2 and FUT3 enzymes, respectively (Lyons et al., 2020). Based on their composition, HMOs are divided into three classes: sialylated, neutral fucosylated, and simple neutral (Dinleyici et al., 2023). Functionally, their resistance to acidic environments allows them to reach the colon, where they are fermented by intestinal bacteria. This evolutionary mechanism offers the newborn direct protection against pathogens and promotes the maturation of the immune system. HMOs also act as "decoy receptors" preventing the adhesion of microorganisms such as *Helicobacter pylori* and *Escherichia coli* to epithelial cells (Urashima et al., 2025). In parallel, HMOs perform a prebiotic function by promoting the growth of Bifidobacteria (*Bifidobacterium breve*, *Bifidobacterium longum infantis*, *Bifidobacterium bifidum*), which metabolize these compounds to produce SCFAs, including butyrate. These metabolites support the integrity of the intestinal barrier and modulate the inflammatory response (Biagioli, Sortino, et al., 2024; Falsaperla et al., 2024). Furthermore, a growing body of evidence suggests that HMOs participate in the regulation of the gut–brain axis, influencing communication between the microbiota and the central nervous system. Sialic acid, abundant in human milk, is involved in neuronal transmission and cognitive development. Recent studies have linked the intake of sialylated and fucosylated HMOs to improved language skills in children (Jorgensen et al., 2021), while research on animal models has highlighted a positive effect on learning and memory (Docq et al., 2020). Finally, HMOs appear to modulate the serotonin system and gamma-aminobutyric acid (GABA) production by promoting bacteria such as *Bifidobacterium adolescentis*, which are capable of synthesizing this neurotransmitter (Duranti et al., 2020). These effects, mediated by the microbiota, suggest a potential role for HMOs in supporting neurodegenerative conditions and neurodevelopmental disorders, such as autism, Parkinson's disease, and Alzheimer's disease (Lechner & Vohr, 2017).

GOS, on the other hand, can be divided into alpha-GOS and beta-GOS; the former is typically found in plants, while the latter is synthetic. GOS are selective for Bifidobacteria and Lactobacilli, counteracting the growth of *Clostridium* (Mei et al., 2022). Their prebiotic effect makes them extremely useful in reducing constipation, obesity, metabolic syndrome, diabetes, atopic dermatitis, psoriasis, and in the metabolism of lipids and carbohydrates (Ambrogi et al., 2023; Mei et al., 2022). FOS are soluble fibers found in asparagus, Jerusalem artichoke, oats, chicory, and garlic. The FOS class also includes inulin, xylooligosaccharides (XOS), and isomaltose oligosaccharides (IMO). FOS appear to play an important role in regulating the sensation of hunger and satiety by reducing ghrelin and upregulating GLP-1 and PYY (Wongkrasant et al., 2020). They also improve insulin sensitivity, reducing insulin resistance, and facilitate intestinal transit (Dou et al., 2022). Furthermore, XOS, present in sprouts, fruit, honey, and vegetables, are selectively fermented by *B. adolescentis* (Li et al., 2021). Finally, IMO are abundant in fermented foods, such as miso, natto, tempeh, kombucha, and honey, and are selectively metabolized by Lactobacilli and Bifidobacteria (Leeuwendaal et al., 2022).

Another class widely present and studied in the literature is polyphenols. The most common are flavonoids, including quercetin and catechins, also known as duplibiotics for their ability to favor commensal symbiotic bacteria such as *Lactobacillus*, *Bifidobacterium*, *Akkermansia*, *Roseburia*, and *Faecalibacterium* spp., and to discourage potential pathogens such as *Clostridium perfringens* and *E. coli* (Plamada & Vodnar, 2021). Quercetin is a flavonol, increasingly being investigated for its potential clinical use, thanks to the antioxidant, anti-inflammatory, and antiviral properties attributed to it. The study by Di Pierro et al. (2021) tested quercetin supplementation as an add-on to standard therapy in patients with early stage viral infection. The study involved outpatients with mild-to-moderate symptoms who were administered a highly bioavailable formulation of quercetin (500 mg/day in the first week, then reduced in the second) in addition to their usual care. Results showed that, compared to standard treatment alone, the quercetin group had a significantly higher number of viral swab negatives after one week, a more rapid resolution of acute symptoms, and a reduction in serum levels of the lactate dehydrogenase (LDH) marker, suggesting a possible favorable effect on viral clearance and modulation of the inflammatory response. A further study investigated quercetin in subjects with hyperuricemia, overweight, and dyslipidemia. The cohort was treated with a daily formulation of quercetin (400 mg/day). The study (Di Pierro et al., 2025), conducted on three separate cohorts, one composed of healthy individuals, one of subjects with mild hyperuricemia, and one of obese subjects with hypercholesterolemia, showed that quercetin led to significant reductions in uric acid levels and a decrease in triglycerides, especially in metabolically compromised subjects. However, it is important to emphasize that many of the studies available in literature are still open-label or conducted in "real-world" settings and therefore should be interpreted with caution pending more rigorous and controlled trials. Moreover, catechins, including epigallocatechin (EGC) gallate (EGCG), epicatechin (EC), EGC, and EC gallate (ECG), are natural compounds found in green tea known for their antioxidant, anti-inflammatory, and potentially anticancer properties. Numerous clinical studies have examined their effects on human health. A systematic review of the literature found that green tea catechin intake can lead to a modest reduction in both systolic and diastolic blood pressure in individuals at high cardiovascular risk (Khalesi et al., 2014). Other studies have suggested that catechins can improve endothelial function, contributing to vascular health (Sagris et al., 2024). Regarding metabolism, green tea catechins appear to influence lipid and sugar metabolism, facilitating weight loss (Patanè et al., 2023). However, the effects on body weight reduction have not always been clinically significant. In the neurological field, green tea catechins have been studied for their potential neuroprotective properties, with the hypothesis that they could prevent or treat neurodegenerative diseases (Farkhondeh et al., 2020; S. Li et al., 2024; Patanè et al., 2023). Despite the promising results for these prebiotic substances, further randomized, double-blind, multicenter, and longitudinal studies are needed to determine optimal doses and long-term safety.

1.1.10.3 Postbiotics

The term postbiotic currently lacks a coherent and systematic definition. The terms tyndallized probiotics, bacterial lysates, and parapsychobiotics are sometimes used, all to refer to non-living microorganisms (Aguilar-Toalá et al., 2021). However, in 2021, ISAPP, convening a panel of experts, defined the term postbiotic as a preparation of inanimate microorganisms or parts thereof that confer a health benefit to the host (Salminen et al., 2021). A postbiotic, like a probiotic or prebiotic, must possess specific characteristics to be marketed. It must be safe, with proven health benefits, and its site of action is not limited to the intestine alone but can contribute to the balance of various microbial niches such as the oral cavity, urogenital tract, and skin. The mechanisms that make a postbiotic beneficial to the host's health are varied, and several have been proposed by the scientific community. Postbiotics may be able to modulate the microbiota, thanks to molecules such as bacteriocins or lactic acid, which possess antimicrobial activity (Liang et al., 2024). Furthermore, postbiotics can compete with resident microorganisms for available adhesion sites. They are also able to modulate immune responses; for example, SCFAs and histamine appear to induce the suppression of NF-kB, or the LPS from some Gram-positive bacteria, such as *E. coli* Nissle, interacts with TLR4 (Behrouzi et al., 2020). Postbiotics improve intestinal barrier function; for example, EPSs produced by *Bifidobacterium* reduce the functionality and integrity of the intestinal barrier, reducing inflammation, through signaling pathways that are yet to be defined (Amobonye et al., 2025). Recent studies on Caco-2 cell models of LPS-induced inflammation have evaluated the administration of pasteurized strains of *Lacticaseibacillus paracasei* (HK-LP) to the intestinal barrier (Xie et al., 2023). These studies showed that HL-LP strains reduced intestinal permeability by inhibiting pro-inflammatory factors such as TNF-alpha and IL-6, while increasing anti-inflammatory factors such as IL-10 and IL-4 (Y. Li et al., 2024). Finally, postbiotics are being closely investigated for their ability to modulate the interaction between microbiome gut brain axis (MGBA) and systemic metabolism. In particular, we know that microorganisms are capable of producing numerous bioactive compounds and neurotransmitters, such as GABA, serotonin, dopamine, or microbial metabolites such as SCFAs (Lahariya et al., 2026). These, when present in sufficient quantities, can stimulate enterochromaffin cells to produce serotonin. Furthermore, SCFAs promote satiety by promoting anorectic hormones such as PYY and GLP-1. Bile salt hydrolase (BSH), a microbial enzyme capable of initiating the deconjugation of bile acids, thus diversifying the pool of circulating bile acids, has also been investigated. A reduction in BSH is associated with a greater predisposition to recurrent *Clostridioides difficile* infections (Foley et al., 2023). Therefore, numerous postbiotic strains have been studied in animal and human models, such as pasteurized *A. muciniphila* in mice with high-fat diet (HFD)–induced obesity. Postbiotic-supplemented mice not only did not exhibit deterioration of intestinal barrier integrity and LPS endotoxemia but also showed improved insulin sensitivity and did not develop obesity, compared to the unsupplemented control group (Cani et al., 2022). For the pediatric population, the possibility of fermenting infant formula with the addition of postbiotic and probiotic mixtures has been proposed for the management of atopic diseases, gastroenteritis, and infectious diseases. However, in 2007, the Nutrition Committee of the European Society of Pediatric Gastroenterology, Hepatology and Nutrition (ESPGHAN), based on the existing randomized controlled trial (RCTs), concluded that there were insufficient data available to conclude on fermented infant formulas (Agostoni et al., 2007). Regarding fermented infant formulas, it is interesting to mention a study conducted on preterm infants in which a sample of 58 infants (gestational age 30–35 weeks) were started on a formula fermented with *B. breve* and *S. thermophilus*. Following administration, a statistically significant reduction in fecal calprotectin levels ($p = 0.001$) and a reduction in abdominal distension were observed (Campeotto et al., 2011). Another study (Kaila et al., 1995) in infants with acute rotavirus diarrhea, following supplementation with inactivated *Lacticaseibacillus rhamnosus* GG, showed a faster clinical recovery, with results similar to those of ingesting live *L. rhamnosus* GG. The study by Kirjavainen et al. (2003) showed that inactivated or active *L. rhamnosus* GG, added to extensive hydrolyzed whey formula (EHWF), in 35 infants with atopic eczema (average age 5.5 months), following supplementation with EHWF, showed a significant reduction in atopic dermatitis scores after 1 month of treatment.

These results underscore the importance not only of targeted supplementation based on the clinical and diagnostic findings, but also of the potential role of fermented foods as truly living foods, rich in prebiotics, probiotics, and postbiotics, thus capable of improving the microbial ecosystem and consequently the overall health of the host.

1.1.11 Precision Nutrition and the Microbiota: The Future of Personalized Medicine

The latest scientific evidence indicates that there is no one-size-fits-all dietary pattern. Instead, the body's response to nutrients is strongly influenced by individual genetic and epigenetic characteristics, including the composition of the gut microbiota. Diet is the primary factor shaping the microbiota over the course of a lifetime. Changes in macronutrient intake or fiber quality, as well as exposure to sweeteners, probiotics, and prebiotics, and food preparation methods themselves, generate rapid changes in microbial composition and function. However, these effects are highly individual. Numerous experimental evidence indicates that the composition of the gut microbiota can significantly influence an individual's response to dietary interventions. Indeed, some bacterial species demonstrate potential predictive value in determining the metabolic efficacy of specific diets (Kolodziejczyk et al., 2019b). In pediatric irritable bowel syndrome (IBS), for example, responders to a diet low in fermentable oligosaccharides, disaccharides, monosaccharides, and polyols (low-FODMAPs) had a higher abundance of Bacteroidaceae, Erysipelotrichaceae, and Clostridiales, with a high capacity for saccharolytic metabolism, while non-responders harbored higher concentrations of *Turicibacter* (Chumpitazi et al., 2014). Similarly, in children treated with diets low in fermentable substrates, responders showed higher levels of *Sporobacter* and *Subdoligranulum* and a lower abundance of *Bacteroides* (Chumpitazi et al., 2015). Based on these observations, more accurate predictive models have been developed to distinguish responders from non-responders, combining basal microbiome characteristics with physiological and anthropometric parameters.

In a cohort of 800 overweight or obese non-diabetic adults, marked interpersonal variability in the postprandial glycemic response (PPGR) to identical meals was predicted with high accuracy using machine learning models that integrated microbiome data, clinical parameters, dietary habits, and blood profiles. Personalized dietary interventions based on these predictions subsequently showed consistent changes in microbial composition and a significant reduction in PPGR (Zeevi et al., 2015c). Overall, these data support the hypothesis that the effectiveness of a dietary regimen depends not solely on its composition, but on the dynamic interaction between diet, microbiota, and host physiology. To optimize these interactions, it will be necessary to develop sustainable and individualized precision nutrition strategies capable of specifically modulating the gut microbial community and improving the individual's metabolic and inflammatory response.

However, numerous challenges remain, such as the complexity of the interactions between the microbiota, host, and diet, the paucity of longitudinal studies in humans, and the lack of standardization of microbiome analysis methods. Furthermore, most research focuses on Western populations, limiting the generalizability of the findings globally.

Despite these limitations, the microbiota-based nutritional approach marks a decisive step toward tailored and individualized preventive medicine. The growing availability of omics data and the use of advanced computational tools pave the way for dietary strategies capable of specifically regulating microbial function and, consequently, improving individual health.

1.1.12 One Health: Human, Microbial, Animal, and Environmental Health

Human, animal, and environmental health are interconnected. Microbiomes are the common thread in this network, as microorganisms move between soils, plants, animals, and people, influencing ecological balance (or its loss).

Modern agriculture and intensive livestock farming have profoundly transformed ecosystems, often with negative impacts on natural microbiomes. Chemical fertilizers, pesticides, and antibiotics can alter microbial biodiversity in soils, water, and farmed animals, compromising natural processes such as the decomposition of organic matter and nutrient cycling (Garbisu et al., 2026). Animals raised in intensive systems can develop potentially pathogenic microbiomes, favoring the emergence of resistant species. These changes are not confined to livestock farming: they spread through water, soil, and the food chain, impacting human health. Understanding these microbial dynamics is essential to preventing epidemics, containing antibiotic resistance, and promoting healthier production systems. Managing microbial health, therefore, means adopting integrated strategies that consider human, veterinary, and environmental health.

More sustainable solutions include regenerative agriculture practices, crop rotations, pesticide reduction, and responsible use of antibiotics. All these interventions help preserve microbial biodiversity, improving ecosystem resilience and the quality of agricultural products (T. Zhang et al., 2024).

The microbiome, therefore, represents an irreplaceable ecological resource. Microbial diversity can and must be preserved and enhanced through sustainable agricultural practices, including regenerative agriculture practices, crop rotations, pesticide reduction, and responsible use of antibiotics (Ahn & Hayes, 2021). All these interventions help preserve microbial biodiversity, improving ecosystem resilience and the quality of every food on our tables.

The microbiome, therefore, is not just an indicator of health or a nutritional factor: it is a true ecological heritage to be understood, protected, and used responsibly.

1.1.13 Prospects, Limitations, and Conclusions

Microbiota-based nutrition is emerging as a tool to guide personalized therapeutic strategies in numerous clinical settings. The next step in developing personalized nutrition could be to monitor and control the levels of specific metabolites, such as lipids, vitamins, TMAO, SCFAs, and neuropeptides, in the blood, or of multiple molecules simultaneously, combined with metagenomic data (Kolodziejczyk et al., 2019c). However, designing diets that consider multiple characteristics is complex, as certain foods and the microbiota associated with specific metabolites, despite showing numerous correlations, do not always demonstrate causal relationships. Furthermore, the study of the microbiota and the results derived from sequencing techniques can be influenced by sample storage conditions, DNA extraction methods, and sequencing library preparation protocols. Currently, available technologies allow for detailed microbiome analysis; however, their clinical application is still limited by high costs and the lack of standardized tools for data interpretation in healthcare settings. Despite these challenges, recent advances in microbiome research offer promising prospects. With the progressive reduction of costs and the implementation of dedicated training programs for clinicians, a more accurate and clinically relevant interpretation of microbial profiles will be possible. In this context, microbiome analysis has the potential to become a routine practice in preventive and personalized medicine, similar to what happened with the sequencing of the human genome.

Prevention, the promotion of healthy lifestyles, and technological innovations are the fundamental pillars of personalized medicine. Looking to the future means conceiving prevention not only as a clinical tool, but also as a principle of social equity, investing in the health and dignity of each individual. Translating the results of scientific research into clinical practice, therefore, represents an ethical and political commitment to which every healthcare professional is called to contribute.

REFERENCES

Abdollahpour, N., Fard, S. A. M., Salahmanesh, A., Hatamzadeh, H., Moeini, R., Soflaei, S. S., Seifi, N., & Ghayour-Mobarhan, M. (2025). The association between ultra-processed foods and depression, anxiety and sleep in adults: A cross-sectional study in Iran. *Food Science & Nutrition*, 13(7). https://doi.org/10.1002/fsn3.70316

Adeyeye, S. A. O., Sivapriya, T., & Sankarganesh, P. (2025). Formation and mitigation of heterocyclic amines (HCAs) and polycyclic aromatic hydrocarbons (PAHs) in high temperature processed meat products: A review. *Discover Food*, 5(1), 258. https://doi.org/10.1007/s44187-025-00391-w

Adhikari, S., Schop, M., de Boer, I. J. M., & Huppertz, T. (2022). Protein quality in perspective: A review of protein quality metrics and their applications. *Nutrients*, 14(5), 947. https://doi.org/10.3390/nu14050947

Agostoni, C., Goulet, O., Kolacek, S., Koletzko, B., Moreno, L., Puntis, J., Rigo, J., Shamir, R., Szajewska, H., & Turck, D. (2007). Fermented infant formulae without live bacteria. *Journal of Pediatric Gastroenterology and Nutrition*, 44(3), 392–397. https://doi.org/10.1097/01.mpg.0000258887.93866.69

Aguilar-Toalá, J. E., Arioli, S., Behare, P., Belzer, C., Berni Canani, R., Chatel, J.-M., D'Auria, E., de Freitas, M. Q., Elinav, E., Esmerino, E. A., García, H. S., da Cruz, A. G., González-Córdova, A. F., Guglielmetti, S., de Toledo Guimarães, J., Hernández-Mendoza, A., Langella, P., Liceaga, A. M., Magnani, M., ... Zhou, Z. (2021). Postbiotics — When simplification fails to clarify. *Nature Reviews Gastroenterology & Hepatology*, 18(11), 825–826. https://doi.org/10.1038/s41575-021-00521-6

Agus, A., Denizot, J., Thévenot, J., Martinez-Medina, M., Massier, S., Sauvanet, P., Bernalier-Donadille, A., Denis, S., Hofman, P., Bonnet, R., Billard, E., & Barnich, N. (2016). Western diet induces a shift in microbiota composition enhancing susceptibility to Adherent-Invasive E. coli infection and intestinal inflammation. *Scientific Reports*, 6(1), 19032. https://doi.org/10.1038/srep19032

Ahn, J., & Hayes, R. B. (2021). Environmental influences on the human microbiome and implications for noncommunicable disease. *Annual Review of Public Health*, 42(1), 277–292. https://doi.org/10.1146/annurev-publhealth-012420-105020

Amaro, A., Baptista, F. I., & Matafome, P. (2022). Programming of future generations during breastfeeding: The intricate relation between metabolic and neurodevelopment disorders. *Life Sciences*, 298, 120526. https://doi.org/10.1016/j.lfs.2022.120526

Ambrogi, V., Bottacini, F., Cao, L., Kuipers, B., Schoterman, M., & van Sinderen, D. (2023). Galacto-oligosaccharides as infant prebiotics: Production, application, bioactive activities and future perspectives. *Critical Reviews in Food Science and Nutrition*, 63(6), 753–766. https://doi.org/10.1080/10408398.2021.1953437

Amobonye, A., Pillay, B., Hlope, F., Asong, S. T., & Pillai, S. (2025). Postbiotics: An insightful review of the latest category in functional biotics. *World Journal of Microbiology and Biotechnology*, 41(8), 293. https://doi.org/10.1007/s11274-025-04483-8

Anand, R., Sahil, R., Jain, M., Maurya, G. K., & Kharat, A. S. (2026). Plant-based diet as a precursor to human gut diversity. *The Journal of Nutrition*, 156(1), 101251. https://doi.org/10.1016/j.tjnut.2025.11.020

Barends, C., de Vries, J., Mojet, J., & de Graaf, C. (2013). Effects of repeated exposure to either vegetables or fruits on infant's vegetable and fruit acceptance at the beginning of weaning. *Food Quality and Preference*, 29(2), 157–165. https://doi.org/10.1016/j.foodqual.2013.03.008

Bashore, L., Smith, A. M., Johnson, A. H., & Farbo, D. (2025). Gastrointestinal and sleep disorders in children with and without autism. *Gastroenterology Nursing*, 48(5), 346–354. https://doi.org/10.1097/SGA.0000000000000890

Baucells, B. J., Sebastiani, G., Herrero-Aizpurua, L., Andreu-Fernández, V., Navarro-Tapia, E., García-Algar, O., & Figueras-Aloy, J. (2023). Effectiveness of a probiotic combination on the neurodevelopment of the very premature infant. *Scientific Reports*, 13(1), 10344. https://doi.org/10.1038/s41598-023-37393-6

Beghetti, I., Panizza, D., Lenzi, J., Gori, D., Martini, S., Corvaglia, L., & Aceti, A. (2021). Probiotics for preventing necrotizing enterocolitis in preterm infants: A network meta-analysis. *Nutrients*, 13(1), 192. https://doi.org/10.3390/nu13010192

Behrouzi, A., Mazaheri, H., Falsafi, S., Tavassol, Z. H., Moshiri, A., & Siadat, S. D. (2020). Intestinal effect of the probiotic Escherichia coli strain Nissle 1917 and its OMV. *Journal of Diabetes & Metabolic Disorders*, 19(1), 597–604. https://doi.org/10.1007/s40200-020-00511-6

Berg, G., Toledo, G. V., Schierstaedt, J., Hyöty, H., & Adi Wicaksono, W. (2025). Linking the edible plant microbiome and human gut microbiome. *Gut Microbes*, 17(1). https://doi.org/10.1080/19490976.2025.2551113

Biagioli, V., Matera, M., & Striano, P. (2025). How maternal diet, probiotics, prebiotics, and postbiotics during pregnancy influence neurodevelopment in newborns. *Global Pediatrics*, 14, 100301. https://doi.org/10.1016/j.gpeds.2025.100301

Biagioli, V., Sortino, V., Falsaperla, R., & Striano, P. (2024). Role of human milk microbiota in infant neurodevelopment: Mechanisms and clinical implications. *Children*, 11(12), 1476. https://doi.org/10.3390/children11121476

Biagioli, V., Volpedo, G., Riva, A., Mainardi, P., & Striano, P. (2024). From birth to weaning: A window of opportunity for microbiota. *Nutrients*, 16(2), 272. https://doi.org/10.3390/nu16020272

Bonaccio, M., Iacoviello, L., Donati, M. B., & de Gaetano, G. (2022). The tenth anniversary as a UNESCO World Cultural Heritage: An unmissable opportunity to get back to the cultural roots of the Mediterranean diet. *European Journal of Clinical Nutrition*, 76(2), 179–183. https://doi.org/10.1038/s41430-021-00924-3

Borghi, E., Xynomilakis, O., Ottaviano, E., Ceccarani, C., Viganò, I., Tognini, P., & Vignoli, A. (2024). Gut microbiota profile in CDKL5 deficiency disorder patients. *Scientific Reports*, 14(1), 7376. https://doi.org/10.1038/s41598-024-56989-0

Budoff, M. J., de Oliveira Otto, M. C., Li, X. S., Lee, Y., Wang, M., Lai, H. T. M., Lemaitre, R. N., Pratt, A., Tang, W. H. W., Psaty, B. M., Siscovick, D. S., Hazen, S. L., & Mozaffarian, D. (2025). Trimethylamine-N-oxide (TMAO) and risk of incident cardiovascular events in the multi ethnic study of Atherosclerosis. *Scientific Reports*, 15(1), 23362. https://doi.org/10.1038/s41598-025-05903-3

Calcaterra, V., Verduci, E., Milanta, C., Agostinelli, M., Todisco, C. F., Bona, F., Dolor, J., La Mendola, A., Tosi, M., & Zuccotti, G. (2023). Micronutrient deficiency in children and adolescents with obesity—A narrative review. *Children*, 10(4), 695. https://doi.org/10.3390/children10040695

Campeotto, F., Suau, A., Kapel, N., Magne, F., Viallon, V., Ferraris, L., Waligora-Dupriet, A.-J., Soulaines, P., Leroux, B., Kalach, N., Dupont, C., & Butel, M.-J. (2011). A fermented formula in pre-term infants: Clinical tolerance, gut microbiota, down-regulation of faecal calprotectin and up-regulation of faecal secretory IgA. *British Journal of Nutrition*, 105(12), 1843–1851. https://doi.org/10.1017/S0007114510005702

Cani, P. D., Depommier, C., Derrien, M., Everard, A., & de Vos, W. M. (2022). Akkermansia muciniphila: Paradigm for next-generation beneficial microorganisms. *Nature Reviews Gastroenterology & Hepatology*, 19(10), 625–637. https://doi.org/10.1038/s41575-022-00631-9

Canyelles, M., Borràs, C., Rotllan, N., Tondo, M., Escolà-Gil, J. C., & Blanco-Vaca, F. (2023). Gut microbiota-derived TMAO: A causal factor promoting atherosclerotic cardiovascular disease? *International Journal of Molecular Sciences*, 24(3), 1940. https://doi.org/10.3390/ijms24031940

Cao, Y., Liu, H., Qin, N., Ren, X., Zhu, B., & Xia, X. (2020). Impact of food additives on the composition and function of gut microbiota: A review. *Trends in Food Science & Technology*, 99, 295–310. https://doi.org/10.1016/j.tifs.2020.03.006

Chiang, J.Y. L., & Ferrell, J. M. (2020). Bile acid receptors FXR and TGR5 signaling in fatty liver diseases and therapy. *American Journal of Physiology-Gastrointestinal and Liver Physiology*, 318(3), G554–G573. https://doi.org/10.1152/ajpgi.00223.2019

Chouraqui, J.-P. (2023). Risk assessment of micronutrients deficiency in vegetarian or vegan children: Not so obvious. *Nutrients*, 15(9), 2129. https://doi.org/10.3390/nu15092129

Chumpitazi, B. P., Cope, J. L., Hollister, E. B., Tsai, C. M., McMeans, A. R., Luna, R. A., Versalovic, J., & Shulman, R. J. (2015). Randomised clinical trial: Gut microbiome biomarkers are associated with clinical response to a low FODMAP diet in children with the irritable bowel syndrome. *Alimentary Pharmacology & Therapeutics*, 42(4), 418–427. https://doi.org/10.1111/apt.13286

Chumpitazi, B. P., Hollister, E. B., Oezguen, N., Tsai, C. M., McMeans, A. R., Luna, R. A., Savidge, T. C., Versalovic, J., & Shulman, R. J. (2014). Gut microbiota influences low fermentable substrate diet efficacy in children with irritable bowel syndrome. *Gut Microbes*, 5(2), 165–175. https://doi.org/10.4161/gmic.27923

Comerford, K. B., Papanikolaou, Y., Jones, J. M., Rodriguez, J., Slavin, J., Angadi, S., & Drewnowski, A. (2021). Toward an evidence-based definition and classification of carbohydrate food quality: An expert panel report. *Nutrients*, 13(8), 2667. https://doi.org/10.3390/nu13082667

D'Auria, E., Bergamini, M., Staiano, A., Banderali, G., Pendezza, E., Penagini, F., Zuccotti, G. V., & Peroni, D. G. (2018). Baby-led weaning: What a systematic review of the literature adds on. *Italian Journal of Pediatrics*, 44(1), 49. https://doi.org/10.1186/s13052-018-0487-8

Dalile, B., Van Oudenhove, L., Vervliet, B., & Verbeke, K. (2019). The role of short-chain fatty acids in microbiota–gut–brain communication. *Nature Reviews Gastroenterology & Hepatology*, 16(8), 461–478. https://doi.org/10.1038/s41575-019-0157-3

David, L. A., Maurice, C. F., Carmody, R. N., Gootenberg, D. B., Button, J. E., Wolfe, B. E., Ling, A. V., Devlin, A. S., Varma, Y., Fischbach, M. A., Biddinger, S. B., Dutton, R. J., & Turnbaugh, P. J. (2014). Diet rapidly and reproducibly alters the human gut microbiome. *Nature*, 505(7484), 559–563. https://doi.org/10.1038/nature12820

Davis, H., Magistrali, A., Butler, G., & Stergiadis, S. (2022). Nutritional benefits from fatty acids in organic and grass-fed beef. *Foods*, 11(5), 646. https://doi.org/10.3390/foods11050646

De Filippis, F., Pellegrini, N., Vannini, L., Jeffery, I. B., La Storia, A., Laghi, L., Serrazanetti, D. I., Di Cagno, R., Ferrocino, I., Lazzi, C., Turroni, S., Cocolin, L., Brigidi, P., Neviani, E., Gobbetti, M., O'Toole, P. W., & Ercolini, D. (2016). High-level adherence to a Mediterranean diet beneficially impacts the gut microbiota and associated metabolome. *Gut*, 65(11), 1812–1821. https://doi.org/10.1136/gutjnl-2015-309957

De Giorgis, V., Tagliabue, A., Bisulli, F., Brambilla, I., Camerini, A., Cusmai, R., Darra, F., Dianin, A., Domenica, E., Lodi, M. A. M., Matricardi, S., Messana, T., Operto, F., Ragona, F., Russo, E., Varesio, C., Volpi, L., Zanaboni, M. P., Pasca, L., & Veggiotti, P. (2023). Ketogenic dietary therapies in epilepsy: Recommendations of the Italian League against Epilepsy Dietary Therapy Study Group. *Frontiers in Neurology*, 14. https://doi.org/10.3389/fneur.2023.1215618

de Onis, M., & Branca, F. (2016). Childhood stunting: A global perspective. *Maternal & Child Nutrition*, 12(S1), 12–26. https://doi.org/10.1111/mcn.12231

Di Pierro, F., Derosa, G., Maffioli, P., Bertuccioli, A., Togni, S., Riva, A., Allegrini, P., Khan, A., Khan, S., Khan, B. A., Altaf, N., Zahid, M., Ujjan, I. D., Nigar, R., Khushk, M. I., Phulpoto, M., Lail, A., Devrajani, B. R., & Ahmed, S. (2021). Possible therapeutic effects of adjuvant quercetin supplementation against early-stage COVID-19 infection: A prospective, randomized, controlled, and open-label study. *International Journal of General Medicine*, 14, 2359–2366. https://doi.org/10.2147/IJGM.S318720

Di Pierro, F., Rabbani, F., Tareen, M., Nigar, R., Khan, A., Zerbinati, N., Tanda, M. L., Cazzaniga, M., Bertuccioli, A., Falasca, P., Damiani, G., & Villanova, N. (2025). Potential pharmacological effect of Quercetin Phytosome™ in the management of hyperuricemia: Results from real-life clinical studies. *Frontiers in Nutrition*, 12. https://doi.org/10.3389/fnut.2025.1519459

Ding, M., Ross, R. P., Dempsey, E., Li, B., & Stanton, C. (2025). Infant gut microbiome reprogramming following introduction of solid foods (weaning). *Gut Microbes*, 17(1). https://doi.org/10.1080/19490976.2025.2571428

Dinleyici, M., Barbieur, J., Dinleyici, E. C., & Vandenplas, Y. (2023). Functional effects of human milk oligosaccharides (HMOs). *Gut Microbes*, 15(1). https://doi.org/10.1080/19490976.2023.2186115

Docq, S., Spoelder, M., Wang, W., & Homberg, J. R. (2020). The protective and long-lasting effects of human milk oligosaccharides on cognition in mammals. *Nutrients*, 12(11), 3572. https://doi.org/10.3390/nu12113572

Dominguez-Bello, M. G., Costello, E. K., Contreras, M., Magris, M., Hidalgo, G., Fierer, N., & Knight, R. (2010). Delivery mode shapes the acquisition and structure of the initial microbiota across multiple body habitats in newborns. *Proceedings of the National Academy of Sciences*, 107(26), 11971–11975. https://doi.org/10.1073/pnas.1002601107

Dominguez-Bello, M. G., De Jesus-Laboy, K. M., Shen, N., Cox, L. M., Amir, A., Gonzalez, A., Bokulich, N. A., Song, S. J., Hoashi, M., Rivera-Vinas, J. I., Mendez, K., Knight, R., & Clemente, J. C. (2016). Partial restoration of the microbiota of cesarean-born infants via vaginal microbial transfer. *Nature Medicine*, 22(3), 250–253. https://doi.org/10.1038/nm.4039

Dou, Y., Yu, X., Luo, Y., Chen, B., Ma, D., & Zhu, J. (2022). Effect of Fructooligosaccharides supplementation on the gut microbiota in human: A systematic review and meta-analysis. *Nutrients*, 14(16), 3298. https://doi.org/10.3390/nu14163298

Duranti, S., Ruiz, L., Lugli, G. A., Tames, H., Milani, C., Mancabelli, L., Mancino, W., Longhi, G., Carnevali, L., Sgoifo, A., Margolles, A., Ventura, M., Ruas-Madiedo, P., & Turroni, F. (2020). Bifidobacterium adolescentis as a key member of the human gut microbiota in the production of GABA. *Scientific Reports*, 10(1), 14112. https://doi.org/10.1038/s41598-020-70986-z

Elmén, L., Zlamal, J. E., Scott, D. A., Lee, R. B., Chen, D. J., Colas, A. R., Rodionov, D. A., & Peterson, S. N. (2020). Dietary emulsifier sodium stearoyl lactylate alters gut microbiota in vitro and inhibits bacterial butyrate producers. *Frontiers in Microbiology*, 11. https://doi.org/10.3389/fmicb.2020.00892

Estruch, R., Ros, E., Salas-Salvadó, J., Covas, M.-I., Corella, D., Arós, F., Gómez-Gracia, E., Ruiz-Gutiérrez, V., Fiol, M., Lapetra, J., Lamuela-Raventos, R. M., Serra-Majem, L., Pintó, X., Basora, J., Muñoz, M. A., Sorlí, J. V., Martínez, J. A., Fitó, M., Gea, A., … Martínez-González, M. A. (2018). Primary prevention of cardiovascular disease with a Mediterranean diet supplemented with extra-virgin olive oil or nuts. *New England Journal of Medicine*, 378(25). https://doi.org/10.1056/NEJMoa1800389

Fackelmann, G., Manghi, P., Carlino, N., Heidrich, V., Piccinno, G., Ricci, L., Piperni, E., Arrè, A., Bakker, E., Creedon, A. C., Francis, L., Capdevila Pujol, J., Davies, R., Wolf, J., Bermingham, K. M., Berry, S. E., Spector, T. D., Asnicar, F., & Segata, N. (2025). Gut microbiome signatures of vegan, vegetarian and omnivore diets and associated health outcomes across 21,561 individuals. *Nature Microbiology*, 10(1), 41–52. https://doi.org/10.1038/s41564-024-01870-z

Falsaperla, R., Sortino, V., Gambilonghi, F., Vitaliti, G., & Striano, P. (2024). Human milk oligosaccharides and their pivotal role in gut–brain axis modulation and neurologic development: A narrative review to decipher the multifaceted interplay. *Nutrients*, 16(17), 3009. https://doi.org/10.3390/nu16173009

Farkhondeh, T., Pourbagher-Shahri, A., Ashrafizadeh, M., Folgado, S., Rajabpour-Sanati, A., Khazdair, M., & Samarghandian, S. (2020). Green tea catechins inhibit microglial activation which prevents the development of neurological disorders. *Neural Regeneration Research*, 15(10), 1792. https://doi.org/10.4103/1673-5374.280300

Fasano, A. (2025). The physiology of hunger. *New England Journal of Medicine*, 392(4), 372–381. https://doi.org/10.1056/NEJMra2402679

FitzGerald, J., Patel, S., Eckenberger, J., Guillemard, E., Veiga, P., Schäfer, F., Walter, J., Claesson, M. J., & Derrien, M. (2022). Improved gut microbiome recovery following drug therapy is linked to abundance and replication of probiotic strains. *Gut Microbes*, 14(1). https://doi.org/10.1080/19490976.2022.2094664

Foley, M. H., Walker, M. E., Stewart, A. K., O'Flaherty, S., Gentry, E. C., Patel, S., Beaty, V. V., Allen, G., Pan, M., Simpson, J. B., Perkins, C., Vanhoy, M. E., Dougherty, M. K., McGill, S. K., Gulati, A. S., Dorrestein, P. C., Baker, E. S., Redinbo, M. R., Barrangou, R., & Theriot, C. M. (2023). Bile salt hydrolases shape the bile acid landscape and restrict Clostridioides difficile growth in the murine gut. *Nature Microbiology*, 8(4), 611–628. https://doi.org/10.1038/s41564-023-01337-7

Garbisu, C., Unamunzaga, O., & Alkorta, I. (2026). An agricultural perspective on One Health. *Frontiers in Sustainable Food Systems*, 9. https://doi.org/10.3389/fsufs.2025.1706994

García-Vega, Á. S., Corrales-Agudelo, V., Reyes, A., & Escobar, J. S. (2020). Diet quality, food groups and nutrients associated with the gut microbiota in a nonwestern population. *Nutrients*, 12(10), 2938. https://doi.org/10.3390/nu12102938

Gauthier, A., Simic, N., Jones, K. C., & RamachandranNair, R. (2020). Modified Atkins Diet with slow reduction of carbohydrate. *Epilepsy & Behavior Reports*, 13, 100353. https://doi.org/10.1016/j.ebr.2019.100353

Geiker, N. R. W., Bertram, H. C., Mejborn, H., Dragsted, L. O., Kristensen, L., Carrascal, J. R., Bügel, S., & Astrup, A. (2021). Meat and human health—Current knowledge and research gaps. *Foods*, 10(7), 1556. https://doi.org/10.3390/foods10071556

Gibson, G. R., Hutkins, R., Sanders, M. E., Prescott, S. L., Reimer, R. A., Salminen, S. J., Scott, K., Stanton, C., Swanson, K. S., Cani, P. D., Verbeke, K., & Reid, G. (2017). Expert consensus document: The International Scientific Association for Probiotics and Prebiotics (ISAPP) consensus statement on the definition and scope of prebiotics. *Nature Reviews Gastroenterology & Hepatology*, 14(8), 491–502. https://doi.org/10.1038/nrgastro.2017.75

Gracner, T., Boone, C., & Gertler, P. J. (2024). Exposure to sugar rationing in the first 1000 days of life protected against chronic disease. *Science*, 386(6725), 1043–1048. https://doi.org/10.1126/science.adn5421

Grüber, C., van Stuivenberg, M., Mosca, F., Moro, G., Chirico, G., Braegger, C. P., Riedler, J., Yavuz, Y., Boehm, G., & Wahn, U. (2015). Immunoactive prebiotics transiently prevent occurrence of early atopic dermatitis among low-atopy-risk infants.

Journal of Allergy and Clinical Immunology, 136(6), 1696–1698. e1. https://doi.org/10.1016/j.jaci.2015.07.049

Guarino, M., Altomare, A., Emerenziani, S., Di Rosa, C., Ribolsi, M., Balestrieri, P., Iovino, P., Rocchi, G., & Cicala, M. (2020). Mechanisms of action of prebiotics and their effects on gastro-intestinal disorders in adults. *Nutrients*, 12(4), 1037. https://doi.org/10.3390/nu12041037

Hammer, A., Schliep, A., Jörg, S., Haghikia, A., Gold, R., Kleinewietfeld, M., Müller, D. N., & Linker, R. A. (2017). Impact of combined sodium chloride and saturated long-chain fatty acid challenge on the differentiation of T helper cells in neuroinflammation. *Journal of Neuroinflammation*, 14(1), 184. https://doi.org/10.1186/s12974-017-0954-y

Heiman, M. L., & Greenway, F. L. (2016). A healthy gastrointestinal microbiome is dependent on dietary diversity. *Molecular Metabolism*, 5(5), 317–320. https://doi.org/10.1016/j.molmet.2016.02.005

Hickman, B., Salonen, A., Ponsero, A. J., Jokela, R., Kolho, K.-L., deVos, W. M., & Korpela, K. (2024). Gut microbiota wellbeing index predicts overall health in a cohort of 1000 infants. *Nature Communications*, 15(1), 8323. https://doi.org/10.1038/s41467-024-52561-6

Hill, C., Guarner, F., Reid, G., Gibson, G. R., Merenstein, D. J., Pot, B., Morelli, L., Canani, R. B., Flint, H. J., Salminen, S., Calder, P. C., & Sanders, M. E. (2014a). The International Scientific Association for Probiotics and Prebiotics consensus statement on the scope and appropriate use of the term probiotic. *Nature Reviews Gastroenterology & Hepatology*, 11(8), 506–514. https://doi.org/10.1038/nrgastro.2014.66

Horner, D., Jepsen, J. R. M., Chawes, B., Aagaard, K., Rosenberg, J. B., Mohammadzadeh, P., Sevelsted, A., Vahman, N., Vinding, R., Fagerlund, B., Pantelis, C., Bilenberg, N., Pedersen, C.-E. T., Eliasen, A., Brandt, S., Chen, Y., Prince, N., Chu, S. H., Kelly, R. S., ... Rasmussen, M. A. (2025). A western dietary pattern during pregnancy is associated with neurodevelopmental disorders in childhood and adolescence. *Nature Metabolism*, 7(3), 586–601. https://doi.org/10.1038/s42255-025-01230-z

Jorgensen, J. M., Young, R., Ashorn, P., Ashorn, U., Chaima, D., Davis, J. C., Goonatilleke, E., Kumwenda, C., Lebrilla, C. B., Maleta, K., Prado, E. L., Sadalaki, J., Totten, S. M., Wu, L. D., Zivkovic, A. M., & Dewey, K. G. (2021). Associations of human milk oligosaccharides and bioactive proteins with infant growth and development among Malawian mother-infant dyads. *The American Journal of Clinical Nutrition*, 113(1), 209–220. https://doi.org/10.1093/ajcn/nqaa272

Kaila, M., Isolauri, E., Saxelin, M., Arvilommi, H., & Vesikari, T. (1995). Viable versus inactivated lactobacillus strain GG in acute rotavirus diarrhoea. *Archives of Disease in Childhood*, 72(1), 51–53. https://doi.org/10.1136/adc.72.1.51

Kazemi, A., Noorbala, A. A., Azam, K., Eskandari, M. H., & Djafarian, K. (2019). Effect of probiotic and prebiotic vs placebo on psychological outcomes in patients with major depressive disorder: A randomized clinical trial. *Clinical Nutrition*, 38(2), 522–528. https://doi.org/10.1016/j.clnu.2018.04.010

Keys, A., Mienotti, A., Karvonen, M. J., Aravanis, C., Blackburn, H., Buzina, R., Djordjevic, B. S., Dontas, A. S., Fidanza, F., Keys, M. H., Kromhout, D., Nedeljkovic, S., Punsar, S., Seccareccia, F., & Toshima, H. (1986). THE diet and 15-year death rate in the seven countries study. *American Journal of Epidemiology*, 124(6), 903–915. https://doi.org/10.1093/oxfordjournals.aje.a114480

Khalesi, S., Sun, J., Buys, N., Jamshidi, A., Nikbakht-Nasrabadi, E., & Khosravi-Boroujeni, H. (2014). Green tea catechins and blood pressure: A systematic review and meta-analysis of randomised controlled trials. *European Journal of Nutrition*, 53(6), 1299–1311. https://doi.org/10.1007/s00394-014-0720-1

Khoury, N., Martínez, M. Á., Garcidueñas-Fimbres, T. E., Pastor-Villaescusa, B., Leis, R., de Las Heras-Delgado, S., Miguel-Berges, M. L., Navas-Carretero, S., Portoles, O., Pérez-Vega, K. A., Jurado-Castro, J. M., Vázquez-Cobela, R., Mimbrero, G., Andía Horno, R., Martínez, J. A., Flores-Rojas, K., Picáns-Leis, R., Luque, V., Moreno, L. A., ... Babio, N. (2024). Ultraprocessed food consumption and cardiometabolic risk factors in children. *JAMA Network Open*, 7(5), e2411852. https://doi.org/10.1001/jamanetworkopen.2024.11852

Kirjavainen, P. V., Salminen, S. J., & Isolauri, E. (2003). Probiotic bacteria in the management of atopic disease: Underscoring the importance of viability. *Journal of Pediatric Gastroenterology and Nutrition*, 36(2), 223–227. https://doi.org/10.1097/00005176-200302000-00012

Koh, A., De Vadder, F., Kovatcheva-Datchary, P., & Bäckhed, F. (2016a). From dietary fiber to host physiology: Short-chain fatty acids as key bacterial metabolites. *Cell*, 165(6), 1332–1345. https://doi.org/10.1016/j.cell.2016.05.041

Kolodziejczyk, A. A., Zheng, D., & Elinav, E. (2019a). Diet–microbiota interactions and personalized nutrition. *Nature Reviews Microbiology*, 17(12), 742–753. https://doi.org/10.1038/s41579-019-0256-8

Kwon, D., Zhang, K., Paul, K. C., Folle, A. D., Del Rosario, I., Jacobs, J. P., Keener, A. M., Bronstein, J. M., & Ritz, B. (2024). Diet and the gut microbiome in patients with Parkinson's disease. *NPJ Parkinson's Disease*, 10(1), 89. https://doi.org/10.1038/s41531-024-00681-7

Lahariya, R., Anand, G., Kumari, B., & Priyadarshi, K. (2026). Postbiotics and the gut–brain axis: A mechanistic review on modulating neuroinflammation and cognitive aging. *Journal of Neuroimmunology*, 413, 578870. https://doi.org/10.1016/j.jneuroim.2026.578870

Lane, M. M., Gamage, E., Travica, N., Dissanayaka, T., Ashtree, D. N., Gauci, S., Lotfaliany, M., O'Neil, A., Jacka, F. N., & Marx, W. (2022). Ultra-processed food consumption and mental health: A systematic review and meta-analysis of observational studies. *Nutrients*, 14(13), 2568. https://doi.org/10.3390/nu14132568

Latorre, R., Sternini, C., De Giorgio, R., & Greenwood-Van Meerveld, B. (2016). Enteroendocrine cells: A review of their role in brain–gut communication. *Neurogastroenterology & Motility*, 28(5), 620–630. https://doi.org/10.1111/nmo.12754

Lechner, B. E., & Vohr, B. R. (2017). Neurodevelopmental outcomes of preterm infants fed human milk: A systematic review. *Clinical Perinatology*, 44(1), 69–83.

Leeuwendaal, N. K., Stanton, C., O'Toole, P. W., & Beresford, T. P. (2022). Fermented foods, health and the gut microbiome. *Nutrients*, 14(7), 1527. https://doi.org/10.3390/nu14071527

Leo, A., De Caro, C., Mainardi, P., Tallarico, M., Nesci, V., Marascio, N., Striano, P., Russo, E., Constanti, A., De Sarro, G., & Citraro, R. (2021). Increased efficacy of combining prebiotic and postbiotic in mouse models relevant to autism and depression. *Neuropharmacology*, 198, 108782. https://doi.org/10.1016/j.neuropharm.2021.108782

Li, S., Wang, Z., Liu, G., & Chen, M. (2024). Neurodegenerative diseases and catechins: (−)-epigallocatechin-3-gallate is a modulator of chronic neuroinflammation and oxidative stress. *Frontiers in Nutrition*, 11. https://doi.org/10.3389/fnut.2024.1425839

Li, Y., Aoki, T., Iwabuchi, S., Arai, S., Iwabuchi, N., Motobayashi, H., Tanaka, M., & Hashimoto, S. (2024). Immunomodulatory activity of heat-killed *Lacticaseibacillus paracasei* MCC1849 based on the activation of plasmacytoid dendritic cells in the peripheral blood of healthy adults. *Food Science & Nutrition*, 12(5), 3452–3460. https://doi.org/10.1002/fsn3.4009

Li, Z., Li, Z., Zhu, L., Dai, N., Sun, G., Peng, L., Wang, X., & Yang, Y. (2021). Effects of xylo-oligosaccharide on the gut microbiota of patients with ulcerative colitis in clinical remission. *Frontiers in Nutrition*, 8. https://doi.org/10.3389/fnut.2021.778542

Liang, X., Li, Y., Zhao, Z., Ding, R., Sun, J., & Chi, C. (2024). Safety and efficacy of adding postbiotics in infant formula: A systematic review and meta-analysis. *Pediatric Research*, 95(1), 43–51. https://doi.org/10.1038/s41390-023-02813-w

Louis, P., Young, P., Holtrop, G., & Flint, H. J. (2010). Diversity of human colonic butyrate-producing bacteria revealed by analysis of the butyryl-CoA: Acetate CoA-transferase gene. *Environmental Microbiology*, 12(2), 304–314. https://doi.org/10.1111/j.1462-2920.2009.02066.x

Lyons, K. E., Ryan, C. A., Dempsey, E. M., Ross, R. P., & Stanton, C. (2020). Breast milk, a source of beneficial microbes and associated benefits for infant health. *Nutrients*, 12(4), 1039. https://doi.org/10.3390/nu12041039

Ma, D., Wang, A. C., Parikh, I., Green, S. J., Hoffman, J. D., Chlipala, G., Murphy, M. P., Sokola, B. S., Bauer, B., Hartz, A. M. S., & Lin, A.-L. (2018). Ketogenic diet enhances neurovascular function with altered gut microbiome in young healthy mice. *Scientific Reports*, 8(1), 6670. https://doi.org/10.1038/s41598-018-25190-5

Ma, J., Li, Z., Zhang, W., Zhang, C., Zhang, Y., Mei, H., Zhuo, N., Wang, H., Wang, L., & Wu, D. (2020). Comparison of gut microbiota in exclusively breast-fed and formula-fed babies: A study of 91 term infants. *Scientific Reports*, 10(1), 15792. https://doi.org/10.1038/s41598-020-72635-x

Macfarlane, S., & Macfarlane, G. T. (2003). Regulation of short-chain fatty acid production. *Proceedings of the Nutrition Society*, 62(1), 67–72. https://doi.org/10.1079/PNS2002207

Malesza, I. J., Malesza, M., Walkowiak, J., Mussin, N., Walkowiak, D., Aringazina, R., Bartkowiak-Wieczorek, J., & Mądry, E. (2021). High-fat, western-style diet, systemic inflammation, and gut microbiota: A narrative review. *Cells*, 10(11), 3164. https://doi.org/10.3390/cells10113164

Manyi-Loh, C., Mamphweli, S., Meyer, E., & Okoh, A. (2018). Antibiotic use in agriculture and its consequential resistance in environmental sources: Potential public health implications. *Molecules*, 23(4), 795. https://doi.org/10.3390/molecules23040795

Marzorati, M., Ghyselinck, J., Van den Abbeele, P., Maruszak, A., & Harthoorn, L. (2023). Galactooligosaccharide (GOS) reduces branched short-chain fatty acids, ammonium, and pH in a short-term colonic fermentation model. *Applied Microbiology*, 3(1), 90–103. https://doi.org/10.3390/applmicrobiol3010008

Mei, Z., Yuan, J., & Li, D. (2022). Biological activity of galacto-oligosaccharides: A review. *Frontiers in Microbiology*, 13. https://doi.org/10.3389/fmicb.2022.993052

Mengist, B., Lotfaliany, M., Pasco, J. A., Agustini, B., Berk, M., Forbes, M., Lane, M. M., Orchard, S. G., Ryan, J., Owen, A. J., Woods, R. L., McNeil, J. J., & Mohebbi, M. (2025). The risk associated with ultra-processed food intake on depressive symptoms and mental health in older adults: A target trial emulation. *BMC Medicine*, 23(1), 172. https://doi.org/10.1186/s12916-025-04002-4

Mennella, J. A., & Beauchamp, G. K. (1991). The transfer of alcohol to human milk. *New England Journal of Medicine*, 325(14), 981–985. https://doi.org/10.1056/NEJM199110033251401

Mennella, J. A., Jagnow, C. P., & Beauchamp, G. K. (2001). Prenatal and postnatal flavor learning by human infants. *Pediatrics*, 107(6), e88 https://doi.org/10.1542/peds.107.6.e88

Miranda, P. M., De Palma, G., Serkis, V., Lu, J., Louis-Auguste, M. P., McCarville, J. L., Verdu, E. F., Collins, S. M., & Bercik, P. (2018). High salt diet exacerbates colitis in mice by decreasing Lactobacillus levels and butyrate production. *Microbiome*, 6(1), 57. https://doi.org/10.1186/s40168-018-0433-4

Mortensen, A. (2006). Sweeteners permitted in the European Union: Safety aspects. *Food & Nutrition Research*, 50(3). https://doi.org/10.3402/fnr.v50i3.1588

Nohesara, S., Mostafavi Abdolmaleky, H., Pirani, A., & Thiagalingam, S. (2025). Therapeutic horizons: Gut microbiome, neuroinflammation, and epigenetics in neuropsychiatric disorders. *Cells*, 14(13), 1027. https://doi.org/10.3390/cells14131027

Okburan, G., & Kızıler, S. (2023). Human milk oligosaccharides as prebiotics. *Pediatrics & Neonatology*, 64(3), 231–238. https://doi.org/10.1016/j.pedneo.2022.09.017

O'Riordan, K. J., Collins, M. K., Moloney, G. M., Knox, E. G., Aburto, M. R., Fülling, C., Morley, S. J., Clarke, G., Schellekens, H., & Cryan, J. F. (2022). Short chain fatty acids: Microbial metabolites for gut-brain axis signalling. *Molecular and Cellular Endocrinology*, 546, 111572. https://doi.org/10.1016/j.mce.2022.111572

Padhi, S., Sarkar, P., Sahoo, D., & Rai, A. K. (2025). Potential of fermented foods and their metabolites in improving gut microbiota function and lowering gastrointestinal inflammation. *Journal of the Science of Food and Agriculture*, 105(8), 4058–4069. https://doi.org/10.1002/jsfa.13313

Paoli, A., Rubini, A., Volek, J. S., & Grimaldi, K. A. (2013). Beyond weight loss: A review of the therapeutic uses of very-low-carbohydrate (ketogenic) diets. *European Journal of Clinical Nutrition*, 67(8), 789–796. https://doi.org/10.1038/ejcn.2013.116

Park, I., & Mannaa, M. (2025). Fermented foods as functional systems: Microbial communities and metabolites influencing gut health and systemic outcomes. *Foods*, 14(13), 2292. https://doi.org/10.3390/foods14132292

Patanè, G. T., Putaggio, S., Tellone, E., Barreca, D., Ficarra, S., Maffei, C., Calderaro, A., & Laganà, G. (2023). Catechins and proanthocyanidins involvement in metabolic syndrome. *International Journal of Molecular Sciences*, 24(11), 9228. https://doi.org/10.3390/ijms24119228

Pietrzak, D., Kasperek, K., Rękawek, P., & Piątkowska-Chmiel, I. (2022). The therapeutic role of ketogenic diet in neurological disorders. *Nutrients*, 14(9), 1952. https://doi.org/10.3390/nu14091952

Plamada, D., & Vodnar, D. C. (2021). Polyphenols—Gut microbiota interrelationship: A transition to a new generation of prebiotics. *Nutrients*, 14(1), 137. https://doi.org/10.3390/nu14010137

Premkumar, M. H., & Pammi, M. (2025). Probiotics in breast-fed healthy term infants: Imperative or superfluous? *Pediatric Research*, 99(4), 1264–1265. https://doi.org/10.1038/s41390-025-04485-0

Qi, X., Yun, C., Pang, Y., & Qiao, J. (2021). The impact of the gut microbiota on the reproductive and metabolic endocrine system. *Gut Microbes*, 13(1). https://doi.org/10.1080/19490976.2021.1894070

Ramos-Vivas, J. (2020). Microbiología de Hafnia alvei. *Enfermedades Infecciosas y Microbiología Clínica*, 38, 1–6. https://doi.org/10.1016/j.eimc.2020.02.001

Rinninella, E., Tohumcu, E., Raoul, P., Fiorani, M., Cintoni, M., Mele, M. C., Cammarota, G., Gasbarrini, A., & Ianiro, G. (2023). The role of diet in shaping human gut microbiota. *Best Practice & Research Clinical Gastroenterology*, 62–63, 101828. https://doi.org/10.1016/j.bpg.2023.101828

Rondinella, D., Raoul, P. C., Valeriani, E., Venturini, I., Cintoni, M., Severino, A., Galli, F. S., Mora, V., Mele, M. C., Cammarota, G., Gasbarrini, A., Rinninella, E., & Ianiro, G. (2025). The detrimental impact of ultra-processed foods on the human gut microbiome and gut barrier. *Nutrients*, 17(5), 859. https://doi.org/10.3390/nu17050859

Rusch, J. A., Layden, B. T., & Dugas, L. R. (2023). Signalling cognition: The gut microbiota and hypothalamic-pituitary-adrenal axis. *Frontiers in Endocrinology*, 14. https://doi.org/10.3389/fendo.2023.1130689

Ryan, F. J., Clarke, M., Lynn, M. A., Benson, S. C., McAlister, S., Giles, L. C., Choo, J. M., Rossouw, C., Ng, Y. Y., Semchenko, E. A., Richard, A., Leong, L. E. X., Taylor, S. L., Blake, S. J., Mugabushaka, J. I., Walker, M., Wesselingh, S. L., Licciardi, P. V., Seib, K. L., … Lynn, D. J. (2025). Bifidobacteria support optimal infant vaccine responses. *Nature*, 641(8062), 456–464. https://doi.org/10.1038/s41586-025-08796-4

Sagris, M., Vlachakis, P. K., Simantiris, S., Theofilis, P., Gerogianni, M., Karakasis, P., Tsioufis, K., & Tousoulis, D. (2024). From a cup of tea to cardiovascular care: Vascular mechanisms of action. *Life*, 14(9), 1168. https://doi.org/10.3390/life14091168

Salminen, S., Collado, M. C., Endo, A., Hill, C., Lebeer, S., Quigley, E. M. M., Sanders, M. E., Shamir, R., Swann, J. R., Szajewska, H., & Vinderola, G. (2021). The International Scientific Association of Probiotics and Prebiotics (ISAPP) consensus statement on the definition and scope of postbiotics. *Nature Reviews Gastroenterology & Hepatology*, 18(9), 649–667. https://doi.org/10.1038/s41575-021-00440-6

Samtiya, M., Aluko, R. E., Puniya, A. K., & Dhewa, T. (2021). Enhancing micronutrients bioavailability through fermentation of plant-based foods: A concise review. *Fermentation*, 7(2), 63. https://doi.org/10.3390/fermentation7020063

Sanders, M. E., Akkermans, L. M. A., Haller, D., Hammerman, C., Heimbach, J. T., Hörmannsperger, G., & Huys, G. (2010). Safety assessment of probiotics for human use. *Gut Microbes*, 1(3), 164–185. https://doi.org/10.4161/gmic.1.3.12127

Schneeberger, M., Everard, A., Gómez-Valadés, A. G., Matamoros, S., Ramírez, S., Delzenne, N. M., Gomis, R., Claret, M., & Cani, P. D. (2015). Akkermansia muciniphila inversely correlates with the onset of inflammation, altered adipose tissue metabolism and metabolic disorders during obesity in mice. *Scientific Reports*, 5(1), 16643. https://doi.org/10.1038/srep16643

Schöpping, M., Zeidan, A. A., & Franzén, C. J. (2022). Stress response in bifidobacteria. *Microbiology and Molecular Biology Reviews*, 86(4). https://doi.org/10.1128/mmbr.00170-21

Shaaban, S. Y., El Gendy, Y. G., Mehanna, N. S., El-Senousy, W. M., El-Feki, H. S. A., Saad, K., & El-Asheer, O. M. (2018). The role of probiotics in children with autism spectrum disorder: A prospective, open-label study. *Nutritional Neuroscience*, 21(9), 676–681. https://doi.org/10.1080/1028415X.2017.1347746

Shan, Z., Rehm, C. D., Rogers, G., Ruan, M., Wang, D. D., Hu, F. B., Mozaffarian, D., Zhang, F. F., & Bhupathiraju, S. N. (2019). Trends in dietary carbohydrate, protein, and fat intake and diet quality among US adults, 1999-2016. *JAMA*, 322(12), 1178. https://doi.org/10.1001/jama.2019.13771

Sharawat, I. K., Panda, P., Dawman, L., Gupta, D., & Panda, P. K. (2025). Modified Atkins Diet versus low glycemic index treatment in children with drug-resistant epilepsy: A systematic review and meta-analysis. *Seizure: European Journal of Epilepsy*, 131, 471–479. https://doi.org/10.1016/j.seizure.2024.12.001

Shimizu, H., Miyamoto, J., Hisa, K., Ohue-Kitano, R., Takada, H., Yamano, M., Nishida, A., Sasahara, D., Masujima, Y., Watanabe, K., Nishikawa, S., Takahashi, S., Ikeda, T., Nakajima, Y., Yoshida, N., Matsuzaki, C., Kageyama, T., Hayashi, I., Matsuki, A., … Kimura, I. (2025). Sucrose-preferring gut microbes prevent host obesity by producing exopolysaccharides. *Nature Communications*, 16(1), 1145. https://doi.org/10.1038/s41467-025-56470-0

Siddiqui, R., Lloyd, D., Maciver, S. K., & Khan, N. A. (2025). Gut microbiome-derived metabolites and epigenetic modulation as potential countermeasures to acute stress. *Discover Medicine*, 2(1), 280. https://doi.org/10.1007/s44337-025-00490-8

Stewart, C. J., Ajami, N. J., O'Brien, J. L., Hutchinson, D. S., Smith, D. P., Wong, M. C., Ross, M. C., Lloyd, R. E., Doddapaneni, H., Metcalf, G. A., Muzny, D., Gibbs, R. A., Vatanen, T., Huttenhower, C., Xavier, R. J., Rewers, M., Hagopian, W., Toppari, J., Ziegler, A.-G., … Petrosino, J. F. (2018). Temporal development of the gut microbiome in early childhood from the TEDDY study. *Nature*, 562(7728), 583–588. https://doi.org/10.1038/s41586-018-0617-x

Stiemsma, L. T., Nakamura, R. E., Nguyen, J. G., & Michels, K. B. (2020). Does consumption of fermented foods modify the human gut microbiota? *The Journal of Nutrition*, 150(7), 1680–1692. https://doi.org/10.1093/jn/nxaa077

Stoeva, M. K., Garcia-So, J., Justice, N., Myers, J., Tyagi, S., Nemchek, M., McMurdie, P. J., Kolterman, O., & Eid, J. (2021). Butyrate-producing human gut symbiont, *Clostridium butyricum*, and its role in health and disease. *Gut Microbes*, 13(1). https://doi.org/10.1080/19490976.2021.1907272

Sun, E. W. L., Martin, A. M., Young, R. L., & Keating, D. J. (2019). The regulation of peripheral metabolism by gut-derived hormones. *Frontiers in Endocrinology*, 9. https://doi.org/10.3389/fendo.2018.00754

Swidsinski, A., Dörffel, Y., Loening-Baucke, V., Gille, C., Göktas, Ö., Reißhauer, A., Neuhaus, J., Weylandt, K.-H., Guschin, A., & Bock, M. (2017). Reduced mass and diversity of the colonic microbiome in patients with multiple sclerosis and their improvement with ketogenic diet. *Frontiers in Microbiology*, 8. https://doi.org/10.3389/fmicb.2017.01141

Szajewska, H., Canani, R. B., Guarino, A., Hojsak, I., Indrio, F., Kolacek, S., Orel, R., Shamir, R., Vandenplas, Y., van Goudoever, J. B., & Weizman, Z. (2016). Probiotics for the prevention of antibiotic-associated diarrhea in children. *Journal of Pediatric Gastroenterology and Nutrition*, 62(3), 495–506. https://doi.org/10.1097/MPG.0000000000001081

Tan, Q., Orsso, C. E., Deehan, E. C., Kung, J.Y., Tun, H. M., Wine, E., Madsen, K. L., Zwaigenbaum, L., & Haqq, A. M. (2021). Probiotics, prebiotics, synbiotics, and fecal microbiota transplantation in the treatment of behavioral symptoms of autism spectrum disorder: A systematic review. *Autism Research*, 14(9), 1820–1836. https://doi.org/10.1002/aur.2560

Tomova, A., Bukovsky, I., Rembert, E., Yonas, W., Alwarith, J., Barnard, N. D., & Kahleova, H. (2019). The effects of vegetarian and vegan diets on gut microbiota. *Frontiers in Nutrition*, 6. https://doi.org/10.3389/fnut.2019.00047

Troisi, J., Autio, R., Beopoulos, T., Bravaccio, C., Carraturo, F., Corrivetti, G., Cunningham, S., Devane, S., Fallin, D., Fetissov, S., Gea, M., Giorgi, A., Iris, F., Joshi, L., Kadzielski, S., Kraneveld, A., Kumar, H., Ladd-Acosta, C., Leader, G., … Fasano, A. (2020). Genome, environment, microbiome and metabolome in autism (GEMMA) study design: Biomarkers Identification for precision treatment and primary prevention of autism spectrum disorders by an integrated multi-omics systems biology approach. *Brain Sciences*, 10(10), 743. https://doi.org/10.3390/brainsci10100743

Tsigalou, C., Tsolou, A., Stavropoulou, E., Konstantinidis, T., Zafiriou, E., Dardiotis, E., Tsirogianni, A., & Bogdanos, D. (2024). Unraveling the intricate dance of the Mediterranean diet and gut microbiota in autoimmune resilience. *Frontiers in Nutrition*, 11. https://doi.org/10.3389/fnut.2024.1383040

Turnbaugh, P. J., Ley, R. E., Mahowald, M. A., Magrini, V., Mardis, E. R., & Gordon, J. I. (2006). An obesity-associated gut microbiome with increased capacity for energy harvest. *Nature*, 444(7122), 1027–1031. https://doi.org/10.1038/nature05414

Turroni, F., Milani, C., Duranti, S., Mahony, J., van Sinderen, D., & Ventura, M. (2018). Glycan utilization and cross-feeding activities by bifidobacteria. *Trends in Microbiology*, 26(4), 339–350. https://doi.org/10.1016/j.tim.2017.10.001

Urashima, T., Ajisaka, K., Ujihara, T., & Nakazaki, E. (2025). Recent advances in the science of human milk oligosaccharides. *BBA Advances*, 7, 100136. https://doi.org/10.1016/j.bbadva.2024.100136

Veiga, P., Pons, N., Agrawal, A., Oozeer, R., Guyonnet, D., Brazeilles, R., Faurie, J.-M., van Hylckama Vlieg, J. E. T., Houghton, L. A., Whorwell, P. J., Ehrlich, S. D., & Kennedy, S. P. (2014). Changes of the human gut microbiome induced by a fermented milk product. *Scientific Reports*, 4(1), 6328. https://doi.org/10.1038/srep06328

Walsh, C., Owens, R. A., Bottacini, F., Lane, J. A., van Sinderen, D., & Hickey, R. M. (2023). HMO-primed bifidobacteria exhibit enhanced ability to adhere to intestinal epithelial cells. *Frontiers in Microbiology*, 14. https://doi.org/10.3389/fmicb.2023.1232173

Wang, J., Cazzato, E., Ladewig, E., Frattini, V., Rosenbloom, D. I. S., Zairis, S., Abate, F., Liu, Z., Elliott, O., Shin, Y.-J., Lee, J.-K., Lee, I.-H., Park, W.-Y., Eoli, M., Blumberg, A. J., Lasorella, A., Nam, D.-H., Finocchiaro, G., Iavarone, A., & Rabadan, R. (2016). Clonal evolution of glioblastoma under therapy. *Nature Genetics*, 48(7), 768–776. https://doi.org/10.1038/ng.3590

Wang, S., Bao, Z., Li, Z., Zhao, M., Wang, X., & Liu, F. (2025). The impact of very-low-calorie ketogenic diets on gut microbiota in individuals with obesity: A systematic review and meta-analysis. *Gut Microbes*, 17(1). https://doi.org/10.1080/19490976.2025.2566305

Wang, X., Lang, F., & Liu, D. (2024). High-salt diet and intestinal microbiota: Influence on cardiovascular disease and inflammatory bowel disease. *Biology*, 13(9), 674. https://doi.org/10.3390/biology13090674

Wang, Y., Zhang, K., Dai, L., Sun, F., Wang, D., Meng, S., Zhao, J., Liu, Y., Liu, W., Li, C., Wang, Y., Lu, W., & Zhu, Y. (2023). Associations of fruit, whole grain, and total energy intakes with gut microbiome diversity and composition. *Food & Nutrition Research*, 67. https://doi.org/10.29219/fnr.v67.9725

Więckowska-Gacek, A., Mietelska-Porowska, A., Wydrych, M., & Wojda, U. (2021). Western diet as a trigger of Alzheimer's disease: From metabolic syndrome and systemic inflammation to neuroinflammation and neurodegeneration. *Ageing Research Reviews*, 70, 101397. https://doi.org/10.1016/j.arr.2021.101397

Wongkrasant, P., Pongkorpsakol, P., Chitwattananont, S., Satianrapapong, W., Tuangkijkul, N., & Muanprasat, C. (2020). Fructo-oligosaccharides alleviate inflammation-associated apoptosis of GLP-1 secreting L cells via inhibition of iNOS and cleaved caspase-3 expression. *Journal of Pharmacological Sciences*, 143(2), 65–73. https://doi.org/10.1016/j.jphs.2020.03.001

Wu, G. D., Chen, J., Hoffmann, C., Bittinger, K., Chen, Y.-Y., Keilbaugh, S. A., Bewtra, M., Knights, D., Walters, W. A., Knight, R., Sinha, R., Gilroy, E., Gupta, K., Baldassano, R., Nessel, L., Li, H., Bushman, F. D., & Lewis, J. D. (2011). Linking long-term dietary patterns with gut microbial enterotypes. *Science*, 334(6052), 105–108. https://doi.org/10.1126/science.1208344

Xiao, W., Zhang, Q., Yu, L., Tian, F., Chen, W., & Zhai, Q. (2022). Effects of vegetarian diet-associated nutrients on gut microbiota and intestinal physiology. *Food Science and Human Wellness*, 11(2), 208–217. https://doi.org/10.1016/j.fshw.2021.11.002

Xie, Z., Zhang, G., Liu, R., Wang, Y., Tsapieva, A., Zhang, L., & Han, J. (2023). Heat-killed lacticaseibacillus paracasei repairs lipopolysaccharide-induced intestinal epithelial barrier damage via MLCK/MLC pathway activation. *Nutrients*, 15(7), 1758. https://doi.org/10.3390/nu15071758

Xu, R., Gridneva, Z., Payne, M. S., Nicol, M. P., Cheema, A. S., Geddes, D. T., & Stinson, L. F. (2025). Longitudinal profiling of the human milk microbiome from birth to 12 months reveals overall stability and selective taxa-level variation. *Microorganisms*, 13(8), 1830. https://doi.org/10.3390/microorganisms13081830

Yang, M., Qi, X., Li, N., Kaifi, J. T., Chen, S., Wheeler, A. A., Kimchi, E. T., Ericsson, A. C., Rector, R. S., Staveley-O'Carroll, K. F., & Li, G. (2023). Western diet contributes to the pathogenesis of non-alcoholic steatohepatitis in male mice via remodeling gut microbiota and increasing production of 2-oleoylglycerol. *Nature Communications*, 14(1), 228. https://doi.org/10.1038/s41467-023-35861-1

Zafar, M. I., Mills, K. E., Zheng, J., Regmi, A., Hu, S. Q., Gou, L., & Chen, L.-L. (2019). Low-glycemic index diets as an intervention for diabetes: A systematic review and meta-analysis. *The American Journal of Clinical Nutrition*, 110(4), 891–902. https://doi.org/10.1093/ajcn/nqz149

Zeevi, D., Korem, T., Zmora, N., Israeli, D., Rothschild, D., Weinberger, A., Ben-Yacov, O., Lador, D., Avnit-Sagi, T., Lotan-Pompan, M., Suez, J., Mahdi, J. A., Matot, E., Malka, G., Kosower, N., Rein, M., Zilberman-Schapira, G., Dohnalová, L., Pevsner-Fischer, M., … Segal, E. (2015a). Personalized nutrition by prediction of glycemic responses. *Cell*, 163(5), 1079–1094. https://doi.org/10.1016/j.cell.2015.11.001

Zhang, T., Nickerson, R., Zhang, W., Peng, X., Shang, Y., Zhou, Y., Luo, Q., Wen, G., & Cheng, Z. (2024). The impacts of animal agriculture on One Health—Bacterial zoonosis, antimicrobial resistance, and beyond. *One Health*, 18, 100748. https://doi.org/10.1016/j.onehlt.2024.100748

Zhang, W., Zhang, Y., Zhao, Y., Li, L., Zhang, Z., Hettinga, K., Yang, H., & Deng, J. (2024). A comprehensive review on dietary polysaccharides as prebiotics, synbiotics, and postbiotics in infant formula and their influences on gut microbiota. *Nutrients*, 16(23), 4122. https://doi.org/10.3390/nu16234122

Zhu, L., Baker, S. S., Gill, C., Liu, W., Alkhouri, R., Baker, R. D., & Gill, S. R. (2013). Characterization of gut microbiomes in nonalcoholic steatohepatitis (NASH) patients: A connection between endogenous alcohol and NASH. *Hepatology*, 57(2), 601–609. https://doi.org/10.1002/hep.26093

CHAPTER 2

The Intricate Relationship between Food and Gut Microbes

IMPLICATIONS IN HEALTH AND DISEASES

Gopal Khodve, Suparna Roy Sarkar, and Sugato Banerjee

2.1 INTRODUCTION

The human gut microbiome is the most diverse and complex ecosystem within the human body, comprising trillions of microorganisms that influence the host's health and susceptibility to disease. This diverse microbial community, primarily composed of bacteria but also including fungi, archaea, viruses, and protozoans, plays a crucial role as a mediator between dietary intake and various health-related outcomes. Studies have highlighted dietary changes that can induce significant, transient microbial modifications within a day (Leeming et al., 2019). Such rapid responsiveness suggests that food has a profound impact on shaping microbial communities. The gut microbes play a crucial role in modulating the risk of several chronic diseases, including inflammatory bowel diseases (IBDs), obesity, cardiovascular diseases, type 2 diabetes, neurological complications, and cancer (Hou et al., 2022). The vital role played by food in shaping microbial communities opens new, extraordinary therapeutic opportunities. Understanding the link between particular microbes and their effect on microbial populations reveals diverse functions in host metabolism and immunity (Cao et al., 2024) (Figure 2.1). Recent evidence suggests that targeted dietary interventions can play a role in disease prevention and treatment.

Various food items represent the dietary inputs that shape microbial composition and function. One pathway illustrates how the consumption and digestion of food impact microbiome diversity within the gastrointestinal tract. The other pathway (right arrow) indicates that indigestible dietary components undergo microbial fermentation, resulting in metabolites that affect host physiology. At the bottom left, the intestinal microbiome is depicted, emphasizing the rich diversity of microbial species. Two horizontal arrows represent reciprocal communication between the host and its microbiota: microbiome-derived components (such as metabolites, signaling molecules, and microbial products) act on the host to modulate health outcomes, while host-derived components (including immune factors, epithelial secretions, and nutrients) influence microbial community structure and function.

2.2 THE GUT MICROBIOTA: COMPOSITION, STRUCTURE, AND FUNCTION

2.2.1 Basic Characteristics of the Gut Microbiota

The human gut tract is colonized by billions of microbes, primarily composed of bacteria. The microbial ecosystems exhibit remarkable complexity, with composition and density varying significantly along the gastrointestinal tract. The bacterial populations are largely defined by two major phytotypes, Bacteroidetes and Firmicutes.

DOI: 10.1201/9781003638292-2

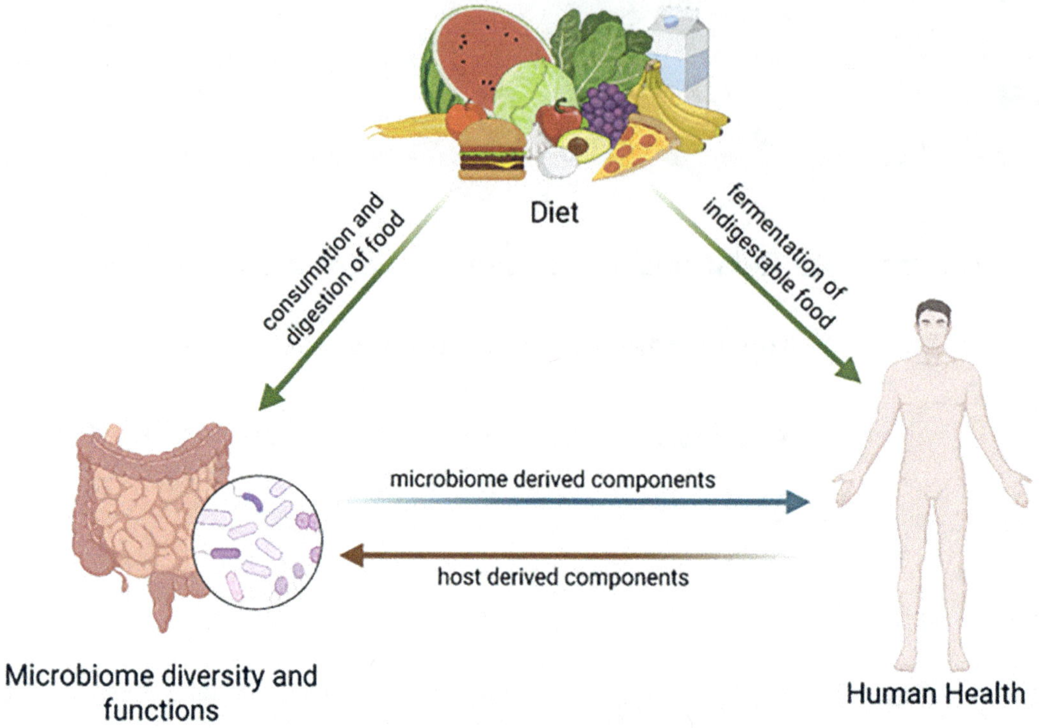

Figure 2.1 The bidirectional relationship between diet, the gut microbiome, and human health.

Proteobacteria, Actinobacteria, *Fusobacteria*, and Verrucomicrobia are also present in relatively lower numbers (Thursby & Juge, 2017). The most outstanding characteristic of the microbiota is its genomic capacity. The metagenome is 150 times larger than the human genetic code because the collective genomes of gut microorganisms, known as the microbiome, encode about 100 times as many genes as the human genome. This extensive gene catalogue facilitates the microbial community to perform metabolic functions far beyond those possible by human cells alone, effectively functioning as an auxiliary organ that modulates numerous aspects of host physiology (Dinan et al., 2015). The composition of microbes is not uniform among all individuals, and interindividual variation exists in microbiota. However, recent research has identified distinct enterotypes, characterized by microbial community structures that appear to be more conserved across populations than initially estimated. Enterotype identification is crucial for clinical and dietary decision-making, as it enables the tailoring of nutritional strategies to individual microbiota profiles. This personalized approach can enhance health outcomes by aligning dietary interventions with the specific microbial compositions found in different people. Research comparing groups with different eating habits has shown that the population consuming a Mediterranean diet, which is rich in plant-based foods, is largely colonized by the *Prevotella* enterotype. In contrast, those who consume a Western diet, characterized by high levels of animal protein, fats, and processed carbohydrates, are mainly associated with the *Bacteroides* enterotype. This finding highlights the significant impact of dietary patterns on the development of these enterotypes (Khaledi et al., 2024).

2.2.2 Fundamental Microbial Genera and Their Functions

The functional capacity of the gut microbiota depends critically on the specific bacterial genera present and their metabolic capabilities. *Bifidobacteria* represent one of the most extensively studied genera, with numerous functions attributed to them, comprising the degradation of non-digestible carbohydrates, defense against pathogens, production of vitamin B and antioxidants, and stimulation of the immune system. These bacteria are especially prevalent in babies; in vaginally delivered, breastfed infants, they can make up as much as 90% of the entire colon microbiota. However, their numbers decline significantly with age to less than 5% in healthy adults. The functional capacity of the gut microbiota largely depends on the specific bacterial genera present and their metabolic capabilities (Rivière et al., 2016). Butyrate-producing bacteria, particularly species such as *Faecalibacterium prausnitzii*, *Roseburia*, *Eubacterium rectale*, and *Anaerostipes*, play a dynamic conservational role due to their ability to generate butyrate. This essential metabolite serves as the primary energy source for intestinal epithelial cells. Fiber-degrading bacteria from genera such as *Prevotella*, *Bacteroides*, *Ruminococcus*, and *Oscillibacter* possess the enzymatic tools essential to ferment complex dietary polysaccharides, making them crucial for converting dietary fiber into beneficial short-chain fatty acids (SCFAs) (Güler et al., 2025). For clinicians and dietitians, understanding these microbial roles underscores the importance of recommending fiber-rich and fermented foods to support a healthy gut environment and enhance patient health outcomes. The occurrence and richness of specific bacterial taxa have been linked to health outcomes, with some bacteria producing beneficial effects while others are responsible for harmful effects in pathological conditions. For example, *Akkermansia muciniphila* has been responsible for its anti-inflammatory action. Conversely, pro-inflammatory bacteria, such as the *Ruminococcus* and *Blautia* genera, have been associated with dysbiosis and disease states (Kumar S et al., 2025).

2.3 DIETARY COMPONENTS AND THEIR EFFECTS ON MICROBIOTA COMPOSITION

2.3.1 Dietary Fiber and Complex Carbohydrates

In recent decades, people have been eating a more Western diet, but fiber intake has decreased. This occurs because most of the population consumes ultra-processed food that is low in fiber. These elements work together to cause dysbiosis and other metabolic issues, which frequently lead to an increase in the number of beneficial microbial flora and their metabolic effects, especially those that can ferment complex carbs into SCFAs. Over the past few decades, Western diets have undergone significant changes, with people consuming less fiber and more ultra-processed foods, which are typically low in dietary fiber. This has led to dysbiosis and other metabolic disorders (Clemente-Suárez et al., 2023). The different types of diets and structural dietary carbohydrates have a profound influence on which bacterial community becomes more dominant within the microbiota. Complex carbohydrates, such as resistant starch, non-starch polysaccharides, and inulin-type fructans, selectively support the growth of specific bacterial groups (Lee et al., 2024). In carefully controlled feeding studies, volunteers consuming diets high in resistant starch experienced significant increases in bacteria related to *Ruminococcus bromii*. Notably, the structural characteristics of resistant starch, including the amylose-to-amylopectin ratio, granule morphology, and crystalline type, have a significant impact on microbial fermentation dynamics. High-amylose, B-type resistant starch selectively boosts the population of butyrate-producing gut bacteria. In comparison, retrograded resistant starch tends to stimulate other microbial communities, such as Bacteroides, thereby altering the relative quantities of SCFAs produced. Interestingly, individuals have varying abilities to ferment different types of dietary fiber, which is largely influenced by their initial microbiota composition, particularly their dominant enterotype. This finding has significant implications for personalized nutrition, as it suggests that differences in baseline microbiota composition can influence how a person metabolically responds to specific dietary interventions (Jarrett & Ashworth, 2018).

2.3.2 Proteins and Amino Acid Metabolism

The effect of protein ingestion and amino acid metabolism on gut microbial populations is a complex subject. Dietary proteins serve dual roles as both energy sources and building blocks for bacterial growth. A comparative study between individuals following Mediterranean diets rich in plant-based proteins and those consuming Western diets high in animal protein revealed distinct microbial signatures. Following a Mediterranean diet was associated with a lower Firmicutes-to-Bacteroidetes ratio and a greater presence of Bacteroidetes, indicating that protein intake has a positive influence on microbial diversity. However, it was also observed that high protein consumption could decrease overall diversity. This suggests that both the source and quantity of protein intake are important for maintaining healthy microbiota (Liu et al., 2024). Microbes break down amino acids and make different end products, some of which might be bad for your health. Studies show that people who follow a Mediterranean diet, which contains less animal protein, have lower levels of 1-methylhistamine, a marker for allergic reactions, compared to those who consume a diet high in animal protein. High-protein, high-fat Western diets, on the other hand, create an environment in the stomach where amino acids and substances that aid in breaking down fats are abundant. In these diets, there are more microbial genes that help break down proteins, make vitamins, and get iron (de Jesús Rodríguez-Romero et al., 2022). According to recent studies, the gut microbiota regulates the transport and absorption of amino acids through several reliable processes. Microbiota-derived proteases aid in protein digestion by breaking down dietary proteins into absorbable amino acids and peptides. Some bacterial strains can also degrade dietary immunogenic peptides, which enhances the bioavailability of amino acids while reducing inflammatory responses. Furthermore, microbial metabolites, especially SCFAs, affect transporter activity by acidifying the intestinal lumen, thereby enhancing the efficiency of amino acid transport (Trautmann et al., 2024).

2.3.3 Dietary Fats and Lipid Metabolism

The composition and function of gut microbiota can be influenced by the type and quantity of dietary fats. Diets that are high in saturated fats and low in plant-based foods, characteristic of Western eating patterns, have been consistently linked to dysbiosis and increased inflammation. These high-fat diets encourage the growth of bacteria that can metabolize lipids. This shift in microbial composition and functionality can contribute to the development of chronic diseases, such as food allergies, IBD, and metabolic disorders (Soldán et al., 2024). The introduction of omega-3 polyunsaturated fatty acids has shown promising effects in addressing dysbiosis caused by high-fat diets. A systematic investigation of preclinical models demonstrated that interventions with omega-3 polyunsaturated fatty acids consistently reduced weight gain and fat accumulation associated with high-fat diets. More importantly, omega-3 supplementation significantly altered the composition of the gut microbiota, notably by decreasing the Firmicutes-to-Bacteroidetes ratio, which is a key indicator of dysbiosis induced by high-fat diets (Kumar V et al., 2025). Additionally, omega-3 supplementation was associated with the enhancement of helpful bacterial taxa, such as *A. muciniphila*, *Bifidobacterium*, and *Lactobacillus*. This enrichment was correlated with increased production of SCFAs, improved gut barrier integrity, and reduced systemic inflammation (Cao et al., 2025).

2.3.4 Polyphenols and Bioactive Compounds

Plant-derived polyphenols, found abundantly in foods such as berries, red wine, tea, and various vegetables, are another important class of dietary compounds that influence the composition and function of the microbiota. These bioactive substances regulate the gut microbiota by promoting the growth of beneficial bacteria and inhibiting the growth of pathogenic ones. Plant-based polyphenol-rich diets encourage the growth of bacteria, such as *Lactobacillus* and *Bifidobacterium*, which possess anti-inflammatory and anti-pathogenic properties, thereby improving cardiovascular health. Meta-analytical evidence indicates that polyphenol supplementation significantly increases the abundance of *Lactobacillus* by 220% and *Bifidobacterium* by 56%, while also inhibiting the growth of pathogenic *Clostridium* species (Wang et al., 2024). Typically, this substantial rise in *Lactobacillus* abundance is observed with a daily polyphenol intake equivalent to consuming two cups of mixed berries or two glasses of red wine. Providing such a concrete dosing context empowers clinicians to translate these findings into practical dietary advice. The mechanisms through which polyphenols influence the microbiota are complex, involving both direct antimicrobial effects and indirect support of beneficial bacteria via selective fermentation patterns. The structural features of polyphenols and their dietary levels affect gut microbiota growth and metabolic activity. When ingested, polyphenols tend to promote the growth of Gram-positive bacteria in the gut relative to Gram-negative bacteria, due to differences in cell wall structure. These bioactive compounds lead to the production of crucial microbiota-derived metabolites, including SCFAs, bile acid derivatives, and tryptophan metabolites, which are essential for gut homeostasis and influence gut barrier function, immune responses, energy metabolism, and anti-inflammatory processes (Plamada & Vodnar, 2021).

2.4 MICROBIAL METABOLITES: THE MEDIATORS OF HEALTH AND DISEASE

2.4.1 Short-Chain Fatty Acids

The main byproducts of gut bacteria fermenting dietary fiber and resistant starch are SCFAs, primarily acetate, propionate, and butyrate, which normally make up 90–95% of total SCFA in a ratio of 3:1:1. These volatile fatty acids are vital links between diet, gut microbiota, and overall host health, with butyrate serving as the preferred energy source for intestinal epithelial cells, influencing their proliferation and differentiation, and affecting specific subpopulations such as enteroendocrine cells that contribute to gastrointestinal motility (Den Besten et al., 2013). The physiological importance of SCFAs extends far beyond their role in nourishing intestinal epithelial cells. These metabolites bolster the intestinal barrier through mechanisms that preserve epithelial cell junctions and enhance their structural integrity, thereby preventing the translocation of pathogenic bacteria. Recent research has shown that butyrate and other SCFAs have immunomodulatory functions, with dietary fiber and its fermentation products proven to strengthen barrier integrity, regulate glucose and lipid metabolism, and reduce inflammatory responses. However, it is important to note that recent studies have also highlighted instances where SCFA overproduction is linked to certain types of cancer, suggesting that the health benefits of SCFAs must be interpreted within a broader clinical context. The production of SCFAs relies heavily on the availability of fermentable substrates and the metabolic capacity of specific bacterial populations (Silva et al., 2020). Notably, not all fermentable fibers are equally capable of stimulating SCFA production, and individual microbiota composition plays a critical role in determining response to specific dietary supplements. In response to resistant starch, increased butyrate production can necessitate the use of *R. bromii* or *Clostridium chartatabidum*. Although they are adept at breaking down resistant starch and inulin, *Bifidobacteria* could not be directly responsible for the short-term butyrogenic impact of those fermentable fibers. However, by interacting with other bacteria and exchanging nutrients, they promote the production of butyrate (Fusco et al., 2023). The mechanism by which SCFAs promote health involves their interaction with metabolite-sensing receptors GPR43 and GPR109A, located on non-hematopoietic cells, which helps protect against the onset of colitis. A deficiency or low intake of fiber leads to a reduction in SCFA levels, thereby worsening the development of colitis. In contrast, a high consumption of the SCFA acetate offers protection against colitis by promoting potassium efflux and hyperpolarization, ultimately inhibiting the activation of the NLRP3 inflammasome (Macia et al., 2015).

2.4.2 Bile Acid Metabolites and Secondary Metabolites

In addition to SCFAs, the gut microbiota produces a range of other bioactive metabolites that impact host health. Bile acid metabolites are a significant category of microbial products that play a role in lipid regulation and metabolic control. The microbial transformation of bile acids results in the formation of bioactive compounds that interact with receptors, such as the farnesoid X receptor and G protein-coupled receptor 1, thereby affecting lipid and glucose metabolism both locally and systemically throughout the body (Liu et al., 2022). Important dietary components, such as specific dietary fats and fibers, can significantly influence the composition of bile acid pools, thereby establishing a critical link between nutrient input and metabolite output in the food–microbe–metabolite narrative. Additional newly discovered factors, including endocannabinoids, bioactive lipids, phenolic-derived chemicals, and advanced glycation end products, are also produced from dietary components as secondary metabolites. These substances and their receptors, including aryl hydrocarbon receptors, peroxisome proliferator-activated receptors alpha and gamma, and various G protein-coupled receptors (GPR41, GPR43, GPR119), represent additional mechanisms by which metabolites derived from the microbiota regulate host metabolism and immunity (De Vos et al., 2022).

2.4.3 Tryptophan Metabolites

Tryptophan metabolism by the gut microbiota results in metabolites that have a significant impact on host health and disease, particularly in relation to immunological and neurological processes. The microbiota and the central nervous system communicate in both directions through the gut–brain axis, and microbial metabolites of tryptophan play a crucial role in the production of neurotransmitters and the regulation of mood. An increase in plasma tryptophan, which serves as a precursor to serotonin, a vital neurotransmitter within the gut–brain axis, occurs due to the microbial breakdown of dietary tryptophan, affecting pathways associated with psychological well-being and responses to stress (Shaw et al., 2023). Here, an intriguing question arises: How do specific dietary interventions targeting the gut microbiota influence tryptophan metabolism and, consequently, mental health outcomes? Future research might explore this area to uncover novel therapeutic strategies.

2.5 DIET QUALITY AND SPECIFIC DIETARY PATTERNS INFLUENCING INTESTINAL MICROBIOTA

2.5.1 The Mediterranean Diet and Plant-Based Diets

The Mediterranean diet, characterized by a high intake of plant-based foods, monounsaturated fats (mainly from extra-virgin olive oil), and polyphenols, has been extensively studied for its ability to promote the growth of beneficial gut bacteria. This dietary pattern encourages greater microbial diversity and reduces the presence of pro-inflammatory bacteria compared to other nutritional approaches. Both clinical and preclinical studies have consistently shown that following a Mediterranean diet is associated with improved markers of insulin sensitivity, lipid metabolism, and cognitive function (Perrone & D'Angelo, 2025). The specific mechanisms through which Mediterranean diet components influence the microbiota have been progressively elucidated. The Mediterranean diet promotes the growth of beneficial bacteria, including *Bifidobacterium*, *F. prausnitzii*, and *Roseburia*, which produce SCFAs that enhance gut barrier integrity, reduce inflammation, and improve metabolic homeostasis (Abrignani et al., 2024). Studies examining the impact of Mediterranean diet adherence have found that specific nutrients and food components significantly affect microbiota composition and diversity. Higher consumption of plant-based nutrients, such as vegetable proteins and polysaccharides, is associated with higher bifidobacterial counts and total SCFA production (Garcia-Mantrana et al., 2018). Plant-based diets, such as vegetarian and vegan eating, help create a more diverse and stable gut microbiome. People who follow these diets

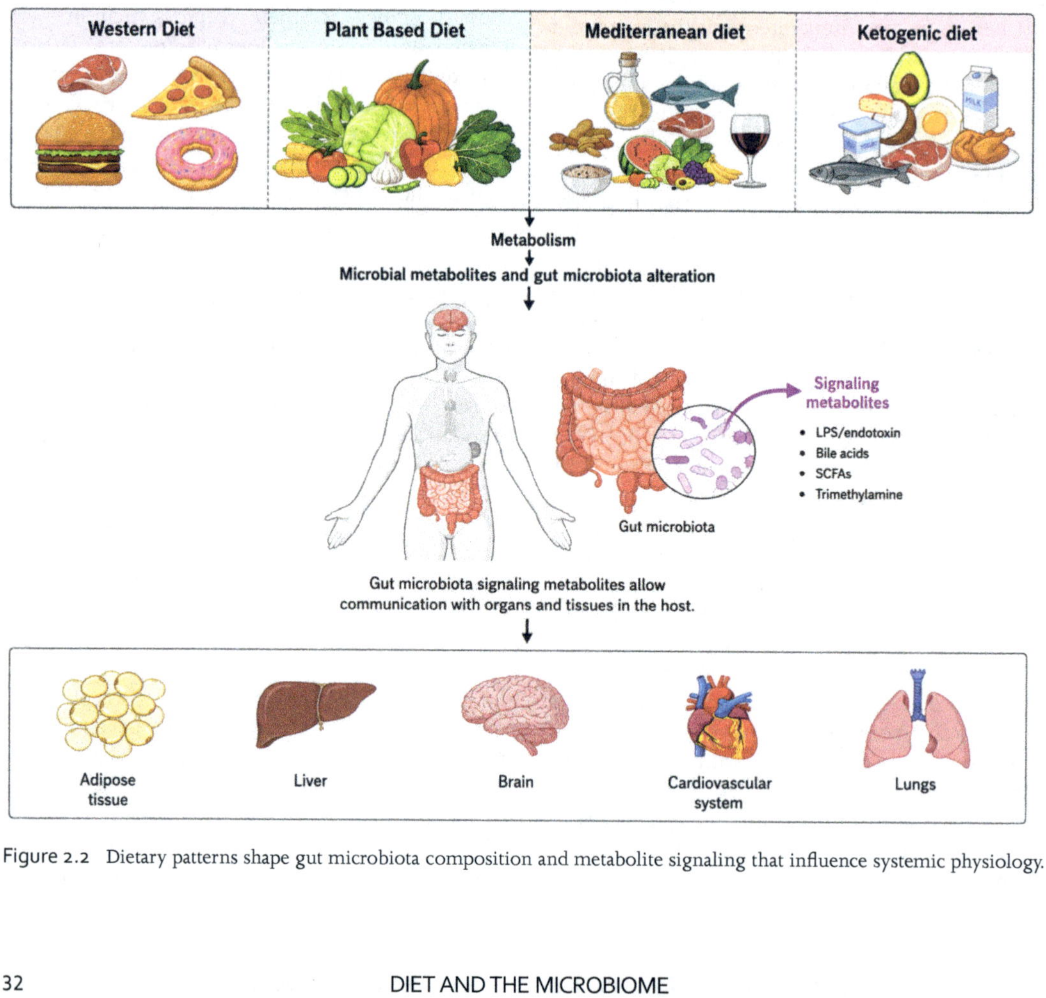

Figure 2.2 Dietary patterns shape gut microbiota composition and metabolite signaling that influence systemic physiology.

have higher levels of certain Bacteroidetes-related bacteria than those who eat meat. Fiber is the primary reason for the increase in beneficial bacteria, such as *Ruminococcus*, *E. rectale*, and *Roseburia*, and it also reduces levels of *Clostridium* and *Enterococcus*. Recent studies have shown that adhering to a consistent, high-quality diet is crucial for maintaining gut health. Diets rich in vegetables, fruits, nuts, and micronutrients lead to a more diverse gut microbiome and improved stool quality, whereas consuming a high amount of fast food has the opposite effect. Regularly eating healthy foods appears to matter most, and being consistent with your diet can have an even greater impact on gut health than just the quantity consumed (Tomova et al., 2019).

2.5.2 Western Diet and Dysbiosis

Unlike Mediterranean and plant-based diets, Western diets are high in calories, animal proteins, saturated fats, and simple sugars. These features are linked to a higher risk of obesity, diabetes, cancer, and heart disease. Western diets also promote dysbiosis, a persistent imbalance in microbial composition and function, in several ways, including a shift toward a Firmicutes-dominant microbiota and a reduction in bacterial diversity (Severino et al., 2024). Dysbiosis caused by the Western diet is characterized by reduced microbial diversity, lower levels of *Bifidobacterium* and *A. muciniphila*, and a higher Firmicutes-to-Bacteroidetes ratio. This microbial imbalance is consistently linked to insulin resistance, chronic inflammation, and metabolic syndrome across diverse populations. The underlying mechanisms encompass the proliferation of pro-inflammatory bacteria, including Proteobacteria, the suppression of beneficial microbial strains, and a reduction in the synthesis of protective SCFAs. Additionally, heightened intestinal permeability promotes the translocation of bacterial endotoxins into the bloodstream, thereby triggering inflammatory responses (Menafra et al., 2024) (Figure 2.2).

Different dietary regimes, including Western, plant-based, Mediterranean, and ketogenic diets, drive distinct metabolic processes that modulate gut microbial composition and the production of key microbial metabolites. These signaling metabolites (e.g., lipopolysaccharide (LPS)/endotoxin, bile acids, SCFAs, and trimethylamine) interact with host tissues and organs. Through this bidirectional communication, gut microbiota-derived signals influence multiple physiological systems, including adipose tissue, liver, brain, cardiovascular system, and lungs.

2.6 PREBIOTICS, PROBIOTICS, AND SYNBIOTICS: FUNCTIONAL FOODS FOR MICROBIOTA MODULATION

2.6.1 Prebiotics: Dietary Nourishment for Beneficial Bacteria

Prebiotics, non-digestible carbohydrates, selectively promote the growth of beneficial gut bacteria by serving as a nutrient source for the microbiota. These compounds are fermented by probiotics, aiding their colonization in the gastrointestinal tract. Examples include inulin and oligosaccharides found in foods like artichokes, onions, garlic, leeks, legumes, chicory root, and various fruits.The bifidogenic effects of inulin-type fructans and arabinoxylan-oligosaccharides result from strain-specific yet complementary carbohydrate utilization mechanisms within cooperating bifidobacterial communities (Obayomi et al., 2024). Recent clinical research shows that inulin supplementation offers multiple health benefits beyond microbiota modulation. In randomized controlled trials, inulin has been shown to significantly promote the growth of Bifidobacterium and increase fat-free mass in obese children, through mechanisms such as the production of SCFAs and anti-inflammatory effects (Visuthranukul et al., 2024). Notably, these prebiotic fibers have also been demonstrated to produce butyrogenic effects in the colon, meaning they boost butyrate production beyond direct fermentation. This is a crucial finding, as the cross-feeding interactions between butyrate-producing bacteria, including *F. prausnitzii* from clostridial cluster IV and species from cluster XIVa, such as *Anaerostipes*, *Eubacterium*, and *Roseburia*, may be enhanced through prebiotic-driven community changes. Prebiotics include inulin and fructooligosaccharides (FOS) (from chicory root, onions, and bananas), which promote *Bifidobacteria* growth; galactooligosaccharides (GOS) (found in breast milk), which strengthens immunity; resistant starch (in green bananas and cooked-cooled potatoes), which boosts butyrate production; beta-glucans (from oats and barley), which improve metabolic health; and pectin (from apples and citrus), which enhances gut integrity. These prebiotics help improve digestion, immunity, and overall gut function (Amin et al., 2025; Singh et al., 2023). Additionally, prebiotics can impact host phenotypes by influencing satiety hormones and body composition. For instance, increased satiety from higher production of SCFAs can lead to reduced calorie intake, while shifts in body composition, such as increased lean mass, are measurable benefits that extend beyond the gut lumen.

2.6.2 Probiotics: Live Beneficial Organisms

Probiotics are live microorganisms that are reported to confer health benefits when consumed in adequate amounts. Commonly utilized strains include species from the genera *Lactobacillus* and *Bifidobacterium*. These microorganisms must survive passage through the gastrointestinal tract to reach the intestine in a viable state and establish functional populations. Fermented foods such as kefir, yogurt, miso, tempeh, and sauerkraut are rich sources of probiotics; however, not all commercially available fermented foods contain sufficient viable microbes to provide health benefits (Amin et al., 2025). Numerous clinical trials have demonstrated that probiotics can alter the composition of the microbiota and enhance metabolic outcomes. Strain-specific effects are essential, as various probiotic strains exhibit unique therapeutic properties that are affected by the individual's baseline microbiota composition and health status (Manan, 2025). For instance, *Lactobacillus plantarum* has been noted for its role in improving lipid profiles by reducing cholesterol levels, while *Bifidobacterium bifidum* is linked to enhancing immune responses. *Lactobacillus rhamnosus* GG and *Bifidobacterium longum* are two strains that help restore microbial balance, improve the intestinal barrier, and reduce inflammation in gastrointestinal illnesses such as irritable bowel syndrome (IBS) and IBD. Probiotics, such as *Lactobacillus gasseri* and *A. muciniphila*, have been shown to increase insulin sensitivity, regulate lipid metabolism, and reduce body weight by altering gut-derived metabolites in metabolic disorders like type 2 diabetes and obesity (Lau & Quek, 2024). Recent clinical evidence suggests that probiotic and synbiotic supplementation can significantly improve insulin resistance, as indicated by decreases in HOMA-IR, fasting glucose, and insulin levels, along with improvements in lipid profiles and hormonal balance. Personalizing probiotic treatments is a new area of research. The initial microbial profile is a key factor in figuring out how well a person will respond to live probiotic treatments (Martinez Guevar et al., 2024).

2.6.3 Synbiotics and Postbiotics: Emerging Therapeutic Approaches

Synbiotics are defined as a combination of prebiotics and probiotics designed to work synergistically to enhance immune function and gut health. The integration of prebiotics, which selectively promote the growth of beneficial bacteria, with probiotics adapted to this enriched environment increases the likelihood of successful probiotic colonization and ongoing metabolic benefits. For instance, symbiotic pairings, such as *L. rhamnosus* GG and inulin or *B. longum* and FOS, support the growth, survival, and improved function of beneficial bacteria in the gut. Other pairings that improve digestion, promote immunity, and increase beneficial metabolites include *Lactobacillus acidophilus* with GOS and *Bifidobacterium breve* with resistant starch. By providing both the helpful microbes and their preferred nourishment, synbiotics offer stronger and more sustained health benefits than probiotics or prebiotics alone. Recent clinical trials suggest that synbiotics have more pronounced effects than either probiotics or prebiotics alone, resulting in significantly improved stool frequency, consistency, and gastrointestinal symptom scores after eight weeks of treatment in patients with chronic functional constipation (Wang et al., 2025). Probiotic fermentation produces bioactive molecules known as postbiotics, which include SCFAs, exopolysaccharides, enzymes, peptides, and cell wall components like glycoproteins and peptidoglycans. These molecules have antimicrobial, anti-inflammatory, and immunomodulatory properties even when live bacteria are not present. By preventing pathogen adherence and biofilm development on the intestinal epithelium, parabiotics, which are the non-viable remnants of probiotics, also support gut health after they have completed their life cycle. Compared to live probiotics, these postbiotic components offer several benefits, including increased stability, enhanced bioavailability, colonization-independent and standardized bioactivity, and therapeutic promise for immunological, metabolic, and gut–brain diseases (Al-Habsi et al., 2024) (Table 2.1).

TABLE 2.1

Preclinical and clinical evidence: Functional foods for microbiota modulation

Functional food/intervention	Study type	Model/population	Main findings on microbiota modulation	Health implications/outcomes	References
Fungal polysaccharides (from edible and medicinal mushrooms)	Preclinical and clinical	Animal and human studies	Significantly altered gut microbial composition; increased beneficial bacteria and microbial metabolites	Improved metabolic profiles, neuroprotection, and anticancer activity	Barcan et al. (2024)
Tea polyphenols and extracts	Preclinical and clinical	In vitro, animal, and human studies	Acted as prebiotics; reduced dysbiosis induced by high-fat diet; modulated key bacterial taxa	Supported gut health and reduced inflammation	Yang et al. (2025)
Berry polyphenols	Preclinical and clinical	Animal and human trials	Promoted beneficial microbiota diversity; influenced SCFA production	Improved cardiovascular health and reduced chronic inflammation	Bouyahya et al. (2022)
Probiotics, prebiotics, diet in rheumatoid arthritis	Preclinical and clinical	Mouse models and RA patients	Modulated intestinal microbiota composition and immune pathways	Reduced inflammatory markers and disease incidence	Ferro et al. (2021)
Dietary modulation and probiotics in liver disease	Preclinical and clinical	Mouse models and NAFLD/ALD patients	Altered microbial diversity; reduced pathogenic taxa; improved gut barrier function	Decreased liver inflammation and improved hepatic outcomes	Lang and Schnabl (2020)
Microbiota-targeted diet and probiotics in liver cancer	Preclinical and clinical	Animal and human studies	Restored gut–liver axis balance; modulated bile acid metabolism	Reduced inflammation and inhibited tumor growth	Rajapakse et al. (2023)
Gut microbiota modulation in cancer immunotherapy (diet, probiotics, FMT)	Preclinical and early clinical	Mouse models and oncology patients	Enhanced T-cell infiltration and antitumor immune response	Improved response to immunotherapy	Kang et al. (2024)
Diet and supplementation in epilepsy	Preclinical and clinical	Animal models and patients	Modified gut microbial taxa and metabolite production	Influenced seizure susceptibility via gut–brain axis	Yan et al. (2025)
Pre-/Probiotics in pediatric gut–lung axis	Preclinical and clinical	Animal studies and pediatric populations	Increased SCFA production; modulated respiratory microbiota	Improved lung immunity and reduced infection risk	Su et al. (2024)
Stressor-related diet modulation (nutrition-based)	Preclinical	Animal studies	Environmental and psychological stress altered microbiota composition; dietary modulation reversed dysbiosis	Suggested nutritional strategies to mitigate stress effects	Herselman et al. (2022)

2.7 DISEASE PREVENTION AND TREATMENT THROUGH MICROBIOTA MODULATION

2.7.1 Metabolic Disorders and Glucose Homeostasis

The relationship between diet-induced microbiota changes and metabolic health is one of the most extensively characterized disease–microbiota associations. Dysbiosis is characterized by a reduction in microbial diversity and an alteration in bacterial composition. It has been consistently associated with insulin resistance, type 2 diabetes, and metabolic syndrome. Several mechanisms underlie this association. These include reduced production of SCFAs, impaired gut barrier function, increased intestinal permeability, and elevated circulating lipopolysaccharides (endotoxemia). Endotoxemia activates toll-like receptors, promoting systemic inflammation (Shen et al., 2025). SCFAs produced through microbial fermentation regulate anti-inflammatory and immune pathways. A reduction in these metabolites during dysbiosis contributes to chronic inflammation and metabolic dysfunction. Dietary interventions that restore beneficial bacteria and increase SCFA production have demonstrated potential for improving glycemic control and insulin sensitivity. Specific dietary components, including fiber, promote the growth of beneficial bacteria and enhance the synthesis of SCFAs. Additionally, polyphenols support anti-inflammatory microbial populations, providing a comprehensive strategy for the intervention of metabolic diseases (Du et al., 2024).

2.7.2 Inflammatory Bowel Disease and Gastrointestinal Health

The gut microbiota plays a crucial role in maintaining intestinal homeostasis and preventing IBD. Dietary interventions, particularly those high in fiber and low in fats and sugars compared to Western diets high in fats and sugars, have demonstrated health benefits.These benefits include promoting the growth of beneficial bacteria, enhancing mucus barrier function and immune tolerance, and suppressing pro-inflammatory responses and their subsequent effects (He et al., 2022). Long-term dietary patterns are associated with the pro-inflammatory and anti-inflammatory characteristics of the gut microbiota in both individuals with gastrointestinal diseases and healthy populations. Processed animal-derived foods are consistently linked to increased abundances of pro-inflammatory bacteria, such as Firmicutes, *Ruminococcus*, and *Blautia* genera, as well as enhanced endotoxin synthesis pathways. Conversely, consumption of plant-based foods and fish is positively correlated with SCFA-producing commensals and improved nutrient metabolism. These findings indicate that specific dietary components can directly modulate the inflammatory potential of the gut microbiota (Soldán et al., 2024). Recent clinical evidence suggests that fecal microbiota transplantation, which restores dysbiotic microbiota by transplanting healthy donor stool, yields robust evidence of efficacy in ulcerative colitis and Crohn's disease, with 37% of patients achieving clinical remission and 54% exhibiting a clinical response. Multiple fecal microbiota transplantation administrations demonstrated superior efficacy compared to single administrations in attaining clinical remission rates exceeding 44% (Bénard et al., 2024).

2.7.3 Immune Function and Allergy Prevention

The development of immune tolerance and the prevention of allergic responses depend critically on the composition of the microbiota and its secretion of immunomodulatory metabolites. Food allergy has become a major public health problem, with evidence demonstrating that allergic reactions induced by food proteins often lead to disturbances in the gut microbiota. The microbiota plays an important role in maintaining the balance between intestinal immune tolerance and allergic reactions, making dietary intervention and microbiota modulation through prebiotics and probiotics potentially effective adjuvant treatment measures for allergic diseases (Yu et al., 2025). The gut–brain axis and its function in immune regulation exemplify a significant domain where microbiota-mediated effects are apparent. The intricate interplay among microbiota, stress response, and immune function encompasses various mechanisms, including direct endocrine signaling via the secretion of bioactive compounds by microbiota, as well as indirect activation through toll-like receptors and the synthesis of immune modulators, cytokines, and chemokines (O'Riordan et al., 2025).

2.8 ADVANCED INTERVENTIONS AND THERAPEUTIC APPLICATIONS

2.8.1 Fecal Microbiota Transplantation

Fecal microbiota transplantation is a sophisticated method for restoring gut health by modifying the gut's microbial community. In this procedure, doctors transfer fecal matter from healthy donors to patients with gut dysbiosis to help bring back microbial balance. This treatment is particularly effective for recurrent *Clostridioides difficile* infection, with a reported cure rate of 95.56% in several meta-analyses (Cha & Sonu, 2025). Lean-donor fecal microbiota transplantation and supplementation with *A. muciniphila* have been shown in clinical data to improve insulin sensitivity and lipid metabolism. Clinical remission rates for ulcerative colitis achieved through fecal microbiota transplantation are substantially improved when higher stool dosages are used, with delivery via the lower gastrointestinal tract achieving higher cure rates. These interventions represent important options when dietary modifications alone prove insufficient, though they require careful donor screening and standardization to ensure safety and efficacy (Porcari et al., 2023).

2.8.2 Colonization Resistance and Pathogen Prevention

The gut microbiota provides multiple mechanisms of colonization resistance against exogenous microorganisms, including the secretion of antimicrobial products, nutrient competition, support of gut barrier integrity, and the deployment of bacteriophages. These mechanisms work synergistically to prevent pathogenic bacterial colonization and maintain microbiota homeostasis. Dysbiotic conditions, whether induced by antibiotics, altered diet, or other factors, significantly reduce colonization resistance and increase susceptibility to enteric infections (Ducarmon et al., 2019).

2.8.3 Integration of Precision Nutrition and Digital Health

The advancement of microbiota-based interventions is increasingly characterized by precision nutrition strategies that are informed by individual microbiota composition, genetic factors, and comprehensive dietary monitoring. Precision nutrition, a personalized approach grounded in individual characteristics, has demonstrated potential in directly influencing gut microbiota composition. The integration of machine learning techniques with temporal nutrition data, microbiota profiling, and advanced analytical methods offers significant promise for elucidating the gut microbiome's dietary responses and for generating tailored lifestyle recommendations (Liu et al., 2025).

2.9 CONCLUSION

The relationship between food and gut microbes shows one of the most compelling and therapeutically promising areas of advanced biomedical research. The widespread evidence demonstrates that specific dietary materials, including fibers, protein, fats, and polyphenols, shape diverse microbial communities. Therapeutic implications span a wide range of disease states, including metabolic disorders, gastrointestinal conditions, immune-mediated diseases, and responses to cancer immunotherapy. SCFAs, especially butyrate, serve as key mediators of the positive effects associated with fiber-rich diets. These compounds influence energy metabolism, immune homeostasis, and neurological function through various receptor-mediated mechanisms. Precision nutrition, guided by individual microbiota profiling and advanced analytical techniques, is poised to advance beyond general dietary guidelines and enable personalized interventions tailored to each individual's microbiota composition and metabolic profile. To integrate precision nutrition tools effectively into routine clinical practice, a concrete first step could be the establishment of a collaborative initiative between healthcare providers and technological innovators. This initiative can focus on developing user-friendly digital platforms that allow for comprehensive microbiota profiling and nutritional tracking in clinical settings. By implementing these tools, healthcare professionals can offer personalized dietary recommendations that are more aligned with individual patient needs, thereby enhancing treatment outcomes and preventative care strategies. Embracing these advancements can pave the way for more precise and personalized medical care, setting a new standard for preventive and therapeutic dietary interventions.

REFERENCES

Abrignani V, Salvo A, Pacinella G, Tuttolomondo A. The Mediterranean diet, its microbiome connections, and cardiovascular health: a narrative review. *Int J Mol Sci*. 2024;25(9):4942.

Al-Habsi N, Al-Khalili M, Haque SA, Elias M, Olqi NA, Al Uraimi T. Health benefits of prebiotics, probiotics, synbiotics, and postbiotics. *Nutrients*. 2024;16(22):3955.

Amin MR, Biswas AP, Tasnim M, Islam MN, Azam MS. Probiotics and their applications in functional foods: a health perspective. *Appl Food Res*. 2025;101193.

Barcan AS, Barcan RA, Vamanu E. Therapeutic potential of fungal polysaccharides in gut microbiota regulation: implications for diabetes, neurodegeneration, and oncology. *J Fungi (Basel)*. 2024;10(6):394. doi:10.3390/jof10060394.

Bénard MV, de Goffau MC, Blonk J, Hugenholtz F, van Buuren J, Paramsothy S, et al. Gut microbiota features in relation to fecal microbiota transplantation outcome in ulcerative colitis: a systematic review and meta-analysis. *Clin Gastroenterol Hepatol*. 2024;23(10):1719–1736.

Bouyahya A, Omari NE, El Hachlafi N, Jemly ME, Hakkour M, Balahbib A, et al. Chemical compounds of berry-derived polyphenols and their effects on gut microbiota, inflammation, and cancer. *Molecules*. 2022;27(10):3286. doi:10.3390/molecules27103286.

Cao B, Sun Y, Lam C, Chen Y, Dri CE, McIntyre RS. Interaction between dietary omega-3 polyunsaturated fatty acids, obesity and gut microbiota in preclinical models: a systematic review of randomized controlled trials. *Diabetes Obes Metab*. 2025;27(9):4643–4661.

Cao C, Yue S, Lu A, Liang C. Host-gut microbiota metabolic interactions and their role in precision diagnosis and treatment of gastrointestinal cancers. *Pharmacol Res*. 2024;207:107321.

Cha RR, Sonu I. Fecal microbiota transplantation: present and future. *Clin Endosc*. 2025;58(3):352.

Clemente-Suárez VJ, Beltrán-Velasco AI, Redondo-Flórez L, Martín-Rodríguez A, Tornero-Aguilera JF. Global impacts of western diet and its effects on metabolism and health: a narrative review. *Nutrients*. 2023;15(12):2749.

de Jesús Rodríguez-Romero J, Durán-Castañeda AC, Cárdenas-Castro AP, Sánchez-Burgos JA, Zamora-Gasga VM, Sáyago-Ayerdi SG. What we know about protein gut metabolites: implications and insights for human health and diseases. *Food Chem X*. 2022;13:100195.

den Besten G, van Eunen K, Groen AK, Venema K, Reijngoud DJ, Bakker BM. The role of short-chain fatty acids in the interplay between diet, gut microbiota, and host energy metabolism. *J Lipid Res*. 2013;54(9):2325–2340.

De Vos WM, Tilg H, Van Hul M, Cani PD. Gut microbiome and health: mechanistic insights. *Gut*. 2022;71(5):1020–1032.

Dinan TG, Stilling RM, Stanton C, Cryan JF. Collective unconscious: how gut microbes shape human behavior. *J Psychiatr Res*. 2015;63:1–9.

Du Y, He C, An Y, Huang Y, Zhang H, Fu W, et al. The role of short-chain fatty acids in inflammation and body health. *Int J Mol Sci*. 2024;25(13):7379.

Ducarmon QR, Zwittink RD, Hornung BVH, Van Schaik W, Young VB, Kuijper EJ. Gut microbiota and colonization resistance against bacterial enteric infection. *Microbiol Mol Biol Rev*. 2019;83(3):e00007-19.

Ferro M, Charneca S, Dourado E, Guerreiro CS, Fonseca JE. Probiotic supplementation for rheumatoid arthritis: a promising adjuvant therapy in the gut microbiome era. *Front Pharmacol*. 2021;12:711788. doi:10.3389/fphar.2021.711788.

Fusco W, Lorenzo MB, Cintoni M, Porcari S, Rinninella E, Kaitsas F, et al. Short-chain fatty-acid-producing bacteria: key components of the human gut microbiota. *Nutrients*. 2023;15(9):2211.

Garcia-Mantrana I, Selma-Royo M, Alcantara C, Collado MC. Shifts on gut microbiota associated to Mediterranean diet adherence and specific dietary intakes on general adult population. *Front Microbiol*. 2018;9:890.

Güler MS, Arslan S, Ağagündüz D, Cerqua I, Pagano E, Canani RB, Capasso R. Butyrate: a potential mediator of obesity and microbiome via different mechanisms of actions. *Food Res Int*. 2025;199:115420.

He P, Yu L, Tian F, Zhang H, Chen W, Zhai Q. Dietary patterns and gut microbiota: the crucial actors in inflammatory bowel disease. *Adv Nutr*. 2022;13(5):1628–1651.

Herselman MF, Bailey S, Bobrovskaya L. The effects of stress and diet on the brain–gut and gut–brain pathways in animal models of stress and depression. *Int J Mol Sci*. 2022;23(4):2013. doi:10.3390/ijms23042013.

Hou K, Wu ZX, Chen XY, Wang JQ, Zhang D, Xiao C, et al. Microbiota in health and diseases. *Signal Transduct Target Ther*. 2022;7(1):135.

Jarrett S, Ashworth CJ. The role of dietary fibre in pig production, with a particular emphasis on reproduction. *J Anim Sci Biotechnol*. 2018;9(1):59.

Kang X, Lau HCH, Yu J. Modulating gut microbiome in cancer immunotherapy: harnessing microbes to enhance treatment efficacy. *Cell Rep Med*. 2024;5(4):101478. doi:10.1016/j.xcrm.2024.101478.

Khaledi M, Poureslamfar B, Alsaab HO, Tafaghodi S, Hjazi A, Singh R, et al. The role of gut microbiota in human metabolism and inflammatory diseases: a focus on elderly individuals. *Ann Microbiol*. 2024;74(1):1.

Kumar S, Mukherjee R, Gaur P, Leal É, Lyu X, Ahmad S, et al. Unveiling roles of beneficial gut bacteria and optimal diets for health. *Front Microbiol*. 2025;16:1527755.

Kumar V, Rohilla A, Ahire JJ. Omega-3 fatty acids and the gut microbiome: a new frontier in cardiovascular disease prevention. *Discover Med*. 2025;2(1):1–17.

Lang S, Schnabl B. Microbiota and fatty liver disease—the known, the unknown, and the future. *Cell Host Microbe*. 2020;28(2):233–244. doi:10.1016/j.chom.2020.07.007.

Lau LYJ, Quek SY. Probiotics: health benefits, food application, and colonization in the human gastrointestinal tract. *Food Bioeng*. 2024;3(1):41–64.

Lee H, Song J, Lee B, Cha J, Lee H. Food carbohydrates in the gut: structural diversity, microbial utilization, and analytical strategies. *Food Sci Biotechnol*. 2024;33(9):2123–2140.

Leeming ER, Johnson AJ, Spector TD, Le Roy CI. Effect of diet on the gut microbiota: rethinking intervention duration. *Nutrients*. 2019;11(12):2862.

Liu J, Tan Y, Cheng H, Zhang D, Feng W, Peng C. Functions of gut microbiota metabolites, current status and future perspectives. *Aging Dis*. 2022;13(4):1106–1122.

Liu X, Xu M, Wang H, Zhu L. Integrating precision medicine and digital health in personalized weight management: the central role of nutrition. *Nutrients*. 2025;17(16):2695.

Liu Z, Liu M, Meng J, Wang L, Chen M. A review of the interaction between diet composition and gut microbiota and its impact on associated disease. *J Future Foods*. 2024;4(3):221–232.

Macia L, Tan J, Vieira AT, Leach K, Stanley D, Luong S, et al. Metabolite-sensing receptors GPR43 and GPR109A facilitate dietary fibre-induced gut homeostasis through regulation of the inflammasome. *Nat Commun*. 2015;6:6734.

Manan MA. Comprehensive review: the role of probiotics in personalized therapeutics—advances in gut microbe-driven interventions. *Microbe*. 2025;8:100497.

Martinez Guevara D, Vidal Cañas S, Palacios I, Gómez A, Estrada M, Gallego J, Liscano Y. Effectiveness of probiotics, prebiotics, and synbiotics in managing insulin resistance and hormonal imbalance in women with polycystic ovary syndrome: a systematic review of randomized clinical trials. *Nutrients*. 2024;16(22):3916.

Menafra D, Proganò M, Tecce N, Pivonello R, Colao A. Diet and gut microbiome: impact of each factor and mutual interactions on prevention and treatment of type 1, type 2, and gestational diabetes mellitus. *Hum Nutr Metab*. 2024;38:200286.

Obayomi OV, Olaniran AF, Owa SO. Unveiling the role of functional foods with emphasis on prebiotics and probiotics in human health: a review. *J Funct Foods*. 2024;119:106337.

O'Riordan KJ, Moloney GM, Keane L, Clarke G, Cryan JF. The gut microbiota–immune–brain axis: therapeutic implications. *Cell Rep Med*. 2025;6(3):101982.

Perrone P, D'Angelo S. Gut microbiota modulation through Mediterranean diet foods: implications for human health. *Nutrients*. 2025;17(6):948.

Plamada D, Vodnar DC. Polyphenols–gut microbiota interrelationship: a transition to a new generation of prebiotics. *Nutrients*. 2021;14(1):137.

Porcari S, Benech N, Valles-Colomer M, Segata N, Gasbarrini A, Cammarota G, et al. Key determinants of success in fecal microbiota transplantation: from microbiome to clinic. *Cell Host Microbe*. 2023;31(5):712–733.

Rajapakse J, Khatiwada S, Akon AC, Yu KL, Shen S, Zekry A. Unveiling the complex relationship between gut microbiota and liver cancer: opportunities for novel therapeutic interventions. *Gut Microbes*. 2023;15(2):2240031. doi:10.1080/19490976.2023.2240031.

Rivière A, Selak M, Lantin D, Leroy F, De Vuyst L. Bifidobacteria and butyrate-producing colon bacteria: importance and strategies for their stimulation in the human gut. *Front Microbiol*. 2016;7:979.

Severino A, Tohumcu E, Tamai L, Dargenio P, Porcari S, Rondinella D, et al. The microbiome-driven impact of western diet in the development of noncommunicable chronic disorders. *Best Pract Res Clin Gastroenterol*. 2024;72:101923.

Shaw C, Hess M, Weimer BC. Microbial-derived tryptophan metabolites and their role in neurological disease: anthranilic acid and anthranilic acid derivatives. *Microorganisms*. 2023;11(7):1825.

Shen Y, Fan N, Ma SX, Cheng X, Yang X, Wang G. Gut microbiota dysbiosis: pathogenesis, diseases, prevention, and therapy. *MedComm*. 2025;6(5):e70168.

Silva YP, Bernardi A, Frozza RL. The role of short-chain fatty acids from gut microbiota in gut–brain communication. *Front Endocrinol (Lausanne)*. 2020;11:508738.

Singh V, Lee G, Son H, Koh H, Kim ES, Unno T, Shin JH. Butyrate producers, "the sentinel of gut": their intestinal significance with and beyond butyrate, and prospective use as microbial therapeutics. *Front Microbiol*. 2023;13:1103836.

Soldán M, Argalášová Ľ, Hadvinová L, Galileo B, Babjaková J. The effect of dietary types on gut microbiota composition and development of non-communicable diseases: a narrative review. *Nutrients*. 2024;16(18):3134.

Su Z, Ma C, Ru X, Zhang S, Wu C, Huang Y, et al. Effects of probiotic treatment on patients and animals with chronic obstructive pulmonary disease: a systematic review and meta-analysis of randomized controlled trials. *Front Cell Infect Microbiol*. 2024;14:1411222.

Thursby E, Juge N. Introduction to the human gut microbiota. *Biochem J*. 2017;474(11):1823–1836.

Tomova A, Bukovsky I, Rembert E, Yonas W, Alwarith J, Barnard ND, Kahleova H. The effects of vegetarian and vegan diets on gut microbiota. *Front Nutr.* 2019;6:447652.

Trautmann D, Suazo F, Torres K, Simón L. Antitumor effects of resveratrol opposing mechanisms of *Helicobacter pylori* in gastric cancer. *Nutrients.* 2024;16(13):2141.

Visuthranukul C, Leelahavanichkul A, Tepaamorndech S, Chamni S, Mekangkul E, Chomtho S. Inulin supplementation exhibits increased muscle mass via gut–muscle axis in children with obesity: double evidence from clinical and in vitro studies. *Sci Rep.* 2024;14(1):11181.

Wang Q, Huang H, Yang Y, Yang X, Li X, Zhong W, et al. Reinventing gut health: leveraging dietary bioactive compounds for the prevention and treatment of diseases. *Front Nutr.* 2024;11:1491821.

Wang Y, Tian L, Fabi JP, de Vos P. The potential of prebiotics, probiotics, and synbiotics for ameliorating intestinal barrier dysfunction and modulating inflammatory responses as dietary supplements in diabetes mellitus management. *Food Biosci.* 2025;72:107539.

Yan R, Zhang L, Chen Y, Zheng Y, Xu P, Xu Z. Therapeutic potential of gut microbiota modulation in epilepsy: a focus on short-chain fatty acids. *Neurobiol Dis.* 2025;209:106880.

Yang J, Chen W, Chen J, Xie D, Wang Y, Zhou J. Tea polyphenol epigallocatechin gallate and the gut–health axis: unraveling structural characteristics, metabolic pathways, and systemic benefits. *Adv Nutr.* 2025;16(12):100545.

Yu G, Zhang Q, Zhao L, van Ree R, Fu L. Risk and protective factors for food allergy: an in-depth analysis of dietary patterns and specific dietary components. *Allergy Med.* 2025;6:100076.

CHAPTER 3

The Role of Fiber-Rich Diet in Modulating the Gut Microbiome and Health Outcomes

Alex Muppasani and Sunil Thomas

3.1 INTRODUCTION

The human gut microbiome comprises an estimated 30 trillion resident microorganisms, including bacteria, viruses, fungi, and protozoa, that coexist symbiotically within the intestinal tract. Among these, bacteria are the most extensively studied and will serve as the primary focus of this review. The predominant bacterial phyla within the human gut are Firmicutes (Gram-positive) and Bacteroidetes (Gram-negative). Recent research has revealed that the gut microbiota can be classified into distinct enterotypes, each enriched with particular bacterial genera but exhibiting a remarkable degree of functional uniformity across individuals, regardless of factors such as age, sex, body mass index, or nationality (Magne et al., 2020).

Most microorganisms reside in the distal regions of the digestive tract, where they play critical roles in maintaining host health. These microbes contribute to the biosynthesis of vitamins and essential amino acids and generate key metabolic by-products from dietary components that escape digestion in the small intestine. Among these metabolites, short-chain fatty acids (SCFAs)—notably butyrate, propionate, and acetate—serve as major energy sources for intestinal epithelial cells, reinforcing the mucosal barrier and supporting gut integrity. Evidence from germ-free mouse studies further indicates that the microbiota enhance local intestinal immunity through modulation of toll-like receptor (TLR) expression, antigen-presenting cells, T-cell differentiation, and lymphoid follicle development. Moreover, the microbiota appear to influence systemic immunity by increasing splenic $CD4^+$ T cells and systemic antibody production (Thomas et al., 2017).

The recognized health benefits of the gut microbiota have spurred growing interest in strategies to modulate microbial composition through diet. Remarkably, even acute dietary changes—such as switching to an entirely animal-based or plant-based diet—can alter microbial composition within 24 hours, with reversion to baseline observed within 48 hours after discontinuation. Additionally, high-fat or high-sugar diets have been shown to disrupt the circadian rhythm of the gut microbiome (Singh et al., 2017).

Dietary composition exerts profound effects on the intestinal microbiome, which in turn influences overall health, either positively or negatively, depending on the identity and abundance of microbial taxa. For instance, high-fat diets have been associated with a reduction in *Akkermansia muciniphila* and *Lactobacillus*—bacteria linked to healthy metabolic states. This underscores how dietary interventions might serve as tools for managing complex metabolic disorders such as obesity and diabetes. Moreover, advances in microbiome research have opened new therapeutic avenues for diseases previously difficult to treat. Notably, fecal microbiota transplantation (FMT) has

DOI: 10.1201/9781003638292-3

demonstrated success in treating ulcerative colitis, *Clostridium difficile*–associated colitis, irritable bowel syndrome (IBS), and even obesity. Emerging evidence also suggests that re-engineering the gut microbiota may hold promise for dermatologic conditions such as psoriasis and atopic dermatitis.

The enteric nervous system (ENS) is a complex and highly organized network of neurons embedded within the walls of the gastrointestinal tract. Often referred to as the "second brain," the ENS contains hundreds of millions of neurons—comparable in number to those found in the spinal cord—and is capable of coordinating digestive processes independently of the central nervous system (CNS). It regulates key physiological functions such as intestinal motility, secretion, blood flow, and communication with immune and endocrine cells, thereby playing an essential role in maintaining gut homeostasis (Avetisyan et al., 2015). The health and proper functioning of the ENS are intimately connected to the gut microbiome, the diverse community of microorganisms residing in the digestive tract. These microbes produce a wide range of neuroactive compounds, including neurotransmitters such as serotonin, dopamine, and gamma-aminobutyric acid (GABA), which can influence ENS signaling and, consequently, gastrointestinal and emotional well-being. The gut–brain axis, a bidirectional communication system linking the gut, ENS, and CNS, facilitates this interaction—allowing microbial and dietary signals from the intestine to affect mood, cognition, and behavior. Emerging evidence highlights that diet plays a pivotal role in maintaining the health of both the microbiome and the ENS. Nutritional patterns rich in fiber, polyphenols, and essential fatty acids promote beneficial microbial communities that support neuronal integrity and reduce inflammation within the gut. Conversely, diets high in processed foods and saturated fats may disrupt this delicate balance, leading to altered neurotransmission and increased susceptibility to gastrointestinal and neuropsychiatric disorders (Thomas et al., 2023; Tarasiuk-Zawadzka and Fichna, 2025).

Most studies investigating the microbiome have employed 16S rRNA amplicon sequencing, which targets hypervariable regions of the bacterial 16S rRNA gene to identify microbial taxa. This approach remains the most widely used due to its cost-effectiveness and relatively straightforward workflow. However, 16S sequencing primarily reveals microbial identity, not function. To address this limitation, researchers increasingly utilize shotgun metagenomic sequencing, which profiles entire microbial genomes, providing insights into both taxonomic composition and gene function. Despite higher costs and greater computational demands, metagenomics allows for a deeper understanding of microbial roles in human health. Continued improvements in next-generation sequencing, sample preparation, and bioinformatics tools are making this approach increasingly accessible. Furthermore, integrating metagenomic data with host genomic, transcriptomic, and immunophenotypic datasets through meta-analyses represents a promising frontier for elucidating host–microbe interactions (Wang et al., 2025).

An emerging and transformative concept within this field is precision medicine, which seeks to design and optimize medical treatments according to an individual's unique genetic, epigenetic, and microbial characteristics. Rather than applying a one-size-fits-all approach, precision medicine integrates data from the host genotype and microbiome composition to predict responses to therapies and dietary interventions. The host's genetic background profoundly influences the structure and function of the gut microbiome, shaping microbial diversity, metabolic potential, and immune interactions. Consequently, a deeper understanding of host–microbe relationships is fundamental to promoting health, preventing disease, and developing personalized therapeutic strategies.

One of the most remarkable features of the gut microbiome is its resilience and adaptability. Although microbial communities can be disrupted by factors such as poor diet, antibiotic use, or chronic stress—resulting in a state of dysbiosis—they retain a remarkable capacity for recovery. Evidence suggests that a dysbiotic gut microbiome can often be restored to a more balanced and beneficial state through sustained dietary modifications, particularly the adoption of nutrient-rich, fiber-based, and plant-centered diets (Thomas et al., 2023). This adaptive flexibility underscores the dynamic interplay between environmental factors, diet, and host genetics in maintaining gut homeostasis.

Overall, the recognition that diet can modulate host–microbe interactions represents a powerful new paradigm in health science. By elucidating how specific dietary components influence microbial composition and metabolic output, researchers can uncover mechanisms linking nutrition, microbiome function, and systemic health. This chapter therefore explores in detail how beneficial dietary patterns shape the gut microbiome, support physiological well-being, and contribute to the prevention of diseases.

3.2 THE FORAGER–FARMER TRANSITION: HUMAN EXPANSION AND THE RESHAPING OF CIVILIZATION

The "Out of Africa" theory postulates that modern humans (*Homo sapiens*) originated in Africa before dispersing across the globe. Anthropological and genetic data derived from fossils, archaeological findings, and climatic records (Lopez et al., 2016) indicate that the African continent was the principal cradle of anatomically modern humans (Tassi et al., 2015). Molecular evidence further refines this model, showing that early human populations diversified as they spread out of Africa. Genetic and anthropological analyses suggest that Australo-Melanesians were among the first to diverge from African and other regional populations, followed later by additional regional lineages. Thus, the observed genetic diversity across human populations cannot be explained by a single, uniform dispersal event but rather by multiple waves of migration and complex patterns of gene flow (Tassi et al., 2015).

Understanding why these early humans migrated is as important as determining when and where they did so. Early human groups were hunter-gatherers, relying entirely on their surrounding ecosystems for food and resources (Padilla-Iglesias and Bischoff., 2024). Their survival depended on mobility—moving across vast landscapes in search of game, edible plants, and freshwater sources. This nomadic way of life gave rise to what anthropologists call central-place foraging (CPF)—a behavioral strategy where individuals or groups operated from a "home base" or central site to which they regularly returned after foraging expeditions (Garg et al., 2021). CPF not only optimized the use of spatial resources but also fostered social cohesion and communication between dispersed groups. Although they lacked permanent settlements, these early societies maintained intricate networks that facilitated the exchange of knowledge, tools, and survival strategies—effectively mitigating the challenges of mobility.

The hunter-gatherer lifestyle shaped human health, diet, and physiology. Though continuous walking by hunter-gatherers shaped physiology, early humans had poor health and longevity due to infectious diseases (Goldman, 2018). However, during this period, chronic diseases such as obesity, diabetes, and cardiovascular disorders were virtually absent. Average body fat percentages remained low (24%–28% in women, 9%–18% in men), reflecting a lifestyle that required over 100 minutes of moderate to vigorous physical activity per day (World Health Organization, 2024). Their diet, derived directly from the natural environment, was nutrient-rich but low in energy density—composed primarily of fibrous plants, lean meats, and naturally occurring carbohydrates. This dietary balance and constant movement sustained their physical endurance and metabolic stability. Unlike the modern world, ease of living was not a given; survival depended on continuous exertion and adaptability.

However, around 10,000 years ago, a profound transformation reshaped human life: the Neolithic Revolution. This period marked humanity's transition from a nomadic, foraging existence to a sedentary, agricultural lifestyle, representing one of the most significant milestones in human history. The shift did not occur uniformly or simultaneously across regions but resulted from a convergence of independent innovations—agricultural viability, religious expression, artistic development, and climatic opportunity. The earliest and best-documented site of early farming emerged in the Fertile Crescent of the Middle East, where communities began cultivating cereal grains such as emmer wheat, einkorn wheat, and barley, alongside legumes like lentils and chickpeas (Preece et al., 2017; Allen, 2024). Around 10,000 years ago, these agricultural practices were accompanied by the domestication of animals such as sheep, goats, and pigs. Simultaneously, in East Asia, rice and millet were independently cultivated, while Indigenous peoples in the Americas domesticated squash and maize-like crops (Cucchi and Arbuckle, 2021).

The driving forces behind the Neolithic transition remain a matter of debate, but mounting evidence suggests a combination of climatic and ecological pressures. The end of the last Ice Age ushered in a period of global warming and increased rainfall, producing lush, resource-rich environments that initially favored foraging. Yet this stability was abruptly disrupted by the Younger Dryas, a climatic reversal characterized by colder and drier conditions. Populations, now larger due to previous abundance, were forced into smaller, resource-dense regions, creating intense competition and scarcity (Carey, 2023). Faced with diminishing returns from foraging, humans began experimenting with cultivation and selective breeding, laying the groundwork for sustained agriculture.

While agriculture catalyzed population growth, technological advancement, and the birth of civilization, it also introduced social hierarchies, specialization of labor, and new health challenges. Permanent settlements fostered population density, surplus food production, and labor diversification—allowing individuals to specialize in crafts, trade, and governance. However, this newfound stability came at a cost: individual health declined. Agricultural diets—high in starch but low in nutritional diversity—replaced the varied diets of hunter-gatherers. Living in close-knit, settled communities heightened exposure to waste and pathogens, creating ideal conditions for the spread of infectious diseases and the emergence of epidemics (Fuchs et al., 2019). Thus, the Neolithic Revolution marked both collective advancement and personal compromise, intertwining progress with vulnerability.

Centuries later, another transformative wave swept across human civilization—the Second Agricultural Revolution, occurring between the 17th and 19th centuries, particularly in Britain. Closely tied to the Industrial Revolution, this era introduced mechanized farming, crop rotation, and chemical fertilizers, transforming agriculture into a commercial, globally integrated enterprise (Herrera and Garcia-Bertrand., 2018). Increased productivity led to surplus labor in rural areas, fueling the expansion of urban industrial centers. Food systems became increasingly mechanized, globalized, and chemically dependent, incorporating synthetic fertilizers and pesticides that redefined what was considered "natural."

In retrospect, the human journey—from forager to farmer to factory worker—represents a multistage evolutionary process driven by adaptation, necessity, and innovation. Each revolution brought profound societal gains but also new costs, reshaping the relationship between humans, their environment, and their health. The legacies of these transitions remain deeply embedded in modern life. The same forces that once spurred survival now fuel urbanization, technology, and industrial growth—continuing the delicate balance between collective progress and individual well-being. Humanity's story is thus not a straightforward narrative of advancement but a complex interplay of choices, trade-offs, and transformations that continue to define our species.

3.3 FOUNDER CROPS AND FIBER DIET

The concept of "founder crops" was first introduced by Zohary and Hopf in their seminal work *Domestication of Plants in the Old World* (1988). This concept refers to the original suite of plant species that formed the foundation of early Neolithic agriculture during the Pre-Pottery Neolithic B period in Southwest Asia. These crops represent the earliest known instances of systematic plant cultivation and domestication, marking a pivotal transition from foraging to farming societies. By identifying these key species, Zohary and Hopf provided an essential framework for understanding the origins of agriculture and the subsequent rise of complex civilizations in the Fertile Crescent.

According to Zohary and Hopf (1988), early Neolithic farmers cultivated three principal cereal crops: emmer wheat (*Triticum turgidum* subsp. *dicoccum*), einkorn wheat (*Triticum monococcum* subsp. *monococcum*), and barley (*Hordeum vulgare*). These grains were among the first to be domesticated due to their favorable traits, including high yield potential, storability, and nutritional value. Their successful cultivation laid the groundwork for stable food supplies and the development of permanent settlements.

In addition to cereals, several leguminous crops were consistently found alongside them, serving as vital sources of protein and nitrogen for both humans and soils. The most frequently encountered pulses in early Neolithic archaeological contexts of Southwest Asia are lentil (*Lens culinaris*) and pea (*Pisum sativum*). Two additional local legume species—bitter vetch (*Vicia ervilia*) and chickpea (*Cicer arietinum*)—also appear in early farming assemblages. It is probable that these four legumes were domesticated either concurrently with or shortly after the cereals, reflecting a diversified cropping system that balanced nutritional and ecological needs.

Finally, flax (*Linum usitatissimum*) is also included among the Near Eastern founder crops. Beyond its role as a food source, flax provided valuable fibers for textile production and oil-rich seeds, highlighting the growing sophistication and versatility of early agricultural economies. Together, these eight founder crops—three cereals, four legumes, and one oil/fiber plant—represent the cornerstone of the Agricultural Revolution that transformed human societies and laid the biological and cultural foundations of civilization.

The founder crops of wheat, barley, and legumes are a rich source of fiber diet that influenced the health of the early humans.

3.4 WHEAT AND BARLEY ARE A RICH SOURCE OF FIBER

In pre-industrial societies, people consumed grains in their whole form, making full use of all the nutritional and structural components of the kernel. A cereal grain is composed of three main parts: the embryo (or germ), the endosperm, and the outer kernel layers, collectively known as the bran. The starchy endosperm constitutes the largest portion—approximately 80%–85% of the grain's total weight—and serves primarily as an energy reserve, rich in starch and protein. The bran, accounting for 12%–18% of the grain, and the germ, representing about 2%–3%, provide essential vitamins, minerals, lipids, and dietary fiber (DF) that are often lost during modern refining processes.

The embryo is the vital reproductive structure of the grain, responsible for germination and the formation of a new plant. It contains the embryonic axis and scutellum and possesses the highest concentration of lipids and lipid-soluble vitamins among the grain's components. The endosperm, on the other hand, is of greatest economic significance as it provides the primary raw material for flour production. This portion is largely composed of insoluble nutrients, primarily starch and proteins, which act as the plant's energy source during germination. The outermost layer of the endosperm, known as the aleurone layer, typically consists of one to three cell layers. In some cereals, pigmentation in this layer imparts distinctive colors to the grains. Although botanically part of the endosperm, much of the aleurone layer is removed during roller milling, making it absent from refined white flour (An et al., 2020).

The bran fraction itself is a complex structure made up of several distinct layers, including the outer and inner pericarp, testa, and nucellar epidermis (or hyaline layer). The pericarp layers are particularly rich in crosslinked polysaccharides such as cellulose, lignin, and heteroxylan, which provide mechanical strength and protection to the seed. The testa, or seed coat, varies among cereal species—appearing as a single layer in barley, oats, and rice, but as a double layer in wheat and rye. The nucellar epidermis, a maternal tissue covering the endosperm, is not equally prominent in all cereals (Prasadi and Joye, 2020).

Cereal grains are also one of the most important dietary sources of fiber, contributing roughly 50% of total fiber intake in Western diets. Vegetables supply about 30%–49%, while fruits contribute around 16% (Prasadi and Joye, 2020). The total DF content of wheat varies between 9% and 20% on a dry weight basis, comprising both soluble and insoluble components. Within the wheat endosperm, the primary fiber constituents are arabinoxylan (AX) and β-D-glucan, while minor components such as cellulose and glucomannans are also present. Although cellulose, a linear polymer of β-(1→4)–linked glucose units, forms insoluble networks in cell walls, its concentration in wheat endosperm is relatively low (<5%). Hemicelluloses, a key group of non-cellulosic polysaccharides, are another significant component of cereal DF. These heterogeneous molecules include xylans, xyloglucans, glucomannans, and mixed-linkage β-glucans, varying in solubility based on their molecular size, branching, and degree of crosslinking.

In wheat, AX and β-glucan together make up about 70% and 20% of the total DF, respectively (Yang et al., 2024). AX consists of a linear backbone of β-(1→4)-linked D-xylopyranosyl (Xyl) residues, with α-L-arabinofuranosyl (Ara) side chains attached at the O-2 and O-3 positions. Structural variations—including non-substituted, monosubstituted, and disubstituted xylosyl residues—contribute to AX's functional diversity. Ferulic acid groups, esterified to the arabinose residues at the O-5 position, can form crosslinks between AX chains, increasing molecular weight while decreasing solubility. This structural complexity influences the physicochemical behavior of cereal fibers and their functional role in food systems.

3.4.1 Dietary Fiber Composition of Barley

Barley (*H. vulgare*), one of the earliest domesticated grains, exists in both hulled and hulless forms. In hulled varieties, the outer hull adheres tightly to the pericarp, making dehulling challenging, whereas hulless barley naturally separates from the kernel upon threshing. The barley caryopsis is composed of the pericarp, testa, aleurone layer, endosperm, and embryo, much like other cereals. Barley serves as an excellent source of both soluble and insoluble DF, as well as various bioactive compounds. Soluble fiber, primarily β-glucan, is concentrated in the endosperm cell walls, whereas insoluble fibers such as cellulose, AX, and lignin are predominantly found in the bran layers.

The total DF content of dehulled barley typically ranges between 10% and 28% (Prasadi and Joye, 2020). The dominant non-starch polysaccharide in barley is β-glucan, while AX occurs in smaller proportions. In general, β-glucan and AX together constitute approximately 70% and 20% of the total DF in barley, respectively. The structure of β-glucan consists of repeating cellotriosyl and cellotetraosyl units linked by β-(1→3) bonds. These linkages introduce bends in the polymer chain, allowing water molecules to penetrate and hydrate the structure. This property explains why β-glucan is significantly more soluble than cellulose, which is composed exclusively of β-(1→4)–linked D-glucose units forming tightly packed, insoluble fibers. The high solubility and viscosity of β-glucan contribute to its well-documented health benefits, including cholesterol reduction, glycemic control, and promotion of gut health—making barley an important grain in both traditional diets and modern functional foods.

3.5 THE BENEFITS OF DIETARY FIBER

A high intake of DF offers numerous health benefits. People who consume more fiber have a significantly lower risk of developing coronary heart disease, stroke, hypertension, diabetes, obesity, and various gastrointestinal disorders. Increased fiber intake helps lower blood pressure and serum cholesterol levels, while soluble fiber improves blood glucose control and insulin sensitivity in both diabetic and non-diabetic individuals. In those with obesity, fiber supplementation can enhance weight loss. Higher fiber consumption also supports digestive health, reducing symptoms of conditions such as gastroesophageal reflux disease, duodenal ulcers, diverticulitis, constipation, and hemorrhoids. Additionally, prebiotic fibers may strengthen immune function. The health benefits of DF extend to children as well as adults (Anderson et al., 2009; Barber et al., 2020; Prasadi and Joye, 2020).

3.5.1 Gut Motility

DF is best known for improving bowel regularity and preventing constipation. Randomized controlled trials and systematic reviews confirm that fiber supplementation—such as through vegetable or grain-based products—enhances stool consistency and frequency and reduces straining. Evidence also supports fiber as an effective treatment and preventive measure for constipation and IBS (Barber et al., 2020).

3.5.2 Body Weight and Abdominal Fat

Fiber may modestly aid weight loss by promoting satiety and reducing meal frequency. Meta-analyses show small but consistent reductions in body weight and waist circumference with higher fiber or pulse intake. While effects on fat mass are minor, fiber can help with long-term weight maintenance and supports metabolic health, especially in individuals with obesity.

3.5.3 Insulin Sensitivity and Metabolic Health

High-fiber diets improve insulin sensitivity, glucose control, and lipid profiles. Controlled trials show cereal fiber enhances insulin response compared with high-protein diets. Observational studies link greater fiber intake with lower HbA1C and reduced risk of type 2 diabetes (T2D). Both soluble and insoluble fibers contribute, though insoluble cereal fiber appears particularly protective.

3.5.4 Gut Microbiota and Metabolites

Fiber nourishes beneficial gut bacteria, promoting production of SCFAs such as butyrate, acetate, and propionate. These metabolites enhance gut barrier function, regulate glucose and lipid metabolism, reduce appetite, and may influence mood and cognition through the gut–brain axis. Fiber deficiency, by contrast, can erode the intestinal mucus layer and increase disease susceptibility.

3.5.5 Chronic Inflammation

Low-fiber intake is linked with gut dysbiosis, reduced SCFA production, and increased inflammation. Butyrate, a key SCFA, suppresses pro-inflammatory pathways and oxidative stress. Population studies show higher fiber intake correlates with lower levels of inflammatory markers (CRP, PAI-1, resistin), possibly mediated by lower body fat.

3.5.6 Depression and Mental Health

Higher fiber intake associates with lower risk of depression, possibly through reduced inflammation and improved gut–brain signaling. Clinical trials support that dietary improvements—including fiber-rich diets like the Mediterranean diet (MD)—can reduce depressive symptoms. The gut microbiota likely plays a central role in this relationship.

3.5.7 Cardiovascular Disease (CVD)

Meta-analyses of large cohort studies show that every 7 g/day increase in fiber intake reduces cardiovascular disease (CVD) and coronary heart disease risk by about 9% (Threapleton et al., 2013). High-fiber diets improve lipid and glucose metabolism and may reduce trimethylamine-N-oxide (TMAO) levels, a gut-derived compound linked to CVD. Low-fiber, ultra-processed diets show the opposite pattern.

3.5.8 Colorectal Cancer (CRC)

Consistent evidence links higher DF—especially from vegetables and cereals—with lower colorectal cancer (CRC) risk. Meta-analyses indicate about a 25% reduction in CRC incidence among high-fiber consumers. While fiber may not prevent recurrence of pre-existing polyps, it likely protects against initial tumor formation.

3.5.9 Mortality

Prospective studies suggest an 11% reduction in all-cause mortality per 10 g/day increase in fiber intake, particularly from cereal sources. While causality cannot be confirmed, high-fiber consumption typically aligns with other healthy lifestyle behaviors that contribute to longevity.

3.6 DIETARY INTERVENTION AND MICROBIOME MODULATION

Given the central role of the gut microbiome in regulating host physiology, metabolism, and immunity, as well as its strong association with numerous diseases, there is growing scientific interest in strategies to intentionally modulate the gut ecosystem. Among the most effective, accessible, and sustainable of these strategies is dietary intervention.

Diet represents the most significant environmental determinant shaping the structure, diversity, and functionality of the gut microbiome. The components of food that escape enzymatic digestion and absorption in the small intestine—particularly non-digestible carbohydrates and fibers—serve as primary energy sources for colonic microbes. The type, quantity, and quality of these substrates dictate which microbial taxa flourish and which metabolites they produce. For instance, the fermentation of complex carbohydrates by beneficial microbes supports a saccharolytic metabolism that yields health-promoting metabolites such as SCFAs, whereas the putrefaction of undigested proteins leads to potentially harmful products like ammonia and phenolic compounds (Peled and Livney, 2021). Thus, the balance between these metabolic pathways is highly dependent on dietary composition and directly affects gut and systemic health.

A diet abundant in plant-based foods and DF fosters a favorable microbial community structure. Fiber-rich diets promote the growth of beneficial bacteria such as *Bifidobacterium* and *Lactobacillus*, which are associated with saccharolytic fermentation and enhanced SCFA production. Conversely, a diet high in animal protein and low in fiber encourages proteolytic fermentation by bacteria such as *Clostridium* and *Bacteroides*, generating metabolites that can disrupt gut homeostasis, increase intestinal permeability, and trigger inflammatory responses. The SCFAs—primarily acetate, propionate, and butyrate—produced through fermentation of complex carbohydrates are central to maintaining gut health. SCFAs nourish colonocytes, fortify the intestinal barrier, and exert potent anti-inflammatory and immunomodulatory effects by inhibiting histone deacetylases and promoting the activity of regulatory T cells (De Luca and Shoenfeld, 2019).

In contrast, a low-fiber diet deprives fermentative microbes of their preferred substrates, forcing them to degrade host-derived glycans from the mucus layer produced by goblet cells. Over time, this process thins the mucus barrier, increases intestinal permeability ("leaky gut"), and allows microbial antigens and toxins to reach the epithelium. The result is a heightened risk of local and systemic inflammation, which may contribute to metabolic and autoimmune disorders.

3.7 THE HIGH-FIBER DIET: FUELING THE GUT ECOSYSTEM

A high-fiber diet emphasizes the consumption of complex carbohydrates indigestible by human enzymes but readily fermentable by gut microbes. These carbohydrates are abundant in plant-derived foods such as legumes (beans, lentils, chickpeas), whole grains (oats, barley, quinoa), vegetables (broccoli, carrots, leafy greens), fruits (apples, berries, bananas), and nuts and seeds. DFs are broadly classified as soluble (which dissolve in water to form viscous gels, found in oats, apples, and beans) and insoluble (which increase stool bulk and accelerate intestinal transit, found in wheat bran, nuts, and whole grains) (Dhingra et al., 2012).

The fermentation of these fibers by colonic bacteria triggers a cascade of metabolic and ecological benefits. SCFA production enhances intestinal barrier integrity by strengthening epithelial tight junctions and stimulating mucus production. Butyrate, in particular, serves as the preferred energy substrate for colonocytes, maintaining mucosal health and reducing inflammation. Furthermore, the acidic environment generated by SCFA production suppresses pH-sensitive pathogenic bacteria such as *Escherichia coli* and *C. difficile*, thereby stabilizing the gut microbial ecosystem (Canani et al., 2011).

The advantages of a high-fiber diet extend beyond the gastrointestinal tract. By reinforcing the gut barrier, SCFAs prevent lipopolysaccharide (LPS)—a potent pro-inflammatory molecule from Gram-negative bacteria—from translocating into the bloodstream. This reduces chronic, low-grade systemic inflammation implicated in metabolic syndrome, insulin resistance, and CVD. Numerous studies have linked high-fiber dietary patterns to lower risks of obesity, T2D, cardiovascular disorders, and CRC, highlighting the far-reaching benefits of a well-nourished microbiome (Veronese et al., 2018).

In essence, dietary intervention through increased fiber intake is one of the most effective and natural methods to maintain microbial balance, enhance intestinal resilience, and protect systemic health. By feeding the right microbes, humans, in turn, sustain a harmonious relationship with their microscopic partners—an essential foundation of long-term wellness.

3.7.1 Dietary Fiber: The Primary Fuel for a Healthy Gut Microbiome

DF exemplifies the profound influence of diet on the gut microbiome, acting as the primary fuel for the trillions of microorganisms that reside in the colon. Fiber is composed of plant-based carbohydrates that humans cannot digest due to the absence of the specific enzymes required to break their complex bonds. Consequently, fiber passes largely intact through the small intestine and reaches the colon, where it serves as a microbiota-accessible carbohydrate (MAC)—a critical energy source for the resident microbial community. Far from being a passive component of our diet, fiber acts as a form of ecological engineering, shaping the composition, diversity, and metabolic activity of the gut microbiota.

The anaerobic fermentation of MACs by colonic bacteria produces a suite of beneficial metabolites, most notably SCFAs such as acetate, propionate, and butyrate (Nagpal et al., 2019). These molecules are not merely by-products of microbial metabolism; they are powerful signaling molecules that mediate many of the health benefits associated with a high-fiber diet. Butyrate, in particular, serves as the preferred energy source for colonocytes, the epithelial cells lining the colon, and plays a central role in maintaining the integrity of the gut barrier. By reinforcing tight junctions and promoting mucus production, SCFAs prevent the translocation of pro-inflammatory molecules into the bloodstream, thereby reducing chronic, low-grade systemic inflammation (Zhang, 2023). Beyond the gut, SCFAs enter the circulation, where they contribute to the regulation of glucose and lipid metabolism and modulate immune function, typically promoting an anti-inflammatory state that supports overall health (Nagpal et al., 2019).

DF also selectively nurtures beneficial commensal bacteria, an effect known as the bifidogenic effect. Certain fibers reliably increase the abundance of *Bifidobacterium* species, while others enhance *Faecalibacterium prausnitzii*, a key butyrate producer with potent anti-inflammatory properties. Intervention studies suggest that a daily intake of roughly 7–10 g of specific fibers is sufficient to elicit measurable microbial effects. However, the diversity of fiber sources is as important as the total quantity. Data from the American Gut Project reveal that individuals who consumed more than 30 distinct types of plant foods in a single week exhibited significantly higher gut microbiome diversity than those who consumed fewer than 10 types (Oliver et al., 2021). This finding underscores the importance of providing a wide array of MACs, as each fiber type creates unique metabolic niches that support a more complex and resilient microbial community. Therefore, the most effective dietary strategy is not merely increasing fiber intake but also consuming a broad variety of fiber-containing plant foods.

In contrast, the adoption of a Western-style diet—high in processed foods, simple sugars, and saturated fats, and low in fiber, fruits, and vegetables—is a primary driver of the shift from gut eubiosis to dysbiosis in industrialized nations. This dietary pattern reduces microbial diversity, diminishes beneficial fiber fermentation, and promotes the growth of Proteobacteria, a phylum that includes many enteric pathogens, while decreasing the abundance of Firmicutes that produce health-promoting SCFAs (Nagpal et al., 2019). The result is a gut ecosystem prone to inflammation, metabolic dysfunction, and chronic disease.

Translating these mechanistic insights into practical dietary approaches, certain traditional diets have emerged as validated models for promoting gut health. The MD and the Blue Zones (BZ) diet exemplify holistic, ecosystem-level interventions that provide a rich and diverse array of substrates for the gut microbiota. Both emphasize high intake of whole grains, legumes, vegetables, fruits, nuts, and seeds—delivering not only quantity but diversity of fiber. By fostering a robust, SCFA-producing microbiome, these dietary patterns support metabolic health, immune regulation, and longevity, illustrating the transformative potential of DF as the primary fuel for a thriving gut ecosystem.

3.8 SIGNIFICANCE OF FIBER DIET ON HEALTH

DF plays a fundamental role in maintaining intestinal health and systemic homeostasis through its interactions with the gut microbiota and the intestinal mucosal barrier. The gut epithelium is protected by a thick mucus layer that separates luminal bacteria from direct contact with epithelial cells, thus serving as a physical and biochemical defense mechanism against microbial invasion and infection. A well-structured and intact mucus layer is essential for preventing pathogenic infiltration and maintaining immune tolerance. Both diet and gut microbiota profoundly influence the production and integrity of this mucus layer. Diets deficient in fiber can lead to the degradation of the mucus barrier, exposing epithelial surfaces to pathogenic bacteria and increasing susceptibility to infections, inflammation, and chronic diseases such as inflammatory bowel disease and metabolic syndrome (Makki et al., 2018).

DFs and their fermentation products—SCFAs—stimulate mucus production and secretion, thereby maintaining epithelial integrity. Acetate and butyrate play particularly important roles in regulating mucus homeostasis. For instance, *Bacteroides thetaiotaomicron*, a producer of acetate and propionate, promotes goblet cell differentiation and enhances the expression of mucin-related genes. Conversely, *F. prausnitzii*, a butyrate-producing bacterium, consumes acetate and modulates mucus production to prevent excessive accumulation, ensuring an optimal mucus layer thickness (Wrzosek et al., 2013). In addition to microbial and chemical stimulation, DFs also provide mechanical stimulation to the intestinal epithelium, triggering mucus secretion through physical contact (Makki et al., 2018).

A prolonged deficiency in DF disrupts this delicate equilibrium. Low-fiber diets encourage the proliferation of mucin-degrading bacteria such as *A. muciniphila*, which degrade host mucins to obtain nutrients, leading to thinning of the mucus barrier. Under such fiber-deprived conditions, gut bacteria shift their metabolism toward the utilization of mucin glycans, upregulating mucin-degrading enzymes. Animal studies demonstrate that mice fed Western-style, low-fiber diets develop thinner mucus layers, increased mucosal penetrability, and a higher risk of intestinal infection and inflammation. Interestingly, supplementation with inulin, a prebiotic fiber, or administration of *Bifidobacterium longum* can restore mucus integrity. Low concentrations of inulin (1%) correct mucus penetrability, while *B. longum* restores mucus growth rate, highlighting distinct but complementary roles. However, only high inulin intake (around 20%) improves metabolic parameters in obese mice, suggesting that low-fiber levels protect local gut functions, whereas higher doses are required for systemic metabolic benefits (Schroeder et al., 2018). Nevertheless, such high inulin concentrations are unlikely to be tolerated in humans, pointing to a dose-dependent, species-specific response.

Beyond mucus regulation, DF provides numerous health benefits through microbial fermentation processes in the colon. Intestinal bacteria ferment non-digestible carbohydrates to produce monosaccharides, gases (methane, hydrogen, carbon dioxide), and SCFAs—chiefly acetate (60%), propionate (25%), and butyrate (15%). These SCFAs are central to intestinal physiology: they supply energy to colonocytes, regulate fluid and electrolyte transport, and contribute to intestinal motility. Acetate serves as a substrate for cholesterol and fatty acid synthesis; propionate functions as a gluconeogenic precursor; and butyrate, the preferred energy source for colon cells, enhances barrier integrity, modulates immune responses, and regulates gene expression through epigenetic mechanisms. The ratio and quantity of SCFAs produced depend on both the type of DF consumed and the composition of the gut microbiota (Makki et al., 2018).

SCFAs produced in the colon are absorbed into the bloodstream via specific transporters and circulate to various organs, where they act as both energy substrates and signaling molecules. Studies show that SCFAs influence lipid, glucose, and cholesterol metabolism across tissues. In colonocytes—the primary absorptive cells of the large intestine—SCFA transport occurs through passive diffusion of undissociated acids and active transport via monocarboxylate transporters (MCTs) and sodium-coupled MCTs (SMCTs). MCT1, located on the apical membrane, facilitates proton-coupled SCFA uptake, while SMCT1 cotransports SCFAs with sodium ions, promoting sodium and water absorption. On the basolateral side, transporters such as MCT4 and MCT5 export SCFAs into circulation, linking gut microbial metabolism directly to host systemic metabolism (Fu et al., 2022; den Besten et al., 2013).

Once absorbed, SCFAs serve as crucial energy sources. They provide approximately 10% of human daily caloric needs, with colonocytes deriving up to 70% of their energy from SCFA oxidation. Butyrate, in particular, fuels colonocytes, supports mitochondrial respiration, and prevents autophagy. In germ-free mice, the absence of butyrate-producing bacteria results in impaired colonocyte energy metabolism and tissue atrophy—effects that can be reversed by *Butyrivibrio fibrisolvens* or exogenous butyrate supplementation. Acetate and propionate also play vital systemic roles: acetate, which constitutes the majority of circulating SCFAs, is primarily metabolized by the liver for energy production and lipogenesis, while propionate acts as a precursor for hepatic gluconeogenesis, contributing to glucose homeostasis. The liver clears most propionate and butyrate from the portal vein to prevent excessive systemic accumulation, underscoring the organ's central role in SCFA metabolism.

Collectively, these mechanisms demonstrate that DF is not only a structural component of plant-based foods but also a key regulator of host–microbe interactions and systemic health. A high-fiber diet sustains a balanced microbiome, strengthens the intestinal mucus barrier, supports metabolic and immune functions, and protects against chronic diseases. Conversely, fiber deficiency disrupts these symbiotic relationships, leading to inflammation, metabolic disorders, and heightened infection risk. Therefore, regular consumption of diverse DFs—such as inulin, resistant starches (RSs), and pectins—is essential for maintaining gastrointestinal and overall physiological well-being, making DF one of the most important determinants of long-term human health (den Besten et al., 2013).

A diet deficient in DF is increasingly recognized as a major driver of intestinal inflammation and impaired mucosal health. Research using murine models demonstrates that the absence of fiber promotes a pro-inflammatory baseline environment in the colon and heightens the host's vulnerability to subsequent inflammatory insults. In one study, mice maintained on a no-fiber diet for 14 days experienced profound shifts in the composition and function of their gut microbiota. These alterations were accompanied by a marked increase in neutrophil–endothelial interactions within the colonic microvasculature, indicating early activation of inflammatory pathways even before overt symptoms appeared. Although the mice consuming a fiber-free diet did not initially display classical signs of colitis, they became extraordinarily susceptible to colonic injury when exposed to a low dose (0.5%) of dextran sodium sulfate (DSS), a commonly used chemical inducer of experimental colitis. This heightened sensitivity underscores the critical role of DF in preserving epithelial integrity, maintaining microbial balance, and preventing inappropriate immune activation (Shen et al., 2021).

Importantly, supplementation with acetate—the most abundant SCFA produced by microbial fermentation of fiber—was sufficient to counteract many of the detrimental effects of fiber deprivation. Acetate administration reduced the enrichment of colonic neutrophils and protected the mice from developing severe DSS-induced colitis, suggesting that SCFAs act as key mediators linking DF intake to immune regulation and tissue homeostasis.

Overall, these findings highlight that DF, primarily through its microbial fermentation products such as acetate, plays a pivotal role in modulating neutrophil recruitment, regulating inflammatory responses, and safeguarding the host against colonic damage. The study reinforces the concept that inadequate fiber intake compromises gut resilience and predisposes the colon to exaggerated inflammatory disease (Shen et al., 2021).

3.9 INFLUENCES OF DIETARY FIBER ON DIFFERENT GUT MICROBES

DF plays a central role in shaping the structure and function of the gut microbiota, and its consumption has been repeatedly linked to increases in SCFA-producing bacteria. However, the effects of fiber are highly type-specific, as different fiber substrates selectively stimulate the growth of distinct microbial groups. Interventions using inulin, guar gum, RS, galacto-oligosaccharides (GOS), fructo-oligosaccharides (FOS), and AX oligosaccharides (AXOS) consistently promote the proliferation of *Bifidobacterium*. At the same time, certain fibers preferentially stimulate *Faecalibacterium*, *Ruminococcus* (especially with RS), *Lactobacillus* (notably with galactose- or fructose-containing fibers), *Akkermansia*, and *Roseburia*. These microbial changes typically become evident within one to two weeks of dietary supplementation and often remain stable throughout the entire intervention period (Fu et al., 2022).

3.9.1 *Bifidobacterium*

The well-established bifidogenic effect of DFs is largely attributed to their ability to selectively increase multiple species within the *Bifidobacterium* genus. Numerous studies indicate that inulin is a particularly potent stimulator of bifidobacteria. For example, Healey et al. (2018) reported that inulin supplementation increased *Bifidobacterium* levels from 6.69% to 15.07%. Similarly, Kiewiet et al. (2021) found that inulin primarily elevated *Bifidobacterium adolescentis* and induced detectable levels of *Bifidobacterium angulatum* and *Bifidobacterium ruminantium*. Inulin-rich foods have also produced a threefold increase in *B. longum*. Partially hydrolyzed guar gum, taken for just two weeks, increased bifidobacterial abundance from 8% to 12%, whereas no significant change occurred in the placebo group. RS from potatoes raised the abundance of *Bifidobacterium faecale/adolescentis/stercoris* sequences by more than sixfold. GOS and FOS exhibit similar bifidogenic potential. GOS increased *Bifidobacterium* relative abundance from 7.0% to 34.8%, and another study found that GOS supplementation elevated bifidobacterial counts from 7.2 to 7.8 log10 CFU/g. Adults treated with both GOS and FOS showed significantly higher *Bifidobacterium* levels, with LDA effect sizes around 4.0. AXOS supplementation also enriched *Bifidobacterium*, with two operational taxonomic units (OTUs) identified as major drivers of the pre- to post-intervention shift (Fu et al., 2022).

3.9.2 *Faecalibacterium*

Several long-chain fibers have been shown to increase the abundance of *Faecalibacterium*, a key butyrate-producing genus associated with anti-inflammatory effects and gut health. Inulin increased *Faecalibacterium* from 0.41% to 0.61%, while partially hydrolyzed guar gum produced sustained increases during both intervention and washout periods (Fu et al., 2022). Whole-grain wheat rich in RS and total fiber more than doubled levels of *Faecalibacterium* spp. Similarly, RS2-enriched wheat significantly elevated *Faecalibacterium* levels compared to baseline and control groups, as demonstrated by Hughes et al. (2021). These findings underscore that RSs are particularly effective in promoting this beneficial genus.

3.9.3 *Ruminococcus*

The proliferation of *Ruminococcus*, especially *Ruminococcus bromii*, is strongly linked to the consumption of RS2. Numerous studies show that RS2 acts as a selective substrate for this key primary degrader of RS. Baxter et al. documented a 2.5-fold increase in *R. bromii* following supplementation with native maize RS2. Martínez et al. (2010) reported that individuals consuming maize RS2 exhibited a mean *R. bromii* abundance of 4.1%, compared to 1.0% at baseline, and substantially higher levels relative to both placebo and RS4 groups. RS2-enriched wheat and whole-grain wheat also supported increases in the *Ruminococcus* genus. Other fibers produce similar effects. Arabinogalactan supplementation increased an uncultured *Ruminococcus* species nearly eightfold. Partially hydrolyzed guar gum, in multiple studies, consistently promoted *Ruminococcus* growth. In contrast, inulin appears to suppress *R. bromii*; one trial demonstrated a reduction from 2.11% to 1.15% following inulin-type fructan (ITF) supplementation. Yeast mannan, another fiber-rich gum, likewise reduced *Ruminococcus* abundance compared to controls (Fu et al., 2022).

3.9.4 *Lactobacillus*

Fibers rich in fructose or galactose units—such as inulin, FOS, and GOS—are particularly effective in stimulating the growth of *Lactobacillus*. Very-long-chain inulin (containing 50–103 fructose units) increased lactobacilli by 2.42-fold compared to baseline and by nearly sixfold relative to placebo. In another study involving healthy adults, inulin supplementation elevated *Lactobacillus* abundance from 0.26% to 1.26%; individuals with lower DF intake at baseline experienced even larger increases (0.6%–3.0%). Additional evidence comes from interventions using Deshipu stachyose granules (a GOS mixture derived from *Lycopus lucidus*), which raised lactobacilli counts from 6.8 to 7.5 log10 CFU/g after 14 days. Gum arabic and AXOS also demonstrated significant lactobacilli-promoting effects, confirming that multiple fiber types can support this beneficial group (Fu et al., 2022).

3.9.5 *Prevotella*

Observational research shows that high-fiber diets in traditional or rural populations—such as the Hadza hunter-gatherers of Tanzania or individuals in Papua New Guinea—are associated with markedly elevated *Prevotella* levels. These populations typically consume diverse, carbohydrate-rich diets based on unprocessed plant foods. However, many controlled dietary interventions fail to replicate these increases. This discrepancy likely stems from the broad carbohydrate-fermenting capabilities of *Prevotella*. Beyond indigestible fiber, *Prevotella* efficiently breaks down digestible carbohydrates, oligosaccharides, and monosaccharides that are abundant in starchy plant–based diets common in non-industrialized settings. Therefore, long-term habitual intake of diverse carbohydrates, rather than short-term supplementation with a single fiber type, appears necessary to establish a *Prevotella*-dominant microbiome (Fu et al., 2022).

In addition, geographic, genetic, and lifestyle differences among populations contribute to the contrasting microbial patterns observed between industrialized and traditional societies.

3.10 SIGNIFICANCE OF MEDITERRANEAN AND BLUE ZONE DIETS

Nutrition is a foundational pillar of overall wellness and is strongly associated with numerous determinants of healthy aging and longevity. Although no single dietary pattern guarantees optimal health for every individual, certain eating styles have gained widespread recognition for their consistent links to reduced chronic disease risk and extended lifespan. Among the most celebrated are the Blue Zone diet and the MD—two approaches rooted in long-standing cultural traditions and supported by growing scientific evidence for their contributions to well-being, resilience, and longevity.

Both the Blue Zone and MDs emphasize plant-forward eating, prioritizing fruits, vegetables, legumes, whole grains, nuts, and seeds as core components of daily nutrition. However, they differ in the foods that take center stage, largely reflecting the unique geography, climate, and cultural customs from which they emerged. The MD, inspired by countries such as Greece, Italy, and Spain, highlights the abundant use of olive oil, fresh produce, whole grains, seafood, and moderate wine consumption. In contrast, the Blue Zone dietary patterns—derived from the world's longest-living populations in Okinawa (Japan), Sardinia (Italy), Nicoya (Costa Rica), Ikaria (Greece), and Loma Linda (California)—place stronger emphasis on beans as a staple protein source, minimal consumption of processed foods, and simple, minimally altered ingredients that reflect traditional lifestyles.

While these diets share a common foundation of plant-based nutrition, their distinctions illustrate how diverse cultural foodways can support similar health outcomes. The MD is rich in monounsaturated fats, antioxidants, and omega-3 fatty acids from fish and olive oil, which contribute to heart health and reduced inflammation. Blue Zone dietary habits, on the other hand, are shaped by local staples like sweet potatoes in Okinawa or chickpeas in Ikaria and are complemented by lifestyle practices such as regular physical activity, strong social networks, and mindful eating. Together, these patterns highlight that longevity is not solely a product of the foods consumed, but also of the cultural rhythms and environmental contexts surrounding them.

Ultimately, the overlap between these diets demonstrates that a plant-centered, minimally processed, nutrient-dense eating pattern—regardless of regional variations—supports long-term health and vitality.

3.10.1 The Mediterranean Diet: A Paradigm of Microbial Restoration

The MD is widely regarded as one of the healthiest and most sustainable dietary patterns in the world, renowned for its extensive benefits to cardiovascular, metabolic, and cognitive health. Increasingly, scientific evidence indicates that many of these benefits are mediated through the diet's profound influence on the gut microbiome—the complex community of microorganisms that resides in the human gastrointestinal tract (Perrone and D'Angelo, 2025). Rather than representing a rigid set of dietary rules, the MD embodies a flexible and holistic way of eating, grounded in the traditional food culture of countries bordering the Mediterranean Sea.

At its core, the MD emphasizes the consumption of a wide variety of plant-based foods, including vegetables, fruits, legumes, nuts, seeds, and whole grains. Extra-virgin olive oil serves as the principal source of fat, providing abundant monounsaturated fatty acids (MUFAs) and polyphenolic compounds with potent antioxidant properties. Moderate amounts of fish and poultry are encouraged, supplying essential omega-3 fatty acids, while dairy products—mainly yogurt and cheese—are consumed in small quantities. Red meat and processed foods are eaten sparingly. Collectively, this composition makes the MD naturally rich in DF (approximately 33 g/day), MUFAs, omega-3 fatty acids, polyphenols, and other bioactive compounds that reduce oxidative stress and inflammation (Contaldo et al., 2003).

One of the most remarkable features of the MD is its role in microbial restoration—the process of reestablishing a healthy and balanced gut microbiota. Human clinical studies have demonstrated that adherence to the MD can lead to rapid and measurable improvements in gut microbial diversity. In a controlled feeding trial, participants who followed a two-week MD intervention showed a significant increase in gut bacterial diversity compared to those consuming a typical Western or American diet (Rejeski et al., 2022). On a broader scale, a multicountry study conducted across five European nations found that a year-long MD intervention in older adults not only enhanced microbiome composition but also produced systemic benefits. Participants exhibited reduced frailty, lower inflammatory markers, and improved cognitive function. Mechanistically, these outcomes were linked to a shift in microbial metabolism—specifically, an increase in SCFA production and a decrease in pro-inflammatory compounds such as LPSs (Ghosh et al., 2020).

Preclinical research further strengthens the causal link between the MD and microbial health. In long-term studies involving non-human primates, consistent consumption of an MD led to a more balanced and diverse gut microbiome characterized by increased abundance of beneficial bacterial species (Nagpal et al., 2019). Similarly, mouse model experiments have shown that Mediterranean-style diets induce profound microbiome-mediated effects that protect against a spectrum of diseases—including Alzheimer's disease, CRC, and inflammatory bowel disease (Park et al., 2024).

Collectively, these findings highlight the MD as a powerful dietary strategy for cultivating an anti-inflammatory gut environment. Its high content of fiber, polyphenols, and unsaturated fats promotes the proliferation of SCFA-producing bacteria such as *Bifidobacterium*, *F. prausnitzii*, and *Roseburia*, all of which contribute to intestinal barrier integrity and immune regulation (Perrone and D'Angelo, 2025). Through this microbiome-centered mechanism, the MD exemplifies how traditional dietary patterns can serve as modern interventions for restoring microbial balance, supporting longevity, and protecting against chronic disease.

3.10.2 Blue Zone Diets: Integrating Nutrition and Lifestyle for Healthy Aging

The concept of "Blue Zones" (BZ) refers to specific geographic regions across the world where people live significantly longer and healthier lives, often reaching 100 years or more with remarkably low rates of chronic disease. The five validated BZ include Ogliastra in Sardinia (Italy), Ikaria (Greece), the Nicoya Peninsula (Costa Rica), Okinawa (Japan), and Loma Linda (California, USA)—home to a large community of Seventh-day Adventists known for their longevity (Santacroce et al., 2024). While each region has its own cultural and environmental context, they all share strikingly similar dietary and lifestyle characteristics that collectively promote health, resilience, and longevity.

Although the cuisines of these regions differ in specific ingredients and culinary traditions, the core nutritional philosophy across all BZ closely parallels that of the MD. A meta-analysis of dietary surveys from all five BZ revealed that their traditional diets are overwhelmingly plant-based—comprising 90%–100% of total food intake—and emphasize whole, minimally processed foods such as whole grains, legumes, beans, nuts, seeds, fruits, and a variety of leafy greens (Mohol et al., 2025). Meat consumption is rare, typically limited to small portions eaten only a few times per month, while added sugars and refined foods are almost entirely absent. These diets are naturally rich in complex carbohydrates, DF, polyphenols, β-glucans, and unsaturated fatty acids, all of which contribute to their profound metabolic and anti-inflammatory benefits (Santacroce et al., 2024).

Each Blue Zone showcases a distinctive local expression of these shared principles. For example, the Okinawan diet has historically centered around sweet potatoes, soy products such as tofu and miso, seaweeds, and a diverse array of vegetables—foods that are dense in nutrients and fiber but low in calories. Similarly, Sardinians consume a variety of legumes, sourdough bread made from whole grains, goat's milk, and olive oil, while the Nicoyan diet features corn tortillas, beans, and tropical fruits. The Adventists of Loma Linda often follow a vegetarian or vegan lifestyle, with a focus on nuts, whole grains, and legumes. Across all these regions, such fiber-rich and phytonutrient-dense diets provide ideal substrates for the maintenance of a balanced and diverse gut microbiota, which is increasingly recognized as a cornerstone of healthy aging.

Emerging research suggests that the link between Blue Zone diets, gut microbiota composition, and longevity may be mediated through a reduction in chronic, low-grade inflammation—often termed "inflammaging." Foods abundant in antioxidants and anti-inflammatory compounds, such as flavonoids, carotenoids, and omega-3 fatty acids, help modulate inflammatory signaling pathways and enhance immune regulation through the activation of regulatory T cells (Santacroce et al., 2024). In parallel, a healthy gut microbiome—nourished by high-fiber plant foods—produces beneficial metabolites such as SCFAs, especially butyrate. These compounds reinforce the integrity of the intestinal barrier, reduce systemic inflammation, and regulate energy metabolism. Together, these effects slow biological aging and protect against chronic diseases such as CVD, diabetes, cancer, and neurodegeneration.

However, the Blue Zone model illustrates that diet alone does not account for exceptional longevity. Equally important are the complementary lifestyle factors that interact synergistically with nutrition to sustain overall health. Individuals in BZ engage in regular, natural physical activity—such as walking, gardening, and manual labor—rather than structured exercise routines. They maintain a strong sense of purpose ("ikigai" in Okinawa or "plan de vida" in Nicoya), practice daily stress-reduction rituals such as prayer, meditation, or afternoon rest, and nurture deep social connections within their families and communities. Moderate alcohol consumption, particularly red wine with meals in some regions, is common but not excessive (Cronin et al., 2021).

These intertwined factors—nutrient-rich diets, physical movement, emotional well-being, and social support—create a holistic ecosystem of health that sustains vitality well into advanced age. The Blue Zone experience thus provides a compelling blueprint for modern societies: longevity is not achieved through diet alone but through the harmonious integration of nutrition, lifestyle, and community. This model underscores the idea that true health is cultivated not merely at the table, but through daily living in connection with others and the natural world.

3.11 CANCER AND DIETARY FIBER

A total of 416,588 participants (54% women) from the UK Biobank cohort were included in a comprehensive investigation exploring the relationship between diet and lung cancer risk. Using baseline food-frequency questionnaire (FFQ) data, researchers identified three major dietary patterns through principal component analysis. To determine the associations between these dietary patterns, specific food groups, and lung cancer incidence, the study employed Cox proportional hazards models, a standard approach for analyzing time-to-event outcomes.

Over a median follow-up period of 7.13 years, 1782 new cases of lung cancer were recorded. Analysis revealed a clear divergence between foods associated with increased risk and those offering potential protection. Higher consumption of red meat and processed meat was linked to a significantly elevated lung cancer risk (HR per 50 g/day: 1.36; 95% CI: 1.13–1.65 for red meat; HR per 25 g/day: 1.30; 95% CI: 1.10–1.53 for processed meat). In contrast, dietary components rich in fiber and micronutrients—including fruits, vegetables, breakfast cereals, and DF overall—were inversely associated with lung cancer risk. For example, each 5 g/day increase in total fiber intake was associated with a 24% reduction in lung cancer risk (HR: 0.76; 95% CI: 0.69–0.84).

When dietary patterns were assessed across quartiles, individuals with the highest adherence to a prudent dietary pattern—characterized by high intake of plant-based foods, fiber, and whole grains—exhibited a significantly lower risk of lung cancer compared with those in the lowest quartile (HRQ4 vs. Q1: 0.84; 95% CI: 0.73–0.96). Conversely, participants who most strongly adhered to a Western dietary pattern, rich in processed foods, meats, and refined grains, showed an increased risk (HRQ4 vs. Q1: 1.27; 95% CI: 1.11–1.46). Collectively, these findings suggest that diets emphasizing fiber-rich plant foods and minimizing red and processed meats may offer substantial protective benefits against lung cancer (Wei et al., 2021).

Breast cancer is the most prevalent cancer among women, representing nearly 30% of all cancer diagnoses, whereas it accounts for only about 1% of cases in men. Incidence and mortality vary widely across populations, influenced by factors such as ethnicity, geographic region, and socioeconomic status. Because male breast cancer is rare and research in this population is limited, exercise recommendations for men are frequently extrapolated from studies involving women. A growing body of evidence demonstrates that physical activity plays a critical role in the prevention, treatment, and post-treatment recovery of breast cancer. Exercise not only helps reduce sedentary behavior but also supports maintenance of a healthy body weight, regulation of metabolic health, and reduction of systemic inflammation—all key components in lowering breast cancer risk. In addition to regular exercise, a balanced diet rich in fruits, vegetables, whole grains, and DF, combined with limited alcohol intake and reduced consumption of red and processed meats, is strongly recommended. Beyond cancer-specific benefits, such lifestyle patterns are known to reduce the incidence of CVDs, improve overall functional capacity, and lower all-cause and cardiovascular mortality (Campos et al., 2022).

Extensive research supports the protective effects of DF against CRC. Aune et al. (2011) reported that high-fiber intake—particularly from cereal grains and whole grains—is associated with a significantly reduced risk of CRC. Fiber is believed to influence carcinogenesis through multiple mechanisms, including dilution of carcinogens in the intestinal tract, modulation of the gut microbiome, improvement of insulin sensitivity, and reduction in chronic inflammation.

Supporting these findings, a large prospective analysis within a population-based colorectal screening trial demonstrated that individuals consuming the highest levels of DF had substantially lower risks of developing incident colorectal adenomas and distal colon cancer. Importantly, the protective effect appeared strongest for fiber derived from cereals and fruits, suggesting that different fiber sources may contribute uniquely to colorectal health. The study further indicated that the benefits of a high-fiber diet may emerge early in the carcinogenic process, highlighting the importance of sustained fiber intake throughout adulthood (Kunzmann et al., 2015).

3.12 MODULATION OF IMMUNOTHERAPY BY DIETARY FIBERS

Gut bacteria play a central role in shaping the response to immune checkpoint blockade (ICB) therapies in cancer, yet the influence of diet and supplements on these interactions has historically received limited attention. In an effort to clarify these relationships, researchers analyzed fecal microbiota profiles, dietary habits, and probiotic supplement use in melanoma patients, while also conducting parallel preclinical experiments. Their findings revealed that higher DF intake was significantly associated with improved progression-free survival (PFS) among 128 patients receiving ICB. Notably, the strongest benefits were observed in patients who consumed sufficient DF without using commercially available probiotics. This suggests that diet and probiotic supplementation may interact in ways that influence therapeutic outcomes.

Preclinical studies helped validate these clinical observations. Mice fed a low-fiber diet or given probiotic supplements showed impaired responses to anti–programmed cell death 1 (anti–PD-1) therapy. These mice also displayed reduced frequencies of interferon-γ–producing cytotoxic T cells within the tumor microenvironment—cells essential for robust antitumor immunity. Together, these results provide compelling evidence that DF supports the immune response during ICB treatment, while certain probiotic formulations may inadvertently hinder it. This work has meaningful clinical implications for how dietary guidance should be integrated into cancer care (Spencer et al., 2021).

Further clinical research has identified specific gut bacterial taxa that are enriched in patients who respond favorably to immunotherapy, including *A. muciniphila*, Ruminococcaceae, *Faecalibacterium*, and Lachnospiraceae. A high-fiber diet promotes the growth of these bacteria by providing substrates for fermentation. During fermentation, these microbes produce SCFAs—notably acetate, propionate, and butyrate. These metabolites nourish intestinal epithelial cells, maintain gut barrier integrity, and enter the circulation to modulate systemic immunity. SCFAs can activate DC8+ cytotoxic T cells, enhancing their ability to kill cancer cells. This mechanism helps explain why high-fiber intake is associated with lower risks of disease progression or death during checkpoint immunotherapy.

Dietary patterns that support a diverse and metabolically active gut microbiome appear to be especially beneficial for patients undergoing ICB. High-fiber, plant-based diets such as the MD have been shown to enhance microbial diversity and increase concentrations of SCFA-producing bacteria. In contrast, antibiotics and proton pump inhibitors can disrupt the microbiota, negatively influencing immunotherapy outcomes. A narrative review of the literature emphasizes that both the composition of the microbiota and its metabolic outputs are strongly associated with favorable immunotherapy responses. However, prospective clinical trials are needed to determine whether specific dietary interventions can be reliably used to improve cancer treatment outcomes (Gamrath et al., 2025).

The success of ICB therapy in advanced melanoma varies widely, despite its transformative impact on survival. Between 40% and 60% of patients experience durable responses, but others gain little benefit or develop immune-related adverse events of varying severity. In this context, nutrition represents a promising but understudied modifier of treatment efficacy. Because diet modulates both immune function and the gut microbiome, it may serve as a practical intervention to enhance patient outcomes. To explore this possibility, the PRIMM multicenter cohort study examined 91 ICB-naïve melanoma patients from the Netherlands and the United Kingdom who began ICB therapy between 2018 and 2021. Researchers collected baseline dietary data using FFQs prior to treatment initiation.

The study population included 44 Dutch and 47 British patients, ranging in age from their late 50s to mid-60s. Clinical and dietary data were prospectively gathered to evaluate how eating patterns might influence ICB outcomes. Statistical modeling using logistic generalized additive models revealed strong positive associations between adherence to a Mediterranean dietary pattern and immunotherapy success. Patients with higher intake of whole grains, fish, nuts, fruits, and vegetables had significantly greater odds of achieving an objective response rate (ORR) and maintaining PFS at 12 months (PFS-12). These findings highlight the potential value of dietary quality as a modifiable predictor of treatment response.

Importantly, the PRIMM study demonstrated that the MD—a model widely endorsed by public health organizations—not only promotes general health but may also enhance the effectiveness of cancer immunotherapy. However, because diet varies substantially across regions and cultural contexts, larger and more geographically diverse studies are needed to validate these findings. Such research would help clarify whether the observed benefits apply broadly across populations and cancer types (Bolte et al., 2023).

The mechanisms through which diet influences immunotherapy response likely involve the gut microbiome. The MD, characterized by high intake of plant-derived foods and minimal consumption of processed and red meats, promotes the growth of SCFA-producing bacteria. These microbes generate metabolites that support immune regulation and antitumor activity. Preclinical studies have shown that fiber, polyphenols, and antioxidants exert immunomodulatory effects via microbial metabolism, helping to shape the tumor microenvironment. In a cohort of 52 ICB-treated patients with various solid tumors, high fecal SCFA concentrations were strongly associated with prolonged PFS. This growing body of evidence suggests that targeting the gut microbiome through diet may represent an effective approach to improving patient outcomes during checkpoint immunotherapy.

Overall, the emerging research underscores the profound influence of dietary patterns—particularly fiber-rich, Mediterranean-style diets—on the gut microbiome and, subsequently, the effectiveness of ICB therapy (Bolte et al., 2023). As scientists continue to unravel the complex relationships among diet, microbial ecology, and immune function, dietary interventions may become a valuable complement to existing cancer treatments. Further clinical trials will be essential to determine how best to integrate nutritional strategies into routine immunotherapy care.

3.13 CONCLUSION

Diet is a powerful and modifiable determinant of human health, with far-reaching effects on metabolism, immunity, and the gut microbiome. The evidence clearly demonstrates that dietary patterns rich in diverse, fiber-containing plant foods, unsaturated fats, and bioactive compounds promote a balanced and resilient gut ecosystem, enhance SCFA production, strengthen intestinal barrier function, and reduce systemic inflammation. In contrast, diets high in processed foods, refined sugars, and saturated fats disrupt microbial diversity, favor pathogenic bacteria, and contribute to chronic disease risk.

Holistic dietary approaches, such as the Mediterranean and Blue Zone diets, illustrate that optimal health and longevity are achieved not solely through nutrition but through the integration of diet with lifestyle factors including physical activity, social engagement, and stress management. By emphasizing nutrient diversity, fiber variety, and minimally processed foods, these diets create a supportive environment for a healthy microbiome, which in turn mediates numerous systemic health benefits.

Ultimately, strategic dietary interventions offer a feasible and effective means to enhance gut health, prevent chronic disease, and promote healthy aging. Prioritizing fiber-rich, plant-based, and diverse diets represents a cornerstone of modern nutritional strategies, highlighting the profound interplay between what we eat, the microbial communities within us, and our long-term health outcomes.

ACKNOWLEDGMENTS

The author (ST) acknowledges Wawa Foundation, Sharpe-Strumia Research Foundation, W.W. Smith Charitable Trust and Abraham Thomas Foundation for providing the resources for this work.

REFERENCES

Allen RC. The Neolithic revolution in the middle East. *The Economic History Review*. 2024;77:1154–1196.

An L, Tao Y, Chen H, et al. Embryo-endosperm interaction and its agronomic relevance to rice quality. *Front Plant Sci*. 2020;11:587641.

Anderson JW, Baird P, Davis RH Jr, Ferreri S, Knudtson M, Koraym A, Waters V, Williams CL. Health benefits of dietary fiber. *Nutr Rev*. 2009;67(4):188–205.

Aune D, Chan DS, Lau R, et al. Dietary fibre, whole grains, and risk of colorectal cancer: systematic review and dose-response meta-analysis. *BMJ*. 2011;343:d6617.

Avetisyan M, Schill EM, Heuckeroth RO. Building a second brain in the bowel. *J Clin Invest*. 2015;125(3):899–907.

Barber TM, Kabisch S, Pfeiffer AFH, Weickert MO. The health benefits of dietary fibre. *Nutrients*. 2020;12:3209.

Bolte LA, Lee KA, Björk JR, et al. Association of a Mediterranean diet with outcomes for patients treated with immune checkpoint blockade for advanced melanoma. *JAMA Oncol*. 2023;9(5):705–709.

Campos MDSB, Feitosa RHF, Mizzaci CC, et al. The benefits of exercise in breast cancer. *Arq Bras Cardiol*. 2022;119(6):981–990.

Canani RB, Costanzo MD, Leone L, Bedogni G, Brambilla P, Cianfarani S, Nobili V, Pietrobelli A, Agostoni C. Epigenetic mechanisms elicited by nutrition in early life. *Nutr Res Rev*. 2011 Dec;24(2):198–205. doi: 10.1017/S0954422411000102.

Carey J. Unearthing the origins of agriculture. *Proc Natl Acad Sci U S A*. 2023 Apr 11;120(15):e2304407120.

Contaldo F, Pasanisi F, Mancini M. Beyond the traditional interpretation of Mediterranean diet. *Nutr Metab Cardiovasc Dis*. 2003 Jun;13(3):117–119.

Cronin P, Joyce SA, O'Toole PW, O'Connor EM. Dietary fibre modulates the gut microbiota. *Nutrients*. 2021 May 13;13(5):1655. doi: 10.3390/nu13051655.

Cucchi T, Arbuckle B. Animal domestication: from distant past to current development. *Anim Front*. 2021;11(3):6–9.

De Luca F, ShoenfeldY. The microbiome in autoimmune diseases. *Clin Exp Immunol*. 2019 Jan;195(1):74–85. doi: 10.1111/cei.13158.

den Besten G, van Eunen K, Groen AK, Venema K, Reijngoud DJ, Bakker BM. The role of short-chain fatty acids in the interplay between diet, gut microbiota, and host energy metabolism. *J Lipid Res*. 2013;54(9):2325–2340.

Dhingra D, Michael M, Rajput H, Patil RT. Dietary fibre in foods: a review. *J Food Sci Technol*. 2012 Jun;49(3):255–266. doi: 10.1007/s13197-011-0365-5.

Fu J, Zheng Y, Gao Y, Xu W. Dietary fiber intake and gut microbiota in human health. *Microorganisms*. 2022;10(12):2507.

Fuchs K, Rinne C, Drummer C, Immel A, Kyora BK, Nebel A. Infectious diseases and Neolithic transformations: evaluating biological and archaeological proxies in the German loess zone between 5500 and 2500 BCE. *The Holocene*. 2019;29:1545–1557.

Gamrath L, Pedersen TB, Møller MV, et al. Role of the microbiome and diet for response to cancer checkpoint immunotherapy. *Curr Oncol Rep*. 2025;27(1):45–58.

Garg K, Padilla-Iglesias C, Restrepo Ochoa N, Knight VB. Hunter-gatherer foraging networks promote information transmission. *R Soc Open Sci*. 2021 Dec 22;8(12):211324.

Ghosh TS, Rampelli S, Jeffery IB, Santoro A, Neto M, Capri M, ... O'Toole PW. Mediterranean diet intervention alters the gut microbiome in older people reducing frailty and improving health status: the NU-AGE 1-year dietary intervention across five European countries. *Gut*. 2020 Jul;69(7):1218–1228. doi: 10.1136/gutjnl-2019-319654.

Goldman L. Three stages of health encounters over 8000 human generations. *Am J Public Health*. 2018;108(1):60–62.

Healey G, Murphy R, Butts C, et al. Habitual dietary fibre intake influences gut microbiota response to an inulin-type fructan prebiotic. *Br J Nutr*. 2018;119:176–189.

Herrera RJ, Garcia-Bertrand R. The agricultural revolutions, Ancestral DNA, human origins, and migrations. In: *Ancestral DNA, Human Origins, and Migrations*. Academic Press, United Kingdom, 2018. pp. 475–509.

Hughes RL, Horn WH, Finnegan P, et al. Resistant starch type 2 from wheat reduces postprandial glycemic response. *Nutrients*. 2021;13:645.

Kiewiet MBG, Elderman ME, El Aidy S, et al. Flexibility of gut microbiota in ageing individuals during dietary fiber inulin intake. *Mol Nutr Food Res*. 2021;65:e2000390.

Kunzmann AT, Coleman HG, Huang WY, et al. Dietary fiber intake and risk of colorectal cancer. *Am J Clin Nutr*. 2015;102(4):881–890.

López S, van Dorp L, Hellenthal G. Human dispersal out of Africa: A lasting debate. *Evol Bioinform* [Online]. 2016 Apr 21;11(Suppl 2):57–68. doi: 10.4137/EBO.S33489.

Magne F, Gotteland M, Gauthier L, et al. The Firmicutes/bacteroidetes ratio: a marker of gut dysbiosis. *Nutrients*. 2020;12(5):1474.

Makki K, Deehan EC, Walter J, Bäckhed F. The impact of dietary fiber on gut microbiota in host health and disease. *Cell Host Microbe*. 2018;23(6):705–715.

Martínez I, Kim J, Duffy PR, et al. Resistant starches types 2 and 4 and microbiota composition. *PLoS One*. 2010;5:e15046.

Mohol P. Blue zone dietary patterns and longevity: a critical review. *J. Integrated Health*. 2025;4:433–435.

Nagpal R, Neth BJ, Wang S, Craft S, Yadav H. Modified Mediterranean-ketogenic diet modulates gut microbiome and short-chain fatty acids in association with Alzheimer's disease markers in subjects with mild cognitive impairment. *EBioMedicine*. 2019 Sep;47:529–542. doi: 10.1016/j.ebiom.2019.08.032.

Oliver A, Chase AB, Weihe C, Orchanian SB, Riedel SF, Hendrickson CL, ... & Whiteson K. High-fiber, whole-food dietary intervention alters the human gut microbiome but not fecal short-chain fatty acids. *mSystems*. 2021 Mar 16;6(2):e00115-21.

Padilla-Iglesias C, Bischoff RJ. (2024). Hunter-gatherer mobility patterns influence the reconstruction of social networks from archaeological assemblages. *J Archaeol. Sci.: Rep*. 2024;59:104798.

Park G, Kadyan S, Hochuli N, Pollak J, Wang B, Salazar G, ... Nagpal R. A modified Mediterranean-style diet enhances brain function via specific gut-microbiome-brain mechanisms. *Gut Microbes*. 2024 Jan-Dec;16(1):2323752. doi: 10.1080/19490976.2024.2323752.

Perrone P, D'Angelo S. Gut microbiota modulation through Mediterranean diet foods: implications for human health. *Nutrients*. 2025 Mar 8;17(6):948.

Prasadi NPV, Joye IJ. Dietary fibre from whole grains and metabolic health. *Nutrients*. 2020;12(10):3045.

Preece C, Livarda A, Christin PA, et al. Domestication of fertile crescent crops and yields. *Funct Ecol*. 2017;31(2):387–397.

Rejeski JJ, Wilson FM, Nagpal R, Yadav H, Weinberg RB. The impact of a Mediterranean diet on the gut microbiome in healthy human subjects: a pilot study. *digestion*. 2022;103(2):133–140. doi: 10.1159/000519445.

Santacroce L, Bottalico L, Charitos IA, Haxhirexha K, Topi S, Jirillo E. Healthy diets and lifestyles in the world: Mediterranean and Blue Zone people live longer. Special focus on gut microbiota and some food components. *Endocr Metab Immune Disord Drug Targets*. 2024;24(15):1774–1784. doi: 10.2174/0118715303271634240319054728.

Schroeder BO, Birchenough GMH, Ståhlman M, et al. Bifidobacteria or fiber protects against colonic mucus loss. *Cell Host Microbe*. 2018;23(1):27–40.e7.

Shen S, Prame Kumar K, Wen SW, et al. Deficiency of dietary fiber modulates gut microbiota and colitis. *Front Immunol*. 2021;12:619366.

Singh RK, Chang HW, Yan D, et al. Influence of diet on the gut microbiome. *J Transl Med*. 2017;15:73.

Spencer CN, McQuade JL, Gopalakrishnan V, et al. Dietary fiber and probiotics influence immunotherapy response. *Science*. 2021;374(6575):1632–1640.

Tarasiuk-Zawadzka A, Fichna J. Nutrition and the enteric nervous system in IBD. *J Nutr Biochem*. 2025;144:109959.

Tassi F, Ghirotto S, Mezzavilla M, Vilaça ST, De Santi L, Barbujani G. Early modern human dispersal from Africa: Genomic evidence for multiple waves of migration. *Investig Genet*. 2015 Nov 6;6:13. doi: 10.1186/s13323-015-0030-2.

Thomas S, Dilbarov N, Kelly J, et al. Diet effects on colonic health and immunotherapy. *Sci Rep*. 2023;13:11802.

Thomas S, Izard J, Walsh E, et al. The host microbiome regulates human health. *Cancer Res*. 2017;77(8):1783–1812.

Threapleton DE, Greenwood DC, Evans L, et al. Dietary fibre intake and risk of CVD: meta-analysis. *BMJ*. 2013;347:f6879.

Veronese N, Solmi M, Caruso MG, Giannelli G, Osella AR, Evangelou E, …, & Tzoulaki I. Dietary fiber and health outcomes: an umbrella review of systematic reviews and meta-analyses. *Am J Clin Nutr*. 2018 Mar 1;107(3):436–444.

Wang M, Yuan T, Chen J, et al. Species-level identification for gut microbiota via 16S rRNA. *Front Microbiol*. 2025;16:1553124.

Wei X, Zhu C, Ji M, et al. Diet and risk of lung cancer. *Am J Clin Nutr*. 2021;114(6):2043–2051.

World Health Organization. *Physical activity*. WHO; 2024.

Wrzosek L, Miquel S, Noordine ML, et al. Gut microbes influence mucus and goblet cell development. *BMC Biol*. 2013;11:61.

Yang C, Chen Q, Zhang X, et al. Genetic improvement of dietary fiber in wheat grains. *Seed Biol*. 2024;3:e002.

Zhang D, Jian YP, Zhang YN, et al. Short-chain fatty acids in diseases. *Cell Commun Signal*. 2023;21:212. https://doi.org/10.1186/s12964-023-01219-9.

Zohary D, Hopf M. *Domestication of plants in the Old World*. Clarendon Press; 1988.

CHAPTER 4

The Living Pantry

UNDERSTANDING THE BACTERIAL ECOSYSTEM IN FERMENTED FOODS

Kinjal J. Parmar, Charmy R. Kothari, and Ramesh K. Kothari

4.1 INTRODUCTION TO FERMENTATION

As the population expands, the demand for nutritious, flavorful food also rises. People's eating habits shift as their lifestyles change. People today are so preoccupied with their daily lives that they are unable to look after themselves or their health. Because of the lack of time in today's modern world, many people do not prepare delicious and nutritious meals at home, leading to a shift in readily available cuisine. The expanding worldwide population has boosted the demand for nutritional, natural, safe, and enjoyable food. Today, the market offers a wide range of food options that play a vital part in addressing people's requirements. These foods are widely available, tasty, and high in nutrients, benefiting people's general health, causing no harm, and serving as a daily staple for all of us. Fermented foods are one of the best options to fulfill all these criteria and provide beneficial effect on human health. Fermented foods and fermentation play a vital role in food preparation.

Fermentation is a chemical and metabolic process that transforms organic compounds like sugars into simpler molecules in the absence of oxygen. Several industries, including food, dairy, medicines, drinks, food processing, energy and waste management, and chemical fermentation, are essential. Based on growth rate, the fermentation process is divided into three categories: (1) growth-related products, which are produced directly from the metabolism of carbohydrates; (2) products produced indirectly from the metabolism of carbohydrates; and (3) products unrelated to the oxidation of carbohydrates (Gaden, 2000). The type of raw material utilized, the composition of the fermentation medium, and the metabolism of the fermenting organism are some of the elements that affect the efficiency and positive outcomes of fermentation. For instance, the chemical composition and microbiological diversity of apples used in the manufacturing of cider largely dictate the overall fermentation process outcome and final quality. In a similar vein, producers want fresh and unique strains for fermented beverages in order to produce unique and genuine goods.

For thousands of years, people have used fermentation to increase the organoleptic quality and shelf life of perishable food. Bacteria transform carbohydrates into lactic acid during fermentation, which enhances food's nutritional value, flavor, and texture. Many food products, such as fruits, vegetables, beverages, milk, and grains, are produced through lactic acid fermentation. Sauerkraut, kimchi, fermented cucumbers, olives, and kefir are typical examples. Fermented foods have distinct taste and aroma owing to the formation of active chemicals during fermentation (Wieczorek & Drabińska, 2022).

DOI: 10.1201/9781003638292-4

Due to its beneficial health effects and sustainable methods of food production, fermentation has become more and more popular in recent years. Probiotic bacteria, prebiotics, and postbiotics found in fermented foods help boost immunity and guard against pathogen infections. Additionally, fermentation has become more well-known due to its capacity to turn rejected or unsightly fruits and vegetables into useful foods and ingredients (Salas-Millán & Aguayo, 2024).

The nineteenth-century scientist Louis Pasteur postulated that microorganisms like bacteria, yeast, and some live cells that are invisible to the human eye are mostly responsible for fermentation, a natural process. He also talked about the numerous kinds of fermentation, which are primarily based on how well particular bacteria work. This also determines the various fermentation-derived end products (Taveira et al., 2021). For many years, fermentation has been used as a bioprocess to increase nutritional value, preserve food, and create a variety of useful compounds.

A tried-and-true method for enhancing the flavor, safety, appearance, functionality, and nutrition of cereal-based products is lactic acid fermentation (Petrova & Petrov, 2020). Traditional cuisine or antiquated methods of preparation come to mind when we discuss fermentation. However, fermentation is currently used for a variety of purposes, such as the production of industrial and agricultural byproducts. For instance, whey is an important byproduct of the cheese business that is fermented by bacteria and yeast to produce a range of healthful dietary, industrial, and agricultural products (Pescuma et al., 2015). Similar to this, some fruits and vegetables' byproducts are fermented to create bioactive compounds and boost their nutritional content (Sabater et al., 2020).

In conclusion, we know that fermentation is a multifaceted process with a wide range of uses in various industries. Careful control and optimization management is essential to producing a highly useful, flawless, and economical product (Chai et al., 2022). Understanding the basic principles and techniques of fermentation, as well as microbial interactions, substrate composition, environmental factors, and other aspects that are crucial to process improvement and the creation of new fermented products, is the first step toward comprehending the fermentation process.

4.1.1 History of Fermentation: From God's Magic to the Industrial Revolution

For thousands of years, fermentation has been used to aid digestion and preserve food, and the practice is recognized worldwide. In many regions, fermentation is deeply rooted in cultural heritage and traditional knowledge. These fermented foods harbor diverse bacteria with vast genetic potential, yet many of the underlying processes and microbial interactions remain poorly understood. Beyond its role in food preparation, fermentation has profoundly influenced the development of civilizations and the growth of international relationships through trade and shared practices.

Ancient civilizations such as the Sumerians and Egyptians used fermentation to produce a wide variety of foods and beverages. Although they successfully harnessed the process, they were unaware of the role microorganisms played in transforming raw ingredients. Instead, fermentation was perceived as a mysterious occurrence, often attributed to divine intervention or miraculous forces (Taveira et al., 2021).

Although meals and nutrition remain the primary focus, fermented foods have evolved from traditional preservation techniques into versatile bioprocesses with wide-ranging industrial applications. Modern consumers are increasingly attracted to fermented foods and beverages because of their use of natural raw materials, perceived freshness, and potential health benefits. Beyond food, fermentation is central to the production of biofuels, biodegradable polymers, functional foods, and many other high-value products. The development of improved products can be achieved by integrating diverse fermentation-based innovation strategies, including biotechnological approaches, sensory and consumer sciences, and advanced multi-omics technologies (Wang et al., 2023).

The ancient practice of fermentation is gaining increasing importance in biotechnology and food science as ongoing research continues to uncover the health benefits of fermented foods and the broader potential of fermentation processes. Long before any scientific understanding existed, humans relied on fermentation to produce staples such as bread and cheese. Traditional fermented beverages also played an important role in daily life, serving as drinks for enjoyment, social gatherings, celebrations, and religious ceremonies. These beverages are commonly produced from raw materials such as millet, rice, sorghum, and maize, using two main fermentation approaches: spontaneous fermentation and controlled industrial fermentation (Madilo et al., 2024).

The production of alcoholic beverages depends heavily on a diverse microbial community, which develops over time to produce distinctive regional flavors and preparation techniques.

It's interesting to note that the conventional fermentation method, which does not meet the requirements of contemporary industrial scale and standards, was employed for a longer time. A decrease in product stability is caused by numerous hazardous substances, disagreeable smells, and nutritional inhibitors. Researchers have employed synthetic microbial communities to address this issue and enhance the quality of fermented meals (Jin et al., 2024).

In biotechnology, the transition from early to industrial-scale fermentation is crucial. Chaim Weizmann, one of the first large-scale industrial fermenters of the twentieth century with worldwide significance, found certain significant events, such as acetone–butanol–ethanol fermentation (Sauer, 2016). The revolution in the pharmaceutical sector starting in 1950 led to the production of pharmacological products, particularly antibiotics, through large-scale fermentation (Davies, 2013). Without comprehending the natural role and function of the chemicals created during fermentation, the fermentation process was industrialized. The true function of metabolites produced during fermentation, as well as their potential and uses, is becoming increasingly clear as research on this topic advances (Dzialo et al., 2017).

In summary, scientific knowledge and concepts served as the foundation for the early fermentation process. Food safety, quality, and consistency are altered when a traditionally uncontrolled approach is replaced with a scientifically motivated, controlled, and regulated fermentation process (Jin et al., 2024; Niyigaba et al., 2025). The gap between early fermentation and industrialization was filled in part by knowledge of microbiological processes, technological innovation, and the commercial potential of fermented items. This shift has produced a wide range of industrial applications, from food to pharmaceuticals, proving that fermentation is an essential and crucial biotechnology activity.

4.2 MAJOR ROLE OF MICROBES IN FERMENTATION AND THEIR DIVERSITY

Microorganisms are the key agents of fermentation, driving the breakdown of complex molecules into simpler compounds. Although these microbes are ubiquitous, their microscopic size makes them invisible to the human eye. Despite this, they play an indispensable role in fermentation. Microorganisms contribute in multiple ways, including decomposing complex substrates, generating beneficial metabolites, producing valuable end products, and enhancing the flavor, quality, and overall value of foods. In the food and beverage industries, microbial diversity is especially important, as fermentation occurs in environments where diverse microbial communities metabolically transform raw materials into final products. This diversity strongly influences the flavor, aroma, and quality of fermented foods.

Fungal species including *Pichia*, *Saccharomyces*, and *Monascus* are used in traditional fermentation procedures, such as the creation of Baijiu, to enhance metabolic profiles and create distinct flavors. The microbial network becomes more modular as a result of increased variety, which enhances product quality and glucose-mediated carbon metabolism (Zhang et al., 2022). Through a variety of fermentable substrates and processes, the microbial diversity in vinegar fermentation influences metabolic products and product quality. To guarantee fermentative stability and product homogeneity, it is essential to comprehend these predominant bacteria. Microbial diversity in non-sterile environments is essential for continuous fermentation. While stable microbial populations are essential for economic sustainability, extremophiles help to process stability and lessen contamination problems. The periodic table of fermented foods demonstrates the great diversity of fermented meals according to local customs (Gänzle, 2022).

A sophisticated microbial ecosystem can be found in fermented foods. LAB (lactic acid bacteria) which contributes acidity to lacto-fermented food and is utilized in preservation. Alcohol is converted to vinegar by AAB (acetic acid bacteria), which also helps to improve product qualities by combining with other microorganisms to build dynamic communities. The microbial ecosystem in fermented foods influences its taste, quality, and functionality. These ecosystems are home to a

TABLE 4.1

Major role played by microbes in fermented foods

Sr. No	Role/function	Description and mechanisms	Key microbes/examples	Selected references
1	Preservation of foods	Lactic acid bacteria (LAB) are beneficial microbes that produce lactic acid and other metabolites (organic acids, alcohols, CO_2, bacteriocins, antifungal peptides, and H_2O_2) that reduce pH, suppress rotting and pathogens, and improve shelf life. LAB operates as a natural biopreservative by competing for nutrients and producing antibacterial compounds.	Lactic acid bacteria (*Lactobacillus*, *Leuconostoc*, *Pediococcus*)	Reis et al. (2012) and Lahiri et al. (2022)
2	Enhancement and development of flavor and aroma	Microbes produce flavor and fragrance molecules (esters, alcohols, organic acids, and terpenes). Yeasts and fungi produce complex flavors by breaking down macromolecules using enzymes such as proteases, lipases, and glycosidases. Microbial fermentation of vegetable waste can produce fruity, flowery, and cheesy flavors. Advances in cell factory development have increased the production of natural-tasting chemicals.	Yeasts (*Saccharomyces cerevisiae*), LAB, molds (*Aspergillus*, *Penicillium*)	Chen et al. (2023) and Melini and Melini (2024)
3	Improvement of nutritional value	Fermentation improves the nutritional value of food by generating bioactive molecules, lowering antinutrient levels, and promoting gut health. LAB are starter cultures that turn raw substrates into useful meals. Rhizospheric bacteria improve plant nutrient availability, boosting crop output and nutritional quality.	LAB (*Lactobacillus*, *Streptococcus*), rhizospheric bacteria (*Azospirillum*, *Rhizobium*)	Karlund et al. (2020), Raj et al. (2021), and Sawant et al. (2025)
4	Safety of foods	LAB and other beneficial microorganisms improve food safety by producing organic acids and bacteriocins that inhibit pathogens. Controlled fermentations with omics-guided starter selection ensure stability and safety. *Bacillus* and acetic acid bacteria contribute to competitive inhibition and metabolite formation.	LAB (*Lactococcus lactis*, *Lactobacillus* spp.), *Bacillus marcorestinctum*, acetic acid bacteria	Mokoena et al. (2021), Zhong et al. (2022), Wang et al. (2022), and Han et al. (2024)
5	Production of industrial products	Microbes enable the large-scale synthesis of chemicals, fuels, and additives through fermentation. Its applications include bioethanol, ABE solvents, pigments, and enzymes. Metabolic engineering and open fermentation systems have improved sustainability and production efficiency.	Bacteria (*Clostridium acetobutylicum*, *Zymomonas mobilis*), yeasts (*Saccharomyces* spp.), fungi (*Aspergillus*, *Monascus*)	Seo et al. (2020), Nielsen et al. (2022), Ramesh et al. (2022), Bilal et al. (2025), and Slimane and El-Hafid (2024)
6	Probiotic health benefits	Probiotic microorganisms, such as *Lactobacillus* and *Bifidobacterium*, improve gut microbiota, boost immunological response, and create bioactive substances (vitamins, peptides, and phenolics) that have antioxidant, antihypertensive, and antidiabetic properties. They help prevent lactose intolerance, obesity, and inflammatory bowel disease. Strains must be carefully selected to prevent the spread of antibiotic resistance.	*Lactobacillus* spp., *Bifidobacterium* spp.	Garcia-Gonzalez et al. (2021), Soemarie et al. (2021), Shah et al. (2023), and Saleem et al. (2024)

wide variety of microorganisms, such as molds, bacteria, yeasts, and phages.

The main organisms of fermentation are presented in Table 4.1 along with their roles and research techniques. Microorganisms that enhance the taste and safety of fermented meat products include yeasts, Lactobacilli, and Staphylococci. The microbial composition and product characteristics are influenced by raw materials and technology (Wang et al., 2021). By utilizing advantageous interactions and metabolic capacities, an understanding of microbial diversity improves product quality, which in turn improves fermentation technology and company viability.

4.3 TYPES OF FERMENTATION

Microorganisms like yeast and bacteria convert carbohydrates into organic acids or alcohol through fermentation. Generally, fermentation types are categorized according to the products they produce. Here is a thorough explanation given below.

4.3.1 Types of Fermentation Based on the Microorganisms

The production and preservation of food and beverages are just two benefits of microorganism involvement in fermentation. The employment of microorganisms and the supply of the substrate they ferment are the main factors that determine the many types of microbial fermentation.

Alcoholic fermentation: It is a type of fermentation that is carried out by yeast, specifically *Saccharomyces cerevisiae*. This yeast is a favorite for fermentation because of its resistance to high ethanol and other difficult circumstances. The manufacture of wine, beer, and bread is largely dependent on the conversion of sugar into CO_2 and ethanol. Microbe interactions impact the overall process and contribute to the final product's sensory qualities (Torres-Guardado et al., 2021).

Lactic acid fermentation: LAB are responsible for this kind of fermentation. In this kind of fermentation, bacteria aid in the conversion of carbohydrates into lactic acid, boosting shelf life, improving flavor and texture, and offering a host of health advantages. Probiotic-rich functional meals are made utilizing both conventional and contemporary biotechnology approaches (Sionek et al., 2023).

Acetic acid fermentation: This process is carried out by AAB, which transform ethanol into acetic acid, which is useful for making vinegar and enhances the flavor of other fermented foods and beverages. By interacting with other microbes, these bacteria improve the product's flavor and complexity (Han et al., 2024).

Mixed culture fermentation: A variety of microbial species, including yeasts and LAB, contribute to the fermentation of various foods and drinks. To improve product quality and stop undesirable fungal development, a combination of yeast and fungi is utilized (Assad et al., 2023; Holguín-Sterling et al., 2023).

In Daqu, a Chinese liquor, complex microflora such as bacteria, fungi, and yeasts provide distinctive flavors. The final product's quality and fermentation process might be impacted by the synergistic or antagonistic fermentation of various microorganisms. In spontaneous fermentation, when these natural microbial communities drive the process without the inclusion of a starting culture, the interaction of these bacteria is crucial (Torres-Guardado et al., 2021). Optimizing the fermentation process and enhancing the safety and quality of fermented food products require an understanding of these microbial interactions.

4.3.2 Types of Fermentation Based on End Products

Alcoholic fermentation: This method primarily uses the yeast *S. cerevisiae* to convert sugar into ethanol and CO_2. When making alcoholic beverages like wine and beer, yeast is used in the brewing process. Secondary byproducts including succinic acid, acetic acid, and glycerol are produced during this process. When these secondary byproducts build up in large quantities, yeast activity is suppressed (Zentou et al., 2021).

Lactic acid fermentation: In this kind of fermentation, microorganisms convert carbohydrates to lactic acid, with *Lactobacillus* bacteria being a key player. This kind of fermentation is frequently used in the dairy industry to produce goods like cheese and yogurt. This fermentation is valued for its low reliance on artificial processes and is widely known for its ability to enhance the nutritional and sensory aspects of food (Praveen & Brogi, 2025).

Acetic acid fermentation: It is the process of turning alcohol into acetic acid, mostly for the production of vinegar. The primary function of AAB is to oxidize ethanol into acetic acid and water, which are necessary for vinegar's acidic flavor and preservation properties.

Malolactic fermentation: Malic acid is transformed into lactic acid and carbon dioxide during the wine-making process, which improves the wine's flavor and lowers its acidity. This procedure is carried out by the LAB *Oenococcus oeni* type, which also helps to stabilize the microbial ecology in wines (Neto et al. 2016).

Propionic acid fermentation: The primary bacteria that aid in the formation of propionic acid in this kind of fermentation are *Propionibacterium*. This fermentation's primary function in the dairy business is to provide goods like Swiss cheese their distinct flavor and gas bubble qualities.

Butyric acid fermentation: This kind of fermentation takes place in anaerobic settings, including the intestines of animals, where butyric acid is created along with gasses like CO_2 and hydrogen. Products like rancid butter have a distinct smell due to the generation of gasses and acids. This fermentation demonstrates a range of techniques and applications, each influenced by substrate composition and operation circumstances (Bernardes et al., 2024).

4.3.3 Types of Fermentation by Physical State

Solid-state fermentation (SSF): In this kind of fermentation, microorganisms are grown on solid substrates like sawdust, grains, and agricultural waste without the presence of free water. Traditional techniques are used to ferment soybeans, and SSF is a key component. The nutritional and sensory qualities of soy sauce are greatly enhanced by *Bacillus* species or filamentous fungi (Elhalis et al., 2023).

Submerged fermentation: In industrial settings with a liquid environment, this kind of fermentation is often used. This process involves fermenting molds, yeast, and bacteria in liquid broth. This fermentation procedure is frequently used in the manufacturing of alcoholic beverages like wine and beer (Albergaria & Arneborg, 2016).

4.3.4 Types of Fermentation by Process

Batch fermentation: This fermentation introduces microbes into a closed environment that is controlled by nutrients. It is advantageous to do experimental research on the kinetics of fermentation processes, growth influence, and rates of product creation (Gaden, 2000).

Continuous fermentation: By continuously supplying nutrients, the process is maintained in a steady state while products are collected on a regular basis. This approach enables high product yields. For example, food waste can be efficiently converted into high-purity lactic acid using this method (Wang et al., 2020).

4.3.5 Specialized and Modern Types of Fermentation

Electro-fermentation (EF): It is a bioprocess technique that combines conventional fermentation with electrochemical principles to control microbial metabolism. Electrodes are employed as donors or acceptors to promote electron and proton transfer in microorganisms like *Geobacter* and *Shewanella* species, hence increasing their bioelectric activity (Pilania et al., 2025). It is beneficial to produce hydrogen, methane, and biopolymers like biofuels and biochemicals. The primary goal of adding electrodes to fermentation is to improve efficiency and scalability by allowing for more control over redox reactions (Salar-García et al., 2024). Additionally, this technique supports the circular economy and offers sustainable alternatives to the fossil fuel industry by converting trash into valuable chemicals and fuels through microbial electrosynthesis (Chandrasekhar et al., 2021).

Precision fermentation: In the fields of biotechnology and food production, precision fermentation creates a novel method of producing proteins utilizing bacteria. It also aids in resolving important problems like food security and environmental sustainability. This approach is different from traditional animal-based agriculture, which can be detrimental and unsustainable (Nielsen et al., 2023). Animal sources, such as those found in milk and eggs, are typically the source of genetically engineered microorganisms employed in precision fermentation to create proteins. Large-scale production is made possible by the use of these proteins in food products. These are then utilized in a method that should be economical for large-scale production. Compared to regular farming, this method uses fewer resources, such as land and water. It also helps to make food that is nutritious, safe, and good for animal welfare (Knychala et al., 2024).

Inoculated fermentation: This type of fermentation uses targeted microorganisms to regulate and improve the fermentation process. This procedure differs slightly from spontaneous fermentation, in which microbes naturally carry out the process. Starter cultures are certain kinds of bacteria that are utilized in this kind of fermentation to enhance the quality, safety, and uniformity of the fermented products. As an example, pomegranate fermentation is used to make wine, and *S. cerevisiae*, a yeast culture, is crucial to controlling the entire fermentation process and enhancing flavor through interactions with local bacteria (Wang et al., 2020). Similar to this, LAB like *Lactobacillus plantarum* improve sourdough fermentation by reducing various saccharides and polyols by up to 91% (Pejcz et al., 2021).

An understanding of how various fermentation processes affect the fermentation sector can be gained from the types of fermentation. The function of microbial fermentation in food growth is covered in the next section.

4.4 VARIETIES OF FERMENTED FOOD

Fermented foods are gaining popularity because of their benefits to human health, their ability to meet consumer preferences, and their reliance on natural ingredients. Microorganisms play a central role in fermentation, transforming raw materials into nutritious, safe, and edible products. During this process, certain antinutritional compounds are degraded, enhancing both flavor and nutritional value (Wang et al., 2022). While fermented foods may not dominate any single region, they are recognized worldwide and hold strong cultural significance. Traditional products such as yogurt and kefir in Turkey and fermented maize and cassava foods in Latin America have gained wider acceptance largely due to their deep roots in local traditions.

These foods offer antioxidant and immunostimulatory qualities that support intestinal health. Numerous elements, including vitamins, minerals, and antioxidants, are present in food derived from vegetable fermentation and aid in preventing oxidative stress (Ampemohotti et al., 2025). Fermentation is a key factor in prolonging food's shelf life and improving its nutritional value in places where fresh items are scarce (Obafemi et al., 2022). This technique has the potential to improve health by producing bioactive molecules (Sharma et al., 2020). Additionally, it produces novel ingredients that support culinary innovation. The field of fermentation is constantly developing, focusing on and enhancing conventional techniques, and investigating the possibilities of probiotics in fermented foods (Sivamaruthi et al., 2018).

Table 4.2 lists several fermented food varieties according to their source, origin, ingredients, microorganisms, and functional or health characteristics.

TABLE 4.2
Types of fermented foods

No.	Examples	Origin/region	Main ingredients	Microorganisms involved	Function/health benefits	References
A.	Dairy-based					
1.	Yogurt	Global	Milk	*Lactobacillus bulgaricus*, *Streptococcus thermophilus*	Supports gut health, improves lactose tolerance, antioxidant effects	Sarıtaş et al. (2024)
2.	Kefir	Eastern Europe	Milk (cow, goat, etc.)	Lactic acid bacteria, yeasts	Antimicrobial, antidiabetic, and gastrointestinal benefits	Farag et al. (2020)
3.	Cheese	Global	Milk	*Lactococcus lactis*, yeasts, molds	Rich in calcium	Kechagia et al. (2013)
4.	Buttermilk	South Asia	Fermented cream or milk	Lactic acid bacteria	Aids digestion, supports gut microbiota	Saleem et al. (2024)
5.	Lassi/ayran	South Asia, Turkey	Yogurt with water and salt	Lactic acid bacteria	Improves gut and metabolic health	Kechagia et al. (2013)
B.	Liquid-based					
1.	Koumiss	Central Asia	Mare's milk	Lactic acid bacteria, yeasts	Slightly alcoholic, provides enzymes and vitamins	Kabak and Dobson (2011)
2.	Boza	Turkey	Millet, corn, wheat	Lactic acid bacteria, yeasts	Provides nutrients and antioxidants	Kabak and Dobson (2011)
3.	Mahewu	Africa	Maize	Lactic acid bacteria	Nutrition rich, non-alcoholic	Odunfa and Oyewole (1998)
4.	Salgam	Turkey	Black carrot, turnip	*Lactobacillus plantarum*	Rich in antioxidants	Kabak and Dobson (2011)
5.	Hardaliye	Turkey	Grape juice, mustard seeds	Lactic acid bacteria, yeasts	Provide antioxidant and probiotic effects	Kabak and Dobson (2011)

(Continued)

Table 4.2 (Continued)

No.	Examples	Origin/region	Main ingredients	Microorganisms involved	Function/health benefits	References
6.	Cauim/caxiri	Latin America	Palm sap, sugarcane juice	Lactic acid bacteria, yeasts	Traditional fermented drinks used in celebrations	Chaves-López et al. (2014)
7.	Cachaca/ tiquira	Brazil	Sugarcane, cassava	Yeasts	Alcoholic beverages with cultural value	Lima et al. (2022)
C.	Grain-based					
1.	Boza	Bulgaria, Balkans	Whole wheat grains or flour	*Lactobacillus* spp., yeast	Nutrient-rich probiotic beverages with mild acidity and sweetness	Gotcheva et al. (2001)
2.	Munkoyo	Zambia	Maize	Streptococcaceae, Leuconostocaceae, Enterobacteriaceae	Spontaneously fermented, rich in lactic acid bacteria	Phiri et al. (2019)
3.	Maize-based foods	Africa, Latin America	Maize	Lactic acid bacteria	Contain phenolic acids and flavonoids, enhance antioxidant potential	Meena et al. (2022)
4.	Rye and wheat breads	Europe	Rye and wheat	Lactic acid bacteria, yeasts	Sour taste, improved digestion ability and nutritional value	Gänzle and Salovaara (2019)
5.	Oat- and buckwheat-fermented foods	Western countries	Oat, buckwheat malt grains	Lactic acid bacteria	Gluten-free, bioactive compounds improve functionality of bakery	Salamon et al. (2023)
D. Vegetable-based						
1.	Sauerkraut	Europe	Cabbage	*Leuconostoc*, *Lactobacillus* spp.	Higher in fiber and probiotics, supports digestion	Lu et al. (2024)
2.	Kimchi	Korea	Cabbage, radish, chili, garlic	Lactic acid bacteria	Rich in vitamins, antioxidants, and probiotics	Yuan et al. (2023)

3.	Pickled vegetables	Global	Carrots, cucumber, beets	Lactic acid bacteria	Preserved flavor, enhanced nutrients	Palmnäs-Bédard et al. (2023)
4.	Turshi	Middle East, North Africa	Mixed vegetables	*Lactobacillus* spp.	Crunchy, tangy flavor, digestive benefits	Dahiya and Nigam (2022)
5.	Gundruk	Nepal	Mustard leaves	*L. plantarum*	Source of dietary fiber and micronutrients	Wieczorek and Drabińska (2022)
6.	Curtido	Central America	Cabbage, onion, carrot	*Leuconostoc mesenteroides*	Tangy flavor, antioxidant potential	Choi et al. (2024)
7.	Fermented beets and carrots	Worldwide	Beets, carrots	Lactic acid bacteria		Thierry et al. (2023)
E.	Meat- and fish-based					
1.	Fish sauce	Southeast Asia	Fish salt	Halotolerant bacteria	High umami, rich in amino acids and peptides	Cha and Yu (2024) and Zang et al. (2019)
2.	Surstromming	Sweden	Baltic herring	Anaerobic halophilic bacteria	Distinct aroma, preserved protein	Zang et al. (2019)
3.	Hongeo (fermented skate)	Korea	Skate fish	Lactic acid bacteria	Unique ammonia-rich flavor, traditional delicacy	Zang et al. (2019)
4.	Salami and sausages	Europe	Processed meat	*Lactobacillus sakei*, *Staphylococcus carnosus*	Preserved meats with probiotic potential	Munekata et al. (2022)
5.	Prosciutto	Italy	Beef	Lactic acid bacteria	Rich flavor, low fat, high protein	Wang et al. (2021)
6.	Bresaola	Italy	Beef	Lactic acid bacteria	Rich flavor, low fat, high protein	Wang et al. (2021)

4.5 MICROBIAL INTERACTIONS DURING FERMENTATION

Both the efficiency of the fermentation process and the quality of the final product are positively impacted by the interaction of bacteria. As demonstrated by both synchronous and asynchronous activities between various bacteria, these interactions can be categorized into two groups: cooperative interactions, in which microbes cooperate, and competitive interactions, in which germs compete with one another.

4.5.1 Cooperative Interactions

Microorganisms including yeast, bacteria, and molds collaborate in a variety of settings where fermentation takes place to produce food and drink. For instance, in fermented foods like kefir, vinegar, and kombucha, AAB favorably interacts with yeasts and LAB to create distinctive tastes and nutritional profiles (Han et al., 2024). Certain bacteria can support the normal functioning of other bacteria, resulting in beneficial modifications to flavor, texture, and production rates.

4.5.2 Competitive Interactions

When bacteria compete for the same resources, these interactions often take place. In alcoholic fermentation, *S. cerevisiae* frequently plays a pivotal role. This is due to its robust fermentation capacity and ability to survive in stressful environments like lower pH and greater alcohol concentrations. *S. cerevisiae* dominates the wine-making process through a variety of mechanisms, including direct contact with cells and the production of antimicrobial peptides that inhibit the growth of other microorganisms, thereby promoting the growth of the necessary organism (Albergaria & Arneborg, 2016).

4.5.3 Biofilm Formation

One crucial factor in the interaction of bacteria during fermentation is the formation of biofilms by various microbes. Under stress situations, microbial cells survive by forming clusters and adhering to surfaces because of the organized environment generated by biofilms. Because they are in close proximity to one another, these biofilms encourage both collaboration and competition. The entire function of microbial interactions during fermentation is impacted by this proximity (Yao et al., 2022).

4.5.4 Metabolic Interactions and Quorum Sensing

Quorum sensing is a method by which microorganisms can interact with one another. In order to maintain the cell density, bacteria alter their behavior and gene expression based on the quantity of microorganisms present. This has an impact on their ability to form biofilms and generate specific metabolic chemicals. For instance, bioethanol production in sugarcane fermentation is mostly caused by the interaction of wild yeast and LAB, which can influence ethanol production and level through cell signaling and metabolic exchanges (Brexó & Sant'Ana, 2017).

4.5.5 Methods of Synthetic Biology

Recent advances in synthetic biology now allow the deliberate design of microbial consortia, providing greater control over and improvement of fermentation processes. By engineering synthetic communities with specific interactions, valuable products such as biofuels and pharmaceuticals can be efficiently produced from low-cost carbon sources (McCarty & Ledesma-Amaro, 2018).

In conclusion, microbial interactions during fermentation are highly complex, involving a range of cooperative and competitive behaviors that significantly influence process outcomes. A deeper understanding of these interactions enables the optimization and innovation of fermentation technologies, ensuring the efficient and high-quality production of fermented products.

4.6 HEALTH BENEFITS OF FERMENTED FOOD

For thousands of years, people have included fermented foods in their diets due to both their ability to preserve food and their positive effects on health. Beneficial microorganisms like LAB, which are well-known for their probiotic properties, are abundant in these foods (Doo et al., 2024).

Digestive health and gut microbiota: Improvements in digestion and the treatment of long-term gastrointestinal problems demonstrate the beneficial effects of fermented food on gut health. The microbial composition of the stomach is changed by the introduction of beneficial microbes through fermented foods (Ampemohotti et al., 2025).

Immune modulation and anti-inflammatory effects: Fermented foods can strengthen the immune system and reduce inflammation.

This reduces the incidence of immune-related disorders and has cancer-reducing effects (Ampemohotti et al., 2025; Jalili et al., 2023).

Nutritional enhancement: Fermentation improves food quality by creating a number of nutritional substances. These modifications contribute to a healthy metabolic state and lower the risk of cardiovascular disease and type 2 diabetes (Meena et al., 2022).

Weight management and obesity risk reduction: Consuming fermented foods on a regular basis aids in weight loss and obesity prevention. According to research, microorganisms contained in fermented vegetables like kimchi and sauerkraut have an important role in weight loss and metabolic health.

Antimicrobial and antioxidant effects: Fermented foods have a variety of health-promoting qualities, including antibacterial, antioxidant, and even anticancer benefits. These peptides also aid in other body processes, providing protection against stressful situations and infections. Fermented foods are beneficial not only to human health, but also to functional and nutritional enhancement, overall well-being, and the natural management of a variety of health disorders. Many studies have demonstrated that fermented foods are good for health. However, several studies have shown no clear link between these foods and health advantages. More study is needed to fully understand the impact (Şanlier et al., 2017).

4.7 APPLICATION OF FERMENTED FOODS

Fermented foods have numerous applications, including improving food qualities, providing health benefits, and increasing food safety and quality.

4.7.1 Health Benefits and Nutritional Enhancements

Fermented foods are well-known for their various health benefits, which stem from the creation of unique chemicals during fermentation. Many protein-rich Asian fermented foods, including soybeans, milk, and fish, include peptides with antihypertensive, antioxidant, antibacterial, antidiabetic, and anticancer characteristics (Kumari et al., 2021). Fermented foods can also improve cognitive performance and protect the brain, which is advantageous in neurodegenerative disorders like Alzheimer's (Kumar et al., 2022).

4.7.2 Starch Stability and Food Structure

Fermentation changes the structural features of grain starches, making them more stable and resistant to retrogradation. This is especially useful for things that can go stale during storage, like bread. This transformation ushers in a new age for the use of fermented grains in the food business, where long-term survival is critical (Yan et al., 2024).

4.7.3 Probiotic and Microbial Benefits

LAB in fermented foods has probiotic properties, including better digestion, immunomodulatory activity, and the generation of bioactive chemicals and vitamins. These advantages make fermented foods high in LAB more valuable for health promotion and disease prevention (Doo et al., 2024).

4.7.4 Quality and Safety Control

Enzymes and their functions have a major role in the quality and safety of fermented foods. Enzymes enhance texture, stability, aroma, and bitterness. They also help to eliminate biologically hazardous compounds produced during fermentation, hence offering useful safety standards (Dai et al., 2024).

4.7.5 Cultural and Commercial Prospects

Fermented foods have long been popular worldwide due to their distinct flavors and nutritional benefits. Fermented foods have grown popular and commercially available due to their functional and nutritional benefits (Gao et al., 2021).

4.7.6 Microbial Diversity and Functional Components

Fermented foods are high in enzymes and bioactive substances, demonstrating the variety of bacteria involved in fermentation processes. These bacteria improve the functional properties of dietary cultures (Qin et al., 2022).

Fermented foods are versatile goods with applications that improve food safety and quality, provide several health advantages, and aid in cognitive function. Their numerous applications and benefits highlight their growing importance in dietary habits and food business applications. Fermentation is widely used in a variety of industries, including food production and biofuel synthesis. Nonetheless, its application comes with both inherent limitations and tremendous prospects for future growth.

4.8 CHALLENGES AND FUTURE OUTLOOK

Process optimization: Difficulties emerge when optimizing fermentation processes, particularly those containing microbes like yeasts and fungi. Common yeast, such as *S. cerevisiae*, lack the traits essential for successful bioprocessing, such as the ability to metabolize diverse carbon sources and survive in demanding environments. This may need the use of specialized non-conventional yeasts designed to help meet adequate fermentation conditions while also improving yield and product concentrations.

Scale-up and engineering complexities: The scale-up stage of industrial fermentation presents major hurdles. Regular chemical processes do not make use of modern technical techniques such as mathematical models and computational fluid dynamics. Other difficulties arise, such as how microbe shape influences liquid flow and mixing, as well as the need for new sensors to monitor process parameters (Formenti et al., 2014).

Enzymatic and microbiological approaches frequently compete with new chemical methods. This is due to a variety of factors, including the proliferation of new energy sources such as shale gas. Industrial biotechnology techniques must be as efficient and competitive as chemical ones. This is accomplished through the processes of synthetic biology and molecular biology (Chen, 2012).

Safety and regulatory issues: Microbial contamination and the formation of biogenic amines are major safety concerns in the fermentation process, particularly in food applications. We urgently want improved methods that can help detect and fix safety concerns while adhering to common rules (Niyigaba et al., 2025).

4.8.1 Future Outlook

Advances in bioprocess engineering are driving significant improvements in fermentation technologies, particularly through real-time monitoring systems and high-density fermentation strategies. Real-time monitoring allows precise control of critical parameters such as pH, temperature, oxygen levels, and nutrient availability, enabling faster responses to process variations and reducing product loss. High-density fermentation increases microbial biomass and productivity, leading to higher yields within smaller reactor volumes. Together, these innovations enhance the scalability of fermentation processes while improving overall efficiency and sustainability by reducing energy consumption, minimizing waste, and optimizing resource utilization (Mendes et al., 2024).

Utilization of non-conventional feedstocks: With the increasing emphasis on sustainability, there is a growing need for renewable carbon sources that do not compete with food supplies. Non-conventional feedstocks such as ethanol have emerged as promising alternative carbon sources for microbial processes, supporting efficient microbial growth and product formation. The use of such substrates reduces reliance on food-based raw materials and contributes to addressing global food security challenges while maintaining industrial productivity (Sun et al., 2024).

Circular bioeconomy: SSF technologies are increasingly being integrated into modern biorefineries, playing a key role in advancing the circular bioeconomy. These approaches enable the conversion of agricultural residues and other low-value byproducts into biofuels, biochemicals, and value-added products. By minimizing waste and maximizing resource efficiency, SSF offers a sustainable and economically viable alternative to conventional processing methods (Abdul Manan & Webb, 2017).

Advanced detection and monitoring technologies: Artificial intelligence is now transforming fermentation and bioprocessing systems through its integration with advanced analytical tools such as high-throughput sequencing, biosensors, and automated monitoring platforms. These technologies enhance process efficiency, safety, and consistency by enabling real-time monitoring of microbial activity, rapid detection of contaminants, and early identification of process deviations. As a result, product quality and safety are improved, strengthening consumer confidence and supporting large-scale industrial applications (Niyigaba et al., 2025).

REFERENCES

Abdul Manan, M., & Webb, C. (2017). Modern Microbial Solid State Fermentation Technology for Future Biorefineries for the Production of Added-Value Products. *Biofuel Research Journal*, 4(4), 730–740. https://doi.org/10.18331/brj2017.4.4.5

Albergaria, H., & Arneborg, N. (2016). Dominance of Saccharomyces Cerevisiae in Alcoholic Fermentation Processes: Role of Physiological Fitness and Microbial Interactions. *Applied Microbiology and Biotechnology*, 100(5), 2035–2046. https://doi.org/10.1007/s00253-015-7255-0

Ampemohotti, T., Golneshin, A., Pillidge, C., Brennan, C., & Hao Van, T. T. (2025). Fermented Vegetables: Their Microbiology and Impact on Gut Microbiota and Overall Health Benefits. *Food Reviews International, ahead-of-print(ahead-of-print)*, 1–24. https://doi.org/10.1080/87559129.2025.2486274

Assad, M., Ashaolu, T. J., Khalifa, I., Baky, M. H., & Farag, M. A. (2023). Dissecting the Role of Microorganisms in Tea Production of Different Fermentation Levels: A Multifaceted Review of Their Action Mechanisms, Quality Attributes and Future Perspectives. *World Journal of Microbiology & Biotechnology*, 39(10). https://doi.org/10.1007/s11274-023-03701-5

Bernardes, P. C., Coelho, J. M., Schwan, R. F., & Martins, P. M. M. (2024). Microbial Ecology and Fermentation of Coffea canephora. *Frontiers in Food Science and Technology*, 4. https://doi.org/10.3389/frfst.2024.1377226

Bilal, M., Ibrahim, A., Saleem, R., Husnain, M., Alam, H. M., Mazhar, M. G., ... & Mushtaq, H. (2025). Microbes and Their Role in Food Sciences. *Indus Journal of Bioscience Research*, 3(4), 283–292. https://doi.org/10.70749/ijbr.v3i4.1098

Brexó, R. P., & Sant'Ana, A. D. S. (2017). Microbial Interactions During Augar Cane Must Fermentation for Bioethanol Production: Does Quorum Sensing Play a Role? *Critical Reviews in Biotechnology*, 38(2), 231–244. https://doi.org/10.1080/07388551.2017.1332570

Cha, Y.-J., & Yu, D. (2024). Health Benefits and Functions of Salt-Fermented Fish. *Journal of Ethnic Foods*, 11(1). https://doi.org/10.1186/s42779-024-00251-5

Chai, W.Y., Teo, K.T. K., Tan, M. K., & Tham, H. J. (2022). Fermentation Process Control and Optimization. *Chemical Engineering & Technology*, 45(10), 1731–1747. https://doi.org/10.1002/ceat.202200029

Chandrasekhar, K., Kim, S.-H., Kumar, G., Raj, T., & Kumar, A. N. (2021). Bioelectrochemical System-Mediated Waste Valorization. *Systems Microbiology and Biomanufacturing*, 1(4), 432–443. https://doi.org/10.1007/s43393-021-00039-7

Chaves-López, C., Serio, A., Paparella, A., Grande-Tovar, C. D., Cuervo-Mulet, R., & Delgado-Ospina, J. (2014). Traditional Fermented Foods and Beverages from a Microbiological and Nutritional Perspective: The Colombian Heritage. *Comprehensive Reviews in Food Science and Food Safety*, 13(5), 1031–1048. https://doi.org/10.1111/1541-4337.12098

Chen, G.-Q. (2012). New Challenges and Opportunities for Industrial Biotechnology. *Microbial Cell Factories*, 11(1), 111. https://doi.org/10.1186/1475-2859-11-111

Chen, L., Li, K., Melini, H., & Li, Z. (2023). Reviewing the Source, Physiological Characteristics, and Aroma Production Mechanisms of Aroma-Producing Yeasts. *Foods*, 12(18), 3501. https://doi.org/10.3390/foods12183501

Choi, Y.-J., Lim, J.-Y., Kang, M.-J., Choi, J.-Y., Yang, J.-H., Chung, Y. B., Park, S. H., Min, S. G., & Lee, M.-A. (2024). Changes in Bacterial Composition and Metabolite Profiles During Kimchi Fermentation with Different Garlic Varieties. *Heliyon*, 10(2), e24283. https://doi.org/10.1016/j.heliyon.2024.e24283

Dahiya, D., & Nigam, P. S. (2022). Use of Characterized Microorganisms in Fermentation of Non-Dairy-Based Substrates to Produce Probiotic Food for Gut-Health and Nutrition. *Fermentation*, 9(1), 1. https://doi.org/10.3390/fermentation9010001

Dai, Y., Chen, Y., Lin, X., & Zhang, S. (2024). Recent Applications and Prospects of Enzymes in Quality and Safety Control of Fermented Foods. *Foods (Basel, Switzerland)*, 13(23), 3804. https://doi.org/10.3390/foods13233804

Davies, J. (2013). Specialized Microbial Metabolites: Functions and Origins. *The Journal of Antibiotics*, 66(7), 361–364. https://doi.org/10.1038/ja.2013.61

Doo, H., Kwak, J., Keum, G. B., Ryu, S., Choi, Y., Kang, J., Kim, H., Chae, Y., Kim, S., Kim, H. B., & Lee, J.-H. (2024). Lactic Acid Bacteria in Asian Fermented Foods and Their Beneficial Roles in Human Health. *Food Science and Biotechnology*, 33(9), 2021–2033. https://doi.org/10.1007/s10068-024-01634-9

Dzialo, M. C., Park, R., Steensels, J., Lievens, B., & Verstrepen, K. J. (2017). Physiology, Ecology and Industrial Applications of Aroma Formation in Yeast. *FEMS Microbiology Reviews*, *41*(Supp_1), S95–S128. https://doi.org/10.1093/femsre/fux031

Elhalis, H., Chin, X. H., & Chow, Y. (2023). Soybean Fermentation: Microbial Ecology and Starter Culture Technology. *Critical Reviews in Food Science and Nutrition*, 64(21), 7648–7670. https://doi.org/10.1080/10408398.2023.2188951

Farag, M. A., El-Wahed, A. A., El-Seedi, A. H. R., & Jomaa, S. A. (2020). The Many Faces of Kefir Fermented Dairy Products: Quality Characteristics, Flavour Chemistry, Nutritional Value, Health Benefits, and Safety. *Nutrients*, 12(2), 346. https://doi.org/10.3390/nu12020346

Formenti, L. R., Gernaey, K. V., Mauricio-Iglesias, M., Hagemann, T., Nørregaard, A., Heins, A., Bolic, A., Larsson, H., Krühne, U., Hernandez, D. Q., & Mears, L. (2014). Challenges in Industrial Fermentation Technology Research. *Biotechnology Journal*, 9(6), 727–738. https://doi.org/10.1002/biot.201300236

Gaden Jr, E. L. (2000). Fermentation Process Kinetics. *Biotechnology and Bioengineering*, 67(6), 629–635. https://doi.org/10.1002/(SICI)1097-0290(20000320)67:6<629::AID-BIT2>3.0.CO;2-P

Gänzle, M. (2022). The Periodic Table of Fermented Foods: Limitations and Opportunities. *Applied Microbiology and Biotechnology*, 106(8), 2815–2826. https://doi.org/10.1007/s00253-022-11909-y

Gänzle, M. G., & Salovaara, H. (2019). *Lactic Acid Bacteria in Cereal-Based Products* (pp. 199–213). CRC Press. https://doi.org/10.1201/9780429057465-13

Gao, Y., Fan, B., Wang, F., Gao, J., Li, S., Tian, Z., Li, D., & Hou, L. (2021). Metabolomics Approaches for the Comprehensive Evaluation of Fermented Foods: A Review. *Foods*, 10(10), 2294. https://doi.org/10.3390/foods10102294

Garcia-Gonzalez, N., Corsetti, A., Battista, N., & Prete, R. (2021). Health-Promoting Role of Lactiplantibacillus plantarum Isolated from Fermented Foods. *Microorganisms*, 9(2), 349. https://doi.org/10.3390/microorganisms9020349

Gotcheva, V., Roshkova, Z., Angelov, A., Pandiella, S. S., & Webb, C. (2001). Monitoring the Fermentation of the Traditional Bulgarian Beverage Boza. *International Journal of Food Science and Technology*, 36(2), 129–134. https://doi.org/10.1046/j.1365-2621.2001.00429.x

Han, D., Zhu, Y., Dai, S., Yu, Z., Wang, Y., Yu, Y., Jiang, M., Rong, C., Guo, Z., Yang, Y., & Wang, K. (2024). A Review on the Interaction of Acetic Acid Bacteria and Microbes in Food Fermentation: A Microbial Ecology Perspective. *Foods (Basel, Switzerland)*, 13(16), 2534. https://doi.org/10.3390/foods13162534

Holguín-Sterling, L., Pérez-Salinas, R., Ortiz, A., Navarro-Escalante, L., Pedraza-Claros, B., & Góngora, C. E. (2023). Physical–Chemical and Metataxonomic Characterization of the Microbial Communities Present during the Fermentation of Three Varieties of Coffee from Colombia and Their Sensory Qualities. *Agriculture*, 13(10), 1980. https://doi.org/10.3390/agriculture13101980

Jalili, M., Magkos, F., & Nazari, M. (2023). Fermented Foods in the Management of Obesity: Mechanisms of Action and Future Challenges. *International Journal of Molecular Sciences*, 24(3), 2665. https://doi.org/10.3390/ijms24032665

Jin, R., Song, J., Liu, C., Lin, R., Liang, D., Aweya, J. J., ... & Yang, S. (2024). Synthetic Microbial Communities: Novel Strategies to Enhance the Quality of Traditional Fermented Foods. *Comprehensive Reviews in Food Science and Food Safety*, 23(4), e13388. https://doi.org/10.1111/1541-4337.13388

Kabak, B., & Dobson, A. D. W. (2011). An Introduction to the Traditional Fermented Foods and Beverages of Turkey. *Critical Reviews in Food Science and Nutrition*, 51(3), 248–260. https://doi.org/10.1080/10408390903569640

Kårlund, A., Gómez-Gallego, C., Korhonen, J., Palo-Oja, O. M., El-Nezami, H., & Kolehmainen, M. (2020). Harnessing Microbes for Sustainable Development: Food Fermentation as a Tool for Improving the Nutritional Quality of Alternative Protein Sources. *Nutrients*, 12(4), 1020. https://doi.org/10.3390/nu12041020

Kechagia, M., Basoulis, D., Konstantopoulou, S., Dimitriadi, D., Gyftopoulou, K., Skarmoutsou, N., & Fakiri, E. M. (2013). Health Benefits of Probiotics: A Review. *ISRN Nutrition*, 2013(5–6), 1–7. https://doi.org/10.5402/2013/481651

Knychala, M. M., Boing, L. A., Ienczak, J. L., Stambuk, B. U., & Trichez, D. (2024). Precision Fermentation as an Alternative to Animal Protein, a Review. *Fermentation*, 10(6), 315. https://doi.org/10.3390/fermentation10060315

Kumar, M. R., Omar, A. R., Alitheen, N. B., Osman, M. A., Khalid, M., Mortadza, S. A. S., Azizi, N. F., Yeap, S. K., Abdullah, J. O., & Leow, A. T. C. (2022). Clinical and Preclinical Studies of Fermented Foods and Their Effects on Alzheimer's Disease. *Antioxidants*, 11(5), 883. https://doi.org/10.3390/antiox11050883

Kumari, R., Sahoo, D., Rai, A. K., & Sanjukta, S. (2021). Functional Peptides in Asian Protein Rich Fermented Foods: Production and Health Benefits. *Systems Microbiology and Biomanufacturing*, 2(1), 1–13. https://doi.org/10.1007/s43393-021-00040-0

Lahiri, D., Nag, M., Sarkar, T., Ray, R. R., Shariati, M. A., Rebezov, M., ... & Domínguez, R. (2022). Lactic Acid Bacteria (LAB): Autochthonous and Probiotic Microbes for Meat Preservation and Fortification. *Foods*, 11(18), 2792. https://doi.org/10.3390/foods11182792

Lima, T. T. M., Hosken, B. D. O., Martin, J. G. P., Lopes, I. L., & Venturim, B. C. (2022). Traditional Brazilian Fermented Foods: Cultural and Technological Aspects. *Journal of Ethnic Foods*, 9(1). https://doi.org/10.1186/s42779-022-00153-4

Lu, Y.-H., Huang, J.-R., Zheng, M.-J., Hong, Z.-Z., Huang, Y.-Y., Manzoor, M. F., Wu, J.-M., & Zeng, X.-A. (2024). Fermented Vegetables in China: Overview, Novel Processes, Influencing Factors, Lactic Acid Bacteria and Industrialisation Status. *International Journal of Food Science and Technology*, 59(7), 4420–4436. https://doi.org/10.1111/ijfs.17222

Madilo, F. K., Parry-Hanson Kunadu, A., Tano-Debrah, K., Saalia, F. K., & Kolanisi, U. (2024). Diversity of Production Techniques and Microbiology of African Cereal-Based Traditional Fermented Beverages. *Journal of food quality*, 2024(1), 1241614. **https://doi.org/10.1155/2024/1241614**

Mccarty, N. S., & Ledesma-Amaro, R. (2018). Synthetic Biology Tools to Engineer Microbial Communities for Biotechnology. *Trends in Biotechnology*, 37(2), 181–197. https://doi.org/10.1016/j.tibtech.2018.11.002

Meena, K. K., Taneja, N. K., Jain, D., Ojha, A., Saravanan, C., & Mudgil, D. (2022). Bioactive Components and Health Benefits of Maize-Based Fermented Foods: A Review. *Biointerface Research in Applied Chemistry*, 13(4), 338.https://doi.org/10.33263/briac134.338

Melini, F., & Melini, V. (2024). Role of Microbial Fermentation in the Bio-Production of Food Aroma Compounds from Vegetable Waste. *Fermentation*, 10(3), 132. **https://doi.org/10.3390/fermentation10030132**

Mendes, A. R., Spínola, M. P., Lordelo, M., & Prates, J. A. M. (2024). Advances in Bioprocess Engineering for Optimising Chlorella vulgaris Fermentation: Biotechnological Innovations and Applications. *Foods (Basel, Switzerland)*, 13(24), 4154. https://doi.org/10.3390/foods13244154

Mokoena, M. P., Omatola, C. A., & Olaniran, A. O. (2021). Applications of Lactic Acid Bacteria and Their Bacteriocins Against Food Spoilage Microorganisms and Foodborne Pathogens. *Molecules*, 26(22), 7055. https://doi.org/10.3390/molecules26227055

Munekata, P. E. S., Santos, E. M., Tomasevic, I., Domínguez, R., Lorenzo, J. M., Da Silva Barretto, A. C., & Pateiro, M. (2022). Functional Fermented Meat Products with Probiotics—A Review. *Journal of Applied Microbiology*, 133(1), 91–103. https://doi.org/10.1111/jam.15337

Neto, R., Mota, M. J., Lopes, R. P., Delgadillo, I., & Saraiva, J. A. Growth and metabolism of Oenococcus oeni for malolactic fermentation under pressure. Lett Appl Microbiol. 2016 Dec;63(6):426-433.

Nielsen, J., Tillegreen, C. B., & Petranovic, D. (2022). Innovation Trends in Industrial Biotechnology. *Trends in Biotechnology*, 40(10), 1160–1172. https://doi.org/10.1016/j.tibtech.2022.03.007

Nielsen, M. B., Meyer, A. S., & Arnau, J. (2023). The Next Food Revolution Is Here: Recombinant Microbial Production of Milk and Egg Proteins by Precision Fermentation. *Annual Review of Food Science and Technology*, 15(1), 173–187. https://doi.org/10.1146/annurev-food-072023-034256

Niyigaba, T., Küçükgöz, K., Kołożyn-Krajewska, D., Królikowski, T., & Trząskowska, M. (2025). Advances in Fermentation Technology: A Focus on Health and Safety. *Applied Sciences*, 15(6), 3001. **https://doi.org/10.3390/app15063001**

Obafemi, Y. D., Ajanaku, K. O., Akinduti, P. A., Leech, J., Cotter, P. D., & Oranusi, S. U. (2022). African Fermented Foods: Overview, Emerging Benefits, and Novel Approaches to Microbiome Profiling. *Npj Science of Food*, 6(1). https://doi.org/10.1038/s41538-022-00130-w

Odunfa, S. A., & Oyewole, O. B. (1998). *African Fermented Foods* (pp. 713–752). Springer Us. https://doi.org/10.1007/978-1-4613-0309-1_23

Palmnäs-Bédard, M., De Santa Izabel, A., Dicksved, J., & Landberg, R. (2023). Characterization of the Bacterial Composition of 47 Fermented Foods in Sweden. *Foods*, 12(20), 3827. https://doi.org/10.3390/foods12203827

Pejcz, E., Lachowicz-Wiśniewska, S., Nowicka, P., Wojciechowicz-Budzisz, A., Spychaj, R., & Gil, Z. (2021). Effect of Inoculated Lactic Acid Fermentation on the Fermentable Saccharides and Polyols, Polyphenols and Antioxidant Activity Changes in Wheat Sourdough. *Molecules*, 26(14), 4193. https://doi.org/10.3390/molecules26144193

Pescuma, M., de Valdez, G. F., & Mozzi, F. (2015). Whey-Derived Valuable Products Obtained by Microbial Fermentation. *Applied Microbiology and Biotechnology*, 99, 6183–6196. https://doi.org/10.1007/s00253-015-6766-z

Petrova, P., & Petrov, K. (2020). Lactic Acid Fermentation of Cereals and Pseudocereals: Ancient Nutritional Biotechnologies with Modern Applications. *Nutrients*, 12(4), 1118. https://doi.org/10.3390/nu12041118

Phiri, S., Schoustra, S. E., Van Den Heuvel, J., Shindano, J., Smid, E. J., & Linnemann, A. (2019). Fermented Cereal-Based Munkoyo Beverage: Processing Practices, Microbial Diversity and Aroma Compounds. *PLOS ONE*, 14(10), e0223501. https://doi.org/10.1371/journal.pone.0223501

Pilania, P., Bhushan, K., & Phutela, U. G. (2025). Electro-Fermentation for Biofuel and Biochemical Production. *Fermentation*, 11(4), 219. https://doi.org/10.3390/fermentation11040219

Praveen, M., & Brogi, S. (2025). Microbial Fermentation in Food and Beverage Industries: Innovations, Challenges, and Opportunities. *Foods*, 14(1), 114. https://doi.org/10.3390/foods14010114

Qin, H., Wu, H., Shen, K., Liu, Y., Li, M., Wang, H., Qiao, Z., & Mu, Z. (2022). Fermented Minor Grain Foods: Classification, Functional Components, and Probiotic Potential. *Foods (Basel, Switzerland)*, 11(20), 3155. https://doi.org/10.3390/foods11203155

Raj, T., Chandrasekhar, K., Kumar, A. N., & Kim, S.-H. (2021). Recent Biotechnological Trends in Lactic Acid Bacterial Fermentation for Food Processing Industries. *Systems Microbiology and Biomanufacturing*, 2(1), 14–40. https://doi.org/10.1007/s43393-021-00044-w

Ramesh, C., Dufossé, L., Prasastha, V. R., & Venkatachalam, M. (2022). Natural Substrates and Culture Conditions to Produce Pigments from Potential Microbes in Submerged Fermentation. *Fermentation*, 8(9), 460. https://doi.org/10.3390/fermentation8090460

Reis, J. A., Paula, A. T., Casarotti, S. N., & Penna, A. L. B. (2012). Lactic Acid Bacteria Antimicrobial Compounds: Characteristics and Applications. *Food Engineering Reviews*, 4, 124–140. https://doi.org/10.1007/s12393-012-9051-2

Sabater, C., Ruiz, L., Delgado, S., Ruas-Madiedo, P., & Margolles, A. (2020). Valorization of Vegetable Food Waste and by-Products Through Fermentation Processes. *Frontiers in Microbiology*, 11, 581997. https://doi.org/10.3389/fmicb.2020.581997

Salamon, A., Ignaczak, A., Kowalska, H., Szafrańska, A., Kowalska, J., & Marzec, A. (2023). Characteristics of Oat and Buckwheat Malt Grains for Use in the Production of Fermented Foods. *Foods*, 12(20), 3747. https://doi.org/10.3390/foods12203747

Salar-García, M. J., Godínez-Seoane, C., Sánchez-Segado, S., Sáez López, A., Valero Sánchez, R., Ortiz-Martínez, V. M., & Lozano Blanco, L. J. (2024). Sustainable Production of Biofuels and Biochemicals via Electro-Fermentation Technology. *Molecules*, 29(4), 834. https://doi.org/10.3390/molecules29040834

Salas-Millán, J. Á., & Aguayo, E. (2024). Fermentation for Revalorisation of Fruit and Vegetable By-Products: A Sustainable Approach Towards Minimising Food Loss and Waste. *Foods*, 13(22), 3680. https://doi.org/10.3390/foods13223680

Saleem, G. N., Gu, R., Qasim, M., Rashid Rajput, I., Chen, X., Bahar Khaskheli, G., & Qu, H. (2024). Therapeutic Potential of Popular Fermented Dairy Products and Its Benefits on Human Health. *Frontiers in Nutrition*, 11. https://doi.org/10.3389/fnut.2024.1328620

Şanlier, N., Gökcen, B. B., & Sezgin, A. C. (2017). Health Benefits of Fermented Foods. *Critical Reviews in Food Science and Nutrition*, 59(3), 506–527. https://doi.org/10.1080/10408398.2017.1383355

Sarıtaş, S., Miranda, J. M., Mondragon Portocarrero, A. D. C., Witkowska, A. M., & Karav, S. (2024). Functional Yogurt: Types and Health Benefits. *Applied Sciences*, 14(24), 11798. https://doi.org/10.3390/app142411798

Sauer, M. (2016). Industrial Production of Acetone and Butanol by Fermentation—100 Years Later. *FEMS Microbiology Letters*, 363(13), fnw134. https://doi.org/10.1093/femsle/fnw134

Sawant, S. S., Park, H. Y., Sim, E. Y., Kim, H. S., & Choi, H. S. (2025). Microbial Fermentation in Food: Impact on Functional Properties and Nutritional Enhancement—A Review of Recent Developments. *Fermentation*, 11(1), 15. https://doi.org/10.3390/fermentation11010015

Seo, S.-O., Park, S.-K., Jung, S.-C., Ryu, C.-M., & Kim, J.-S. (2020). Anti-Contamination Strategies for Yeast Fermentations. *Microorganisms*, 8(2), 274. https://doi.org/10.3390/microorganisms8020274

Shah, A. M., Song, Y., Tarfeen, N., & Mohamed, H. (2023). Fermented Foods: Their Health-Promoting Components and Potential Effects on Gut Microbiota. *Fermentation*, 9(2), 118. https://doi.org/10.3390/fermentation9020118

Sharma, R., Bhatia, S. K., Kulshrestha, S., Garg, P., & Kumar, P. (2020). Microbial Fermentation and Its Role in Quality Improvement of Fermented Foods. *Fermentation*, 6(4), 106. https://doi.org/10.3390/fermentation6040106

Sionek, B., Szydłowska, A., Küçükgöz, K., & Kołożyn-Krajewska, D. (2023). Traditional and New Microorganisms in Lactic Acid Fermentation of Food. *Fermentation*, 9(12), 1019. https://doi.org/10.3390/fermentation9121019

Sivamaruthi, B. S., Chaiyasut, C., & Kesika, P. (2018). Thai Fermented Foods as a Versatile Source of Bioactive Microorganisms-A Comprehensive Review. *Scientia Pharmaceutica*, 86(3), 37. https://doi.org/10.3390/scipharm86030037

Slimane, M., & El-Hafid, N. (2024). Recent Status in Production, Biotechnological Applications, Commercial Aspects, and Future Prospects of Microbial Enzymes: A Comprehensive Review. *International Journal of Agricultural Science and Food Technology*, 10(1), 006–020. https://doi.org/10.17352/2455-815x.000202

Soemarie, Y. B., Barliana, M. I., & Milanda, T. (2021). Fermented Foods as Probiotics: A Review. *Journal of Advanced Pharmaceutical Technology & Research*, 12(4), 335–339. https://doi.org/10.4103/japtr.japtr_116_21

Sun, M., Gao, A. X., Liu, X., Bai, Z., Wang, P., & Ledesma-Amaro, R. (2024). Microbial Conversion of Ethanol to High-Value Products: Progress and Challenges. *Biotechnology for Biofuels and Bioproducts*, 17(1). https://doi.org/10.1186/s13068-024-02546-w

Taveira, I. C., Nogueira, K. M. V., Oliveira, D. L. G. D., & Silva, R. D. N. (2021). Fermentation: Humanitys Oldest Biotechnological Tool. *Frontiers for Young Minds*, 9. https://doi.org/10.3389/frym.2021.568656

Thierry, A., Rué, O., Picard, O., Grondin, C., Madec, M.-N., Marché, L., Mariadassou, M., Bage, A.-S., Chuat, V., & Valence, F. (2023). Microbial Communities of a Variety of 75 Homemade Fermented Vegetables. *Frontiers in Microbiology*, 14. https://doi.org/10.3389/fmicb.2023.1323424

Torres-Guardado, R., Esteve-Zarzoso, B., Reguant, C., & Bordons, A. (2021). Microbial Interactions in Alcoholic Beverages. *International Microbiology*, 25(1), 1–15. https://doi.org/10.1007/s10123-021-00200-1

Wang, X., Li, H., Zou, W., Zhang, L., Peng, X., Sun, Z., Shao, Q., & Ren, X. (2020). Transformation of Microbial Negative Correlations into Positive Correlations by Saccharomyces cerevisiae Inoculation During Pomegranate Wine Fermentation. *Applied and Environmental Microbiology*, 86(24). https://doi.org/10.1128/aem.01847-20

Wang, Y., Zhang, C., Liu, F., Jin, Z., & Xia, X. (2022). Ecological Succession and Functional Characteristics of Lactic Acid Bacteria in Traditional Fermented Foods. *Critical Reviews in Food Science and Nutrition, ahead-of-print(ahead-of-print)*, 63(22), 5841–5855. https://doi.org/10.1080/10408398.2021.2025035

Wang, Y., Zhang, C., Liu, F., Jin, Z., & Xia, X. (2023). Ecological Succession and Functional Characteristics of Lactic Acid Bacteria in Traditional Fermented Foods. *Critical Reviews in Food Science and Nutrition*, 63(22), 5841–5855.https://doi.org/10.1080/10408398.2021.2025035

Wang, Z., Wang, Z., Ji, L., Zhang, J., Zhao, Z., Zhang, R., Bai, T., Hou, B., Zhang, Y., Liu, D., Wang, W., & Chen, L. (2021). A Review: Microbial Diversity and Function of Fermented Meat Products in China. *Frontiers in Microbiology*, 12(108372). https://doi.org/10.3389/fmicb.2021.645435

Wieczorek, M. N., & Drabińska, N. (2022). Flavour Generation During Lactic Acid Fermentation of Brassica Vegetables—Literature Review. *Applied Sciences*, 12(11), 5598. https://doi.org/10.3390/app12115598

Yan, X., Mcclements, D. J., Luo, S., Ye, J., & Liu, C. (2024). A Review of the Effects of Fermentation on the Structure, Properties, and Application of Cereal Starch in Foods. *Critical Reviews in Food Science and Nutrition, ahead-of-print(ahead-of-print)*, 65(12), 2323–2342. https://doi.org/10.1080/10408398.2024.2334269

Yao, S., Zhou, R., Hao, L., Jin, Y., Wu, C., & Huang, J. (2022). Multispecies Biofilms in Fermentation: Biofilm Formation, Microbial Interactions, and Communication. *Comprehensive Reviews in Food Science and Food Safety*, 21(4), 3346–3375. https://doi.org/10.1111/1541-4337.12991

Yuan, Y., Yang, Y., Xiao, L., Qu, L., Zhang, X., & Wei, Y. (2023). Advancing Insights into Probiotics during Vegetable Fermentation. *Foods (Basel, Switzerland)*, 12(20), 3789. https://doi.org/10.3390/foods12203789

Zang, J., Xu, Y., Xia, W., & Regenstein, J. M. (2019). Quality, Functionality, and Microbiology of Fermented Fish: A Review. *Critical Reviews in Food Science and Nutrition*, 60(7), 1228–1242. https://doi.org/10.1080/10408398.2019.1565491

Zentou, H., Zainal Abidin, Z., Yunus, R., Awang Biak, D. R., Abdullah Issa, M., & Yahaya Pudza, M. (2021). A New Model of Alcoholic Fermentation Under a Byproduct Inhibitory Effect. *ACS Omega*, 6(6), 4137–4146. https://doi.org/10.1021/acsomega.0c04025

Zhang, H., Tan, Y., Wei, J., Du, H., & Xu, Y. (2022). Fungal Interactions Strengthen the Diversity-Functioning Relationship of Solid-State Fermentation Systems. *mSystems*, 7(4). https://doi.org/10.1128/msystems.00401-22

Zhong, Y., Zou, Y., Zheng, Z., Chen, Q., Xu, W., Wu, Y., ... & Gao, H. (2022). Impact of Inoculating With Indigenous Bacillus Marcorestinctum YC-1 on Quality and Microbial Communities of Yibin Yacai (Fermented Mustard) During the Fermentation Process. *Foods*, 11(22), 3593. https://doi.org/10.3390/foods11223593

CHAPTER 5

Probiotics and Prebiotics in Gut Health

Olivia Lutz and Sunil Thomas

5.1 INTRODUCTION

The human gastrointestinal tract is home to a remarkably complex and dynamic ecosystem of microorganisms collectively known as the gut microbiome. This community, estimated to comprise over 38 trillion microbial cells spanning thousands of bacterial, viral, fungal, and archaeal species, has co-evolved with the human host over millennia (Sender et al., 2016). Far from being a passive passenger, the gut microbiome performs an extraordinary array of functions essential to host physiology, influencing digestion, metabolism, immune regulation, and overall health (Thomas et al., 2017).

Among its critical roles, the gut microbiome contributes to nutrient metabolism, synthesis of essential vitamins, maintenance of intestinal barrier integrity, and protection against pathogenic organisms (Valdes et al., 2018). It also produces neurotransmitters and bioactive metabolites that participate in systemic signaling, forming the foundation of the gut–brain axis—a bidirectional communication network linking intestinal and neurological function. This ecosystem is highly responsive to environmental and host-related factors, including diet, medications, stress, and lifestyle, highlighting its dynamic nature and adaptability.

Disruption of the gut microbial balance, commonly referred to as dysbiosis, has been increasingly associated with a broad spectrum of disorders. These range from gastrointestinal diseases such as inflammatory bowel disease (IBD) and irritable bowel syndrome (IBS) to systemic conditions including obesity, type 2 diabetes, cardiovascular disease, and autoimmune disorders. Emerging evidence also implicates dysbiosis in neuropsychiatric and neurodegenerative conditions, including depression, anxiety, and Parkinson's disease (Rinninella et al., 2019; Cryan et al., 2019).

Given the centrality of the gut microbiome to human health, strategies to modulate its composition and function have gained substantial attention. Among these, probiotics—live microorganisms that confer health benefits when administered in adequate amounts—and prebiotics—dietary substrates that selectively stimulate the growth or activity of beneficial microbes—have emerged as promising interventions. This chapter explores the scientific foundations, mechanisms, clinical applications, and limitations of probiotics and prebiotics, providing a comprehensive overview of how targeted microbiome modulation can contribute to health maintenance and disease prevention.

5.2 MODULATING THE MICROBIOME: PROBIOTICS, PREBIOTICS, AND FERMENTED FOODS

Growing recognition of the microbiome's central role in human physiology has catalyzed intense interest in strategies to beneficially modulate gut microbial composition and function. Among the most extensively researched interventions are probiotics and prebiotics, often accompanied by

DOI: 10.1201/9781003638292-5

a resurgence in the popularity of fermented foods (Sánchez et al., 2017).

Probiotics are defined as live microorganisms that, when administered in adequate amounts, confer a health benefit on the host (Hill et al., 2014). These typically include specific strains of *Lactobacillus*, *Bifidobacterium*, and *Saccharomyces*, among others. Prebiotics, in contrast, are non-digestible substrates, commonly dietary fibers or oligosaccharides, that are selectively utilized by beneficial host microbes to improve health (Gibson et al., 2017).

Fermented foods now occupy a unique and expanding niche at the intersection of culinary tradition, nutritional science, and clinical research. While often valued for their taste and preservation properties, they also present opportunities to influence gut microbiota in beneficial ways. Modern studies are beginning to catalog the microbial diversity in fermented products and investigate how regular consumption might reshape the gut microbiome, enhance metabolic health, and support immune resilience (Chilton et al., 2015; Swer et al., 2024).

The extent to which microbes from fermented foods colonize the gut, interact with existing microbial communities, or produce long-term health benefits is still under investigation (Marco et al., 2021; Mukherjee et al., 2024; Chan et al., 2023).

Products such as yogurt, kefir, sauerkraut, kimchi, miso, tempeh, and kombucha have been dietary staples in various cultures for centuries. These foods undergo microbial fermentation processes, typically involving lactic acid bacteria (LAB) or yeasts, which enhance shelf life, flavor, nutritional value, and potential health benefits (Marco et al., 2021; Septembre-Malaterre et al., 2018). Importantly, fermented foods can serve as natural delivery systems for live microbes and bioactive compounds, blurring the lines between nutrition and therapeutic intervention (Marco et al., 2021; Mukherjee et al., 2024; Chan et al., 2023).

5.3 HISTORICAL FOUNDATIONS AND MODERN ADVANCES IN PROBIOTICS

The scientific inquiry into probiotics and microbial health dates back over a century. In the early 1900s, Élie Metchnikoff (Ilya Ilyich Mechnikov) hypothesized that the exceptional longevity of Bulgarian peasants was attributable to their regular consumption of fermented milk rich in LAB (Shreiner et al., 2015). His work laid out the conceptual groundwork for modern probiotic science, although the term "probiotic" itself was only coined decades later.

Through the 20th century, research gradually uncovered the mechanisms by which specific bacterial strains influence host physiology—such as by competing with pathogens, modulating immune responses, and producing antimicrobial or anti-inflammatory compounds. Yet it was not until the genomic era that the full complexity of the microbiome began to emerge.

The launch of the Human Microbiome Project (HMP) by the National Institutes of Health (NIH) in 2007 marked a transformative shift. This large-scale initiative mapped the microbial communities residing across different body sites in healthy individuals, revealing both remarkable diversity and significant inter-individual variation (Turnbaugh et al., 2007; Thursby and Juge, 2017). Subsequent advances in high-throughput sequencing, metagenomics, metabolomics, and systems biology have deepened our understanding of how microbial metabolites interact with host signaling pathways, immune cells, and epithelial barriers (Zhang et al., 2024a).

5.4 CHALLENGES AND KNOWLEDGE GAPS IN MICROBIOME-BASED INTERVENTIONS

Despite increasing public interest and widespread marketing of probiotic supplements and fermented food products, substantial scientific and regulatory challenges persist. Clinical trial results are often heterogeneous, with outcomes varying based on strain selection, dose, delivery format, duration of administration, and individual microbiome profiles (Office of Dietary Supplements, 2024; Zmora et al., 2019).

Moreover, product quality and labeling accuracy vary considerably across commercial formulations. Issues include incorrect or missing strain identification, insufficient viable cell counts, contamination, and poor survival of microbes through the acidic environment of the stomach (Patro-Golab et al., 2020; Jackson et al., 2019). These limitations highlight the need for rigorous quality control, standardized clinical protocols, and better regulatory oversight, especially when products are targeted at vulnerable populations such as infants, the elderly, or immunocompromised individuals.

5.5 STRAIN ISOLATION AND EARLY PROBIOTIC APPLICATIONS

The first half of the 20th century saw an increasing focus on isolating specific microbial strains with therapeutic potential. In 1917, German physician Alfred Nissle isolated a strain of *Escherichia coli* from a soldier who remained healthy during a severe shigellosis outbreak. This strain, *E. coli* Nissle 1917, demonstrated protective effects against gastrointestinal pathogens and continues to be used clinically today for conditions such as ulcerative colitis (UC) (Lynch et al., 2021).

In the 1930s, Japanese microbiologist Minoru Shirota developed a strain of *Lactobacillus casei* (later named *L. casei* Shirota) with potential gut health benefits. He incorporated this strain into a fermented milk drink, founding Yakult, one of the first globally marketed probiotic brands that are still consumed widely today.

The term "probiotic" has evolved over time (Shreiner et al., 2015). In 1965, Lilly and Stillwell first used it to describe substances produced by one microorganism that stimulate the growth of another, in contrast to the inhibitory action of antibiotics. The modern definition—"live microorganisms that, when administered in adequate amounts, confer a health benefit on the host"—was formalized in 2001 by an FAO/WHO expert panel (Hill et al., 2014).

5.6 THE GENOMIC REVOLUTION AND THE HUMAN MICROBIOME PROJECT

The turn of the 21st century marked a revolutionary shift in microbiome research, driven by breakthroughs in DNA sequencing and bioinformatics. Traditional culture–based microbiology was limited because many gut microbes are obligate anaerobes, making them unculturable in standard laboratory settings (Thursby and Juge, 2017). The advent of culture-independent methods, such as 16S ribosomal RNA (rRNA) gene sequencing and shotgun metagenomics, enabled scientists to identify, quantify, and characterize the vast diversity of microorganisms inhabiting the human body without the need for cultivation.

In 2007, the NIH launched the HMP to systematically map microbial communities across body sites including the gut, skin, mouth, nasal passages, and urogenital tract (Turnbaugh et al., 2007; Thursby and Juge, 2017). HMP Phase I revealed that the human microbiome contains over 100 times more genes than the human genome, varies significantly between individuals and body sites, yet generally remains stable over time unless perturbed by antibiotics, illness, or diet.

Building on these insights, subsequent initiatives such as the Integrative HMP (iHMP) and international collaborations have explored how microbial communities develop, respond to environmental changes, and influence health and disease (Zhang et al., 2024a,b). Research has shifted from cataloging microbial species to understanding their functional traits and metabolic outputs, emphasizing how microbial metabolites regulate immunity, which pathways are protective or pathogenic, and how interventions like diet, probiotics, or prebiotics can beneficially modulate microbial functions. These emerging insights underpin the growing fields of personalized nutrition, precision probiotics, and microbiome-targeted therapeutics, signaling a new era in which understanding and manipulating the microbiome may play a central role in disease prevention and health optimization.

5.7 THE HUMAN GUT MICROBIOME: COMPOSITION, DIVERSITY, AND FUNCTIONAL SIGNIFICANCE

The human gut microbiome is one of the most intricate and metabolically dynamic ecosystems known, consisting of trillions of microorganisms that collectively shape human physiology, metabolism, and immune function. This vast microbial community influences nearly every aspect of health—from digestion and nutrient absorption to immune education and protection against pathogens (Thursby and Juge, 2017; Valdes et al., 2018; Rinninella et al., 2019). Far from being a passive collection of microbes, the gut microbiome acts as a highly coordinated biological network that communicates continuously with the host, contributing to homeostasis and, when imbalanced, to disease.

5.7.1 Taxonomic Composition and Diversity of the Microorganisms in the Human Gut

The human gut harbors a remarkable diversity of microorganisms, including bacteria, archaea, fungi, viruses, and protozoa, with bacteria being the most abundant and functionally dominant members. Estimates suggest the gut contains approximately 10^{13}–10^{14} microbial cells, comparable in number to human somatic and germ cells.

Collectively, these microbes encode millions of genes—forming what is often called the "second genome"—that provides metabolic capabilities far beyond those of the human genome (Ma et al., 2024).

At the phylum level, the gut bacterial community is typically dominated by Firmicutes and Bacteroidetes, which together account for 80–90% of the total bacterial population. Other important contributors include Actinobacteria, Proteobacteria, and Verrucomicrobia. However, such high-level classifications obscure the immense taxonomic richness observed at the genus and species levels, as well as substantial inter-individual variability. Even among healthy individuals, the relative abundance of key genera such as *Bacteroides*, *Faecalibacterium*, *Prevotella*, and *Ruminococcus* may differ dramatically, reflecting unique combinations of diet, lifestyle, genetics, and environment (Goodrich et al., 2014; Machiels et al., 2014; Suez et al., 2018).

The notion of a "core microbiome" shared among all humans remains controversial. While some taxa appear consistently across individuals, it is increasingly recognized that microbial functions—such as short-chain fatty acid (SCFA) production or bile acid metabolism—may be more conserved than specific taxa. This has led to the emerging concept of a "core functional microbiome," emphasizing metabolic potential rather than taxonomic uniformity.

Spatially, the gut microbiome exhibits striking heterogeneity along the gastrointestinal tract. The stomach and duodenum, with their acidic environment and rapid content turnover, contain relatively sparse microbial populations dominated by acid-tolerant species. In contrast, microbial density and diversity increase progressively through the small intestine and peak in the colon, reaching up to 10^{11}–10^{12} cells per gram of content. Moreover, the mucus layer that lines the intestinal epithelium harbors distinct communities, including mucin-degrading bacteria such as *Akkermansia muciniphila*, which play key roles in maintaining gut barrier integrity and metabolic health (McCallum and Tropini, 2024; Hishida and Iwasa, 2021).

5.7.2 Early Life Colonization of Microorganisms

The composition and function of the gut microbiome are shaped by a complex interplay of genetic, environmental, and lifestyle factors. Understanding these determinants is crucial for developing strategies to manipulate microbiomes for health benefits (Goodrich et al., 2014).

The initial establishment of the gut microbiota begins at birth and sets the foundation for future microbial and immune development. The mode of delivery plays a critical role: vaginally delivered infants acquire microbes resembling their mother's vaginal and intestinal microbiota—particularly *Lactobacillus* and *Bacteroides* species—whereas cesarean-delivered infants are initially colonized by skin-associated taxa such as *Staphylococcus* and *Corynebacterium*. Breastfeeding further shapes this ecosystem through the supply of human milk oligosaccharides (HMOs), which selectively nourish beneficial *Bifidobacterium* species capable of metabolizing these complex sugars. During weaning, the introduction of solid foods leads to a diversification of the microbial community, and by around three years of age, the microbiome resembles that of an adult (Moore and Townsend, 2019).

5.7.3 Dietary Influences

Diet exerts one of the most profound influences on gut microbiome structure and function (Valdes et al., 2018). Diets rich in dietary fiber and resistant starch foster the growth of saccharolytic bacteria that ferment carbohydrates to produce SCFAs such as acetate, propionate, and butyrate—metabolites essential for colon health, immune regulation, and energy homeostasis. Conversely, diets high in animal protein, fat, or processed foods can reduce microbial diversity and favor bile-tolerant, potentially pro-inflammatory taxa. Notably, even short-term dietary interventions can cause rapid shifts in microbiome composition within days, but long-term dietary habits exert more stable and enduring effects.

5.7.4 Antibiotics and Medications

Antibiotic exposure is among the most disruptive factors affecting the gut microbiome. Even brief antibiotic courses can dramatically reduce microbial diversity, eliminate beneficial taxa, and allow opportunistic pathogens to thrive. Although partial recovery often occurs after treatment cessation, some microbial shifts can persist for months or years, potentially influencing metabolic and immune function. Other commonly used drugs—including proton pump inhibitors (PPIs), metformin, and non-steroidal anti-inflammatory drugs—also modulate microbial communities through direct antimicrobial effects or changes in gut physiology (Le Bastard et al., 2018).

5.7.5 Host Genetics and Environmental Interactions

While host genetics play a role in shaping the gut microbiome, their influence is modest compared to environmental and lifestyle factors. Twin and family studies suggest that certain microbial taxa are heritable, often those linked to host immune and metabolic genes. However, shared environmental exposures—particularly diet, hygiene practices, and cohabitation—tend to have stronger and more consistent effects. Thus, while genetics may set the stage, environmental factors largely determine the composition and functional dynamics of the gut microbiome (Goodrich et al., 2014).

5.7.6 Microbial Functions and Host Interactions

The human gut microbiome performs a vast array of functions that are essential to maintaining health, influencing not only digestion and nutrient absorption but also immune, metabolic, and even neurological processes (Valdes et al., 2018; Rinninella et al., 2019). Through the production of metabolites and molecular signals, the gut microbiota communicates continuously with host cells, thereby modulating systemic physiology and disease susceptibility. The microbiome can thus be viewed as a "metabolic organ" that works in concert with the host to sustain homeostasis.

5.7.7 Nutrient Metabolism and Energy Harvest

One of the most fundamental roles of microbiomes is the fermentation of indigestible dietary components such as fibers and resistant starches (RS) that escape digestion in the upper gastrointestinal tract. This fermentation process yields SCFAs—primarily acetate, propionate, and butyrate—which serve as major signaling molecules and energy sources. Butyrate is the preferred energy substrate for colonocytes, supporting intestinal barrier integrity and exerting potent anti-inflammatory and anticancer effects through histone deacetylase inhibition and G protein–coupled receptor activation (Lin and Medeiros, 2023).

Beyond fermentation, gut microbes contribute to the synthesis of essential nutrients, including several B vitamins (B_{12}, biotin, folate, and riboflavin) and vitamin K, which are absorbed and utilized by the host. The microbiome also plays a critical role in bile acid metabolism, transforming primary bile acids synthesized by the liver into secondary bile acids that influence lipid absorption, cholesterol homeostasis, and signaling through nuclear receptors such as Farnesoid X receptor (FXR) and Takeda G protein-coupled receptor 5 (TGR5). Additionally, microbial enzymes enhance the bioavailability and transformation of polyphenols and other dietary bioactives, amplifying their antioxidant and anti-inflammatory effects (Park and Mannaa, 2025).

5.7.8 Immune System Development and Regulation

The gut microbiome serves as a master regulator of immune system development and function. Early microbial exposure is essential for the proper maturation of gut-associated lymphoid tissue (GALT) and systemic immune competence. Commensal microorganisms provide continuous, low-level stimulation of the immune system through molecular patterns such as lipopolysaccharides, flagellin, and peptidoglycan fragments. These microbial molecules interact with host pattern recognition receptors (PRRs), including Toll-like receptors (TLRs) and NOD-like receptors (NLRs), guiding the development of immune tolerance and promoting the expansion of regulatory T cells (Tregs) (Brodin, 2022; Donald and Finlay, 2023).

When microbial composition becomes imbalanced due to dysbiosis, immune homeostasis can be disrupted, predisposing individuals to inflammatory, allergic, and autoimmune diseases. For example, loss of SCFA-producing bacteria can reduce Treg function, contributing to diseases like IBD, asthma, and type 1 diabetes. Maintaining a diverse and balanced microbiome is therefore vital to immune resilience and inflammation control (Fusco et al., 2023).

5.7.9 Pathogen Resistance

A healthy gut microbiome acts as a natural defense barrier against invading pathogens—a phenomenon known as colonization resistance. Resident microbes compete with pathogens for nutrients and adhesion sites on the intestinal epithelium, secrete antimicrobial peptides (bacteriocins, lactic acid, hydrogen peroxide), and stimulate mucosal immunity. Disruption of these communities—such as through antibiotic use—can create ecological niches that allow pathogens like *Clostridioides difficile*, *Salmonella*, or *E. coli* to proliferate. Restoration of the microbiome, through dietary interventions or fecal microbiota transplantation (FMT), can reestablish colonization resistance and prevent recurrent infections (Seekatz et al., 2022; Ducarmon et al., 2019).

5.7.10 Gut–Brain Axis

The gut microbiome communicates bidirectionally with the central nervous system via neural, endocrine, and immune pathways—a system referred to as the gut–brain axis (Cryan et al., 2019). Microbes produce a variety of neuroactive compounds, including SCFAs, tryptophan metabolites, γ-aminobutyric acid (GABA), and serotonin, which can influence mood, cognition, and behavior. Approximately 90% of the body's serotonin is produced in the gut, largely under microbial influence. Experimental studies in germ-free animals demonstrate that the absence of a microbiome alters stress responses, anxiety-like behavior, and neurogenesis, underscoring the microbiome's critical role in neurodevelopment and mental health. Although human studies remain ongoing, emerging evidence links dysbiosis to conditions such as depression, anxiety, and autism spectrum disorders (ASDs).

5.7.11 Metabolic Regulation

The gut microbiome exerts profound effects on host metabolism and energy balance. Certain microbial configurations have been associated with obesity, insulin resistance, and metabolic syndrome. Mechanistically, microbes influence lipid metabolism, glucose homeostasis, and appetite regulation by modulating bile acid profiles and producing metabolites that interact with host endocrine pathways. For instance, propionate and butyrate can stimulate the release of peptide YY (PYY) and glucagon-like peptide-1 (GLP-1), hormones that promote satiety and improve insulin sensitivity (Kabahizi et al., 2022). Intriguingly, some therapeutic effects of the diabetes drug metformin appear to depend on alterations in the gut microbiome, highlighting the reciprocal relationship between microbial metabolism and pharmacological response (Geng et al., 2024).

5.8 PROBIOTICS: DEFINITION, MECHANISMS, AND CLINICAL IMPLEMENTATION

Probiotics are live microorganisms that, when administered in adequate amounts, confer a health benefit on the host (Hill et al., 2014). These beneficial microbes—most commonly species of *Lactobacillus*, *Bifidobacterium*, and *Saccharomyces*—can influence gut ecology, enhance barrier function, and modulate immune and metabolic processes. The global interest in probiotics has grown dramatically, fueled by their potential to prevent or manage conditions ranging from antibiotic-associated diarrhea (AAD) to IBS, metabolic disorders, and even mental health conditions. However, translating preclinical findings into consistent clinical outcomes remains challenging due to strain-specific differences, inconsistent dosing, and variable product quality (Zmora et al., 2019; Office of Dietary Supplements, 2024).

5.8.1 Mechanisms of Action of Probiotics

Probiotics exert their effects through multiple, complementary mechanisms. These mechanisms act at the interface of the gut microbiota, immune system, and host metabolism, and collectively contribute to maintaining or restoring health. Because different probiotic strains have distinct biological properties, the mechanisms involved are often highly strain-specific, and no single probiotic strain can exert all potential health benefits (Plaza-Diaz et al., 2019).

One of the fundamental ways probiotics protect the host is through competitive exclusion of pathogens. Probiotic strains can adhere to mucosal surfaces within the gastrointestinal tract, thereby occupying receptor sites that might otherwise be exploited by harmful microorganisms. By doing so, they effectively block pathogens from attaching and colonizing the intestinal epithelium. In addition, probiotics compete with these microbes for essential nutrients, creating an environment that is less favorable for the survival of harmful bacteria. Some probiotic strains also produce antimicrobial substances such as organic acids (e.g., lactic acid), hydrogen peroxide, and bacteriocins, which directly inhibit the growth of pathogenic bacteria (Buffie and Pamer, 2013; Theriot and Young, 2014).

Another key mechanism involves the modulation of the host immune system. Probiotics interact with immune cells and epithelial receptors, leading to the production of anti-inflammatory cytokines such as interleukin-10 (IL-10) and the downregulation of pro-inflammatory cytokines like TNF-α. They also support the differentiation of regulatory T cells (Tregs), which play a critical role in maintaining immune tolerance and preventing excessive inflammatory responses. Furthermore, probiotics enhance the integrity of the intestinal epithelial barrier by promoting the expression of tight junction proteins, thereby reducing intestinal permeability (commonly referred to as "leaky gut") and limiting the translocation of microbial toxins and antigens into systemic circulation (Yan and Polk, 2011).

In addition to their immune-modulating effects, probiotics also have important metabolic and enzymatic activities that benefit the host. Many strains are capable of fermenting non-digestible dietary fibers into SCFAs such as butyrate, acetate, and propionate. These SCFAs serve as energy sources for colonocytes, reduce inflammation, and contribute to the regulation of lipid and glucose metabolism. Probiotics also assist in the synthesis of essential vitamins, particularly B-group vitamins and vitamin K, and can influence bile acid metabolism by deconjugating bile salts. This activity not only affects fat absorption but also alters the composition of the gut microbiota and impacts cholesterol homeostasis.

Finally, certain probiotic strains participate in neuroendocrine signaling via the gut–brain axis. These microorganisms can produce or influence the availability of neuroactive compounds such as GABA, dopamine, and serotonin precursors like tryptophan. Through these biochemical signals, probiotics can affect mood, behavior, and stress responses, likely by interacting with the vagus nerve or modulating systemic inflammation that impacts brain function. This emerging field, often referred to as "psychobiotics," highlights the potential of specific probiotic strains in supporting mental health and cognitive function (Liu et al., 2018; Pirola and Fröjdö, 2008).

Taken together, these diverse mechanisms underscore why the efficacy of probiotics is highly dependent on the specific strain used. While one strain may excel in enhancing immune regulation, another may be more effective at modulating metabolic functions or interacting with the nervous system. For this reason, probiotic interventions must be tailored to the health condition being targeted and supported by robust clinical evidence demonstrating the unique benefits of each strain (Plaza-Diaz et al., 2019).

5.8.2 Regulatory and Quality Considerations

According to the FAO/WHO definition, three criteria must be met for an organism to be considered probiotic: it must be alive, administered in adequate amounts, and proven to confer a health benefit (Hill et al., 2014). Furthermore, probiotic strains must be genetically characterized, shown to survive passage through the gastrointestinal tract, and supported by robust clinical evidence.

Regulatory frameworks for probiotics vary widely across regions. In the European Union, health claims are strictly reviewed by the European Food Safety Authority (EFSA), which demands high-level evidence of efficacy and safety. In contrast, in the United States, most probiotics are marketed as dietary supplements or foods under the oversight of the Food and Drug Administration (FDA), which imposes less stringent premarket evaluation. Only when a probiotic is promoted for treating or preventing disease is it regulated as a drug. This uneven regulatory landscape has contributed to inconsistencies in labeling accuracy, strain identification, and potency across commercial products (Office of Dietary Supplements, 2024).

5.8.3 Strain Specificity and Non-Interchangeability

One of the most critical yet frequently misunderstood principles in probiotic research and application is strain-level specificity (Zmora et al., 2019; McFarland et al., 2018). Although microorganisms are taxonomically categorized through hierarchical ranks—kingdom, phylum, class, order, family, genus, and species—the beneficial effects attributed to probiotics are not conserved across entire species, or even within them. Instead, efficacy is highly dependent on the specific strain, which refers to a genetically distinct isolate of a species that may differ in genome content, metabolic functions, and health-promoting capabilities (Goodrich et al., 2014).

This principle can be illustrated through well-characterized examples within the *Lactobacillus* genus. *Lactobacillus rhamnosus* GG (often abbreviated as LGG) is one of the most extensively studied probiotic strains and is supported by strong clinical evidence showing that it reduces both the incidence and duration of acute infectious diarrhea and helps prevent AAD (Szajewska and Kołodziej, 2015). However, other *L. rhamnosus* strains—even those closely related—do not necessarily exhibit the same effects. The therapeutic properties demonstrated by LGG cannot be extrapolated to other strains within the same species without empirical evidence. Similarly, certain *Bifidobacterium* strains improve intestinal barrier function and alleviate symptoms of IBS through mechanisms such as tight junction reinforcement, while other strains within the *Bifidobacterium* genus show minimal or entirely different physiological effects (Whorwell et al., 2006; Yuan et al., 2017; Wilson et al., 2020).

At the molecular level, this variation arises from strain-specific genomic differences. Individual strains possess unique sets of genes that determine their metabolic capabilities—such as the enzymes used to break down dietary substrates, the adhesins that enable epithelial attachment, and the production of bioactive molecules that modulate immune responses. Even minor genetic variations can profoundly influence phenotypic behavior and, consequently, the clinical outcomes observed. Thus, probiotic efficacy cannot be generalized to a species or genus; it must always be evaluated at the strain level through well-designed, strain-specific clinical trials (Goodrich et al., 2014).

The implications for commercial probiotic products are substantial and often misunderstood by both consumers and healthcare practitioners (Patro-Golab et al., 2020). Many commercial yogurts, supplements, and fermented foods either fail to disclose the exact probiotic strains used or list only the species name (e.g., *Lactobacillus acidophilus*). This lack of specificity prevents consumers from verifying whether the included strain has any documented clinical benefits. Even when strain identification is provided, many formulations contain strains that have not been tested in controlled trials, making any claimed health benefit scientifically uncertain. Consequently, a product's label may imply benefits based on general probiotic research while lacking evidence for the specific strain it contains. This gap between strain-validated science and marketing-driven labeling represents one of the most persistent challenges in probiotic commercialization and regulation.

5.8.4 Dosage Requirements and Viability Thresholds

Probiotic efficacy depends not only on which strain is administered but also on how much of it reaches the gut in a viable, metabolically active form (Office of Dietary Supplements, 2024). The FAO/WHO definition of probiotics emphasizes that benefits occur only when they are consumed in "adequate amounts." These amounts are typically expressed as colony-forming units (CFU)—a measure of the number of live microorganisms capable of replication. The required dose varies by strain and health indication, and most evidence-based benefits have been demonstrated only at specific CFU levels tested in clinical trials.

For example, LGG has consistently shown therapeutic efficacy for reducing acute diarrhea at doses around 10^{10} CFU per day, whereas other strains may require higher or lower thresholds to exert comparable effects (Li et al., 2019). The challenge, however, lies in ensuring that these CFU counts remain viable from production to consumption—a task complicated by multiple environmental and logistical factors.

During manufacturing, storage, and transportation, probiotic viability naturally declines. Temperature fluctuations, humidity, oxygen exposure, and prolonged storage time can all reduce bacterial survival rates. Even when products are manufactured with the correct CFU count, the number of live cells at the point of consumption may be far lower. Pharmaceutical-grade probiotics employ technologies such as microencapsulation, lyophilization (freeze-drying), and controlled-release coatings to maintain cell viability under varying conditions. However, most over-the-counter or food-grade probiotics lack such protective measures, making them particularly vulnerable to degradation (Jannah et al., 2022).

A study by Jackson et al. (2019) found that many consumer probiotic products contained significantly fewer viable cells than stated on their labels—sometimes by several orders of magnitude. Additionally, viability loss accelerates near expiration dates or when products are stored improperly, such as at room temperature instead of refrigeration. As a result, consumers may unknowingly ingest doses well below the effective therapeutic threshold, nullifying potential benefits despite accurate initial manufacturing.

5.8.5 Clinical Evidence Requirements and Strain-Specific Documentation

For a microorganism to be legitimately classified as a probiotic under modern scientific and regulatory standards, it must be supported by robust human clinical evidence demonstrating that the specific strain, administered at a defined dose, confers measurable and clinically meaningful health benefits (Office of Dietary Supplements, 2024; Sánchez et al., 2017). This requirement moves beyond the broad or generalized claims often associated with probiotic marketing and instead emphasizes a precision-based approach to probiotic validation. Only those strains that have undergone rigorous, controlled human trials can be considered evidence-based probiotics. By contrast, microorganisms supported solely by in vitro experiments or animal studies fail to meet the evidentiary threshold required to establish safety and efficacy in human use.

This stringent requirement stems from the recognition that mechanistic data from laboratory or animal models rarely translate directly to human outcomes. While in vitro studies may demonstrate that a bacterial strain produces beneficial metabolites, modulates immune signaling, or enhances epithelial integrity, such findings occur in highly controlled systems that exclude the complexity of the human gastrointestinal environment. Factors such as host genetics, baseline microbiome diversity, diet, health status, immune response, and medication use can profoundly alter how a probiotic behaves once administered to humans. For instance, a strain that upregulates tight junction proteins in a cell culture may not exert the same effect in a living human with an already dynamic intestinal ecosystem. Therefore, human trials remain indispensable to confirm that a strain's purported effects occur in vivo and result in meaningful clinical improvements (Goodrich et al., 2014).

Moreover, probiotic science must adhere to the hierarchy of clinical evidence, wherein randomized, double-blind, placebo-controlled trials (RCTs) represent the highest standard. Such studies minimize bias, control for confounding variables, and allow reproducible evaluation of cause-and-effect relationships. Trials should also include pre-registered protocols, appropriate control arms, well-defined endpoints, adequate sample sizes, and transparent reporting. In contrast, evidence from non-randomized studies, open-label trials, case reports, or mechanistic investigations—while valuable for hypothesis generation—provides limited confidence in efficacy claims. Regulatory agencies have increasingly recognized this distinction: for example, the EFSA applies rigorous criteria requiring strain-level RCT data to substantiate specific health claims. Consequently, many probiotic products have failed to meet EFSA's approval threshold due to insufficient strain-specific evidence. Conversely, regulatory leniency in other jurisdictions—including the United States—has allowed marketing of probiotics with broad, nonspecific claims that often extend beyond the available evidence base. This uneven regulatory environment has resulted in a proliferation of commercial probiotic products marketed with overstated or indirect scientific justification (Patro-Golab et al., 2020).

Product labels frequently invoke general research on "probiotics" or cite studies conducted with unrelated strains or at different doses, creating an illusion of scientific validation. Efficacy demonstrated for one strain cannot be extrapolated to another—even within the same species—nor can results obtained at one dosage be assumed to hold at a lower concentration. Such practices blur the line between evidence-based medicine and marketing rhetoric, leaving both consumers and healthcare professionals vulnerable to misinterpretation of probiotic efficacy. Ultimately, ensuring that probiotic claims rest on strain- and dose-specific clinical documentation is essential for advancing probiotic science from anecdotal assertion to reproducible medical evidence.

5.8.6 Commonly Used Probiotic Strains and Their Mechanisms of Action

Probiotics encompass a diverse group of microorganisms that, when administered in adequate amounts, confer specific health benefits to the host. Among the thousands of microbial species identified in the human microbiome, only a select few have been sufficiently characterized and validated through human clinical research. The most widely studied and commercially utilized probiotics belong to the genera *Lactobacillus*, *Bifidobacterium*, *Streptococcus*, and the yeast *Saccharomyces* (Sánchez et al., 2017; Office of Dietary Supplements, 2024). Each genus contains strains with unique genetic, metabolic, and immunological attributes that underpin their strain-specific effects on host health (Goodrich et al., 2014).

5.8.6.1 Lactobacillus Species

Lactobacillus species are Gram-positive, lactic acid-producing bacteria commonly found in fermented foods, the gastrointestinal tract, and mucosal surfaces. They are among the most extensively studied probiotic organisms. LGG remains one of the most clinically validated strains, with numerous randomized controlled trials demonstrating its efficacy in preventing and treating acute infectious diarrhea, particularly in pediatric populations (Szajewska and Kołodziej, 2015). *L. acidophilus* NCFM has been investigated for its role in improving lactose digestion and supporting general digestive comfort, while *L. casei* Shirota is recognized for its immunomodulatory effects and potential to mitigate constipation and reduce respiratory tract infections. *Lactobacillus plantarum*, naturally present in fermented vegetables, exhibits anti-inflammatory properties and shows therapeutic potential in IBD through modulation of mucosal immunity and epithelial barrier integrity. Collectively, these findings highlight the diversity of functions even within a single genus and reinforce the concept that probiotic effects are strain-specific.

5.8.6.2 *Bifidobacterium* Species

Members of the *Bifidobacterium* genus dominate the gut microbiota of breastfed infants and play critical roles in nutrient metabolism, immune maturation, and gut barrier maintenance. *Bifidobacterium animalis* subsp. *lactis* (BB-12) has been widely studied for enhancing bowel regularity, improving stool consistency, and reducing AAD. *Bifidobacterium longum* strains exhibit promising results in clinical studies addressing IBS and UC, where they may reduce abdominal discomfort and mucosal inflammation. *Bifidobacterium infantis* (35,624), highly adapted to metabolize HMOs, contributes to early life gut colonization and immune development and is used in certain infant formulas to mimic the microbiota of breastfed infants. These species collectively support gastrointestinal and immune health across the lifespan, although their benefits depend on strain selection, dosing, and host characteristics.

5.8.6.3 Other Bacterial Probiotics

Beyond *Lactobacillus* and *Bifidobacterium*, other bacterial species have been explored for probiotic potential. *Streptococcus thermophilus*, traditionally employed in yogurt fermentation, has been shown to enhance lactose digestion and exert mild immunomodulatory effects (del Carmen et al. 2014). *Lactococcus lactis* strains, another lactic acid bacterium, have demonstrated potential in modulating inflammation and supporting mucosal immunity (Saleena et al. 2023). Recently, research attention has shifted toward next-generation probiotics—commensal microbes from less traditional genera that are abundant in healthy individuals but often depleted in disease states. Examples include *A. muciniphila*, which strengthens the mucus layer and modulates glucose metabolism; *Faecalibacterium prausnitzii*, a butyrate-producing species associated with anti-inflammatory properties (Sokol et al. 2008); and specific *Clostridium* cluster IV and XIVa strains that regulate immune tolerance. While promising, these next-generation candidates are still in early phases of safety and efficacy evaluation and have yet to reach widespread commercial availability.

5.8.6.4 Yeast Probiotics

Unlike bacterial probiotics, yeast-based probiotics such as *Saccharomyces boulardii* possess distinct biological and therapeutic advantages. Originally isolated from lychee fruit, *S. boulardii* is resistant to antibiotics, making it particularly useful during or after antibiotic therapy. Extensive clinical research supports its role in preventing and treating AAD, traveler's diarrhea, and recurrent *C. difficile* infection (CDI) (McFarland, 2010). Mechanistically, *S. boulardii* enhances intestinal enzyme activity, inhibits pathogen adhesion, and modulates immune signaling pathways that help restore gut homeostasis following dysbiosis.

5.8.7 Clinical Evidence for Probiotic Efficacy

Probiotics have been investigated for a wide range of health conditions, with clinical evidence varying from robust and well-replicated findings to preliminary or conflicting data (Office of Dietary Supplements, 2024; Sánchez et al., 2017). The strength of evidence depends heavily on factors such as strain specificity, dose, study design, population characteristics, and clinical endpoints. High-quality randomized controlled trials (RCTs) and meta-analyses provide the most reliable insights, while observational studies or mechanistic research often offer supportive but non-definitive information.

5.8.7.1 Acute Infectious Diarrhea

The most compelling evidence for probiotic efficacy exists for acute infectious diarrhea, particularly in children (Szajewska and Kołodziej, 2015; Office of Dietary Supplements, 2024). Multiple meta-analyses demonstrate that LGG and *S. boulardii* can shorten the duration of diarrhea by approximately one day and reduce the likelihood of prolonged episodes exceeding four days. While effect sizes are modest, they are clinically meaningful, especially in resource-limited settings where diarrheal diseases significantly contribute to childhood morbidity and mortality. These benefits appear strain-specific and are less consistent with other *Lactobacillus* or *Bifidobacterium* strains not tested in rigorous trials.

5.8.7.2 Antibiotic-Associated Diarrhea

Antibiotic therapy can disrupt the gut microbiome, leading to diarrhea in 5–35% of patients. Several probiotics—including *S. boulardii*, LGG, and multi-strain formulations—have demonstrated significant reductions in the incidence of AAD (Goldenberg et al., 2017; Office of Dietary Supplements, 2024). A 2017 Cochrane review, including over 12,000 participants, reported that probiotics reduce the risk of AAD by approximately 60%, with a number needed to treat 13. Yeast probiotics like *S. boulardii* are particularly advantageous in this context because they remain viable and active even during antibiotic therapy.

5.8.7.3 Clostridioides difficile Infection

CDI is a severe and potentially life-threatening consequence of antibiotic-induced microbiome disruption. Evidence suggests that concurrent probiotic administration may lower the risk of CDI, though effect sizes are smaller than for general AAD (Goldenberg et al., 2017). For recurrent or severe CDI, FMT currently demonstrates superior efficacy compared to probiotic supplementation, representing a more comprehensive intervention targeting the entire gut microbial ecosystem.

5.8.7.4 Irritable Bowel Syndrome

IBS is a heterogeneous functional gastrointestinal disorder characterized by abdominal pain, bloating, and altered bowel habits. Clinical studies and meta-analyses indicate modest benefits from probiotics, particularly for symptom relief related to bloating and gas (Ford et al., 2018). Multi-strain preparations and *Bifidobacterium* species show promise, but heterogeneity in trial design, strain selection, dosing, and patient phenotypes contributes to variable outcomes. The complexity of IBS pathophysiology—including visceral hypersensitivity, dysmotility, and microbiome variability—likely underpins these inconsistent results.

5.8.7.5 Inflammatory Bowel Disease

Probiotics have been investigated in both Crohn's disease and UC with mixed results (Derwa et al., 2017). In UC, certain multi-strain formulations—most notably VSL#3, containing eight bacterial strains—have demonstrated efficacy in inducing and maintaining remission in select studies. Evidence of Crohn's disease is weaker and less reproducible, limiting recommendations for routine probiotic therapy. Consequently, probiotics are generally considered adjunctive therapies rather than primary treatments for IBD.

5.8.7.6 Lactose Intolerance

Probiotic strains that produce lactase, including certain *Lactobacillus* species and *S. thermophilus*, can improve lactose digestion and reduce symptoms such as bloating and diarrhea (Savaiano and Hutkins, 2021). Fermented dairy products containing live cultures are often better tolerated than unfermented milk, highlighting the functional benefit of microbial enzymatic activity.

5.8.7.7 Necrotizing Enterocolitis

Necrotizing enterocolitis (NEC) is a serious intestinal disease primarily affecting preterm infants. Clinical trials and meta-analyses suggest that specific probiotics can reduce the incidence and severity of NEC, with some studies reporting risk reductions exceeding 50% (Aceti et al., 2015). Despite these promising findings, safety concerns remain in this vulnerable population, and variability in probiotic formulations necessitates careful institutional protocols and selection of evidence-based strains.

5.8.7.8 Allergic Conditions

Probiotics have been studied for preventing and managing allergic diseases such as atopic dermatitis, allergic rhinitis, and food allergies (Cuello-Garcia et al., 2015). Results are mixed: some trials report reduced incidence of eczema when probiotics are administered to pregnant women or infants, whereas others show minimal or no effect. Efficacy appears strain-specific and may depend on timing of administration, host genetics, and immune development, leaving the role of probiotics in allergy management unresolved (Goodrich et al., 2014).

5.8.7.9 *Metabolic Health*

Emerging evidence suggests that select probiotics may influence body weight, insulin sensitivity, and lipid metabolism (Vallianou et al., 2019). Some studies report modest improvements in fasting glucose, HbA1c, and cholesterol levels with specific *Lactobacillus* or *Bifidobacterium* strains. Mechanisms may involve modulation of gut permeability, inflammation, and microbial metabolites that influence metabolic signaling pathways. However, observed effects are generally small, and larger, longer-duration trials are needed to clarify the role of probiotics in obesity and metabolic disease management.

5.8.7.10 *Mental Health and Psychobiotics*

The gut–brain axis has spurred interest in "psychobiotics," probiotics that may influence mood, anxiety, depression, and stress (Cryan et al., 2019; Liu et al., 2019). Small-scale trials have reported improvements in mood and stress resilience with specific strains, yet evidence remains preliminary. Large, well-controlled trials with standardized psychiatric outcomes are necessary before psychobiotic interventions can be widely recommended.

5.8.7.11 *Autism Spectrum Disorder*

Alterations in gut microbiota and frequent gastrointestinal symptoms in children with ASD have prompted research into probiotic interventions. Early pilot studies suggest potential improvements in behavior and gut function, but evidence is limited and preliminary. Larger, rigorously controlled trials are required to determine whether probiotics offer meaningful clinical benefits in ASD (Tabouy et al., 2018).

5.8.8 Quality Assurance, Stability, and Labeling Accuracy of Probiotic Products

In addition to strain specificity and dosing, quality assurance, product stability, and labeling accuracy are critical factors that determine the real-world effectiveness of probiotic interventions (Jackson et al., 2019; Patro-Golab et al., 2020). Independent analyses of commercial probiotic products have consistently identified systematic discrepancies between label claims and actual product content. Common issues include the following:

- **Strain misidentification**: Products may contain different microbial strains than those listed on the label.
- **Low viable counts**: The number of live microorganisms is often below the advertised CFU, potentially undermining efficacy.
- **Contaminants**: Some products harbor unintended microbial species not disclosed in product information, raising potential safety concerns (Rinninella et al., 2019; Boyle et al., 2006).
- **Premature viability loss**: Inadequate stabilization during manufacturing, improper shipping conditions, or suboptimal storage at retail and in consumer homes can result in significant reductions in live microbial content.

These issues reflect manufacturing inconsistencies, insufficient quality control measures, and environmental challenges during distribution and storage. Even products leaving the factory with verified CFU counts may experience progressive loss of viability during transit and while stored in typical kitchen environments, where temperature, humidity, and oxygen exposure are rarely controlled to optimal levels. Consumers often lack guidance on proper storage, and expiration dates may not align with the actual window of optimal probiotic viability.

5.8.9 Implications of Quality and Labeling Variability

Quality and labeling discrepancies carry important practical and clinical consequences. A consumer selecting a probiotic product based on advertised strains and CFU counts is often uncertain whether the product contains the correct organisms at effective doses, potentially compromising health outcomes. Healthcare providers face similar challenges when recommending probiotics, as the lack of reliable quality control introduces variability that is independent of strain-specific efficacy. Third-party certification programs—such as U.S. Pharmacopeia (USP), National Sanitation Foundation (NSF), or ConsumerLab—can provide additional verification of strain identity, viable counts, and absence of contaminants. However, the availability of such certifications is limited, and even certified products may experience viability loss if storage conditions are not maintained.

5.8.10 Limitations and Considerations in Probiotic Use

Despite promising evidence for certain clinical applications, several inherent limitations temper the widespread adoption of probiotics (Zmora et al., 2019; Office of Dietary Supplements, 2024).

- **Strain specificity**: Benefits demonstrated for a specific strain cannot be extrapolated to other strains, even within the same species. This underscores the necessity of selecting strains validated through human clinical trials.
- **Transient colonization**: Most probiotic strains do not permanently engraft in the gut. Their beneficial effects are typically observed only during active supplementation, and they diminish after cessation.
- **Inter-individual variability**: Responsiveness to probiotics varies widely among individuals, influenced by baseline microbiome composition, diet, genetics, health status, and environmental exposures (Goodrich et al., 2014).
- **Product quality inconsistency**: Many commercial formulations fail to meet label claims, contain insufficient viable microbes, or include strains lacking evidence for the claimed health benefit. This variability introduces an additional layer of uncertainty beyond strain-specific efficacy and dosing considerations.

5.9 PREBIOTICS: TARGETED NUTRITION FOR BENEFICIAL GUT MICROBES

Prebiotics offer a strategic and complementary method for modulating the gut microbiome by providing nutrients that selectively support the growth and activity of beneficial microorganisms. Unlike probiotics, which introduce exogenous strains of live bacteria, prebiotics act as a form of "selective fuel," nourishing the host's existing microbial populations. This endogenous support potentially offers a more stable and sustainable means of influencing microbiome composition and function (Gibson et al., 2017).

The concept of prebiotics has evolved significantly since it was first introduced. Originally defined in 1995 as non-digestible food components that confer health benefits by selectively stimulating the growth or activity of beneficial bacteria in the colon, the definition was later revised in 2016 to encompass a broader and more mechanistic understanding. The updated definition reads, "A substrate that is selectively utilized by host microorganisms conferring a health benefit." This modern definition emphasizes function over chemical structure and recognizes that prebiotic activity is not confined to the colon but may occur throughout the gastrointestinal tract. Importantly, it shifts the focus toward host–microbe interactions and measurable health outcomes (Hughes et al., 2022; Wilson et al., 2020; Maier et al., 2017).

To be classified as a prebiotic, a compound must meet several well-established criteria:

- **Resistance to digestion**: It must withstand gastric acidity, enzymatic hydrolysis, and absorption in the upper gastrointestinal tract.
- **Fermentability**: It must be fermented by the host's intestinal microbiota.
- **Selective stimulation**: It must preferentially stimulate the growth and/or activity of beneficial bacteria.
- **Health benefit**: Its effects must translate into measurable benefits for the host's health.

5.9.1 Major Classes of Prebiotics

A variety of compounds have been identified as prebiotics, with some of the most researched including dietary fibers, oligosaccharides, RS, and select polyphenols. Below are the primary classes and their distinctive features (Hughes et al., 2022; Wilson et al., 2020; Maier et al., 2017).

5.9.1.1 Inulin and Fructo-Oligosaccharides

Inulin-type fructans, naturally occurring polysaccharides composed of β-linked fructose units, resist digestion in the upper gastrointestinal tract and are found in foods such as chicory root, Jerusalem artichoke, garlic, onions, and leeks. Fructo-oligosaccharides (FOS) are shorter-chain forms of inulin, and both inulin and FOS are selectively fermented by beneficial gut bacteria, including *Bifidobacterium* and *Lactobacillus* species, producing SCFAs like acetate and butyrate that support gut health. Clinical studies indicate that these compounds can improve bowel regularity, enhance calcium absorption, modulate lipid metabolism, and promote satiety (Mitmesser and Combs, 2017).

5.9.1.2 Galacto-Oligosaccharides

Galacto-oligosaccharides (GOS), composed of galactose chains ending in glucose, occur naturally in human milk or are synthetically produced from lactose using β-galactosidase enzymes. They selectively promote the growth of *Bifidobacterium* species, particularly in infants, and are commonly added to infant formulas to mimic the beneficial effects of HMOs. GOS have also been shown to modulate immune responses and reduce the risk of infections and allergic diseases during early life (Hu et al., 2024; Mei et al., 2022).

5.9.1.3 Resistant Starches

RS are types of dietary starch that escape digestion in the small intestine and undergo fermentation in the colon (Hughes et al., 2022; Wilson et al., 2020; Maier et al., 2017). There are four main types of RS:

- **RS1**: Physically inaccessible starch (e.g., whole or coarsely ground grains)
- **RS2**: Native granular starch (e.g., raw potato, green banana)
- **RS3**: Retrograded starch (formed when cooked starchy foods are cooled)
- **RS4**: Chemically modified starches

RS is fermented by a broader range of microbes, including important butyrate-producing species such as *F. prausnitzii* and *Roseburia*. Butyrate is especially beneficial as an energy source for colonocytes and is known for its anti-inflammatory and anti-carcinogenic properties.

5.9.1.4 Human Milk Oligosaccharides

HMOs are structurally diverse carbohydrates found in high concentrations in human breast milk—over 200 distinct forms have been identified. They serve as a primary prebiotic source for neonates, particularly stimulating *B. longum* subsp. *infantis*, which has specialized machinery to metabolize HMOs. Beyond prebiotic action, HMOs function as decoy receptors to block pathogen adhesion and play vital roles in shaping the infant immune system and gut barrier integrity (Bode, 2012).

5.9.1.5 Polyphenols as Emerging Prebiotics

Polyphenols are bioactive compounds present in plant-based foods such as fruits, vegetables, tea, coffee, and cocoa. Many polyphenols bypass absorption in the small intestine and reach the colon, where they are metabolized by the gut microbiota into smaller, bioactive metabolites. This bidirectional interaction—the modulation of microbial composition by polyphenols and microbial transformation of polyphenols—suggests a prebiotic-like role. Studies have shown that polyphenol-rich diets can increase beneficial bacteria like *A. muciniphila* and *Lactobacillus*, with implications for metabolic and inflammatory conditions (Gibson et al., 2017).

5.9.2 Mechanisms of Prebiotic Action

Prebiotics confer health benefits through a series of interrelated biological processes, most of which stem from their selective fermentation by beneficial gut microbes. This targeted interaction influences host metabolism, immune responses, and gut environment, underscoring the complexity and systemic relevance of prebiotic function (Gibson et al., 2017; Davani-Davari et al., 2019).

5.9.2.1 Production of Short-Chain Fatty Acids

A central mechanism of prebiotic action is the microbial fermentation of prebiotics in the colon, resulting in the production of SCFAs, primarily acetate, propionate, and butyrate.

- **Butyrate**: It serves as the principal energy source for colonocytes (epithelial cells of the colon), promotes tight junction expression, and supports mucosal barrier integrity. It also exhibits anti-inflammatory and anti-neoplastic properties, making it critical for gut homeostasis and protection against colorectal cancer.
- **Propionate**: Primarily absorbed and metabolized by the liver, propionate may reduce hepatic glucose production (gluconeogenesis) and modulate lipid metabolism. It has also been implicated in satiety regulation and may influence appetite through gut–brain signaling.
- **Acetate**: The most abundant SCFA in circulation, acetate enters systemic circulation and can reach peripheral tissues, including the brain and adipose tissue. It may influence cholesterol metabolism, appetite regulation, and blood pressure control.

Collectively, SCFAs have systemic effects beyond the gut, contributing to metabolic regulation, anti-inflammatory signaling, and immune modulation.

5.9.2.2 *Selective Enrichment of Beneficial Microbes*

Prebiotics are specifically designed to be preferentially metabolized by beneficial microbial taxa, particularly *Bifidobacterium* and *Lactobacillus* species. This selective stimulation enhances colonization resistance against pathogenic bacteria by competing for nutrients and binding sites (Buffie and Pamer, 2013; Theriot and Young, 2014). Enriched beneficial microbes can modulate host immune responses, reduce intestinal inflammation, and produce metabolites with positive physiological effects. Simultaneously, prebiotic fermentation may reduce the relative abundance of potentially harmful bacteria, contributing to a more stable and resilient microbial ecosystem (Hughes et al., 2022; Wilson et al., 2020; Maier et al., 2017).

5.9.2.3 *Modulation of Gut pH and Mineral Absorption*

Fermentation of prebiotics leads to the accumulation of SCFAs and other organic acids, lowering the pH of the colonic environment. Acidification of the colon creates conditions unfavorable for the growth of many pathogenic bacteria, providing an indirect protective mechanism against infection (Buffie and Pamer, 2013; Theriot and Young, 2014). A lower colonic pH also increases the solubility and bioavailability of essential minerals, especially calcium, magnesium, and iron. These changes may contribute to enhanced mineral absorption and improved skeletal health, particularly in populations with increased nutritional needs.

5.9.2.4 *Immune System Modulation*

Prebiotics modulate both local and systemic immune function through direct and indirect mechanisms:

- SCFAs, particularly butyrate, influence the differentiation and function of regulatory T cells (Tregs), dendritic cells, and macrophages.
- Prebiotic-induced increases in beneficial microbes have been associated with elevated production of secretory immunoglobulin A (sIgA), which plays a crucial role in mucosal defense (Hughes et al., 2022; Wilson et al., 2020; Maier et al., 2017).
- Improved epithelial barrier function, mediated by both microbial and SCFA activity, helps prevent translocation of harmful microbes and reduces systemic inflammation.
- Some evidence suggests that prebiotics may modulate cytokine production, leading to reduced pro-inflammatory signaling and improved immune homeostasis.

5.9.2.5 *Clinical Evidence for Prebiotic Benefits*

A growing body of clinical research supports the health-promoting effects of prebiotics, though responses can vary based on individual microbiome composition, dose, and type of prebiotic. Below is a summary of key areas of evidence:

1. **Gastrointestinal health**

- **Bowel regularity**: Inulin and GOS are consistently shown to increase stool frequency and soften stool consistency, making them effective in managing constipation (Hughes et al., 2022; Wilson et al., 2020; Maier et al., 2017).
- **IBS**: Some individuals with IBS report symptom improvement with prebiotic supplementation, likely due to improved gut barrier integrity and reduced visceral hypersensitivity. However, others experience worsened symptoms (e.g., bloating, gas), especially at higher doses, reflecting inter-individual variability (Whorwell et al., 2006; Yuan et al., 2017; Wilson et al., 2020).
- **Microbiome balance**: Clinical trials show that prebiotics increase levels of *Bifidobacterium* and other beneficial taxa, contributing to a healthier microbial profile.

5.9.2.6 *Calcium Absorption and Bone Health*

Inulin-type fructans have been shown in multiple studies, especially in adolescents and postmenopausal women, to enhance calcium absorption, which is a critical factor for maintaining bone health. The proposed mechanisms include increased calcium solubility in the acidic environment of the colon, as well as potential upregulation of calcium transporters in the intestinal epithelium, facilitating more efficient uptake. While short-term clinical trials demonstrate improvements in calcium absorption, evidence linking these effects to long-term outcomes such as increased bone mineral density (BMD) and reduced fracture risk remains limited, highlighting the need for extended studies to fully establish their role in supporting skeletal health over the lifespan (Hughes et al., 2022; Wilson et al., 2020; Maier et al., 2017).

5.9.2.7 Metabolic Health and Weight Management

Prebiotics have garnered significant attention for their potential to support metabolic health and aid in weight management by modulating glucose regulation, lipid metabolism, and body weight. Meta-analyses indicate modest but statistically meaningful benefits, including reduced fasting blood glucose, improved insulin sensitivity as reflected by lower homeostatic model assessment for insulin resistance (HOMA-IR) scores, and decreased triglyceride levels. These effects are thought to arise through several mechanisms, such as SCFA-mediated stimulation of gut hormones like GLP-1 and PYY, which regulate appetite and insulin secretion, as well as reductions in intestinal permeability and systemic inflammation. Additionally, prebiotics can reshape the gut microbiota in ways that influence energy harvest and fat storage. Despite these promising findings, the effects are often small and variable across studies, underscoring the need for further research to clarify optimal prebiotic types, dosing strategies, intervention duration, and individual response factors (Vallianou et al., 2020).

5.9.2.8 Immune Support

Several studies have indicated that prebiotics may enhance immune responses, particularly in populations with immature or compromised immune systems. Observed effects include the following:

- Improved vaccine efficacy, with greater antibody titers following immunization
- Reduced incidence or severity of upper respiratory tract infections
- Lower levels of pro-inflammatory markers such as TNF-α and IL-6

These benefits are most pronounced in infants, older adults, and immunocompromised individuals, suggesting prebiotics may help fortify the immune system in vulnerable groups.

5.10 SYNBIOTICS: SYNERGISTIC PAIRING OF PROBIOTICS AND PREBIOTICS

Synbiotics are formulations that combine probiotics—live beneficial microorganisms—with prebiotics, which are non-digestible substrates that selectively fuel those microbes. The central idea behind synbiotics is to enhance the survival, colonization, and activity of probiotic strains by simultaneously delivering their preferred energy sources. This strategy is intended to optimize the functional efficacy of both components (Swanson et al., 2020).

5.10.1 Mechanistic Rationale

- **Enhanced probiotic viability**: Prebiotics in synbiotic formulations may help buffer probiotics against harsh gastrointestinal conditions, improving survival through the stomach and small intestine.
- **Targeted microbial support**: Pairing specific probiotics with their complementary prebiotics—such as *Bifidobacterium* with FOS—can promote more robust colonization and activity in the gut.
- **Amplified metabolic and immune effects**: By fueling probiotic growth and activity, synbiotics may increase the production of health-promoting metabolites like SCFAs, enhance immune signaling, and modulate inflammation more effectively than either component alone.

5.10.2 Types of Synbiotics

Synbiotics are generally categorized into two main types:

- **Complementary synbiotics**: Combine a probiotic and a prebiotic that are independently beneficial but not necessarily designed to work together.
- **Synergistic synbiotics**: Intentionally match a specific probiotic strain with its known selective substrate to promote targeted effects.

5.10.2.1 *Clinical Evidence and Challenges*

Despite the theoretical promise of synbiotics, clinical trials have yielded mixed results.

- **Positive findings**: Some studies report on synergistic effects, such as improved digestive function, enhanced immune responses, reduced inflammation, or better metabolic outcomes compared to probiotics or prebiotics alone.
- **Neutral findings**: Other trials have found no significant advantage of synbiotics over single-component interventions (Swanson et al., 2020; Ford et al., 2018).

Factors contributing to variability include differences in

- Probiotic strains and prebiotic types used
- Dosages and duration of treatment
- Host microbiome composition and baseline health
- Study design and endpoints

5.11 FERMENTED FOODS: ANCIENT TRADITIONS, MODERN INSIGHTS

Fermented foods are among the oldest forms of biotechnology, with roots extending back thousands of years. Originally developed for preservation, flavor enhancement, and safety, these foods have gained modern scientific attention for their potential to positively influence gut health and overall well-being (Marco et al., 2021).

5.11.1 What Are Fermented Foods?

Fermented foods are produced through controlled microbial growth and enzymatic transformation of food components. These processes involve a diverse array of microorganisms—bacteria, yeasts, and molds—that transform raw ingredients into products with extended shelf life, enhanced taste, and often functional bioactivity (Marco et al., 2021; Mukherjee et al., 2024; Chan et al., 2023).

5.11.1.1 *Types of Fermentation*

Fermentation is a metabolic process in which microorganisms convert organic compounds—primarily carbohydrates—into simpler molecules, producing characteristic flavors, textures, and bioactive compounds. The three main types of fermentation relevant to food production are as follows:

Lactic acid fermentation: Dominated by LAB such as *Lactobacillus, Lactococcus, Leuconostoc,* and *Pediococcus* species. These bacteria convert sugars into lactic acid, lowering pH and creating an acidic environment that preserves food and inhibits pathogenic microorganisms (Buffie and Pamer, 2013; Theriot and Young, 2014). This process is central to yogurt, kefir, sauerkraut, kimchi, and many other fermented vegetables and dairy products.

Alcoholic fermentation: Primarily conducted by yeasts, especially *Saccharomyces cerevisiae,* which metabolize sugars into ethanol and carbon dioxide. This process is fundamental to beer, wine, and certain fermented beverages like kefir and kombucha, where yeasts coexist with bacteria (Marco et al., 2021; Mukherjee et al., 2024; Chan et al., 2023).

Acetic acid fermentation: Performed by acetic acid bacteria (AAB) such as *Acetobacter* and *Gluconacetobacter* species, which oxidize ethanol to acetic acid. This process is essential for vinegar production and contributes to the distinctive tang of kombucha (Marco et al., 2021; Mukherjee et al., 2024; Chan et al., 2023).

5.11.1.2 *Bioactive Components of Fermented Foods*

Fermentation transforms raw ingredients into nutritionally enhanced products containing a variety of bioactive compounds:

- **Live microorganisms**: Viable bacteria and yeasts that may exert probiotic effects if consumed in adequate quantities and survive gastrointestinal transit.
- **Organic acids**: Lactic, acetic, propionic, and butyric acids that contribute to preservation, flavor, and potential metabolic benefits.
- **Bioactive peptides**: Short amino acid sequences released during proteolysis that may exhibit antihypertensive, antioxidant, antimicrobial, and immunomodulatory activities.

- **Vitamins**: Enhanced levels of B vitamins (B_2, B_{12}, folate) and vitamin K_2, particularly in fermented dairy and soy products.
- **Polyphenol metabolites**: Microbial transformation of plant polyphenols into more bioavailable forms with enhanced antioxidant capacity.
- **Exopolysaccharides**: Microbial-produced polysaccharides such as kefiran that may modulate immune function and gut health.
- **SCFAs**: Although primarily produced by colonic fermentation of dietary fibers, some fermented foods may contain preformed SCFAs or substrates that promote their production.

Importantly, not all fermented foods contain live microbes (e.g., pasteurized products, baked goods), and not all live microbes in fermented foods meet the criteria for probiotics. The term "probiotic" should be reserved for strains with documented health benefits in controlled human studies, whereas fermented foods may offer health advantages through mechanisms beyond live microbial delivery.

5.11.1.3 Specific Fermented Foods

5.11.1.3.1 YOGURT: COMPOSITION AND MICROBIOLOGY

Yogurt is among the most widely consumed fermented dairy products worldwide and represents a cornerstone of functional nutrition. It is traditionally produced by fermenting milk with specific thermophilic LAB—*S. thermophilus* and *Lactobacillus delbrueckii* subsp. *bulgaricus*—which operate in a synergistic relationship (Fisberg and Machado, 2015).

During fermentation, *S. thermophilus* initiates rapid growth, generating formic acid and carbon dioxide that stimulate *Lactobacillus bulgaricus*. In turn, *L. bulgaricus* releases amino acids and small peptides from milk proteins, which enhance *S. thermophilus* growth. This cooperative metabolism leads to acidification of the milk, transforming lactose into lactic acid and conferring yogurt's characteristic texture, flavor, and extended shelf life.

Traditional yogurt typically contains 10^7–10^9 CFU/g of viable bacteria, primarily the two starter cultures. However, "probiotic yogurts" are formulated with additional strains chosen for specific health-promoting properties. These often include *L. acidophilus*, *L. casei*, *L. rhamnosus*, *B. animalis* subsp. *lactis*, and *B. longum* (Fisberg and Machado, 2015). The inclusion of such probiotics can enhance the total bacterial load and introduce strains capable of surviving gastric acidity and bile exposure. Nonetheless, as emphasized in probiotic research, strain specificity and dose validation are critical: a product labeled containing probiotic species does not guarantee clinical efficacy unless the exact strains and their effective doses have been verified in well-controlled human studies (Patro-Golab et al., 2020).

Beyond its microbial content, yogurt is a nutrient-dense food providing high-quality protein, calcium, phosphorus, potassium, and essential B vitamins such as B_2 (riboflavin) and B_{12} (cobalamin) (Fisberg and Machado, 2015). Fermentation partially hydrolyzes lactose into glucose and galactose, making yogurt easier to digest for individuals with lactose intolerance. Moreover, proteolytic activity during fermentation generates bioactive peptides that may exert antihypertensive, antioxidant, and immunomodulatory effects, potentially contributing to the health-promoting reputation of yogurt.

A large body of epidemiological research associates regular yogurt consumption with improved metabolic and cardiovascular outcomes, including reduced risk of type 2 diabetes, enhanced weight management, and improved BMD (Fernandez and Marette, 2017). Randomized controlled trials (RCTs) support specific benefits such as enhanced lactose digestion, improved immune function—especially in elderly populations—and decreased incidence of AAD. However, the precise mechanisms remain debated: some benefits may arise from live bacteria, while others may result from nutritional components such as calcium, protein, or fermentation-derived peptides.

Despite these potential benefits, the nutritional quality of commercial yogurts varies widely. Many contain added sugars, thickeners, and flavoring agents that can offset or obscure health effects. Therefore, health-conscious consumers should evaluate product labeling carefully, considering sugar content, bacterial strains, and live culture counts rather than assuming all yogurts confer uniform benefits.

5.11.1.3.2 KEFIR: A COMPLEX MICROBIAL CONSORTIUM

Kefir, a traditional fermented milk drink originating from the Caucasus region, is distinguished by its complex and self-sustaining microbial ecosystem. It is produced by inoculating milk with kefir grains—gelatinous granules composed of bacteria and yeasts embedded in a matrix of proteins and polysaccharides, mainly kefiran (Rosa et al., 2017).

Kefir harbors an exceptionally diverse microbial community, with total bacterial counts of 10^8–10^9 CFU/g and yeast counts of 10^6–10^7 CFU/g. LAB dominate, accounting for roughly 83–90% of the microbiota. Key bacterial species include *Lactobacillus kefiranofaciens* (unique to kefir), *Lactobacillus kefiri*, *L. lactis*, and *Leuconostoc mesenteroides*. Yeasts such as *S. cerevisiae*, *Kluyveromyces marxianus*, *Candida kefyr*, and *Kazachstania unispora* coexist symbiotically, while some formulations also include AAB.

This microbial interplay produces a variety of bioactive compounds, including kefiran, organic acids, vitamins, amino acids, and peptides with antioxidant and immunomodulatory properties. Yeasts contribute mild effervescence and trace ethanol (usually <1%), enriching kefir's sensory complexity.

Emerging clinical and experimental research highlights kefir's multifaceted health effects. Compared with yogurt, kefir may more effectively alleviate lactose intolerance, owing to its diverse microbial lactase activity. Human and animal studies suggest kefir supports immune modulation, anti-inflammatory activity, improved glycemic control, and positive alterations in gut microbiota composition (Rosa et al., 2017; Fernandez and Marette, 2017). Some in vitro studies report antimicrobial and potential anti-carcinogenic effects, although human trials are still limited. The diversity of kefir's microbiota likely contributes to its broad functional range, potentially offering more comprehensive probiotic effects than simpler dairy fermentations like yogurt.

5.11.1.3.3 KOMBUCHA: A FERMENTED TEA BEVERAGE

Kombucha is a fermented tea beverage with origins in East Asia, now globally popular for its purported detoxifying and probiotic properties. It is produced by fermenting sweetened tea—commonly black or green—with a symbiotic culture of bacteria and yeast (SCOBY), forming a cellulose-rich gelatinous pellicle (Kapp and Sumner, 2019).

Kombucha contains 10^6–10^8 CFU/mL of viable microorganisms, with yeasts often outnumbering bacteria. The bacterial component is dominated by AAB, notably *Komagataeibacter xylinus* (formerly *Gluconacetobacter xylinus*), *Gluconacetobacter*, and *Acetobacter aceti*. The yeast community includes *Zygosaccharomyces bailii*, *S. cerevisiae*, and *Brettanomyces bruxellensis*. Unlike dairy cultures, kombucha microbes form a structured biofilm (the SCOBY) that can be propagated indefinitely for repeated fermentations (Marco et al., 2021; Mukherjee et al., 2024; Chan et al., 2023).

In addition to live microbes, kombucha contains organic acids (acetic, gluconic, glucuronic), polyphenols, and their metabolites from tea, B vitamins, amino acids, and low levels of ethanol (0.5–2%). Some commercial varieties are further fermented with fruit juices to enhance flavor and functional properties (Kapp and Sumner, 2019).

Although kombucha has a long history of traditional use, robust clinical evidence for its health benefits remains limited. Proposed mechanisms include antioxidant activity (from tea polyphenols), detoxification via glucuronic acid conjugation, antimicrobial effects, and modulation of gut microbiota. Preclinical studies suggest potential benefits for liver protection, blood glucose regulation, and immune support, but controlled human trials are scarce.

Kombucha's increasing popularity has raised safety concerns, particularly regarding home-brewed versions, which may harbor contaminants or develop excessive acidity and alcohol content. Overconsumption of acidic kombucha may contribute to dental erosion or digestive discomfort. Therefore, moderation and adherence to hygienic fermentation practices are essential for safe consumption (Nummer, 2013; Jayabalan et al., 2014; Kapp and Sumner, 2019).

5.11.1.3.4 SAUERKRAUT AND KIMCHI

Sauerkraut (fermented cabbage from Central and Eastern Europe) and kimchi (a Korean fermented vegetable dish typically made with napa cabbage, radish, garlic, and chili) are rich sources of LAB, primarily *Leuconostoc*, *Lactobacillus*, and *Weissella* species (Plengvidhya et al., 2007; Jung et al., 2014; Zabat et al., 2018).The fermentation process enhances the nutritional value of the vegetables by increasing vitamin C and vitamin K and producing organic acids and antioxidant compounds. These foods are also abundant in dietary fiber and phytochemicals from raw vegetables (Peñas et al., 2017; Park et al., 2014).

Regular consumption of sauerkraut and kimchi has been associated with improved gut health, enhanced immune function, and anti-inflammatory effects in both animal and human studies. Some evidence also suggests beneficial modulation of gut microbiota composition and reduction in intestinal pathogens. However, due to their high sodium content, moderation is recommended for individuals with hypertension or cardiovascular disease risk (Song and Lee, 2014; Kim et al., 2012; Lee et al., 2012).

5.11.1.3.5 FERMENTED SOY PRODUCTS

Fermented soy foods—including tempeh, miso, natto, and fermented tofu—play an important role in Asian diets and represent rich sources of plant-based protein and bioactive compounds (Marco et al., 2021; Mukherjee et al., 2024; Chan et al., 2023).

Tempeh, originating from Indonesia, is produced by fermentation with *Rhizopus oligosporus* and contains live fungi, prebiotic fibers, and isoflavones with antioxidant and estrogenic activity (Hughes et al., 2022; Wilson et al., 2020; Maier et al., 2017).

Miso, a fermented soybean paste inoculated with *Aspergillus oryzae*, *Lactobacillus*, and *Pediococcus* species, is valued for its savory umami flavor and rich amino acid profile.

Natto, fermented with *Bacillus subtilis* var. *natto*, is particularly noteworthy for its high vitamin K_2 content and the enzyme nattokinase, which has been linked to antithrombotic and cardiovascular protective effects.

Fermented tofu (also called preserved or "stinky" tofu) involves mixed bacterial and fungal fermentation, producing peptides and fatty acids with unique flavors and potential antioxidant and antimicrobial properties (Marco et al., 2021; Mukherjee et al., 2024; Chan et al., 2023).

Collectively, these soy-based fermented products offer a combination of functional nutrients, bioactive peptides, and beneficial microbes that contribute to cardiovascular, metabolic, and gastrointestinal health.

5.11.1.3.6 SOURDOUGH BREAD

Sourdough fermentation employs a natural starter culture composed of wild yeasts (commonly *S. cerevisiae* and *Candida milleri*) and LAB (*Lactobacillus sanfranciscensis*, *L. plantarum*, and others). These microbes ferment the dough over several hours, breaking down phytic acid (which binds minerals) and partially hydrolyzing gluten proteins, resulting in improved mineral bioavailability and digestive tolerance.

Although the baking process kills most live microbes, the metabolic byproducts of fermentation—such as organic acids and exopolysaccharides—remain, contributing to the bread's flavor, extended shelf life, and potential postbiotic effects. Thus, while sourdough may not deliver live probiotics, it can still confer digestive and metabolic advantages compared to conventionally leavened bread.

5.11.1.3.7 CHEESE

Cheese fermentation involves complex microbial consortia, including LAB, propionic acid bacteria, *Brevibacterium*, and yeasts, which contribute to flavor, texture, and bioactive compound formation. Although pasteurization and aging processes reduce live bacterial counts in many commercial cheeses, ripened and raw-milk cheeses often retain viable microbes and metabolites with functional properties (Helal and Tagliazucchi, 2023b).

Certain aged cheeses, such as Parmigiano-Reggiano, Gouda, and Cheddar, may exert cardiometabolic benefits beyond their nutrient profile—potentially due to bioactive peptides, conjugated linoleic acid (CLA), and fermentation-derived metabolites. Recent studies suggest that habitual cheese consumption is not associated with increased cardiovascular risk and may, in some cases, be protective, challenging traditional dietary assumptions.

5.11.2 Health Benefits of Fermented Foods

Scientific interest in fermented foods is increasing due to their potential to modulate the gut microbiome and influence immune function, digestive health, and mental well-being. By providing dietary microbial exposure, these foods may support immune education and resilience. Ongoing epidemiological and mechanistic studies are exploring the long-term health impacts of regular fermented food consumption, with some evidence suggesting potential benefits in reducing the risk of type 2 diabetes, obesity, cardiovascular disease, and depression, although more rigorous human trials are needed to confirm these effects.

5.11.2.1 Type 2 Diabetes and Cardiometabolic Health

Among the various chronic disease outcomes associated with fermented food consumption, the evidence for type 2 diabetes prevention is particularly robust. Multiple large-scale prospective cohort studies and meta-analyses demonstrate consistent inverse associations between yogurt intake and type 2 diabetes risk. A comprehensive 2014 meta-analysis of three major U.S. cohorts (Health Professionals Follow-Up Study, Nurses' Health Study, and Nurses' Health Study II) encompassing 194,458 participants and 15,156 incident type 2 diabetes cases found that yogurt intake was significantly associated with reduced type 2 diabetes risk, with a pooled hazard ratio of 0.82 (95% CI: 0.70–0.96) per one serving per day increment (Chen et al., 2014). A subsequent 2016 dose-response meta-analysis of 22 cohort studies including 579,832 individuals and 43,118 type 2 diabetes cases found that at 80 grams per day yogurt intake, the relative risk was 0.86 (95% CI: 0.83–0.90) compared with no yogurt consumption (Gijsbers et al., 2016).

This observational evidence is corroborated by interventional data demonstrating that fermented foods produce significant improvements in metabolic parameters. A 2023 meta-analysis of 18 randomized controlled trials with 843 participants found that fermented food consumption in diabetic and prediabetic patients significantly improved fasting blood glucose, insulin resistance (HOMA-IR), total cholesterol, low-density lipoprotein cholesterol, and diastolic blood pressure (Zhang et al., 2023). Additionally, a systematic review of 16 randomized controlled trials examining LAB fermented foods confirmed significant beneficial effects on hemoglobin A1c, fasting plasma glucose, and fasting serum insulin in adults with prediabetes or type 2 diabetes (Rezazadegan et al., 2022). The mechanisms underlying these metabolic benefits likely involve modulation of gut microbiota composition, production of bioactive peptides during fermentation, improvement of intestinal barrier function, and favorable effects on incretin hormone secretion.

5.11.2.2 Cardiovascular Disease

Evidence for cardiovascular disease benefits demonstrates moderate rather than definitive support. A 2020 narrative review of prospective cohort studies found that fermented milk intake was associated with a 4% reduction in combined risk of stroke, ischemic heart disease, and cardiovascular mortality (Companys et al., 2020). A 2021 dose-response meta-analysis of prospective cohort studies reported that yogurt consumption was associated with reduced cardiovascular disease risk, with the strongest protective effects observed at moderate intake levels (Guo et al., 2021). However, comprehensive reviews emphasize that while certain fermented dairy products demonstrate cardiovascular protection, many mechanistic aspects remain uncertain and require better-designed studies with standardized methodologies to establish definitive causal relationships (Marco et al., 2021).

5.11.2.3 Obesity and Weight Management

The relationship between fermented foods and obesity presents more equivocal findings. While some systematic reviews have reported that probiotic fermented milk products produced significant reductions in body weight and body mass index in intervention studies (Koutnikova et al., 2019), a 2025 meta-analysis specifically examining fermented dairy and abdominal obesity found that while trends toward benefit existed, the pooled effect was not statistically significant (Mirmohammadkhani et al., 2025). Similarly, a 2022 dose-response meta-analysis of cohort studies found only modest associations between dairy consumption and reduced obesity risk, with the effects largely dependent on dairy type and baseline body weight (Feng et al., 2022). The current evidence base suggests that fermented foods may assist with weight management in individuals actively attempting weight loss as part of structured dietary interventions, but their role in obesity prevention at the population level remains unclear and requires further investigation through long-term prospective studies with detailed assessment of dietary patterns and lifestyle factors.

5.11.2.4 Depression and Mental Health

Depression and mental health outcomes present the most conflicting evidence profile. A 2023 meta-analysis of eight cohort studies encompassing 83,533 participants found that fermented dairy food intake was associated with an 11% reduction in depression risk (Godos et al., 2023). However, mechanistic studies examining probiotics, prebiotics, and fermented foods have found only negligible and marginally significant effects on cognitive functioning, suggesting that any mental health benefits may be mediated through indirect pathways rather than direct neurological effects (Reis et al., 2018). Furthermore, the relationship between fermented food consumption and mental health appears complex and potentially dependent on baseline psychiatric status, individual microbiome composition, genetic factors, and other patient-specific characteristics that are not yet fully characterized. Some evidence suggests differential effects based on pre-existing mental health conditions, with potential benefits observed in individuals with diagnosed psychiatric illnesses but unclear or absent effects in psychiatrically healthy populations.

5.11.3 Evidence Quality Summary

The evidence of quality for these health outcomes varies substantially. Type 2 diabetes benefits are supported by multiple large-scale meta-analyses of both observational and interventional studies showing consistent, clinically meaningful effects with plausible biological mechanisms. Cardiovascular benefits demonstrate reasonable but less robust support, with smaller effect sizes, greater heterogeneity across studies, and less certainty regarding optimal dosing and specific fermented food types. For obesity and depression, the evidence remains insufficient to draw definitive conclusions, and more rigorous human trials with longer follow-up periods, standardized fermented food interventions, well-defined outcome measures, and comprehensive assessment of potential confounders are essential to confirm or refute these potential effects. Clinical recommendations should therefore emphasize the established benefits for glycemic control and type 2 diabetes prevention while acknowledging the preliminary and uncertain nature of evidence for other cardiometabolic and mental health outcomes. Future research should focus on identifying specific microbial strains, optimal fermentation processes, dosing strategies, and individual patient characteristics that predict therapeutic response.

5.11.3.1 Considerations for Fermented Food Consumption

While fermented foods provide a rich source of nutrients and bioactive compounds, several factors influence their safety, efficacy, and probiotic potential. The concentration of live microbes varies widely depending on fermentation time, storage conditions, and post-processing. Heat treatments such as pasteurization, common in commercial products, effectively sterilize foods and eliminate probiotic activity, although flavor and shelf life are retained.

Many commercial products, particularly flavored yogurts and beverages, contain high levels of added sugars, artificial sweeteners, and stabilizers. These ingredients can counteract health benefits by contributing to metabolic disorders or altering gut microbiota balance. Fermented vegetables, soy sauces, and miso often contain high sodium levels, which may pose risks for individuals with hypertension or kidney disease. Choosing low-sodium versions or moderating intake is recommended (Marco et al., 2021; Mukherjee et al., 2024; Chan et al., 2023).

Certain individuals—especially those with histamine intolerance, immune compromise, or specific gastrointestinal conditions—may experience adverse reactions such as bloating, headaches, or allergic responses. In such cases, healthcare supervision is advisable before incorporating fermented foods regularly.

5.12 DISEASE INTERACTIONS AND THERAPEUTIC APPLICATIONS

The growing recognition of the gut microbiome's pivotal role in human health has positioned fermented foods and probiotics as promising dietary tools in microbiome-targeted therapy (Marco et al., 2021). Evidence from clinical trials and meta-analyses suggests potential benefits for several conditions, though the strength and consistency of evidence vary considerably across disease states.

5.12.1 Gastrointestinal Disorders

5.12.1.1 Inflammatory Bowel Disease (IBD)

IBD—which includes Crohn's disease and UC—is characterized by chronic, relapsing inflammation of the gastrointestinal tract, driven by complex interactions among genetics, the immune system, environmental factors, and the gut microbiome. Individuals with IBD often exhibit reduced microbial diversity, a decline in beneficial commensals such as *F. prausnitzii*, and an increase in pro-inflammatory or pathogenic taxa, including Enterobacteriaceae (Derwa et al., 2017). This microbial imbalance, or dysbiosis, contributes to intestinal barrier dysfunction, mucosal inflammation, and impaired immune regulation.

Probiotic interventions for IBD have shown mixed and disease-specific results. In UC, multiple randomized controlled trials have demonstrated that the multi-strain probiotic formulation VSL#3 can help induce and maintain remission. Two landmark studies, the 2009 Sood et al. trial (n = 147, India) and the 2010 Tursi et al. trial (n = 144, Italy), found that VSL#3 (3.6 trillion CFU/day) significantly improved clinical response rates and induced remission in mild-to-moderate UC when added to standard therapy (Sood et al.,

2009; Tursi et al., 2010). A pediatric trial by Miele et al. (2009) confirmed similar efficacy in children. The largest contemporary meta-analysis of 67 studies through September 2023 confirmed that probiotics significantly induced clinical remission in UC, with VSL#3 showing effectiveness (RR = 1.74, p = 0.004) (Estevinho et al., 2024). Specific formulations show efficacy: probiotics significantly increase remission rates in active UC (RR = 1.51, p = 0.01) and also reduce clinical relapse in pouchitis (RR = 0.18, p < 0.00001). In UC, only *E. coli* Nissle 1917 for maintenance of remission and *Bifidobacterium* and VSL#3 for induction of remission in mild-to-moderate disease have sufficient clinical evidence. *E. coli* Nissle 1917 also demonstrates efficacy for maintenance of remission in UC, though effect sizes remain modest and inter-individual variability substantial (Kruis et al., 2004; Scaladaferri et al., 2016; Losurdo et al., 2015).

Conversely, in Crohn's disease, most probiotic trials have failed to show significant clinical benefit in adults (p = 0.07), though limited data suggest potential benefits in pediatric CD patients (p < 0.01) (Estevinho et al., 2024; Derwa et al., 2017). Differences in effectiveness between UC and CD may relate to distinct lesion patterns and immune-mediated pathophysiology. Prebiotics that stimulate butyrate-producing bacteria (e.g., *Clostridium* cluster IV and XIVa) show preliminary promise for restoring gut homeostasis, though more research is required to confirm efficacy. Given the multifactorial pathogenesis of IBD and distinct disease mechanisms between UC and CD, single-strain probiotic interventions may be insufficient for some phenotypes, emphasizing the need for personalized approaches based on disease subtype and individual microbiome characteristics.

5.12.1.2 Irritable Bowel Syndrome

IBS encompasses a group of functional gastrointestinal disorders marked by chronic abdominal pain, bloating, and altered bowel habits. Although its pathophysiology is multifactorial—encompassing visceral hypersensitivity, gut–brain axis dysfunction, and altered motility—emerging evidence implicates microbiome alterations in its development. Studies comparing IBS patients and healthy controls reveal reduced microbial stability and shifts in taxa such as *Bifidobacterium*, *Lactobacillus*, and *Faecalibacterium*, though findings remain inconsistent across studies (Herndon et al., 2020; Zhuang et al., 2018).

Probiotic research in IBS is extensive yet variable. A 2024 meta-analysis of 16 randomized controlled trials (1264 IBS patients) found that fermented foods increased symptom relief rates (RR 1.22, 95% CI 1.04–1.42, p = 0.01), with fermented milk showing particular benefit (RR 1.19, 95% CI 1.01–1.39, p = 0.04) (Ding et al., 2024). Multiple systematic reviews confirm that probiotics confer modest but statistically significant improvements in global symptom scores, particularly for bloating, flatulence, and abdominal discomfort (Didari et al., 2015; Yang et al., 2024). Multi-strain formulations and *Bifidobacterium* species (e.g., *B. infantis* 35624) appear most promising.

However, outcomes are confounded by high placebo responses, heterogeneous diagnostic criteria, and differences in probiotic strains and dosing. Some individuals may experience worsening symptoms, reinforcing the need for personalized probiotic therapies based on symptom subtype (diarrhea-predominant, constipation-predominant, or mixed) and individual microbiome profile (Whorwell et al., 2006; Yuan et al., 2017; Wilson et al., 2020). The mechanisms underlying efficacy may include modulation of intestinal permeability, motility, visceral sensitivity, immune function, and removal of fermentable oligosaccharides (FODMAPs) during fermentation (Ding et al., 2024).

5.12.1.3 *Helicobacter pylori* Infection

Helicobacter pylori is a Gram-negative bacterium responsible for chronic gastritis and peptic ulcer disease and is a well-established risk factor for gastric cancer. Standard eradication therapy combines antibiotics and PPIs; however, success rates have declined due to antibiotic resistance and treatment-related gastrointestinal side effects.

Adjunctive probiotic therapy has been extensively studied, with multiple meta-analyses demonstrating benefits. The most comprehensive 2024 network meta-analysis of 91 RCTs (13,680 patients) found that adding probiotics to standard treatment significantly increased *H. pylori* eradication rates (78.75 vs 62.43% in controls, OR = 1.62, 95% CI 1.41–1.87, p < 0.0001) (Ahmed et al., 2024). Another 2015 meta-analysis of 45 RCTs (6997 participants) reported an absolute increase of approximately 10% in eradication rates (82.31 vs 72.08%) (Zhang et al., 2015). Meta-analyses specific to *S. boulardii* (10 RCTs) demonstrate a 9% increase in eradication rates (from 73 to

82%) along with significant reductions in AAD (8.5 vs 21% in controls) (Szajewska et al., 2009; McFarland et al., 2015).

Importantly, probiotics also significantly reduced treatment-related side effects, including diarrhea (RR = 0.49, 95% CI 0.40–0.61), nausea/vomiting (RR = 0.69, 95% CI 0.56–0.83), abdominal pain (RR = 0.68, 95% CI 0.54–0.86), and bad taste (RR = 0.64, 95% CI 0.53–0.78) (Ahmed et al., 2024). Duration of probiotic treatment appears important, with courses ≥10–14 days showing superior effects compared to shorter durations (Zhang et al., 2015; Lu et al., 2023). Network meta-analysis suggests *B. longum* may have the highest efficacy (ITT: 81.06 vs 64.88% placebo, OR = 2.52, 95% CI 1.18–5.49) (Ahmed et al., 2024).

While probiotics alone cannot eradicate *H. pylori*, their co-administration with antibiotics appears to improve patient tolerance and treatment adherence, supporting their use as complementary interventions. However, one contrasting 2016 meta-analysis found no significant benefit when probiotics were compared to placebo plus standard therapy (rather than standard therapy alone), suggesting placebo effects may contribute to observed benefits and warranting cautious interpretation (Lu et al., 2016).

5.12.2 Metabolic Disorders

5.12.2.1 Obesity and Weight Management

The gut microbiome plays a pivotal role in regulating energy metabolism, fat storage, appetite, and inflammation (Vallianou et al., 2019). Obese individuals often display distinct microbial patterns, including a higher Firmicutes-to-Bacteroidetes ratio, though findings are not universally consistent. Mechanistically, gut microbes can influence energy harvest from indigestible polysaccharides, modulate satiety hormones (e.g., GLP-1, PYY), and affect systemic inflammatory signaling.

Clinical trials exploring probiotics for weight management have produced modest and strain-specific effects. Certain *Lactobacillus* strains—such as *L. gasseri*, *L. rhamnosus*, and *L. plantarum*—have been linked to small reductions in body weight, BMI, or fat mass in meta-analyses, but overall effects are limited. Prebiotics, such as inulin and FOS, may improve satiety and lipid metabolism, contributing to weight control. However, both probiotics and prebiotics should be regarded as adjuncts to, not substitutes for, dietary and lifestyle interventions.

5.12.2.2 Type 2 Diabetes Mellitus (T2DM)

Dysbiosis of the gut microbiota has been implicated in glucose intolerance, insulin resistance, and metabolic inflammation in type 2 diabetes (Vallianou et al., 2019). Diabetic individuals often exhibit reduced butyrate-producing bacteria and increased opportunistic pathogens.

Clinical studies suggest that probiotic supplementation can modestly improve glycemic control, HbA1c levels, and insulin sensitivity, while reducing inflammatory cytokines. Similarly, prebiotics that favor SCFA production—particularly butyrate—may enhance glucose metabolism by strengthening intestinal barrier integrity and reducing endotoxemia. Interestingly, metformin, a first-line antidiabetic drug, also modifies gut microbiota composition, suggesting that part of its therapeutic effect may be microbiome-mediated. While these findings are encouraging, larger long-term randomized trials are required to define effective microbial targets and optimal combinations of probiotics and prebiotics.

5.12.2.3 Metabolic Syndrome

A comprehensive 2024 meta-analysis of 24 RCTs (1186 patients) demonstrated that probiotic and synbiotic supplementation produced significant but modest improvements in metabolic syndrome parameters, including reductions in body weight (WMD: −0.79 kg, p = 0.001), waist circumference (WMD: −1.04 cm, p = 0.0007), triglycerides (SMD: −0.25, p = 0.0001), total cholesterol (SMD: −0.14, p = 0.03), fasting blood glucose (SMD: −0.20, p = 0.003), and insulin levels (SMD: −0.17, p = 0.03), with increased HDL cholesterol (SMD: 0.15, p = 0.02) (Liu et al., 2025).

Probiotics also positively affected inflammatory biomarkers including interleukin-6 (IL-6), tumor necrosis factor-α (TNF-α), vascular cell adhesion molecule-1 (sVCAM-1), vascular endothelial growth factor (VEGF), and thrombomodulin. Proposed mechanisms include production of SCFAs, modulation of immune responses, promotion of satiety through gut–brain signaling, and enhancement of oxidative metabolism (Tenorio-Jiménez et al., 2020).

5.12.3 Cardiovascular Disease

The gut microbiome influences cardiovascular physiology through several mechanisms, including the production of trimethylamine N-oxide

(TMAO) from dietary choline and carnitine, bile acid metabolism, and systemic inflammation modulation. Certain probiotic strains—such as *Lactobacillus reuteri* and *L. plantarum*—have been shown to reduce serum cholesterol by deconjugating bile acids or incorporating cholesterol into bacterial cell membranes (Wang et al., 2011).

Epidemiological data link regular consumption of fermented dairy foods, particularly yogurt, with lower cardiovascular risk, potentially mediated through improved lipid metabolism and anti-inflammatory effects (Fernandez and Marette, 2017). However, current evidence for clinically meaningful reductions in cardiovascular events from probiotic supplementation remains limited and inconclusive.

5.12.4 Immune-Related Conditions

5.12.4.1 Allergic Diseases

The hygiene hypothesis proposes that limited microbial exposure during early life contributes to rising rates of asthma, eczema, and allergic diseases. Consequently, probiotics have been explored for immune training and allergy prevention (Cuello-Garcia et al., 2015).

Perinatal probiotic supplementation—administered to pregnant mothers and/or infants—has shown modest benefits in reducing atopic dermatitis incidence, particularly with LGG. However, effects on other allergic conditions, such as asthma, allergic rhinitis, and food allergies, are inconsistent. The variability in outcomes reflects differences in strain selection, dosage, timing, and genetic or environmental background of participants. Overall, probiotics may help modulate immune tolerance in early life, but universal recommendations are premature (Fiocchi et al., 2015; More, 2021; West, 2016; Kim et al., 2013).

5.12.4.2 Upper Respiratory Tract Infections

Probiotics have been investigated to prevent and attenuate common respiratory infections, especially in children and older adults. Meta-analyses show modest reductions in infection incidence, duration, and antibiotic use among probiotic users (King et al., 2014). *Lactobacillus* and *Bifidobacterium* species appear most effective, potentially enhancing mucosal immune defenses and promoting systemic immune resilience. Although probiotics are not substitutes for vaccination or hygiene measures, they may represent a low-risk adjunct to immune support in susceptible populations.

5.12.5 Neuropsychiatric Conditions

5.12.5.1 Gut–Brain Axis and Psychobiotics

The gut–brain axis—a bidirectional communication network linking the intestinal microbiome, immune system, and central nervous system—has spurred research into "psychobiotics," or probiotics that may influence mood and cognition (Cryan et al., 2019; Liu et al., 2019).

Small-scale clinical trials suggest that specific strains such as *Lactobacillus helveticus* R0052 and *B. longum* R0175 may reduce anxiety and depressive symptoms and improve stress responses. Mechanistically, these microbes may modulate serotonin pathways, cortisol regulation, and neuroinflammatory processes. However, most studies are limited by small sample sizes, short durations, and variable outcome measures. While the biological rationale is strong, large, long-term, placebo-controlled trials are needed to validate clinical efficacy and identify responder populations.

5.12.5.2 Autism Spectrum Disorder

Children with ASD frequently present with gastrointestinal disturbances and altered gut microbial profiles, fueling interest in microbiome-based interventions. Pilot studies report improvements in gastrointestinal symptoms and behavioral outcomes with specific probiotic strains, but findings remain preliminary. Rigorous, placebo-controlled trials are essential before recommending probiotics as therapeutic agents in ASD (Tang et al., 2025).

5.12.6 Antibiotic-Associated Conditions

5.12.6.1 Clostridioides difficile Infection

Probiotics may help reduce the incidence and recurrence of CDI, particularly when used alongside antibiotic therapy (Goldenberg et al., 2017). However, for recurrent or refractory CDI, FMT remains significantly more effective, achieving >80–90% cure rates. FMT offers comprehensive microbiome restoration, reintroducing entire microbial ecosystems rather than isolated strains.

5.12.6.2 Antibiotic-Induced Dysbiosis

Antibiotic therapy disrupts microbial ecosystems, sometimes leading to long-term dysbiosis, which may predispose individuals to metabolic, infectious, or inflammatory disorders. Probiotics and prebiotics are often employed to support post-antibiotic recovery, but results are mixed (Suez et al., 2018). Some studies suggest probiotics may delay natural microbial reconstitution, whereas prebiotics may facilitate selective regrowth of beneficial taxa, highlighting the importance of strategic timing and formulation in post-antibiotic interventions.

5.12.6.3 Evidence Synthesis and Clinical Implications

The therapeutic impact of fermented foods and probiotics depends critically on microbial strain composition, dosage, formulation, and individual host factors including baseline microbiome composition, genetics, and diet (Marco et al., 2021; Zmora et al., 2019). Current European guidelines support probiotic use primarily for specific indications, *E. coli* Nissle 1917 and VSL#3 for UC, and VSL#3 for pouchitis, but do not recommend probiotics for Crohn's disease.

Given the limitations of current evidence—including heterogeneity in study design, strain selection, and outcome measures—conclusions should be interpreted with caution. Subgroup analyses suggest that intervention effects may be influenced by patient age, intervention duration, geographical location, and disease severity. This underscores the need for personalized nutrition approaches in microbiome research and clinical practice, where interventions are tailored to individual patient characteristics rather than applied universally (Zmora et al., 2019).

5.12.6.4 Safety, Limitations, and Adverse Effects

In general, probiotics, prebiotics, and fermented foods are safe for healthy individuals, but certain populations—including immunocompromised patients, critically ill individuals, and those with central venous catheters—may face increased risks of bacteremia or fungemia. Other considerations include quality control, as microbial identity and viability often deviate from product labels, and dose standardization, which remains poorly regulated. Furthermore, not all probiotics are benign—some may induce gas, bloating, or histamine-related symptoms.

Despite these caveats, when appropriately selected and used, microbiome-targeted strategies—including fermented foods, probiotics, and prebiotics—represent promising adjuncts to conventional therapy for a range of chronic diseases. Continued large-scale, mechanistic, and personalized studies will be key to translating this potential into reproducible clinical practices (Boyle et al., 2006).

5.12.6.5 Probiotic Safety, Limitations, and Emerging Frontiers

While probiotics are widely regarded as safe for the general population, their use is not without potential risks, particularly in vulnerable groups. As clinical use expands, careful evaluation of safety profiles, host susceptibility, and microbial characteristics become increasingly important.

5.12.7 Infection Risk

The most serious safety concern associated with probiotic use is the potential for systemic infections, though such events remain rare (Boyle et al., 2006).

5.12.7.1 Lactobacillus Bacteremia

Despite the long history of safe consumption of *Lactobacillus* species in fermented foods, documented cases of *Lactobacillus* bacteremia have been reported in vulnerable populations. The prevalence of *Lactobacillus* bacteremia is generally low, comprising 0.1–0.2% of all blood culture isolates in hospitalized patients and 0.5% in immunocompromised patients, with risk factors including severe underlying diseases, immune system suppression, admission to intensive care units, and use of central venous catheters (Salminen et al., 2004; Kullar et al., 2023).

Molecular strain typing has confirmed direct links between consumed probiotics and bloodstream infections in several cases. A 17-year-old boy with UC managed with corticosteroids and infliximab developed fever one week after starting LGG probiotics, with 16S rRNA analysis showing a 99.78% match between the blood isolate and the probiotic capsule strain (Vahabnezhad et al., 2013). Similarly, a 79-year-old immunocompromised patient with multiple comorbidities developed recurrent *L. rhamnosus* bacteremia resistant to antibiotic therapy and ultimately succumbed to complications (Eze et al., 2024). A comprehensive 2023 review identified three probiotic strains (*Lacticaseibacillus rhamnosus* GG, *Lactiplantibacillus plantarum*, and *Lacticaseibacillus paracasei*) directly linked to blood isolates from bacteremia patients using molecular identification assays (Kullar et al., 2023).

Beyond bacteremia, other severe *Lactobacillus* infections have been documented. An 82-year-old woman using probiotics for *Clostridium difficile* treatment developed both liver abscess and bacteremia from *Lactobacillus*, requiring prolonged hospitalization (Meini et al., 2015). A retrospective analysis of liver abscess cases caused by *Lactobacillus* found a mean hospital stay of 48 days compared to 16 days for other pyogenic liver abscesses (Kullar et al., 2023).

5.12.7.2 *Saccharomyces boulardii* Fungemia

The yeast probiotic *S. boulardii*, commonly used to prevent AAD, has been associated with fungemia primarily in critically ill or immunocompromised patients. Population-based studies indicate *S. cerevisiae* fungemia accounts for 0.1–3.6% of all fungemia episodes (Muñoz et al., 2005; Rannikko et al., 2021).

An outbreak investigation documented fungemia in three ICU roommates of patients receiving *S. boulardii* preparations, likely due to central venous catheter contamination, emphasizing environmental transmission risks (Cassone et al., 2003). An 80-year-old patient with osteomyelitis developed *S. cerevisiae* fungemia seven days after starting *S. boulardii*, with blood cultures remaining positive despite antifungal therapy; the patient ultimately died from complications including lung empyema (Landaburu et al., 2020). In a series of seven critically ill ICU patients who developed *S. boulardii* fungemia, all were intubated with central venous catheters, and fever resolved only after discontinuing the probiotic and changing catheters (Lherm et al. 2002). Molecular strain typing using genomic and proteomic methods confirmed the relatedness between probiotic capsule strains and fungemia isolates, even in an immunocompetent patient (Hennequin et al., 2000; Appel-da-Silva et al., 2017).

5.12.7.3 *Clinical Implications*

Despite these documented cases, probiotics derived from traditional fermented foods—particularly *Lactobacillus* and *Bifidobacterium* species—retain generally recognized as safe (GRAS) status given their millennia-long history of human consumption (Boyle et al., 2006). One study of 21,652 ICU patients not taking probiotics found only two cases (0.009%) of *Lactobacillus* bacteremia, suggesting baseline risk even without probiotic supplementation (Salminen et al., 2004). However, the prevalence of *Lactobacillus* bacteremia is more common in patients taking probiotics compared to those not taking probiotics (Kullar et al., 2023).

5.12.8 Current Recommendations

Clinicians should exercise caution and avoid probiotic supplementation in

- Severely immunocompromised patients (chemotherapy, HIV/AIDS, organ transplant recipients)
- Critically ill patients in intensive care settings
- Patients with central venous catheters or indwelling medical devices
- Premature infants with underdeveloped immune systems
- Patients with compromised intestinal barrier function (post-surgical, IBD in acute flare)

When infections occur, treatment requires immediate discontinuation of the probiotic, often removal or replacement of central venous catheters, and antifungal or antibiotic therapy as appropriate.

5.12.9 Antibiotic Resistance

Another area of concern is the potential for probiotic strains to harbor or transfer antibiotic resistance genes to pathogenic bacteria within the gut. Although horizontal gene transfer events are considered rare, genomic screening of probiotic candidates for resistance determinants is now standard in quality assurance protocols. The EFSA and U.S. FDA recommend comprehensive genomic and phenotypic characterization before market approval to mitigate this risk (Buffie and Pamer, 2013; Theriot and Young, 2014).

5.12.10 Adverse Metabolic Effects

Some animal studies have suggested that specific *Lactobacillus* strains could promote weight gain or alter lipid metabolism, raising concerns about possible adverse metabolic consequences. However, human data remain inconsistent—many clinical trials report neutral or even beneficial effects on body weight and metabolic parameters. Differences in host genetics, microbiome composition, and diet are likely to influence these outcomes (Million et al., 2012; Drissi et al., 2017).

5.12.11 Common Side Effects

For most healthy individuals, probiotics and prebiotics are well tolerated, causing only mild and transient side effects, primarily during the initial adjustment period. The most reported reactions are gastrointestinal, including bloating, increased gas production, mild abdominal discomfort or cramping, temporary changes in bowel movements such as diarrhea or constipation, and occasional nausea. These symptoms typically resolve within a few days to weeks as the gut microbiome adapts. Gradual introduction, starting with lower doses, can help minimize discomfort, while high doses of prebiotic fibers—particularly inulin and FOS—may cause more pronounced bloating or flatulence, especially in individuals with IBS or other functional gastrointestinal disorders (Whorwell et al., 2006; Yuan et al., 2017; Wilson et al., 2020).

5.12.12 Next-Generation Probiotics

Traditional probiotics are largely derived from food-fermenting bacteria such as *Lactobacillus* and *Bifidobacterium*. Advances in sequencing and culturing technologies have uncovered novel gut commensals with greater therapeutic potential. These "next-generation probiotics" include the following: *A. muciniphila*, a mucin-degrading bacterium linked to improved metabolic and gut barrier function. *F. prausnitzii*, a major butyrate producer with strong anti-inflammatory effects, typically reduced in IBD. *Clostridium* clusters IV and XIVa, including *Clostridium butyricum*, are known for butyrate production and spore-forming resilience (O'Toole et al., 2017).

Despite their promise, these strains pose challenges in cultivation, formulation stability, and safety validation since they lack long histories of human use. Ongoing clinical trials aim to define their therapeutic potential and regulatory pathways (Rinninella et al., 2019; Chang et al., 2014; Ratajczak et al., 2019; van der Hee and Wells, 2021).

5.12.13 Personalized Microbiome Interventions

Not all individuals respond similarly to probiotics or dietary interventions due to wide inter-individual variation in microbiome composition and host metabolism (Zmora et al., 2019). Personalized microbiome-based interventions, informed by individual microbial, genomic, and metabolomic profiles, could optimize efficacy and minimize side effects.

Companies now offer consumer microbiome sequencing with customized recommendations, but these services remain largely exploration and lack strong clinical validation. Future integration of multi-omic data—linking microbiome, metabolome, and host genomic signatures—could enable tailored therapies for specific health conditions.

5.12.13.1 Engineered Probiotics

Advances in synthetic biology have enabled the development of engineered probiotics designed to perform specialized functions within the gastrointestinal tract. These modified microorganisms can be tailored to enhance colonization and survival in the gut, secrete therapeutic compounds such as anti-inflammatory, antimicrobial, or metabolic molecules, detect disease biomarkers in real time through biosensing, and deliver drugs in a targeted manner. While these innovations hold significant potential for precision microbiome interventions, they also raise important safety, ethical, and regulatory concerns, including the risks of containment failure, horizontal gene transfer, and unintended ecological impacts of releasing engineered strains (Mimee et al. 2018).

5.12.13.2 Fecal Microbiota Transplantation

FMT, the transfer of fecal material from healthy donors to restore gut microbial balance, represents a powerful microbiome–based therapy (Allegretti et al., 2019). Its success in treating recurrent CDI—with cure rates exceeding 85–90%—has inspired investigations into IBD, obesity, autism, and metabolic syndrome.

Current research is transitioning from whole-stool transplants toward defined microbial consortia or "synthetic FMT," offering greater safety, standardization, and mechanistic clarity. These advances may pave the way for precision microbiome therapeutics tailored to disease-specific dysbioses (Quraishi et al., 2017; Suez et al., 2018; Kelly et al., 2021).

5.12.13.3 Dietary Approaches and Fermented Foods

Diet is one of the most influential modulators of the gut microbiome, and traditional fermented foods have received renewed scientific attention for their potential as natural, accessible sources of beneficial microbes and bioactive metabolites (Marco et al., 2021; Septembre-Malaterre et al., 2018). Future research aims to optimize fermentation processes to maximize probiotic enrichment, compare health outcomes across different types of fermented foods—such as dairy vs plant-based products—and understand how an individual's baseline microbiome composition influences their response to fermented food consumption. Additionally, efforts are underway to develop novel fermented foods specifically designed to support gut and metabolic health, leveraging both traditional practices and modern scientific insights.

5.12.13.4 *Microbiome-Based Diagnostics and Multi-Omics Integration*

The next frontier of microbiome science lies in translating microbial data into predictive, diagnostic, and therapeutic insights. Microbiome signatures are being investigated as biomarkers for early detection and monitoring of conditions such as colorectal cancer, IBD, and liver disease (Yao et al., 2021; Zhou et al., 2018; Gasaly et al., 2021).

To fully capture the complexity of host–microbe interactions, researchers are integrating multi-omics platforms—combining genomics, transcriptomics, proteomics, metabolomics, and immune profiling. These systems of biology approaches promise to elucidate causal mechanisms and refine targeted interventions. Ultimately, the convergence of probiotics, diet, engineered microbes, and personalized data-driven approaches will usher in a new era of precision microbiome medicine, aligning gut microbial health with overall human well-being.

5.13 CONCLUSION: INTEGRATIVE SYNTHESIS, EVIDENCE GAPS, AND FUTURE DIRECTIONS

Over the past two decades, our understanding of the human gut microbiome has undergone a revolutionary transformation (Thursby and Juge, 2017). The shift from traditional culture-based microbiology to genomic, metagenomic, and metabolomic methodologies has unveiled the immense diversity and functional complexity of the microbial ecosystems residing in the gastrointestinal tract. These discoveries have illuminated the intricate interdependence between microbes and host physiology, immunity, and metabolism—revealing the microbiome as a key determinant of human health. Yet, this explosion of knowledge has also highlighted the persistent challenges of translating promising laboratory insights into reliable clinical interventions.

The body of evidence supporting probiotics, prebiotics, and fermented foods as health-promoting interventions is both compelling and uneven (Sánchez et al., 2017). Certain probiotic formulations demonstrate clear efficacy for specific conditions, such as the prevention of acute infectious diarrhea in children, mitigation of AAD, and possible management of selected symptoms of IBS (Szajewska and Kołodziej, 2015; Goldenberg et al., 2017; Ford et al., 2018). However, many other claimed benefits remain inadequately substantiated or inconsistent across studies. The discrepancy between verified scientific evidence and the wide range of unverified commercial claims represents a major challenge for both clinicians and consumers (Patro-Golab et al., 2020; Whorwell et al., 2006; Yuan et al., 2017; Wilson et al., 2020).

Translation of mechanistic promises into consistent clinical benefit remains hindered by several obstacles. Chief among these is the strain-level specificity principle—benefits cannot be generalized even within the same bacterial species—combined with variability in dosing, product formulation, and storage stability (Zmora et al., 2019; Jackson et al., 2019). Many commercial probiotics diverge significantly from the rigorously tested formulations used in clinical trials, often differing in strain identity, viability, or labeling accuracy. Consequently, positive research outcomes cannot be extrapolated to all products sold under the same species name. This disconnects between laboratory-controlled research and real-world consumer products remains one of the most serious barriers to reliable clinical translation.

To move the field forward, both scientific and regulatory infrastructures must evolve in tandem. Scientifically, future research should prioritize the discovery of next-generation probiotic strains with novel metabolic and immunological functions; the identification of host factors governing individual responsiveness; and the elucidation of molecular mechanisms through advanced analytical tools such as single-cell transcriptomics, spatial microbiome mapping, and real-time metabolomic tracking (Zmora et al., 2018). Equally important is the need for rigorous clinical trials that assess commercially available products under real-world conditions—evaluating not only efficacy under idealized circumstances but also durability, stability, and user adherence in everyday use.

From a regulatory and manufacturing standpoint, the establishment of comprehensive quality standards is essential. Probiotic manufacturers should implement standardized production processes, perform validated shelf-life stability testing, and ensure transparent labeling with strain-specific identification and viable counts at both manufacture and expiration. Clear regulatory distinctions should be made between strain-verified health claims and those extrapolated from genus-level or theoretical evidence. Adoption of third-party verification and certification systems would further enhance consumer trust and clinical confidence in product integrity.

For clinicians and consumers alike, a nuanced understanding of microbiome-directed interventions is critical. Probiotics and prebiotics should not be viewed as universal solutions, but rather as adjuncts within broader lifestyle frameworks that include fiber-rich diets, physical activity, sleep hygiene, and avoidance of unnecessary antibiotics (Valdes et al., 2018). In contexts where robust, strain-specific evidence exists, well-characterized probiotic formulations can provide genuine benefit. In other cases, evidence remains insufficient, warranting cautious optimism rather than unquestioning acceptance of expansive marketing claims.

The future of microbiome therapeutics lies in personalization—tailoring interventions to an individual's microbiome composition, diet, genetics, and immune status (Goodrich et al., 2014; Zmora et al., 2019). Microbiome composition is partly heritable and influenced by host genetic factors, suggesting that precision approaches accounting for individual genetic variation may optimize therapeutic responses.

Ultimately, the next phase of microbiome research will depend on a cross-disciplinary synthesis integrating microbiology, immunology, metabolomics, neuroscience, and genetics (Cryan et al., 2019). This convergence promises to illuminate how microbial communities influence human health across multiple organ systems and life stages.

However, realizing this promise demands unwavering scientific rigor, transparent communication, and high-quality manufacturing standards that address persistent quality control deficiencies in the commercial probiotic market. Despite the expansion of probiotic research and development, significant discrepancies persist between product labels and actual contents, with multiple independent assessments documenting misidentified strains, inaccurate colony counts, and pill-to-pill variability in commercially available products (Lewis et al., 2016; Morovic et al., 2016; Patro et al., 2016). The evidence-practice gap is further widened by inconsistent terminology use and unsubstantiated marketing claims that exploit consumer and clinician interest in microbiome-directed interventions (Hill et al., 2014; Sanders et al., 2019; Shanahan et al., 2024).

The field stands at a remarkable intersection of ancient wisdom and modern science (Marco et al., 2021). Traditional fermented foods, once valued for preservation and flavor, are now understood through molecular detail as vehicles of symbiotic microbial exchange. The union of cultural knowledge and molecular precision holds immense promise—but only when pursued with intellectual honesty, methodological rigor, and ethical responsibility. The microbiome's profound influence on human well-being calls for the highest standards of science and the most disciplined translation of that science into safe, effective, and evidence-based clinical practice.

ACKNOWLEDGMENTS

The author (ST) acknowledges Wawa Foundation, Sharpe-Strumia Research Foundation, W. W. Smith Charitable Trust and Abraham Thomas Foundation for providing the resources for this work.

REFERENCES

Aceti, A., Gori, D., Barone, G., Callegari, M. L., Di Mauro, A., Fantini, M. P., Indrio, F., Maggio, L., Meneghin, F., Morelli, L., Zuccotti, G. V., & Corvaglia, L. (2015). Probiotics for prevention of necrotizing enterocolitis in preterm infants: Systematic review and meta-analysis. *Italian Journal of Pediatrics, 41*, 89.

Ahmed, K. A., Alqaisi, K. M., Ibrahim, N. A., Ahmed, N. J., Al-Balas, Q. A., Jabbar, A. A., ..., & Al-Qaisi, T. S. (2025). Pterostilbene (grape flavonoid) mitigates gastric ulcer events in vivo: biochemical and histopathological approaches. *Journal of Molecular Histology, 56*(6), 345. doi: 10.1007/s10735-025-10634-w

Allegretti, J. R., Mullish, B. H., Kelly, C., & Fischer, M. (2019). The evolution of the use of faecal microbiota transplantation and emerging therapeutic indications. *The Lancet*, 394(10196), 420–431.

Appel-da-Silva, M. C., Narvaez, G. A., Perez, L. R. R., & Dandrea Martins, A. (2017). Saccharomyces cerevisiae var. boulardii fungemia following probiotic treatment. *Medical Mycology Case Reports*, 18, 15–17.

Bode, L. (2012). Human milk oligosaccharides: Every baby needs a sugar mama. *Glycobiology*, 22(9), 1147–1162.

Boyle, R. J., Robins-Browne, R. M., & Tang, M. L. K. (2006). Probiotic use in clinical practice: What are the risks? *American Journal of Clinical Nutrition*, 83(6), 1256–1264.

Brodin, P. (2022). Immune-microbe interactions early in life: A determinant of health and disease long term. *Science*, 376(6596), 945–950.

Buffie, C. G., & Pamer, E. G. (2013). Microbiota-mediated colonization resistance against intestinal pathogens. *Nature Reviews Immunology*, 13(11), 790–801.

Cassone, M., Serra, P., Mondello, F., Girolamo, A., Scafetti, S., Pistella, E., & Venditti, M. (2003). Outbreak of Saccharomyces cerevisiae subtype boulardii fungemia in patients neighboring those treated with a probiotic preparation of the organism. *Journal of Clinical Microbiology*, 41(11), 5340–5343.

Chan, M., Larsen, N., Baerholm Schnedler, M., Ekstrom, C. T., Cayuelas, L. T., Holm, J. B., Meta, T. M., Hansen, L. H., Ankersen, D. V., Lay, C., Holm, J. C., Vestergaard, H., Pedersen, O., Nielsen, T., Kot, W., & Hansen, T. (2023). The impact of botanical fermented foods on metabolic syndrome and type 2 diabetes: A systematic review of randomised controlled trials. *Nutrition Research Reviews*, 36(2), 268–289.

Chang, P. V., Hao, L., Offermanns, S., & Medzhitov, R. (2014). The microbial metabolite butyrate regulates intestinal macrophage function via histone deacetylase inhibition. *Proceedings of the National Academy of Sciences*, 111(6), 2247–2252.

Chen, M., Sun, Q., Giovannucci, E., Mozaffarian, D., Manson, J. E., Willett, W. C., & Hu, F. B. (2014). Dairy consumption and risk of type 2 diabetes: 3 cohorts of US adults and an updated meta-analysis. *BMC Medicine*, 12, 215.

Chilton, S. N., Burton, J. P., & Reid, G. (2015). Inclusion of fermented foods in food guides around the world. *Nutrients*, 7(1), 390–404.

Companys, J., Pla-Pagà, L., Calderón-Pérez, L., Llauradó, E., Solà, R., Pedret, A., & Valls, R. M. (2020). Fermented dairy products rich in probiotics and cardiometabolic risk factors: A narrative review from prospective cohort studies. *Advances in Nutrition*, 11(4), 834–863.

Cryan, J. F., O'Riordan, K. J., Cowan, C. S. M., Sandhu, K. V., Bastiaanssen, T. F. S., Boehme, M., … , & Dinan, T. G. (2019). The microbiota-gut-brain axis. *Physiological Reviews*, 99(4), 1877–2013.

Cuello-Garcia, C. A., Brożek, J. L., Fiocchi, A., Pawankar, R., Yepes-Nuñez, J. J., Terracciano, L., Gandhi, S., Agarwal, A., Zhang, Y., & Schünemann, H. J. (2015). Probiotics for the prevention of allergy: A systematic review and meta-analysis of randomized controlled trials. *Journal of Allergy and Clinical Immunology*, 136(4), 952–961.

Davani-Davari, D., Negahdaripour, M., Karimzadeh, I., Seifan, M., Mohkam, M., Masoumi, S. J., Berenjian, A., & Ghasemi, Y. (2019). Prebiotics: Definition, types, sources, mechanisms, and clinical applications. *Foods*, 8(3), 92.

Del Carmen, S., de Moreno de LeBlanc, A., Martin, R., Chain, F., Langella, P., Bermúdez-Humarán, L. G., & LeBlanc, J. G. (2014). Genetically engineered immunomodulatory Streptococcus thermophilus strains producing antioxidant enzymes exhibit enhanced anti-inflammatory activities. *Applied and Environmental Microbiology*, 80(3), 869–77.

Derwa, Y., Gracie, D. J., Hamlin, P. J., & Ford, A. C. (2017). Systematic review with meta-analysis: The efficacy of probiotics in inflammatory bowel disease. *Alimentary Pharmacology & Therapeutics*, 46(4), 389–400.

Didari, T., Mozaffari, S., Nikfar, S., & Abdollahi, M. (2015). Effectiveness of probiotics in irritable bowel syndrome: Updated systematic review with meta-analysis. *World Journal of Gastroenterology*, 21(10), 3072–3084.

Ding, L., Duan, J., Yang, T., Yuan, M., Ma, A. H., & Qin, Y. (2024). Efficacy of fermented foods in irritable bowel syndrome: A systematic review and meta-analysis of randomized controlled trials. *Frontiers in Nutrition*, 11, 1494118.

Donald, K., & Finlay, B. B. (2023). Early-life interactions between the microbiota and immune system: Impact on immune system development and atopic disease. *Nature Reviews Immunology*, 23(11), 735–748.

Drissi, F., Raoult, D., & Merhej, V. (2017). Metabolic role of lactobacilli in weight modification in humans and animals. *Microbial Pathogenesis*, 106, 182–194.

Ducarmon, Q. R., Zwittink, R. D., Hornung, B. V., van Schaik, W., Young, V. B., & Kuijper, E. J. (2019). Gut microbiota and colonization resistance against bacterial enteric infection. *Microbiology and Molecular Biology Reviews*, 83(3), e00007-19.

Estevinho, M. M., Yuan, Y., Rodríguez-Lago, I., Sousa-Pimenta, M., Dias, C. C., Barreiro-de Acosta, M., Bertolín-Colilla, M., Calviño-Suárez, C., Carneiro, F., Lopes, S., Macedo, G., & Magro, F. (2024). Efficacy and safety of probiotics in IBD: An overview of systematic reviews and updated meta-analysis of randomized controlled trials. *United European Gastroenterology Journal*, 12(7), 960–981.

Eze, P., Farah, H., Nasir, N., Bakhit, W., Prabhu, A., Altorok, N., & Sheriff, D. S. (2024). Recurrent Lactobacillus rhamnosus bacteremia in an immunocompromised patient: A case report highlighting treatment challenges and fatal outcome. *Cureus*, 16(1), e51234.

Feng, Y., Zhao, Y., Liu, J., Huang, Z., Yang, X., Qin, P., Chen, C., Zhao, X., Shi, D., Huang, Q., & Zhang, M. (2022). Consumption of dairy products and the risk of overweight or obesity, hypertension, and type 2 diabetes mellitus: A dose-response meta-analysis and systematic review of cohort studies. *Advances in Nutrition*, 13(6), 2165–2179.

Fernandez, M. A., & Marette, A. (2017). Potential health benefits of combining yogurt and fruits based on their probiotic and prebiotic properties. *Advances in Nutrition*, 8(1), 155S–164S.

Fiocchi, A., Pawankar, R., Cuello-Garcia, C., Ahn, K., Al-Hammadi, S., Agarwal, A., Beyer, K., Burks, W., Canonica, G. W., Ebisawa, M., Gandhi, S., Kamenwa, R., Lee, B.W., Li, H., Prescott, S., Riva, J. J., Rosenwasser, L., Sampson, H., Spigler, M., Terracciano, L., Vereda-Ortiz, A., Waserman, S., Yepes-Nuñez, J. J., Brożek, J. L., & Schünemann, H. J. (2015). World Allergy Organization-McMaster University guidelines for allergic disease prevention (GLAD-P): Probiotics. *World Allergy Organization Journal*, 8(1), 4.

Fisberg, M., & Machado, R. (2015). History of yogurt and current patterns of consumption. *Nutrition Reviews*, 73(Suppl 1), 4–7.

Ford, A. C., Harris, L. A., Lacy, B. E., Quigley, E. M. M., & Moayyedi, P. (2018). Systematic review with meta-analysis: The efficacy of prebiotics, probiotics, synbiotics and antibiotics in irritable bowel syndrome. *Alimentary Pharmacology & Therapeutics*, 48(10), 1044–1060.

Fusco, W., Lorenzo, M. B., Cintoni, M., Porcari, S., Rinninella, E., Kaitsas, F., Lener, E., Mele, M. C., Gasbarrini, A., Collado, M. C., Cammarota, G., & Ianiro, G. (2023). Short-chain fatty-acid-producing bacteria: Key components of the human gut microbiota. *Nutrients*, 15(9), 2211.

Gasaly, N., Hermoso, M. A., & Gotteland, M. (2021). Butyrate and the fine-tuning of colonic homeostasis: Implication for inflammatory bowel diseases. *International Journal of Molecular Sciences*, 22(6), 3061.

Geng, Y., Wang, Z., Xu, X., Sun, X., Dong, X., Luo, Y., & Sun, X. (2024). Extensive therapeutic effects, underlying molecular mechanisms and disease treatment prediction of Metformin: A systematic review. *Translational Research*, 263, 73–92.

Gibson, G. R., Hutkins, R., Sanders, M. E., Prescott, S. L., Reimer, R. A., Salminen, S. J., Scott, K., Stanton, C., Swanson, K. S., Cani, P. D., Verbeke, K., & Reid, G. (2017). Expert consensus document: The International Scientific Association for Probiotics and Prebiotics (ISAPP) consensus statement on the definition and scope of prebiotics. *Nature Reviews Gastroenterology & Hepatology*, 14(8), 491–502.

Gijsbers, L., Ding, E. L., Malik, V. S., de Goede, J., Geleijnse, J. M., & Soedamah-Muthu, S. S. (2016). Consumption of dairy foods and diabetes incidence: A dose-response meta-analysis of observational studies. *American Journal of Clinical Nutrition*, 103(4), 1111–1124.

Godos, J., Ferri, R., Caraci, F., Cosentino, F. I. I., Castellano, S., Galvano, F., & Grosso, G. (2023). Adherence to the Mediterranean diet is inversely associated with depressive symptoms in older adults: A cross-sectional study. *Nutrients*, 15(3), 675.

Goldenberg, J. Z., Yap, C., Lytvyn, L., Lo, C. K. F., Beardsley, J., Mertz, D., & Johnston, B. C. (2017). Probiotics for the prevention of Clostridium difficile-associated diarrhea in adults and children. *Cochrane Database of Systematic Reviews*, 12, CD006095.

Goodrich, J. K., Waters, J. L., Poole, A. C., Knight, R., & Ley, R. E. (2014). Human genetics shape the gut microbiome. *Cell*, 159(4), 789–799.

Guo, J., Astrup, A., Lovegrove, J. A., Gijsbers, L., Givens, D. I., & Soedamah-Muthu, S. S. (2021). Milk and dairy consumption and risk of cardiovascular diseases and all-cause mortality: Dose-response meta-analysis of prospective cohort studies. *European Journal of Epidemiology*, 36(4), 427–445.

Helal, A., & Tagliazucchi, D. (2023a). Bioactive peptides, probiotics, and prebiotics in nutraceutical products destined to support cardiovascular health: A review. *Foods*, 12(5), 1048.

Helal, A., & Tagliazucchi, D. (2023b). Peptidomics profile, bioactive peptides identification and biological activities of six different cheese varieties. *Biology*, 12(1), 78.

Hennequin, C., Kauffmann-Lacroix, C., Jobert, A., Viard, J. P., Ricour, C., Jacquemin, J. L., & Berche, P. (2000). Possible role of catheters in Saccharomyces boulardii fungemia. *European Journal of Clinical Microbiology & Infectious Diseases*, 19(1), 16–20.

Herndon, C. C., Wang, Y. P., Lu, C. L., & Chen, P. H. (2020). Targeting the gut microbiota for the treatment of irritable bowel syndrome. *Kaohsiung Journal of Medical Sciences*, 36(3), 160–170.

Hill, C., Guarner, F., Reid, G., Gibson, G. R., Merenstein, D. J., Pot, B., Morelli, L., Canani, R. B., Flint, H. J., Salminen, S., Calder, P. C., & Sanders, M. E. (2014). Expert consensus document: The International Scientific Association for Probiotics and Prebiotics consensus statement on the scope and appropriate use of the term probiotic. *Nature Reviews Gastroenterology & Hepatology*, 11(8), 506–514.

Hishida, S., & Iwasa, Y. (2021). Spatial distribution of gut microbes along the intestinal duct. *Journal of Theoretical Biology*, 523, 110732.

Hu, Y., Aljumaah, M. R., & Azcarate-Peril, M. A. (2024). Galacto-oligosaccharides and the elderly gut: Implications for immune restoration and health. *Advances in Nutrition*, 15(8), 2234–2248.

Hughes, R. L., Alvarado, D. A., Swanson, K. S., & Holscher, H. D. (2022). The prebiotic potential of inulin-type fructans: A systematic review. *Advances in Nutrition*, 13(2), 492–529.

Jackson, S. A., Schoeni, J. L., Vegge, C., Pane, M., Stahl, B., Bradley, M., Goldman, V. S., Burguière, P., Atwater, J. B., Sanders, M. E., & Latimer, L. (2019). Improving end-user trust in the quality of commercial probiotic products. *Frontiers in Microbiology*, 10, 739.

Jannah, S. R., Rahayu, E. S., Yanti, R., Suroto, D. A., Wikandari, R. (2022, November 17). Study of viability, storage stability, and shelf life of probiotic instant coffee *Lactiplantibacillus plantarum* subsp. plantarum Dad-13 in vacuum and nonvacuum packaging at different storage temperatures. *International Journal of Food Science*, 2022, 1663772.

Jayabalan, R., Malbaša, R. V., Lončar, E. S., Vitas, J. S., & Sathishkumar, M. (2014). A review on kombucha tea—Microbiology, composition, fermentation, beneficial effects, toxicity, and tea fungus. *Comprehensive Reviews in Food Science and Food Safety*, 13(4), 538–550.

Jung, J. Y., Lee, S. H., & Jeon, C. O. (2014). Kimchi microflora: History, current status, and perspectives for industrial kimchi production. *Applied Microbiology and Biotechnology*, 98(6), 2385–2393.

Kabahizi, A., Wallace, B., Lieu, L., Chau, D., Dong, Y., Hwang, E. S., & Williams, K. W. (2022). Glucagon-like peptide-1 (GLP-1) signalling in the brain: From neural circuits and metabolism to therapeutics. *British Journal of Pharmacology*, 179(4), 600–624.

Kapp, J. M., & Sumner, W. (2019). Kombucha: A systematic review of the empirical evidence of human health benefit. *Annals of Epidemiology*, 30, 66–70.

Kelly, C. R., Yen, E. F., Grinspan, A. M., Kahn, S. A., Atreja, A., Lewis, J. D., Moore, T., Rubin, D. T., Szigethy, E., Proksell, S., Collins, M., Nasser, Y., Gerelus, M., Sagi, S., Allegretti, J. R., & Fischer, M. (2021). Fecal microbiota transplantation is highly effective in real-world practice: Final results from the FMT national registry. *Gastroenterology*, 160(1), 183–192.

Kim, H. J., Kim, H. Y., Lee, S. Y., Seo, J. H., Lee, E., & Hong, S. J. (2013). Clinical efficacy and mechanism of probiotics in allergic diseases. *Korean Journal of Pediatrics*, 56(9), 369–376.

Kim, J. Y., Kwon, J. Y., Kim, S. K., Han, M. D., Kim, H. R., Lee, H. J., Song, Y. R., & Paek, N. S. (2012). Effect of fermented kimchi on body weight and body fat in overweight and obese patients. *Journal of Ethnic Foods*, 1(1), 8–12.

King, S., Glanville, J., Sanders, M. E., Fitzgerald, A., & Varley, D. (2014). Effectiveness of probiotics on the duration of illness in healthy children and adults who develop common acute respiratory infectious conditions: A systematic review and meta-analysis. *British Journal of Nutrition*, 112(1), 41–54.

Koutnikova, H., Genser, B., Monteiro-Sepulveda, M., Faurie, J. M., Rizkalla, S., Schrezenmeir, J., & Clément, K. (2019). Impact of bacterial probiotics on obesity, diabetes and non-alcoholic fatty liver disease related variables: A systematic review and meta-analysis of randomised controlled trials. *BMJ Open*, 9(3), e017995.

Kruis, W., Fric, P., Pokrotnieks, J., Lukás, M., Fixa, B., Kascák, M., Kamm, M. A., Weismueller, J., Beglinger, C., Stolte, M., Wolff, C., & Schulze, J. (2004). Maintaining remission of ulcerative colitis with the probiotic Escherichia coli Nissle 1917 is as effective as with standard mesalazine. *Gut*, 53(11), 1617–1623.

Kullar, R., Goldstein, E. J. C., & Johnson, S. (2023). Risk of bacteremia and mortality associated with Lactobacillus bacteremia in patients receiving probiotics for C. difficile infection: A retrospective cohort study. *Microorganisms*, 11(2), 311.

Landaburu, L. S., Moris, M. V., Cornejo, I. I., & Jordán, R. (2020). Saccharomyces boulardii CNCM I-745: A probiotic that may become a problem. *Revista Argentina de Microbiología*, 52(4), 311–316.

Le Bastard, Q., Al-Ghalith, G. A., Grégoire, M., Chapelet, G., Javaudin, F., Dailly, E., Batard, E., Knights, D., & Montassier, E. (2018). Systematic review: Human gut dysbiosis induced by non-antibiotic prescription medications. *Alimentary Pharmacology & Therapeutics*, 47(3), 332–345.

Lee, S. M., Cho, Y., Chung, H. K., Shin, D. H., Ha, W. K., Lee, S. C., & Shin, M. J. (2012). Effects of kimchi supplementation on blood pressure and cardiac hypertrophy with varying sodium content in spontaneously hypertensive rats. *Nutrition Research and Practice*, 6(4), 315–321.

Lewis, Z. T., Shani, G., Masarweh, C. F., Popovic, M., Frese, S. A., Sela, D. A., Underwood, M. A., & Mills, D. A. (2016). Validating bifidobacterial species and subspecies identity in commercial probiotic products. *Pediatric Research*, 79(3), 445–452.

Lherm, T., Monet, C., Nougière, B., Soulier, M., Larbi, D., Le Gall, C., Caen, D., & Cerf, M. (2002). Seven cases of fungemia with Saccharomyces boulardii in critically ill patients. *Intensive Care Medicine*, 28(6), 797–801.

Li, Y. T., Xu, H., Ye, J. Z., Wu, W. R., Shi, D., Fang, D. Q., Liu, Y., & Li, L. J. (2019). Efficacy of Lactobacillus rhamnosus GG in treatment of acute pediatric diarrhea: A systematic review with meta-analysis. *World Journal of Gastroenterology*, 25(33), 4999–5016.

Lin, D., & Medeiros, D. M. (2023). The microbiome as a major function of the gastrointestinal tract and its implication in micronutrient metabolism and chronic diseases. *Nutrition Research*, 112, 30–45.

Liu, B., He, Y., Wang, M., Liu, J., Ju, Y., Zhang, Y., … , & Li, Q. (2018). Efficacy of probiotics on anxiety —A meta-analysis of randomized controlled trials. *Depression and Anxiety* 35(10), 935–945. doi: 10.1002/da.22811

Liu, R. T., Walsh, R. F. L., & Sheehan, A. E. (2019). Prebiotics and probiotics for depression and anxiety: A systematic review and meta-analysis of controlled clinical trials. *Neuroscience & Biobehavioral Reviews*, 102, 13–23.

Liu, X., Tong, Y., Qin, J., Zhao, Y., & Zhou, Y. (2025). Efficacy and safety of probiotic and synbiotic supplementation in metabolic syndrome: A systematic review and meta-analysis. *Nutrition, Metabolism and Cardiovascular Diseases*, 35(9), 2021–2035.

Losurdo, G., Iannone, A., Contaldo, A., Ierardi, E., Di Leo, A., & Principi, M. (2015). Escherichia coli Nissle 1917 in ulcerative colitis treatment: Systematic review and meta-analysis. *Journal of Gastrointestinal and Liver Diseases*, 24(4), 499–505.

Lu, C., Sang, J., He, H., Wan, X., Lin, Y., Li, L., Li, Y., Yu, C., & Sang, X. (2016). Probiotic supplementation does not improve eradication rate of Helicobacter pylori infection compared to placebo based on standard therapy: A meta-analysis. *Scientific Reports*, 6, 23522.

Lu, M., Yu, S., Deng, J., Yan, Q., Yang, C., Xia, G., & Zhou, X. (2023). Efficacy of probiotic supplementation therapy for Helicobacter pylori eradication: A meta-analysis of randomized controlled trials. *PLoS ONE*, 18(4), e0282963.

Lynch, J. P., Werder, R. B., Simpson, J., Loh, Z., Zhang, V., Haque, A., & Spann, K. (2021). Aeroallergen-induced IL-33 predisposes to respiratory virus-induced asthma by dampening antiviral immunity. *Trends in Pharmacological Sciences*, 43(9), 772–786.

Ma, Z., Zuo, T., Frey, N., Kelvin, D. J., Yu, J., Chan, P. K. S., & Ng, S. C. (2024). A systematic framework for understanding the microbiome in human health and disease: From basic principles to clinical translation. *Signal Transduction and Targeted Therapy*, 9, 237.

Machiels, K., Joossens, M., Sabino, J., De Preter, V., Arijs, I., Eeckhaut, V., Ballet, V., Claes, K., Van Immerseel, F., Verbeke, K., Ferrante, M., Verhaegen, J., Rutgeerts, P., & Vermeire, S. (2014). A decrease of the butyrate-producing species Roseburia hominis and Faecalibacterium prausnitzii defines dysbiosis in patients with ulcerative colitis. *Gut*, 63(8), 1275–1283.

Maier, T. V., Lucio, M., Lee, L. H., VerBerkmoes, N. C., Brislawn, C. J., Bernhardt, J., Lamendella, R., McDermott, J. E., Bergeron, N., Heinzmann, S. S., Morton, J.T., González, A., Ackermann, G., Knight, R., Riedel, K., Krauss, R. M., Goodlett, D. R., & Schmitt-Kopplin, P. (2017). Impact of dietary resistant starch on the human gut microbiome, metaproteome, and metabolome. *mBio*, 8(5), e01343-17.

Marco, M. L., Sanders, M. E., Gänzle, M., Arrieta, M. C., Cotter, P. D., De Vuyst, L., Hill, C., Holzapfel, W., Lebeer, S., Levac, D., Pot, B., Reid, G., Salminen, S., Shortt, C., Slavin, J., Smid, E., Tancredi, D., Vinderola, G., & Hutkins, R. (2021). The International Scientific Association for Probiotics and Prebiotics (ISAPP) consensus statement on fermented foods. *Nature Reviews Gastroenterology & Hepatology*, 18(3), 196–208.

McCallum, G., & Tropini, C. (2024). The gut microbiota and its biogeography. *Nature Reviews Microbiology*, 22, 105–118.

McFarland, L. V. (2010). Systematic review and meta-analysis of Saccharomyces boulardii in adult patients. *World Journal of Gastroenterology*, 16(18), 2202–2222.

McFarland, L. V., Evans, C. T., & Goldstein, E. J. C. (2018). Strain-specificity and disease-specificity of probiotic efficacy: A systematic review and meta-analysis. *Frontiers in Medicine*, 5, 124.

McFarland, L. V., Huang, Y., Wang, L., & Malfertheiner, P. (2015). Systematic review and meta-analysis: Multi-strain probiotics as adjunct therapy for Helicobacter pylori eradication and prevention of adverse events. *United European Gastroenterology Journal*, 4(4), 546–561.

Mei, Z., Yuan, J., & Li, D. (2022). Biological activity of galacto-oligosaccharides: A review. *Frontiers in Microbiology*, 13, 993052.

Meini, S., Laureano, R., Fani, L., Tascini, C., Galano, A., Antonelli, A., & Rossolini, G. M. (2015). Breakthrough Lactobacillus rhamnosus GG bacteremia associated with probiotic use in an adult patient with severe active ulcerative colitis: Case report and review of the literature. *Infection*, 43(6), 777–781.

Miele, E., Pascarella, F., Giannetti, E., Quaglietta, L., Baldassano, R. N., & Staiano, A. (2009). Effect of a probiotic preparation (VSL#3) on induction and maintenance of remission in children with ulcerative colitis. *American Journal of Gastroenterology*, 104(2), 437–443.

Million, M., Angelakis, E., Paul, M., Armougom, F., Leibovici, L., & Raoult, D. (2012). Comparative meta-analysis of the effect of Lactobacillus species on weight gain in humans and animals. *Microbial Pathogenesis*, 53(2), 100–108.

Mimee, M., Nadeau, P., Hayward, A., Carim, S., Flanagan, S., Jerger, L., Collins, J., McDonnell, S., Swartwout, R., Citorik, R. J., Bulović, V., Langer, R., Traverso, G., Chandrakasan, A. P., & Lu, T. K. (2018). An ingestible bacterial-electronic system to monitor gastrointestinal health. *Science*, 360(6391), 915–918.

Mirmohammadkhani, M., Shahraki, H. R., Mehrabi, S., & Karandish, M. (2025). The effects of fermented dairy products on abdominal obesity: A systematic review and meta-analysis. *Nutrition & Metabolism*, 22(1), 15.

Mitmesser, S., & Combs, M. (2017). Prebiotics: Inulin and other oligosaccharides. In Martin H. Floch, Yehuda Ringel, & W. Allan Walker (Eds.), *The Microbiota in Gastrointestinal Pathophysiology* (pp. 201–208). Academic Press.

Moore, R. E., & Townsend, S. D. (2019). Temporal development of the infant gut microbiome. *Open Biology*, 9(9), 190128.

More, D., Shepard, C., More, C., & Mayol-Kreiser, S. (2021). The perinatal use of probiotics, prebiotics, and synbiotics for the primary prevention of allergic diseases in children: A systematic review. *Human Nutrition & Metabolism*, 25, 100127.

Morovic, W., Hibberd, A. A., Zabel, B., Barrangou, R., & Stahl, B. (2016). Genotyping by PCR and high-throughput sequencing of commercial probiotic products reveals composition biases. *Frontiers in Microbiology*, 7, 1747.

Mukherjee, A., Lordan, C., Ross, R. P., & Cotter, P. D. (2024). Fermented foods and gastrointestinal health: Underlying mechanisms. *Nature Reviews Gastroenterology & Hepatology*, 21(4), 248–266.

Muñoz, P., Bouza, E., Cuenca-Estrella, M., Eiros, J. M., Pérez, M. J., Sánchez-Somolinos, M., Rincón, C., Hortal, J., Peláez, T., & Rodríguez-Créixems, M. (2005). Saccharomyces cerevisiae fungemia: An emerging infectious disease. *Clinical Infectious Diseases*, 40(11), 1625–1634.

Nummer, B. A. (2013). Special report: Kombucha brewing under the Food and Drug Administration model food code: Risk analysis and processing guidance. *Journal of Environmental Health*, 76(4), 8–11.

O'Toole, P., Marchesi, J., & Hill, C. (2017). Next-generation probiotics: The spectrum from probiotics to live biotherapeutics. *Nature Microbiology*, 2, 17057.

Office of Dietary Supplements, National Institutes of Health. (2024). Probiotics—Health professional fact sheet. Retrieved from https://ods.od.nih.gov/factsheets/Probiotics-HealthProfessional/

Park, I., & Mannaa, M. (2025). Fermented foods as functional systems: Microbial communities and metabolites influencing gut health and systemic outcomes. *Foods*, 14(13), 2292.

Park, K. Y., Jeong, J. K., Lee, Y. E., & Daily, J. W. 3rd. (2014). Health benefits of kimchi (Korean fermented vegetables) as a probiotic food. *Journal of Medicinal Food*, 17(1), 6–20.

Patro, J. N., Ramachandran, P., Lewis, T., Mammel, M. K., Barnaba, T., & Pfeiler, E. A. (2016). Culture-independent metagenomic surveillance of commercially available probiotics with high-throughput next-generation sequencing. *mSphere*, 1(2), e00057-16.

Patro-Golab, B., Shamir, R., & Szajewska, H. (2020). Yogurt for treating acute gastroenteritis in children: Systematic review and meta-analysis. *Clinical Nutrition*, 39(10), 2967–2975.

Peñas, E., Martinez-Villaluenga, C., & Frias, J. (2017). Chapter 24 – Sauerkraut: Production, composition, and health benefits. In J. Frias, C. Martinez-Villaluenga, & E. Peñas (Eds.), *Fermented foods in health and disease prevention* (pp. 557–576). Academic Press.

Pirola, L., & Fröjdö, S. (2008). Resveratrol: One molecule, many targets. *IUBMB Life*, 60(5), 323–332.

Plaza-Diaz, J., Ruiz-Ojeda, F. J., Gil-Campos, M., & Gil, A. (2019). Mechanisms of action of probiotics. *Advances in Nutrition*, 10(Suppl 1), S49–S66.

Plengvidhya, V., Breidt, F., Lu, Z., & Fleming, H. P. (2007). DNA fingerprinting of lactic acid bacteria in sauerkraut fermentations. *Applied and Environmental Microbiology*, 73(23), 7697–7702.

Quraishi, M. N., Widlak, M., Bhala, N., Moore, D., Price, M., Sharma, N., & Iqbal, T. H. (2017). Systematic review with meta-analysis: The efficacy of faecal microbiota transplantation for the treatment of recurrent and refractory Clostridium difficile infection. *Alimentary Pharmacology & Therapeutics*, 46(5), 479–493.

Rannikko, J., Kerttula, T., Salmenlinna, S., Mäki, M., Stuff, P., Richardson, M., Lyytikäinen, O., & Järvinen, A. (2021). Saccharomyces cerevisiae fungemia: An emerging infectious disease in Finland. *Emerging Infectious Diseases*, 27(5), 1442–1445.

Ratajczak, W., Rył, A., Mizerski, A., Walczakiewicz, K., Sipak, O., & Laszczyńska, M. (2019). Immunomodulatory potential of gut microbiome-derived short-chain fatty acids (SCFAs). *Acta Biochimica Polonica*, 66(1), 1–12.

Reis, D. J., Ilardi, S. S., & Punt, S. E. W. (2018). The anxiolytic effect of probiotics: A systematic review and meta-analysis of the clinical and preclinical literature. *PLoS ONE*, 13(6), e0199041.

Rezazadegan, M., Gans, R. O. B., & Teeuw, W. J. (2022). Effects of lactic acid bacteria fermented foods on obesity, type 2 diabetes and cardiovascular risk factors: A systematic review of randomized controlled trials. *Nutrients*, 14(1), 71.

Rinninella, E., Raoul, P., Cintoni, M., Franceschi, F., Miggiano, G. A. D., Gasbarrini, A., & Mele, M. C. (2019). What is the healthy gut microbiota composition? A changing ecosystem across age, environment, diet, and diseases. *Microorganisms*, 7(1), 14.

Rosa, D. D., Dias, M. M. S., Grześkowiak, Ł. M., Reis, S. A., Conceição, L. L., & Peluzio, M. D. C. G. (2017). Milk kefir: Nutritional, microbiological and health benefits. *Nutrition Research Reviews*, 30(1), 82–96.

Saleena, L. A. K., Teo, M. Y. M., How, Y. H., In, L. L. A., & Pui, L. P. (2023). Immunomodulatory action of Lactococcuslactis. *Journal of Bioscience and Bioengineering*, 135(1), 1–9.

Salminen, M. K., Tynkkynen, S., Rautelin, H., Saxelin, M., Vaara, M., Ruutu, P., Sarna, S., Valtonen, V., & Järvinen, A. (2004). Lactobacillus bacteremia during a rapid increase in probiotic use of Lactobacillus rhamnosus GG in Finland. *Clinical Infectious Diseases*, 35(10), 1155–1160.

Sánchez, B., Delgado, S., Blanco-Míguez, A., Lourenço, A., Gueimonde, M., & Margolles, A. (2017). Probiotics, gut microbiota, and their influence on host health and disease. *Molecular Nutrition & Food Research*, 61(1), 1600240.

Sanders, M. E., Merenstein, D. J., Reid, G., Gibson, G. R., & Rastall, R. A. (2019). Probiotics and prebiotics in intestinal health and disease: From biology to the clinic. *Nature Reviews Gastroenterology & Hepatology*, 16(10), 605–616.

Savaiano, D. A., & Hutkins, R. W. (2021). Yogurt, cultured fermented milk, and health: A systematic review. *Nutrition Reviews*, 79(5), 599–614.

Scaldaferri, F., Gerardi, V., Mangiola, F., Lopetuso, L. R., Pizzoferrato, M., Petito, V., …, & Gasbarrini, A. (2016). Role and mechanisms of action of Escherichia coli Nissle 1917 in the maintenance of remission in ulcerative colitis patients: An update. *World Journal* of Gastroenterology, 22(24), 5505–5511. doi: 10.3748/wjg.v22.i24.5505

Seekatz, A. M., Safdar, N., & Khanna, S. (2022). The role of the gut microbiome in colonization resistance and recurrent Clostridioides difficile infection. *Therapeutic Advances in Gastroenterology*, 15, 17562848221134396.

Sender, R., Fuchs, S., & Milo, R. (2016). Revised estimates for the number of human and bacteria cells in the body. *PLoS Biology*, 14(8), e1002533.

Septembre-Malaterre, A., Remize, F., & Poucheret, P. (2018). Fruits and vegetables, as a source of nutritional compounds and phytochemicals: Changes in bioactive compounds during lactic fermentation. *Food Research International*, 104, 86–99.

Shanahan, F., Stanton, C., Ross, P., & Hill, C. (2024). Gut microbiota in health and disease: An overview. *Journal of Gastroenterology and Hepatology*, 39(1), 1–8.

Shreiner, A. B., Kao, J. Y., & Young, V. B. (2015). The gut microbiome in health and in disease. *Current Opinion in Gastroenterology*, 31(1), 69–75.

Sokol, H., Pigneur, B., Watterlot, L., Lakhdari, O., Bermúdez-Humarán, L. G., Gratadoux, J. J., Blugeon, S., Bridonneau, C., Furet, J. P., Corthier, G., Grangette, C., Vasquez, N., Pochart, P., Trugnan, G., Thomas, G., Blottière, H. M., Doré, J., Marteau, P., Seksik, P., & Langella, P. (2008). Faecalibacterium prausnitzii is an anti-inflammatory commensal bacterium identified by gut microbiota analysis of Crohn disease patients. *Proceedings of the National Academy of Sciences of the United States of America* , 105(43), 16731–16736.

Song, H. J., & Lee, H. J. (2014). Consumption of kimchi, a salt fermented vegetable, is not associated with hypertension prevalence. *Journal of Ethnic Foods*, 1(1), 8–12.

Sood, A., Midha, V., Makharia, G. K., Ahuja, V., Singal, D., Goswami, P., & Tandon, R. K. (2009). The probiotic preparation, VSL#3 induces remission in patients with mild-to-moderately active ulcerative colitis. *Clinical Gastroenterology and Hepatology*, 7(11), 1202–1209.

Suez, J., Zmora, N., Zilberman-Schapira, G., Mor, U., Dori-Bachash, M., Bashiardes, S., Zur, M., Regev-Lehavi, D., Ben-Zeev Brik, R., Federici, S., Horn, M., Cohen, Y., Moor, A. E., Zeevi, D., Korem, T., Kotler, E., Harmelin, A., Itzkovitz, S., Maharshak, N., Shibolet, O., Pevsner-Fischer, M., Shapiro, H., Sharon, I., Halpern, Z., Segal, E., & Elinav, E. (2018). Post-antibiotic gut mucosal microbiome reconstitution is impaired by probiotics and improved by autologous FMT. *Cell*, 174(6), 1406–1423.

Swanson, K. S., Gibson, G. R., Hutkins, R., Reimer, R. A., Reid, G., Verbeke, K., Scott, K. P., Holscher, H. D., Azad, M. B., Delzenne, N. M., & Sanders, M. E. (2020). The International Scientific Association for Probiotics and Prebiotics (ISAPP) consensus statement on the definition and scope of synbiotics. *Nature Reviews Gastroenterology & Hepatology*, 17(11), 687–701.

Swer, T. L., Mukhim, C., Joshi, S. R., & Chauhan, K. (2024). Fermented foods and beverages: Trends and scope. *Current Research in Food Science*, 8, 100691.

Szajewska, H., Albrecht, P., & Topczewska-Cabanek, A. (2009). Randomized, double-blind, placebo-controlled trial: Effect of Lactobacillus GG supplementation on Helicobacter pylori eradication rates and side effects during treatment in children. *Journal of Pediatric Gastroenterology and Nutrition*, 48(4), 431–436.

Szajewska, H., & Kołodziej, M. (2015). Systematic review with meta-analysis: Lactobacillus rhamnosus GG in the prevention of antibiotic-associated diarrhoea in children and adults. *Alimentary Pharmacology & Therapeutics*, 42(10), 1149–1157.

Tabouy, L., Getselter, D., Ziv, O., Karpuj, M., Tabouy, T., Lukic, I., Maayouf, R., Werbner, N., Ben-Amram, H., Nuriel-Ohayon, M., Koren, O., & Elliott, E. (2018). Dysbiosis of microbiome and probiotic treatment in a genetic model of autism spectrum disorders. *Brain, Behavior, and Immunity*, 73, 310–319.

Tang, Y., Wang, T., Li, Y., Zou, W., Chen, X., & Li, Z. (2025). The effect of probiotic intervention on behavioral and gastrointestinal symptoms in children with autism: A systematic review and meta-analysis. *Research in Autism*, 126, 202630.

Tenorio-Jiménez, C., Martínez-Ramírez, M. J., Gil, Á., & Gómez-Llorente, C. (2020). Effects of probiotics on metabolic syndrome: A systematic review of randomized clinical trials. *Nutrients*, 12(1), 124.

Theriot, C. M., & Young, V. B. (2014). Microbial and metabolic interactions between the gastrointestinal tract and Clostridium difficile infection. *Gut Microbes*, 5(1), 86–95.

Thomas, S., Izard, J., Walsh, E., Batich, K., Chongsathidkiet, P., Clarke, G., Sela, D. A., Muller, A. J., Mullin, J. M., Albert, K., Gilligan, J. P., DiGuilio, K., Dilbarova, R., Alexander, W., & Prendergast, G. C. (2017). The host microbiome regulates and maintains human health: A primer and perspective for non-microbiologists. *Cancer Research*, 77(8), 1783–1812.

Thursby, E., & Juge, N. (2017). Introduction to the human gut microbiota. *Biochemical Journal*, 474(11), 1823–1836.

Turnbaugh, P. J., Ley, R. E., Hamady, M., Fraser-Liggett, C. M., Knight, R., & Gordon, J. I. (2007). The human microbiome project. *Nature*, 449(7164), 804–810.

Tursi, A., Brandimarte, G., Giorgetti, G. M., Forti, G., Modeo, M. E., & Gigliobianco, A. (2010). Low-dose balsalazide plus a high-potency probiotic preparation is more effective than balsalazide alone or mesalazine in the treatment of acute mild-to-moderate ulcerative colitis. *Medical Science Monitor*, 16(11), PI123–PI130.

Vahabnezhad, E., Mochon, A. B., Wozniak, L. J., & Ziring, D. A. (2013). Lactobacillus bacteremia associated with probiotic use in a pediatric patient with ulcerative colitis. *Journal of Clinical Gastroenterology*, 47(5), 437–439.

Valdes, A. M., Walter, J., Segal, E., & Spector, T. D. (2018). Role of the gut microbiota in nutrition and health. *BMJ*, 361, k2179.

Vallianou, N., Christodoulatos, G. S., Karampela, I., Tsilingiris, D., Magkos, F., Stratigou, T., Kounatidis, D., & Dalamaga, M. (2020). Understanding the role of the gut microbiome and microbial metabolites in non-alcoholic fatty liver disease: Current evidence and perspectives. *Biomolecules*, 10(10), 1360.

Vallianou, N., Stratigou, T., Christodoulatos, G. S., Tsigalou, C., & Dalamaga, M. (2019). Probiotics, prebiotics, synbiotics, postbiotics, and obesity: Current evidence, controversies, and perspectives. *Current Obesity Reports*, 8(4), 317–332.

van der Hee, B., & Wells, J. M. (2021). Microbial regulation of host physiology by short-chain fatty acids. *Trends in Microbiology*, 29(8), 700–712.

Wang, Z., Klipfell, E., Bennett, B. J., Koeth, R., Levison, B. S., Dugar, B., Feldstein, A. E., Britt, E. B., Fu, X., Chung, Y. M., Wu, Y., Schauer, P., Smith, J. D., Allayee, H., Tang, W. H., DiDonato, J. A., Lusis, A. J., & Hazen, S.L. (2011, April 7). Gut flora metabolism of phosphatidylcholine promotes cardiovascular disease. *Nature*, 472(7341), 57–63.

West, C. E. (2016). Probiotics for allergy prevention. *Beneficial Microbes*, 7(2), 171–179.

Whorwell, P. J., Altringer, L., Morel, J., Bond, Y., Charbonneau, D., O'Mahony, L., Kiely, B., Shanahan, F., & Quigley, E. M. (2006). Efficacy of an encapsulated probiotic Bifidobacterium infantis 35624 in women with irritable bowel syndrome. *American Journal of Gastroenterology*, 101(7), 1581–1590.

Wilson, B., Eyice, Ö., Koumoutsos, I., Lomer, M. C. E., Irving, P. M., & Whelan, K. (2020). Prebiotics in irritable bowel syndrome and other functional bowel disorders in adults: A systematic review and meta-analysis of randomized controlled trials. *American Journal of Clinical Nutrition*, 111(5), 1029–1043.

Yan, F., & Polk, D. B. (2011). Probiotics and immune health. *Current Opinion in Gastroenterology*, 27(6), 496–501.

Yang, R., Jiang, J., Ouyang, J., Zhao, Y., & Xi, B. (2024). Efficacy and safety of probiotics in irritable bowel syndrome: A systematic review and meta-analysis. *Clinical Nutrition ESPEN*, 60, 362–372.

Yao, Y., Jia, R., Chen, L., Cao, Y., Luo, Y., & Yuan, M. (2021). Bifidobacterium longum: Protection against inflammatory bowel disease. *Journal of Immunology Research*, 2021, 8030297.

Yuan, F., Ni, H., Asche, C. V`., Kim, M., Walayat, S., & Ren, J. (2017). Efficacy of Bifidobacterium infantis 35624 in patients with irritable bowel syndrome: A meta-analysis. *Current Medical Research and Opinion*, 33(7), 1191–1197.

Zabat, M. A., Sano, W. H., Wurster, J. I., Cabral, D. J., & Belenky, P. (2018). Microbial community analysis of sauerkraut fermentation reveals a stable and rapidly established community. *Foods*, 7(5), 77.

Zhang, M. M., Qian, W., Qin, Y. Y., He, J., & Zhou, Y. H. (2015). Probiotics in Helicobacter pylori eradication therapy: A systematic review and meta-analysis. *World Journal of Gastroenterology*, 21(14), 4345–4357.

Zhang, Y., Guo, X., Guo, J., He, Q., Li, H., Song, Y., & Zhang, H. (2023). Lactobacillus casei reduces blood glucose and modulates the composition of the gut microbiota in type 2 diabetic mice. *Food & Function*, 14(3), 1512–1524.

Zhou, L., Zhang, M., Wang, Y., Dorfman, R. G., Liu, H., Yu, T., Chen, X., Tang, D., Xu, L., Yin, Y., Pan, Y., Zhou, Q., Zhou, Y., & Li, Y. (2018). Faecalibacterium prausnitzii produces butyrate to maintain Th17/Treg balance and to ameliorate colorectal colitis by inhibiting histone deacetylase 1. *Inflammatory Bowel Diseases*, 24(9), 1926–1940.

Zhuang, X., Xiong, L., Li, L., Li, M., & Chen, M. (2018). Alterations of gut microbiota in patients with irritable bowel syndrome: A systematic review and meta-analysis. *Journal of Gastroenterology and Hepatology*, 33(10), 1751–1759.

Zmora, N., Suez, J., & Elinav, E. (2019). You are what you eat: Diet, health and the gut microbiota. *Nature Reviews Gastroenterology & Hepatology*, 16(1), 35–56.

Zmora, N., Zilberman-Schapira, G., Suez, J., Mor, U., Dori-Bachash, M., Bashiardes, S., Kotler, E., Zur, M., Regev-Lehavi, D., Ben-Zeev Brik, R., Federici, S., Cohen, Y., Linevsky, R., Rothschild, D., Moor, A. E., Shental, N., Harmelin, A., Itzkovitz, S., Maharshak, N., Shibolet, O., Shapiro, H., Pevsner-Fischer, M., Sharon, I., Halpern, Z., Segal, E., & Elinav, E. (2018). Personalized gut mucosal colonization resistance to empiric probiotics is associated with unique host and microbiome features. *Cell*, 174(6), 1388–1405.

CHAPTER 6

Impact of Physical Exercise on the Gut Microbiota

Gabriel Mayer Tossi, Leidiane de Medeiros Oliveira Lima, Maurício da Silva Krause, and Patricia Martins Bock

6.1 INTRODUCTION

Among the various factors capable of modulating the gut microbiota, including surgical, dietary, and pharmacological interventions that have been extensively studied for their metabolic consequences (Bock et al. 2021; Bock et al. 2022), physical exercise has emerged as a powerful non-pharmacological strategy, capable of reshaping the taxonomic composition of intestinal microorganisms and eliciting systemic physiological responses (Mach and Fuster-Botella 2017). In parallel with these established interventions, the growing scientific interest in the gut–muscle axis, together with accumulating evidence of the effects of physical exercise on gut microbial ecology, underscores the role of regular physical activity as a functional modulator of the microbiota, with direct implications for metabolic, immune, and neurological health (Mach and Fuster-Botella 2017; Grosicki, Fielding, and Lustgarten 2018).

A substantial body of research indicates that physical exercise markedly influences both the composition and functionality of the gut microbiota by modulating metabolic pathways and signaling cascades involved in energy metabolism, immune regulation, and neuromuscular function (Ortiz-Alvarez, Xu, and Martinez-Tellez 2020; Zhao et al. 2018; Motiani et al. 2020). This interaction is mediated by complex physiological and molecular mechanisms, in which exercise modality, intensity, volume, and duration serve as key determinants (Suryani et al. 2022; Bonomini-Gnutzmann et al. 2022). Recent investigations further demonstrate that distinct training modalities, such as aerobic and concurrent training, induce specific shifts in microbial structure and diversity, reflecting systemic adaptations to physical stimuli (Taniguchi et al. 2018; Dupuit et al. 2022).

Among the mechanisms underlying this interplay, the regulation of intracellular signaling pathways, modulation of systemic inflammation, and enhanced production of bioactive microbial metabolites stand out as central processes (Zhao et al. 2018). Short-chain fatty acids (SCFA), lipopolysaccharide (LPS), and bile acid derivatives play pivotal roles in gut-to-tissue communication, particularly in mediating cross-talk between the intestine and skeletal muscle (Frampton et al. 2020). Insights into these mechanisms have been advanced through evidence derived from experimental models (Frampton et al. 2020), systematic reviews (Mach and Fuster-Botella 2017), and randomized controlled trials (Motiani et al. 2020), all reinforcing the concept of physical exercise as a functional modulator of the gut microbiota. Nonetheless, ongoing research highlights considerable methodological heterogeneity and persistent conceptual gaps that impede causal inference, underscoring the need for integrative and standardized approaches to deepen the understanding of the physiological links within the gut–muscle axis and the potential effects of exercise on the gut microbiota.

DOI: 10.1201/9781003638292-6

6.1.1 Concepts and Classification of Physical Exercise

Physical activity is defined as any bodily movement produced by skeletal muscles that results in energy expenditure above resting levels. The amount of energy required to perform a given movement, therefore, reflects the intensity of physical activity associated with that action. In contrast, physical exercise represents a planned, structured, and repetitive form of physical effort—characterized by variable intensity—intended to improve or maintain one or more components of physical fitness through the enhancement of overall physiological function (Bishop et al. 2025).

The weekly frequency of muscle contraction, associated with regular physical training acts as a potent stimulus for physiological adaptation (Schumann et al. 2022). Over time, skeletal muscle demonstrates remarkable plasticity, undergoing functional and structural remodeling in response to repeated contractile activity. These training-induced adaptations are manifested through alterations in contractile protein expression and function, mitochondrial performance, metabolic regulation, intracellular signaling, and transcriptional responses (Egan and Sharples 2023).

With regard to different training modalities, particularly in clinical contexts, aerobic training, resistance training, and concurrent training are the most prominent approaches. Aerobic and resistance exercises represent opposite ends of the exercise continuum, whereas combined protocols, that integrate both aerobic and resistance components within the same training session, are classified as concurrent training (Schumann et al. 2022).

From a physiological perspective, aerobic training elicits significant adaptations in oxygen consumption (VO_2), reflecting improvements across the cardiovascular, respiratory, and metabolic systems. These adaptations enhance oxygen uptake, transport, and utilization, thereby resulting in increasing energy efficiency and conferring broad cardiometabolic benefits (Jones and Kirby 2025). In contrast, resistance training induces neuromuscular adaptations characterized by increased electrical conduction in motor neurons, enhanced muscle fiber recruitment, heightened sensitivity to anabolic hormones, and activation of intracellular signaling pathways related to protein synthesis, ultimately promoting muscle hypertrophy (Lim et al. 2022).

Concurrent training has been increasingly investigated for its ability to simultaneously promote cardiometabolic and neuromuscular benefits. Although it may not maximize the specific adaptations associated with each individual modality, this form of training still provides substantial functional gains (Huiberts et al. 2024). However, the literature describes a phenomenon known as "interference", in which the activation of distinct—and occasionally antagonistic—intracellular signaling pathways constrains the overall adaptive potential. Aerobic exercise predominantly activates AMPK (AMP-activated protein kinase), a key regulator of mitochondrial biogenesis and oxidative metabolism, whereas resistance exercise primarily stimulates the mTOR pathway (mammalian target of rapamycin), which governs protein synthesis and muscle hypertrophy. Chronic activation of AMPK can suppress mTOR signaling, thereby attenuating the anabolic environment required for optimal strength and muscle mass development (Coffey and Hawley 2017).

6.2 EXPERIMENTAL STUDY DESIGNS IN EXERCISE AND GUT MICROBIOTA RESEARCH

The interplay between physical exercise and the gut microbiota has emerged as a promising frontier in exercise science and clinical research, supported by evidence from clinical trials (Kern et al. 2020; Liu et al. 2020), quasi-experimental studies (Aragón-Vela et al. 2021), observational investigations (Grosicki et al. 2023), and systematic reviews (Suryani et al. 2022; Bonomini-Gnutzmann et al. 2022). This relationship is inherently complex, as it is shaped by multiple modulators of the gut microbiota, such as diet, genetics, environment, and medication use, and further influenced by the inherent heterogeneity of exercise protocols, which together demand rigorous methodological designs to isolate the specific effects of physical activity (Bonomini-Gnutzmann et al. 2022; Suryani et al. 2022).

The complexity of this relationship has driven the development of diverse research approaches to clarify how exercise influences gut microbial communities. In this field, experimental designs generally follow two main approaches: (i) human intervention trials, involving either single exercise bouts or chronic training programs with fecal or plasma sample collection before and after the intervention, and (ii) observational studies that associate habitual physical activity levels or cardiorespiratory fitness with gut microbiota profiles (Ortiz-Alvarez et al. 2020). This methodological diversity is essential to understand both the acute and chronic effects of exercise on metabolic and inflammatory markers, as well as the long-term adaptations in bacterial diversity and composition, and it also contributes to describing and analyzing, in observational studies, associations between variables captured at a single point in time (Bonomini-Gnutzmann et al. 2022).

In randomized controlled and quasi-experimental trials, continuous aerobic protocols (e.g., cycling, running, walking) are most frequently adopted, while a persistent gap in the literature concerns resistance training and combined exercise interventions (Suryani et al. 2022; Cataldi et al. 2022; Bonomini-Gnutzmann et al. 2022). These studies range from single-session interventions to programs lasting 6–12 weeks, with weekly volumes between 90 and 300 min (Ortiz-Alvarez et al. 2020; Suryani et al. 2022). Exercise intensity is also a central factor, typically prescribed based on maximal oxygen consumption (VO_{2max}), target heart rate, or ratings of perceived exertion (Bonomini-Gnutzmann et al. 2022). In addition to the studies already published, clinical trials are currently underway, further highlighting the growing interest in elucidating the effects of these understudied training modalities on gut microbiota dynamics (Bock et al. 2025).

Another key methodological consideration involves the collection and analysis of biological samples. Most studies use feces as the primary matrix, with microbial profiling commonly performed through 16S ribosomal RNA (rRNA) gene sequencing, although some employ shotgun metagenomics or biochemical assays for markers of intestinal permeability (Bonomini-Gnutzmann et al. 2022; Ortiz-Alvarez et al. 2020). The lack of standardization in sample processing as well as in the taxonomic level of analysis (phylum, genus, or species) remains a major limiting factor for comparisons across studies (Ortiz-Alvarezet al. 2020).

Moreover, reviews underscore the importance of controlling for confounding variables, particularly diet and the use of antibiotics or probiotics (Ortiz-Alvarez et al. 2020; Bonomini-Gnutzmann et al. 2022; Cataldi et al. 2022). Many studies do not standardize dietary intake before fecal collection or fail to statistically adjust for dietary factors, thereby constraining the ability to infer causality between exercise and microbiota alterations (Cataldi et al. 2022; Ortiz-Alvarez et al. 2020). In addition, the recurrently inconclusive or divergent findings across the literature highlight the need for larger sample sizes and longer study durations, since most studies included in systematic reviews involve small samples (<50 participants) and short intervention periods (up to 12 weeks) (Ortiz-Alvarez et al. 2020; Bonomini-Gnutzmann et al. 2022). These methodological limitations reinforce the recommendation for future multicenter randomized trials employing standardized exercise protocols to establish robust guidelines for exercise prescription aimed at beneficial modulation of the gut microbiota (Cataldi et al. 2022).

Progress in this field requires more rigorous designs capable of distinguishing chronic adaptations to exercise from transient effects of the last training session—the so-called last bout effect (Suryani et al. 2022; Bonomini-Gnutzmann et al. 2022). To achieve this, it is essential to employ randomized controlled trials with parallel groups and appropriate controls, as well as longitudinal studies incorporating serial sampling at multiple time points (Bonomini-Gnutzmann et al. 2022; Suryani et al. 2022; Knight et al. 2018; Darragh et al. 2021). Additionally, biological sample collection should be standardized, adhering to appropriate post-exercise time windows, and multimodal molecular approaches, such as metagenomics and metabolomics, should be employed (Darragh et al. 2021; Knight et al. 2018). Larger sample sizes, inclusion of populations with different training backgrounds (sedentary, recreationally active, and athletes), and detailed control of confounding variables such as diet, sleep, and medication use are also recommended (Darragh et al. 2021; Knight et al. 2018; Suryani et al. 2022; Bonomini-Gnutzmann et al. 2022). Together, these methodological refinements, coupled with rigorous standards for reproducibility and transparent reporting, will allow future research at the interface of exercise science and gut microbiota to produce more consistent, generalizable, and clinically applicable evidence (Knight et al. 2018; Darragh et al. 2021).

6.3 EXERCISE-DRIVEN GUT MICROBIOTA TAXONOMIC ALTERATIONS: INFLUENCE OF KEY TRAINING VARIABLES

Physical exercise has been shown to modulate the gut microbiota, with responses varying according to the modality, intensity, volume, and duration of the activity. Controlled human trials show that both aerobic and concurrent training can elicit taxonomic and functional shifts in the microbiome; however, the magnitude and direction of these effects depend on exercise type, session length, intervention duration, and participants' baseline health status (Suryani et al. 2022). However, it is important to emphasize that these variables rarely act in isolation; instead, they interact synergistically in a complex and interdependent manner within each exercise protocol. Consequently, current findings reveal only general trends and do not allow specific effects to be attributed to any single factor. Nonetheless, evaluating the potential contribution of each training component individually remains critical for understanding their specific roles in shaping exercise-induced gut microbiota adaptations (Ghaffar et al. 2024).

Despite this relevance, isolating the specific contribution of any single training variable remains particularly challenging, as most studies manipulate more than one factor simultaneously or do not include direct comparisons across different modalities, intensities, or volumes. Several studies have examined how exercise shapes gut microbiota responses, and the main findings of these investigations are summarized in **Table 6.1**.

6.3.1 Exercise Duration and Temporal Dynamics: Acute vs. Chronic Responses

The effects of physical exercise on the gut microbiota emerge both in the form of immediate shifts and as long-term adaptations that take shape with continued training. While chronic exercise tends to promote more stable and biologically relevant remodeling of the microbial ecosystem, even isolated exercise bouts can provoke temporary taxonomic changes. Compositional analyses have shown, for instance, transient increases in bacterial genera linked to lactate metabolism after single exercise sessions (Grosicki et al. 2023). Although findings vary across studies, the overall pattern suggests that the acute metabolic and hormonal milieu generated by exercise can elicit short-term microbial adjustments (Kern et al. 2020; Grosicki et al. 2023).

Research on exercise-induced microbiota modulation has predominantly focused on chronic training, consistently demonstrating its beneficial effects, whereas evidence on acute exercise remains comparatively scarce. Chronic exercise has been shown to promote consistent increases in butyrate-producing genera, such as *Faecalibacterium*, *Roseburia*, *Lachnospira*, *Clostridiales* spp., and members of Lachnospiraceae, accompanied by an enhanced functional capacity for the production of SCFA, particularly in lean individuals. In individuals with obesity, however, these same taxa exhibit attenuated responses or even relative reductions, illustrating that exercise-induced taxonomic changes are strongly influenced by metabolic status. Notably, these shifts tend to return toward baseline profiles following the reintroduction of sedentary behavior (Aragón-Vela et al. 2021).

In addition to modulating specific bacterial genera, chronic training also reshapes broader ecological features of the gut microbiota. Controlled clinical trials in individuals with overweight and obesity have shown that structured training programs carried out over several months can promote increases in alpha-diversity, as well as marked alterations in beta-diversity. Such modifications reflect a more robust remodeling of the intestinal community, accompanied by inferred functional shifts such as enhanced fermentative capacity and increased SCFA production (Kern et al. 2020).

In the context of acute exercise, a study with cross-country amateur athletes demonstrated that, in a running protocol with a 1% incline at an initial speed of 10 km/h, with increments of 0.3 km/h every 30 s until volitional exhaustion, followed by a 1 km submaximal/maximal sprint test on a track, a single exercise session was able to modulate the gut microbiota, increasing the abundance of the genera *Romboutsia*, *Ruminococcaceae*, *Escherichia coli*, and *Blautia*, while reducing *Ruminiclostridium* and *Clostridium phoceensis* (Tabone et al. 2021). These findings provide evidence that even a single bout of physical exercise can elicit detectable microbial shifts.

6.3.2 Exercise Modalities: Aerobic, Resistance, and Combined Training

The type of physical exercise, broadly categorized as aerobic or anaerobic, appears to elicit distinct modulatory effects on the gut microbiota. Evidence indicates that chronic aerobic training

TABLE 6.1

Key features of exercise trials examining microbial taxonomic remodeling

Study	Design	Intervention	Follow-up	Sample	Microbiota outcome measures	Microbiota effects
Allen et al. (2018)	Quasi-experimental study	3 supervised aerobic exercise sessions per week (30–60 min, 60–75% HRR) using a treadmill or cycle ergometer. Week 1: 30 min at 60% HRR; Week 2: 45 min at 60% HRR; Week 3: 60 min at 60% HRR; Weeks 4–6: intensity increased 5% HRR per week, reaching 75% HRR for 60 min in Week 6. Washout period: after post-training assessments, all participants were instructed to refrain from exercise for the next six weeks.	6 weeks	32 sedentary, lean, and obese participants, aged 20–45 years	Taxonomic composition (relative abundance) α-diversity β-diversity	↔ β-diversity ↔ α-diversity *Collinsella* spp.: ↑ subtle after exercise/↓ after washout in obese; ↔ in lean after exercise/↑ subtle after washout. *Faecalibacterium* spp.: in obese, ↓ after exercise/↑ subtle after washout; in lean, ↑ after exercise/↓ after washout. *Lachnospira* spp.: in obese, ↑ subtle after exercise/↑ after washout; in lean, ↑ after exercise/↓ after washout.
Bycura et al. (2021)	Quasi-experimental study	Cardiorespiratory Exercise (CRE): 3×/week, 60 min/session, 60–90% HRmax; mix of cycling and CRE activities (step, circuit, kickboxing, running) Resistance Training Exercise (RTE): 3×/week, 60 min/session; 70–85% 1RM, 3–6 sets of 6–12 reps; full-body, lower-body, upper-body split; exercises stressing abdominal core musculature	8 weeks	56 students aged 18–33 years	Taxonomic composition (relative abundance)	CRE: ↑ RER associated with *Prevotella*, *Romboutsia*, *Dialister*. ↓ RER associated with *Bacteroides*, *Bacteroides* B, *Parabacteroides*. RTE: ↑ Gain 3RM associated with *Ruminococcus*, Lachnospiraceae, *Turicibacter*, *Clostridium*. ↓ Gain 3RM associated with *Siccibacter*, *Bacteroides*, *Bacteroides* B, *Alistipes*, *Oscillibacter*, ER4.
Craven et al. (2022)	Quasi-experimental study	3 weeks normal training (NormTr), 3 weeks high-volume training (HVolTr, +10–30% weekly), and 1-week taper (TaperTr, −55% volume). Participants underwent fecal sample collection before and after each phase.	7 weeks	14 competitive middle-distance runners	Taxonomic composition (relative abundance) α-diversity	↔ OTU counts or α-diversity; After HVolTr: ↑ *Ruminococcus callidus* ↓ *Pasteurellaceae* ↓ *Lachnoclostridium* ↓ *Haemophilus parainfluenzae* ↓ *Streptococcus parasanguinis*

Dupuit et al. (2022)	Randomized controlled study	Control group HIIT + RT 3×/week. Sessions approximately 45 min each. HIIT: repeated cycles of sprinting/speeding for 8 s followed by slow pedaling (30–40 rpm) for 12 s on a bicycle. Resistance was controlled to reach ~85% of each participant's HRmax during the 20-min session. RT: included two different training circuits with ten exercises each.	12 weeks	17 postmenopausal women with overweight or obesity	Taxonomic composition (relative abundance) α-diversity	↔ α-diversity HIIT +RT: ↑ *Bifidobacteriaceae* ↑ *Enterobacteriaceae* ↑ *Verrucimicrobiaceae* ↓ *Desulfovibrionaceae* Paraprevotellaceae and Prevotellaceae: negative association with abdominal fat and positive association with muscle mass. Streptococcaceae and Desulfovibrionaceae: negative correlation with total cholesterol/HDL-C. Alcaligenaceae: positive correlation with fasting blood glucose, total cholesterol, and LDL-C. Prevotellaceae: positive correlation with PPO.
Hampton-Marcell et al. (2020)	Observational study	Athletes monitored during peak training and taper. Fecal samples collected every two weeks. Daily swimming distance and duration recorded; training intensity and calorie expenditure estimated from distance/time.	Peak training through taper (~2–4 weeks, with biweekly sampling)	13 collegiate Swimmers (8 women and 5 men) aged 18–24 years	Taxonomic composition (relative abundance) α-diversity	Reduced training volume: ↓ α-diversity ↓ Firmicutes: Bacteroidetes (~2:1 → ~1:1) ↓ *Coprococcus* and *Faecalibacterium*.

(*Continued*)

Table 6.1 (Continued)

Study	Design	Intervention	Follow-up	Sample	Microbiota outcome measures	Microbiota effects
Kern et al. (2020)	Randomized controlled study	Randomization 1:2:2:2 to: Habitual living (CON) Active commuting by bike (BIKE) Leisure-time exercise of either moderate (MOD, 50% of VO_2peak-reserve) or vigorous intensity (VIG, 70% of VO_2peak-reserve), five days/week of training. All tests were repeated three and six months after the initiation of exercise interventions.	6 month	88 participants (physically inactive, women and men aged 20–45 years)	Taxonomic composition (relative abundance) α-diversity β-diversity ASV counts	Leisure exercise: ↑ α-diversity ↔ β-diversity MOD ↑ ASV richness at 3 months, and VIG at 6 months. ↑ α-diversity for VIG at 3 months.
Liu et al. (2020)	Randomized controlled study	Sedentary control Combined aerobic and strength training. 3×/week. 70 min per session. Warm-up: 10 min 3 stations of 10 min: Treadmill: 3–4 intervals of 2 min running at 85–95% VO_{2max}, with active recovery Bicycle: 4–5 intervals of 45–60 s at 90–95% peak, with active recovery (60–75 s at 30% peak) Calisthenics/Resistance: 2–3 sets of squats, kettlebell swings, planks, and burpees, with 30 s rest between set. Cool-down: 10–15 min Intensity: Adjusted according to HRMax (80–95%), with individualized progression.	12 weeks	39 Obese men aged 20–60 years Responders (n = 14): defined as those who demonstrated a decrease in HOMA-IR greater than twice the technical error, which is considered a threshold for a true physiological adaptation.	Taxonomic composition (relative abundance) α-diversity β-diversity	↔ α or β diversity before and after exercise. Participant Classification: Responders: ↓ *Bacteroides xylanisolvens* ↑ *Streptococcus mitis* ↓ *Alistipes putredinis* ↑ Lachnospiraceae ↓*Alistipes shahii*. ↓ replication rate of *Prevotella copri*. ↑ growth rate of various *Bacteroides* species. Non-responders (n = 6): ↓ *Ruminococcus gnavus*. ↑ *A. shahii*.

Moitinho-Silva et al. (2021)	Randomized controlled study	Control: maintain usual physical inactivity Endurance: running 3×/week ≥30 min; 1 session supervised/week; intensity guided by Borg RPE; Strength: full-body hypertrophy training 3×/week; 2 sessions supervised/week; 6 exercises/session for major muscle groups; warm-up set + load progression to allow 8 maximal reps; In addition, 13 elite athletes (mainly cyclists and triathletes) provided fecal samples as a high-exercise comparison group.	6 weeks	42 healthy, physically inactive adults (men and women), aged 20–45 years	Taxonomic composition (relative abundance) α-diversity β-diversity ASV abundance/occurrence	α-diversity: ↓ Chao1 in the resistance group; no change in Inverse Simpson ↔ β-diversity ↔ ASV abundance/occurrence Elite athletes vs. physically inactive: ↔ α-diversity ↔ β-diversity ↑ *Coprococcus*, *Parasutterella*, Ruminococcaceae (athletes) ↑ *Dialister*, *Odoribacter*, *Phascolarctobacterium* (inactive) ↔*Veillonella*
Motiani et al. (2020)	Randomized controlled study	6 supervised sessions: Sprint interval (SIT): 4–6 × 30 s all-out cycling sprints with 4 min recovery, progressive from 4→5→6 sprints. Moderate-intensity continuous training (MICT): 40–60 min moderate-intensity cycling (60% VO_2peak), progressive duration 40→50→60 min.	2 weeks	18 sedentary middle-age insulin-resistant subjects	Taxonomic composition (relative abundance) α-diversity β-diversity	↔α-diversity and β-diversity between the training modes. ↓ F/B ratio, ↓ *Blautia* and ↓*Clostridium* spp. in both groups SIT: ↑ *Lachnospira* MICT: ↑ *Veillonella*, ↑ *Faecalibacterium* (*F. prausnitzii*) ↑ *Veillonella dispar* (OTU 4034)
Resende et al. (2021)	Randomized controlled study	Cycle ergometer training, 3×/week, 50-min sessions. During the first 2 weeks: continuous exercise at 60 rpm (50 min). In the following weeks: progressive resistance (+15–25 W) to maintain 60–65% of VO_2peak, with sessions consisting of 5 min warm-up, 40 min exercise, and 5 min cool-down.	10 weeks	28 healthy men, aged 20–45 years	Taxonomic composition (relative abundance) α-diversity β-diversity	↔ α- or β-diversity (between or within groups). ↑ *Streptococcus* (genus) ↓ *Clostridiales* (genus)

(*Continued*)

Table 6.1 (Continued)

Study	Design	Intervention	Follow-up	Sample	Microbiota outcome measures	Microbiota effects
Tabone et al. (2021)	Quasi-experimental study	Warm-up: 10 min of continuous treadmill running at 60% of maximal heart rate. Incremental test: Treadmill running with a 1% incline, starting at 10 km/h and increasing by 0.3 km/h every 30 s until voluntary exhaustion. Additional maximal effort: After the treadmill test, participants performed a 1-km track run at maximal speed, with the time to complete the distance recorded.	Acute exercise bout	40 male endurance cross-country runners	Taxonomic composition (relative abundance) between athletes and inatives participants α-diversity β-diversity	↔ α- or β-diversity pre- vs. post-exercise Post-exercise changes: ↑ *Romboutsia*, *Ruminococcaceae* UCG-005, TOP498, *Blautia*; ↓ *Ruminiclostridium* 9, *Clostridium phoceensis*
Taniguchi et al (2018)	Randomized crossover trial	5-week supervised progressive aerobic cycling program or a control period, then crossed over after 5 weeks. Exercise was performed 3×/week, intensity increased from 60% VO_2peak (week 1) to 75% VO_2peak (weeks 4–5), and duration from 30 min (weeks 1–2) to 45 min (weeks 3–5).	5 weeks	33 healthy men, aged 62–76 years	Taxonomic composition (relative abundance) α-diversity β-diversity	↔ α- or β-diversity after 5-week resistance exercise (between or within periods) ↑ *Oscillospira* (genus) ↓ *Clostridium difficile* (species)
Zhao et al (2018)	Quasi-experimental study	Half marathon (21.1 km), completion time: 92–160 min Fecal samples: before race, after race	Half marathon	20 health amateur runners (16 males and 4 females) with an average age of 31.3 years	Taxonomic composition (relative abundance) α-diversity	↔ α-diversity Post-run: 20 bacterial clades enriched; key genera: *Pseudobutyrivibrio*, *Coprococcus_2*, *Collinsella*, *Mitsuokella* 7 OTUs increased, highest in *Coprococcus_2* (~3-fold); other genera: *Romboutsia*, *Pseudobutyrivibrio*; phyla Lentisphaerae and Acidobacteria detected only post-run.

Notes: ↑: increased; ↓: decreased; ↔: no differences F/B: Firmicutes/Bacteroidetes ratio; HRR: Heart Rate Reserve; HIIT: high-intensity interval training; RT: resistance training; CRE: Cardiorespiratory Exercise; RTE: Resistance Training Exercise; OTUs: operational taxonomic units.; RER: Respiratory Exchange Ratio; 3RM: Three-Repetition Maximum; SIT: sprint interval; MICT: moderate-intensity continuous training; ASV: Amplicon Sequence Variants; RPE: Rating of Perceived Exertion; PPO: Potência de pico (expressa em watts ou watts por quilograma).

induces changes in bacterial groups associated with host health (Allen et al. 2018). In an aerobic training protocol conducted over ten weeks using a cycle ergometer, participants trained for 50 min, three times per week. During the first two weeks, the exercise was performed at a constant speed of 60 rpm. In the following weeks, the resistance of the cycle ergometer was progressively increased by adding a load between 15 and 25 W to maintain the training intensity between 60 and 65% of each participant's VO_2peak. During this period, each session consisted of 40 min of exercise, preceded by a 5-min warm-up and followed by a 5-min recovery. This ten-week aerobic training led to a reduction in the relative abundance of bacteria from the order Clostridiales, along with an increase in the genus *Streptococcus*, which may be associated with beneficial metabolic effects (Resende et al. 2021).

Complementarily, a decrease in *Clostridium difficile* species, a microorganism known for its pathogenic potential, was reported after a supervised and progressive five-week aerobic exercise program compared with control group. The study included the use of a cycle ergometer, with exercise intensity gradually increased so that participants trained at a power output designed to elicit 60% of pre-exercise capacity during week 1, 70% during weeks 2 and 3, and 75% during weeks 4 and 5. The exercise duration was set at 30 min for weeks 1 and 2, and 45 min for weeks 3–5. Despite differences in the taxonomic levels used in the analyses, which range from order to species, the results converge on a trend of reduced undesirable microorganisms in response to aerobic exercise (Taniguchi et al. 2018). Interestingly, short-term endurance training (30 min, three times per week for six weeks) leads to a slight reduction in gut microbiota diversity, possibly due to the redistribution of gastrointestinal blood flow during prolonged exercise (Moitinho-Silva et al. 2021).

Other interventions have demonstrated distinct functional responses. In an aerobic training protocol lasting six weeks, with three weekly sessions of 30–60 min at moderate-to-vigorous intensity, increases were observed in butyrate-producing genera such as *Faecalibacterium*, *Roseburia*, and *Lachnospira*, alongside elevated fecal SCFA concentrations, particularly in lean individuals (Allen et al. 2018). Complementing these findings, a 12-week concurrent training program, combining high-intensity interval training, using repeated 8-s sprints interspersed with 12 s of light cycling at ~85–90% HRmax, with resistance exercise performed to volitional fatigue; although α-diversity remained unchanged, this intervention increased β-diversity and revealed negative correlations with reductions in visceral adiposity and positive correlations with increases in muscle mass (Dupuit et al. 2022).

In contrast, strength training did not result in detectable changes in gut microbiota composition when performed for 30 min, three times per week over six weeks, with sessions comprising six exercises (two for the legs, two for the chest, and two for the back) using a load that allowed up to eight repetitions (Moitinho-Silva et al. 2021). Similarly, no appreciable alterations were observed following an eight-week protocol involving 60-min sessions, three times per week, with exercises targeting all major upper- and lower-body muscle groups (Bycura et al. 2021). Together, these findings suggest that resistance training may exert a more stable, or comparatively less pronounced impact, on gut microbial composition relative to aerobic modalities.

6.3.3 Exercise Intensity and Dose–Response Effects

Building on the evidence that both exercise duration and metabolic status modulate microbial responses, the role of training intensity adds another layer of complexity to this interaction. Evidence remains limited regarding the specific effects of exercise intensity, as an isolated training variable, on gut microbiota composition and function. Reviews indicate that higher-intensity efforts, particularly in endurance athletes, may be linked with unfavorable gastrointestinal outcomes, including increased intestinal permeability and exercise-related gastrointestinal symptoms (Bonomini-Gnutzmann et al. 2022), whereas moderate training loads tend to support greater microbial diversity and an increased abundance of SCFA-producing bacteria (Suryani et al. 2022).

In line with this complexity, evidence from clinical and experimental studies further illustrates that exercise intensity does not exert uniform effects on the gut microbiota. Several studies have reported that aerobic exercise may be a beneficial strategy for modulating gut microbiota composition in individuals with metabolic diseases, particularly when performed at moderate or vigorous intensity (Silva et al. 2022). However, findings across the literature are not fully consistent, as some studies report favorable microbiota shifts while others describe neutral or even adverse effects under similar intensity conditions. Studies have demonstrated that high-intensity exercise may reduce intestinal inflammation through modifications in the microbial profile (Motiani et al. 2020). An increase in *Bacteroidetes* has also been observed at 80–90% maximal heart rate (Motiani et al. 2020). Another study reported that high-intensity exercise enhances mitochondrial function and promotes the growth of bacteria involved in urease production and lactate metabolism (Suryani et al. 2022).

However, despite these potentially beneficial effects, higher-training intensities can also impose physiological stress that drives the gut microbiota in less favorable directions. High-intensity exercise can activate stress pathways, increasing catabolic hormones and pro-inflammatory cytokines that enhance intestinal permeability and drive taxonomic shifts—such as increases in *Ruminococcus gnavus*, *Butyrivibrio*, *Coprococcus*, and *Oscillospira* and reductions in *Turicibacter* spp.—highlighting that the nature of the effort is decisive, since voluntary exercise tends to attenuate inflammation and preserve microbial ecology, whereas forced or stress-inducing exercise can exacerbate inflammatory responses and favor the enrichment of mucolytic, barrier-disrupting taxa (Clark and Mach, 2016). Finally, a randomized clinical trial in humans with overweight and obesity observed a reduction in microbial heterogeneity in the high-intensity exercise group compared with the control group (Kern et al. 2020).

6.3.4 Exercise Volume: Frequency, Session Duration, and Weekly Load

Exercise volume has been identified as a key factor in maintaining a healthy gut microbiota. In a study with competitive runners, a seven-week intervention was divided into three phases: three weeks of training at habitual volume (72.0 ± 20.7 km/week for men and 53.1 ± 15.0 km/week for women); three weeks of progressive volume increase (with weekly increments of 10, 20, and 30%); and a final taper week, characterized by approximately a 55% reduction in volume relative to the high-volume phase. The authors found that high exercise volumes were associated with a reduction in the genus *Lachnoclostridium*, belonging to the phylum Bacillota. Additionally, the study reported a significant decrease in *Haemophilus* (often associated with pathogenic bacteria), along with an increase in the abundance of *Ruminococcus callidus*, a species involved in the degradation of complex polysaccharides (Craven et al. 2022).

This relationship between training load and taxonomic shifts is further supported by findings in swimmers. In a longitudinal study with swimmers, it was observed that a lower training volume, measured by the distance covered per week (32.6 ± 4.8 km/week at peak training and 11.3 ± 8.1 km/week during the reduction period), was associated with a decrease in two genera: *Coprococcus* and *Faecalibacterium* (Hampton-Marcell et al. 2020). These results support the hypothesis that higher volumes of physical exercise contribute to a more diverse, metabolically active, and functionally robust microbiota, with potential systemic benefits for the individual.

Beyond total training volume, the duration of each exercise session also appears to play a meaningful role in shaping gut microbiota responses. Physical exercise sessions of varying lengths—such as 30 s in sprint interval training (SIT) in which each session had an average total duration of 22.5 min and between 40 and 60 min in moderate-intensity continuous training (MICT)—both performed with the same frequency (three times per week) over two weeks, have been shown to elicit similar effects on the gut microbiota. In both methods, a reduction in the Bacillota (previously *Firmicutes*)/*Bacteroidota* (previously *Bacteroidetes*) (Berg et al. 2020) ratio, which is generally elevated in obesity, was observed, along with a decrease in the genera *Clostridium* and *Blautia*, the latter often associated with inflammation. However, an increase in the abundance of the genus *Faecalibacterium* (especially *Faecalibacterium prausnitzii*) occurred specifically after MICT, a change not found following SIT (Motiani et al. 2020).

Longer exercise bouts appear to elicit yet another layer of microbial responses, particularly during prolonged endurance efforts. Endurance exercise (a half marathon lasting between 92 and 160 min) was shown to increase the abundance of certain uncommon bacterial phyla, such as Lentisphaerae and Acidobacteria, whose functions in the human gut remain incompletely understood. Additionally, a significant genus-level increase was noted in *Pseudobutyrivibrio*, *Coprococcus_2*, *Collinsella*, and *Mitsuokella*, indicating a distinct functional modulation of the gut microbiota induced by prolonged exercise (Zhao et al. 2018).

Regarding microbial diversity, it has been observed that alpha-diversity indices, such as Shannon and Chao1, tend to remain stable following isolated exercise bouts, whereas more pronounced alterations are typically reported under conditions of extreme or prolonged exercise (Grosicki et al. 2023; Kern et al. 2020). Beta-diversity, in contrast, appears to be more sensitive to exercise stimuli, indicating transient shifts in the relative balance of dominant bacterial groups (Grosicki et al. 2023).

Taken together, current evidence indicates that exercise intensity modulates gut microbial composition in a context-dependent manner, interacting with training duration, modality, and volume. Moderate to vigorous aerobic efforts generally favor microbiota profiles enriched in SCFA-producing taxa and improved fermentative and anti-inflammatory capacity, whereas very high intensities may induce stress-related alterations characterized by transient permeability increases, inflammatory signaling, and shifts toward less stable, mucolytic communities. Thus, microbial remodeling does not follow a linear intensity–response pattern, reinforcing the need for controlled studies capable of disentangling intensity-specific effects within broader training parameters.

6.4 EXERCISE–GUT MICROBIOTA CROSSTALK: PHYSIOLOGICAL MECHANISMS AND EFFECTS

Exercise modulates the gut microbiota through multiple interrelated mechanisms that extend beyond taxonomic composition shifts. Evidence from intervention studies shows that even single exercise bouts or short training periods can elicit functional shifts in microbial metabolism, despite the absence of detectable changes in bacterial taxonomy. In contrast, sustained training promotes more stable and biologically meaningful microbial adaptations, increasingly associated with clinically relevant improvements in metabolic and inflammatory homeostasis (Grosicki et al. 2023; Kern et al. 2020).

Key pathways potentially modulated by physical exercise include the regulation of microbial metabolites that act as systemic signaling molecules. Among these, SCFAs, microbiota-derived bile acids, and trimethylamine N-oxide (TMAO) emerge as central mediators linking microbial function to host metabolic and inflammatory responses. These signaling molecules can enhance gut barrier integrity, attenuate immune activation and reduce metabolic endotoxemia (Bock et al. 2024). Within this mechanistic framework, we discuss how exercise-induced pathways interact and converge to shape the exercise–gut microbiota axis.

6.4.1 Short-Chain Fatty Acids (SCFAs) as Mediators of Exercise Effects

From a functional perspective, SCFAs (acetate, propionate, and butyrate), produced through the fermentation of dietary fibers by intestinal bacteria, represent the most consistent communication pathway between exercise and the gut microbiota (Varghese et al. 2024; Allen et al. 2018; Alvarez-Herms and Odriozola 2024). Acetate acts in peripheral tissues as a lipogenic precursor and modulator of autonomic nervous system signaling, influencing appetite regulation and overall energy homeostasis. Butyrate serves as the primary energy substrate for colonocytes, promoting epithelial integrity and reducing the translocation of LPSs into systemic circulation. Moreover, butyrate activates AMPK and peroxisome proliferator-activated receptor gamma coactivator 1-alpha (PGC-1α) signaling pathways, thereby stimulating mitochondrial biogenesis and oxidative metabolism in skeletal muscle (den Besten et al. 2013; Min et al. 2024; Aya et al. 2023). Propionate, in turn, participates in hepatic gluconeogenesis, contributing to energy balance during prolonged exercise, and appetite regulation (den Besten et al. 2013; Alvarez-Herms and Odriozola 2024; Varghese et al. 2024). The elevation of fecal and plasma levels of these metabolites in response to exercise reinforces the existence of a functional gut–muscle axis that directly depends on microbial plasticity (Allen et al. 2018; den Besten et al. 2013; Alvarez-Herms and Odriozola 2024; Varghese et al. 2024).

The microbial and SCFA-driven metabolic shifts may translate into clinical and performance gains (Aragón-Vela et al. 2021; Allen et al. 2018; Mach and Fuster-Botella 2017). In older adults, even short-term interventions that increase SCFA-producing bacteria have been associated with the preservation of lean mass and greater muscle strength, suggesting that the gut microbiota may mediate the link between exercise and protection against sarcopenia (Aragón-Vela et al.

2021; Giron et al. 2022). Longitudinal studies have shown that supervised aerobic training not only enhances microbial diversity in sedentary adults but also enhances fecal SCFA production in parallel with improvements in cardiorespiratory capacity (VO_{2max}), indicating a synergistic interaction between gut microbiota and aerobic fitness. However, the reversibility of these effects after a period of detraining underscores the need for sustained exercise engagement to maintain these beneficial adaptations (Allen et al. 2018).

Complementarily, six weeks of aerobic exercise have been shown to increase the abundance of butyrate-producing bacteria in lean individuals, a finding associated with improved insulin sensitivity, enhanced mitochondrial biogenesis via AMPK and PGC-1α activation, and a more favorable modulation of muscle protein synthesis. However, these responses appear blunted in individuals with obesity, likely due to low-grade chronic inflammation and metabolic resistance that limit microbiota plasticity (Aragón-Vela et al. 2021). Together, these findings reinforce that the baseline metabolic milieu critically shapes the magnitude of exercise-induced microbiota and SCFA shifts, modulating their downstream functional and clinical effects.

Extending this context-dependent pattern, studies in metabolically at-risk individuals demonstrate that the microbiota's functional capacity is a decisive determinant of exercise effectiveness. In prediabetic adults, improvements in insulin sensitivity occurred primarily in participants whose microbiota displayed greater potential for SCFA biosynthesis and branched-chain amino acid (BCAA) catabolism, metabolic signatures that aligned with enhanced glycemic control. In contrast, non-responders lacked these functional traits and showed minimal metabolic gains. Notably, fecal microbiota transplantation from responders to rodents reproduced the benefits, supporting causal evidence that microbial functional programming governs the metabolic adaptability to exercise (Liu et al. 2020).

Building on this evidence, experimental findings further strengthen this link. Fecal microbiota transplantation from individuals with greater physical capacity has been shown to increase muscle mass and strength and in animal models, reinforcing the concept of a gut–muscle axis as an active regulator of exercise-induced adaptations (Giron et al. 2022). Consistently, the transfer of microbiota from trained to sedentary mice reproduced hallmark benefits of exercise, such as enhanced mitochondrial biogenesis and upregulated oxidative gene expression in skeletal muscle, suggesting that microbial signals may contribute to the physiological remodeling triggered by physical training (Liu et al. 2020).

Taken together, these causal insights from animal models find strong parallels in human research. Clinical trials have consolidated evidence that structured exercise can functionally remodel the gut microbiota and its metabolites in humans. A randomized trial in overweight individuals demonstrated that 12 weeks of aerobic training, which, although not reporting the exact session duration, corresponded to approximately 45–55 min/session in the moderate-intensity group and 30–40 min/session in the vigorous-intensity group, significantly increased the abundance of *Bacteroides*, *Akkermansia*, and *Prevotella*, alongside elevated fecal SCFA production and improved insulin sensitivity (Kern et al. 2020). Another trial evaluated short-term resistance training, in which the exercise protocols differed in structure and session duration. The SIT consisted of four to six bouts of 30 s of all-out cycling, each followed by 4 min of recovery, totaling 18–26 min per session. In contrast, the MICT involved 40–60 min of continuous cycling. Both increased *Bacteroides* spp. and decreased Bacillota, with concomitant increases in plasma butyrate and propionate concentrations (Motiani et al. 2020).

6.4.2 Secondary Bile Acids as Mediators of Exercise Effects

Another key physiological pathway through which exercise influences host metabolism involves the interplay between microbiota-derived bile acids and skeletal muscle function. The microbiota catalyzes the conversion of primary to secondary bile acids, predominantly by genera such as *Clostridium* and *Bacteroides*, thereby enhancing the activation of the farnesoid X receptor (FXR) and the G protein–coupled bile acid receptor 1 (TGR5). These nuclear and membrane receptors orchestrate central metabolic processes, including glucose and lipid homeostasis, energy expenditure, and inflammatory regulation (Mancin et al. 2023).

FXR activation induces the production of fibroblast growth factor 19 (FGF19), an enterokine that acts on the liver and skeletal muscle, modulating glucose and lipid metabolism and stimulating anabolic signaling pathways involved in muscle mass maintenance. Conversely, TGR5 activation enhances thermogenesis and systemic energy expenditure and stimulates the secretion of glucagon-like peptide 1 (GLP-1), a hormone with insulinotropic and anabolic effects on muscle (Lefevre and Bindels 2022). Thus, exercise-driven shifts in microbial composition and function that reshape the bile acid pool indirectly influence muscle metabolism, strengthening the concept of a bile acid–dependent gut–muscle axis as a mechanistic contributor to training-induced physiological remodeling (Qiu et al. 2021).

6.4.3 Trimethylamine N-Oxide (TMAO) as Mediator of Exercise Effects

Extending this bile acid–dependent regulatory network, exercise also modulates another key microbiota-derived metabolic axis: the production of TMAO. Exercise exerts a regulatory role in the microbial metabolism of choline, L-carnitine, and betaine, precursors of TMAO. The formation of TMA is driven by the enzymatic activity of intestinal bacteria such as *Desulfovibrio*, *Clostridium*, and *Eggerthella*, whose abundance is modulated by dietary patterns and training status. Consistently, evidence suggests that regular physical exercise can reduce circulating TMAO (Longoria et al. 2022; Gerdes et al. 2020). TMAO has emerged as a gut microbiota–derived biomarker linked to cardiovascular risk, inflammation, and adiposity indicators such as BMI and waist circumference (Iorra et al. 2025), yet its responsiveness to structured exercise interventions remains insufficiently explored.

TMAO is associated with endothelial dysfunction and the progression of atherosclerosis by promoting oxidative stress and decreasing the bioavailability of nitric oxide (Longoria, Guers, and Campbell 2022). In animal models, TMAO supplementation has been shown to increase arterial stiffness and myocardial collagen deposition, while aerobic exercise attenuated these alterations even under conditions of high-fat diets (Rivera et al. 2024; Theodoridis et al. 2025). Consistently, exercise-trained mice display not only lower circulating TMAO but also an enrichment of beneficial taxa such as *Faecalibacterium* and *Akkermansia*, both of which are linked to improved vascular function and enhanced mitochondrial efficiency (Rivera et al. 2024; Theodoridis et al. 2025; Longoria et al. 2022).

From a functional standpoint, exercise may modulate the gut microbiota-TMAO axis through two complementary pathways: (i) reducing the availability of lipotropic microbial substrates (such as choline and L-carnitine) partly due to their greater metabolic utilization during muscle contraction, and (ii) increasing microbial diversity and the proportion of non TMA–producing species. Together, these adaptations contribute to lower circulating TMAO levels, improving endothelial function, tissue perfusion, and skeletal muscle contractile efficiency, thereby reinforcing the anti-atherogenic and cardioprotective role of the gut microbiota in response to exercise (Gerdes et al. 2020; Rivera et al. 2024; Theodoridis et al. 2025).

6.4.4 Phenolic and Indolic Derivatives as Mediators of Exercise Effects

Another relevant group of metabolites modulated by the gut microbiota and influenced by physical exercise comprises phenolic and indolic derivatives of tryptophan, such as indole, indoxyl sulfate, and indole-3-propionic acid (IPA). These compounds are primarily produced by bacterial genera such as *Clostridium*, *Bacteroides*, *Peptostreptococcus*, and *Lactobacillus*, whose abundance tends to increase in response to regular exercise training programs (Nikkhah et al. 2023). Indole derivatives act as agonists of the aryl hydrocarbon receptor (AhR) and the pregnane X receptor (PXR), modulating signaling pathways that regulate inflammation, energy metabolism, and muscle protein synthesis (Nikkhah et al. 2023; Grosicki, Fielding, and Lustgarten 2018).

These metabolites participate in a functional gut–muscle axis, regulating protein synthesis and mitochondrial turnover through the activation of AMPK, the mTOR, and PGC-1α-mediated pathways. In addition, IPA and other phenolic derivatives preserve intestinal barrier integrity, thereby limiting LPS translocation and dampening the systemic inflammatory tone that accelerates muscle protein breakdown (Nikkhah et al. 2023; Liu et al. 2021). Building on this mechanistic framework, alterations in microbial taxa that produce these phenolic and indolic metabolites have been directly linked to clinically relevant muscle outcomes. Thus, maintaining a eubiotic microbiota through physical exercise supports the balance between inflammation, oxidative stress, and anabolism, establishing a bidirectional metabolic circuit in which gut-derived metabolites modulate skeletal muscle adaptation while muscle activity shapes microbial composition and function (Liu et al. 2021; Grosicki et al. 2018; Nikkhah et al. 2023).

Consistently, studies using models of sarcopenia and cachexia demonstrate a reduction in families such as Lachnospiraceae and Ruminococcaceae—producers of both SCFAs and phenolic compounds—and an increase in *Enterobacteriaceae* and *Eggerthella*, which are associated with inflammation and anabolic resistance. Exercise counteracts these detrimental shifts by restoring the abundance of *Roseburia*, *Lachnospira*, and *F. prausnitzii*, promoting an increased release of indoles with antioxidant and anti-inflammatory properties that are capable of preserving lean mass and improving insulin sensitivity (Nikkhah et al. 2023; Grosicki et al. 2018; Liu et al. 2021).

6.4.5 Exercise, Gut Barrier Function, and Immune-Inflammatory Regulation

Because many of the previously discussed metabolites exert their effects through the preservation of epithelial integrity and the attenuation of low-grade inflammation, their actions naturally converge with another major pathway through which exercise modulates host physiology: the reinforcement of gut barrier function and immune-inflammatory regulation.

Under moderate training protocols, there is a predominance of SCFA-producing bacteria, such as *Roseburia hominis*, *Eubacterium rectale*, and *Akkermansia muciniphila*, which are associated with improved intestinal permeability and enhanced microbial diversity. Conversely, high-intensity exercise can lead to transient increases in genera such as *Enterobacter* and *Escherichia*, accompanied by elevated intestinal permeability and increased luminal LPS concentrations, reflecting an adaptive response to acute physiological stress (Suryani et al. 2022; Bonomini-Gnutzmann et al. 2022).

Broadly, structured aerobic-based programs tend to increase the relative abundance of Bacteroidota and reduce Bacillota, while enhancing genera such as *Akkermansia*, *Faecalibacterium*, and *Roseburia*, which are linked to improved SCFA production, anti-inflammatory activity, and maintenance of intestinal barrier integrity. Collectively, these findings reinforce that exercise functions as a robust physiological stimulus capable of reshaping the gut ecosystem in ways that support metabolic regulation, dampen inflammatory processes, and enhance overall physiological resilience, particularly throughout aging (Varghese et al. 2024).

Extending this integrative framework, the modulation of systemic inflammation constitutes a key component of the exercise-microbiota interaction. Exercise-induced shifts are associated with an increased abundance of bacteria such as *F. prausnitzii* and *Roseburia* spp., which are recognized butyrate-producing taxa with well-established anti-inflammatory properties, along with a reduction in potentially pathogenic microorganisms. Together, these changes contribute to decreased intestinal permeability, reduced LPS translocation, and consequent attenuation of metabolic endotoxemia (Mach and Fuster-Botella 2017).

At the immunological level, this microbial balance promotes higher expression of anti-inflammatory cytokines (e.g., IL-10) and the suppression of pro-inflammatory mediators (TNF-α, IL-6), favoring a more stable metabolic environment conducive to muscle recovery. Such immunometabolic modulation, in turn, enhances insulin sensitivity and limits protein degradation, both critical for maintaining lean mass. In older adults, a population marked by chronic, low-grade inflammation (inflammaging), the combined effects of exercise and microbiota remodeling emerge as a synergistic strategy to counteract sarcopenia and preserve functional capacity (Mach and Fuster-Botella 2017; Aragón-Vela et al. 2021).

A crucial point in the interface between the microbiota and exercise is the modulation of metabolic endotoxemia through the reduction of LPS production and translocation, a major pro-inflammatory component derived from the cell wall of Gram-negative bacteria. Regular exercise increases the abundance of Gram-positive bacteria and decreases that of Gram-negative species, thereby lowering luminal LPS availability and dampening the activation of Toll-like receptor 4 (TLR4), a canonical inflammatory signaling pathway (Allen et al. 2018; Doyle et al. 2011). Chronic TLR4 activation is associated with protein degradation mediated by the ubiquitin–proteasome and autophagy–lysosome systems, whereas its inhibition, facilitated by exercise, preserves muscle tissue integrity and reduces catabolism. Collectively, these adaptations support redox homeostasis and maintain bioenergetic efficiency within muscle fibers (Doyle et al. 2011).

Taken together, current evidence indicates that physical exercise functions as a multifaceted regulator of the gut microbiota, inducing taxonomic and functional shifts that enhance the production of bioactive metabolites such as SCFAs and secondary bile acids. These metabolites integrate with host energy, inflammatory, and anabolic pathways, contributing to metabolic homeostasis and skeletal muscle function. Importantly, interindividual variability in microbiota composition and responsiveness underscores the need to consider baseline microbial profiles when evaluating exercise-induced adaptations. Deepening our understanding of these interactions may enable the development of personalized, microbiota-informed exercise strategies to optimize intestinal and systemic health.

REFERENCES

Allen, J. M., L. J. Mailing, G. M. Niemiro, R. Moore, M. D. Cook, B. A. White, H. D. Holscher, and J. A. Woods. 2018. "Exercise Alters Gut Microbiota Composition and Function in Lean and Obese Humans." *Med Sci Sports Exerc* 50 (4): 747–757. https://doi.org/10.1249/MSS.0000000000001495. www.ncbi.nlm.nih.gov/pubmed/29166320.

Alvarez-Herms, J., and A. Odriozola. 2024. "Microbiome and Physical Activity." *Adv Genet* 111: 409–450. https://doi.org/10.1016/bs.adgen.2024.01.002. www.ncbi.nlm.nih.gov/pubmed/38908903.

Aragón-Vela, J., P. Solis-Urra, F. J. Ruiz-Ojeda, A. I. Álvarez-Mercado, J. Olivares-Arancibia, and J. Plaza-Diaz. 2021. "Impact of Exercise on Gut Microbiota in Obesity." *Nutrients* 13 (11). https://doi.org/10.3390/nu13113999. www.ncbi.nlm.nih.gov/pubmed/34836254.

Aya, V., P. Jimenez, E. Muñoz, and J. D. Ramírez. 2023. "Effects of Exercise and Physical Activity on Gut Microbiota Composition and Function in Older Adults: A Systematic Review." *BMC Geriatr* 23 (1): 364. https://doi.org/10.1186/s12877-023-04066-y. www.ncbi.nlm.nih.gov/pubmed/37308839.

Berg, G., D. Rybakova, D. Fischer, T. Cernava, M. C. Vergès, T. Charles, X. Chen, L. Cocolin, K. Eversole, G. H. Corral, M. Kazou, L. Kinkel, L. Lange, N. Lima, A. Loy, J. A. Macklin, E. Maguin, T. Mauchline, R. McClure, B. Mitter, M. Ryan, I. Sarand, H. Smidt, B. Schelkle, H. Roume, G. S. Kiran, J. Selvin, R. S. C. Souza, L. van Overbeek, B. K. Singh, M. Wagner, A. Walsh, A. Sessitsch, and M. Schloter. 2020. "Microbiome Definition Re-Visited: Old Concepts and New Challenges." *Microbiome* 8 (1): 103. https://doi.org/10.1186/s40168-020-00875-0. www.ncbi.nlm.nih.gov/pubmed/32605663.

Bishop, D. J., B. Beck, S. J. H. Biddle, K. L. Denay, A. Ferri, M. J. Gibala, S. Headley, A. M. Jones, M. Jung, M. J. Lee, T. Moholdt, R. U. Newton, S. Nimphius, L. S. Pescatello, N. J. Saner, and C. Tzarimas. 2025. "Physical Activity and Exercise Intensity Terminology: A Joint American College of Sports Medicine (ACSM) Expert Statement and Exercise and Sport Science Australia (ESSA) Consensus Statement." *Med Sci Sports Exerc* 57 (11): 2599–2613. https://doi.org/10.1249/MSS.0000000000003795. www.ncbi.nlm.nih.gov/pubmed/41085254.

Bock, P. M., L. S. Kowalewski, L. R. Ayres, M. K. B. Russo, G. T. Leites, A. F. Martins, ÁR Oliveira, and M. Krause. 2025. "Effect of Heat Therapy Compared with Strength Training on Metabolic Profile, Heat Shock Response, Inflammation, Cardiovascular Responses and Microbiota in Individuals with Type 2 Diabetes: Study Protocol of a Randomized Trial." *Sao Paulo Med J* 143 (3): e2024040. https://doi.org/10.1590/1516-3180-2024.0040.R1.13082024. www.ncbi.nlm.nih.gov/pubmed/40465937.

Bock, P. M., A. F. Martins, R. Ramalho, G. H. Telo, G. Leivas, C. K. Maraschin, and B. D. Schaan. 2022. "The Impact of Dietary, Surgical, and Pharmacological Interventions on Gut Microbiota in Individuals with Diabetes Mellitus: A Systematic Review." *Diabetes Res Clin Pract* 189: 109944. https://doi.org/10.1016/j.diabres.2022.109944. www.ncbi.nlm.nih.gov/pubmed/35697155.

Bock, P. M., A. F. Martins, and B. D. Schaan. 2024. "Understanding How Pre- and Probiotics Affect the Gut Microbiome and Metabolic Health." *Am J Physiol Endocrinol Metab* 327 (1): E89–E102. https://doi.org/10.1152/ajpendo.00054.2024. www.ncbi.nlm.nih.gov/pubmed/38809510.

Bock, P. M., G. H. Telo, R. Ramalho, M. Sbaraini, G. Leivas, A. F. Martins, and B. D. Schaan. 2021. "The Effect of Probiotics, Prebiotics or Synbiotics on Metabolic Outcomes in Individuals with Diabetes: A Systematic Review and Meta-Analysis." *Diabetologia* 64 (1): 26–41. https://doi.org/10.1007/s00125-020-05295-1. www.ncbi.nlm.nih.gov/pubmed/33047170.

Bonomini-Gnutzmann, R., J. Plaza-Díaz, C. Jorquera-Aguilera, A. Rodríguez-Rodríguez, and F. Rodríguez-Rodríguez. 2022. "Effect of Intensity and Duration of Exercise on Gut Microbiota in Humans: A Systematic Review." *Int J Environ Res Public Health* 19 (15). https://doi.org/10.3390/ijerph19159518. www.ncbi.nlm.nih.gov/pubmed/35954878.

Bycura, D., A. C. Santos, A. Shiffer, S. Kyman, K. Winfree, J. Sutliffe, T. Pearson, D. Sonderegger, E. Cope, and J. G. Caporaso. 2021. "Impact of Different Exercise Modalities on the Human Gut Microbiome." *Sports*

(*Basel*) 9 (2). https://doi.org/10.3390/sports9020014. www.ncbi.nlm.nih.gov/pubmed/33494210.

Cataldi, S., V. Bonavolontà, L. Poli, F. M. Clemente, M. De Candia, R. Carvutto, A. F. Silva, G. Badicu, G. Greco, and F. Fischetti. 2022. "The Relationship between Physical Activity, Physical Exercise, and Human Gut Microbiota in Healthy and Unhealthy Subjects: A Systematic Review." *Biology (Basel)* 11 (3). https://doi.org/10.3390/biology11030479. www.ncbi.nlm.nih.gov/pubmed/35336852.

Clark, A., and N. Mach. 2016. "Exercise-Induced Stress Behavior, Gut-Microbiota-Brain Axis and Diet: A Systematic Review for Athletes." *J Int Soc Sports Nutr* 13: 43. https://doi.org/10.1186/s12970-016-0155-6. www.ncbi.nlm.nih.gov/pubmed/27924137.

Coffey, V. G., and J. A. Hawley. 2017. "Concurrent Exercise Training: Do Opposites Distract?" *J Physiol* 595 (9): 2883–2896. https://doi.org/10.1113/JP272270. www.ncbi.nlm.nih.gov/pubmed/27506998.

Craven, J., A. J. Cox, P. Bellinger, B. Desbrow, C. Irwin, J. Buchan, D. McCartney, and S. Sabapathy. 2022. "The Influence of Exercise Training Volume Alterations on the Gut Microbiome in Highly-Trained Middle-Distance Runners." *Eur J Sport Sci* 22 (8): 1222–1230. https://doi.org/10.1080/17461391.2021.1933199. www.ncbi.nlm.nih.gov/pubmed/34034615.

Darragh, I. A. J., L. O'Driscoll, and B. Egan. 2021. "Exercise Training and Circulating Small Extracellular Vesicles: Appraisal of Methodological Approaches and Current Knowledge." *Front Physiol* 12: 738333. https://doi.org/10.3389/fphys.2021.738333. www.ncbi.nlm.nih.gov/pubmed/34777006.

den Besten, G., K. van Eunen, A. K. Groen, K. Venema, D. J. Reijngoud, and B. M. Bakker. 2013. "The Role of Short-Chain Fatty Acids in the Interplay Between Diet, Gut Microbiota, and Host Energy Metabolism." *J Lipid Res* 54 (9): 2325–2340. https://doi.org/10.1194/jlr.R036012. www.ncbi.nlm.nih.gov/pubmed/23821742.

Doyle, A., G. Zhang, E. A. Abdel Fattah, N. T. Eissa, and Y. P. Li. 2011. "Toll-Like Receptor 4 Mediates Lipopolysaccharide-Induced Muscle Catabolism via Coordinate Activation of Ubiquitin-Proteasome and Autophagy-Lysosome Pathways." *FASEB J* 25 (1): 99–110. https://doi.org/10.1096/fj.10-164152. www.ncbi.nlm.nih.gov/pubmed/20826541.

Dupuit, M., M. Rance, C. Morel, P. Bouillon, A. Boscaro, V. Martin, E. Vazeille, N. Barnich, B. Chassaing, and N. Boisseau. 2022. "Effect of Concurrent Training on Body Composition and Gut Microbiota in Postmenopausal Women with Overweight or Obesity." *Med Sci Sports Exerc* 54 (3): 517–529. https://doi.org/10.1249/MSS.0000000000002809. www.ncbi.nlm.nih.gov/pubmed/34628447.

Egan, B., and A. P. Sharples. 2023. "Molecular Responses to Acute Exercise and Their Relevance for Adaptations in Skeletal Muscle to Exercise Training." *Physiol Rev* 103 (3): 2057–2170. https://doi.org/10.1152/physrev.00054.2021. www.ncbi.nlm.nih.gov/pubmed/36395350.

Frampton, J., K. G. Murphy, G. Frost, and E. S. Chambers. 2020. "Short-Chain Fatty Acids as Potential Regulators of Skeletal Muscle Metabolism and Function." *Nat Metab* 2 (9): 840–848. https://doi.org/10.1038/s42255-020-0188-7. www.ncbi.nlm.nih.gov/pubmed/32694821.

Gerdes, V., M. Gueimonde, L. Pajunen, M. Nieuwdorp, and K. Laitinen. 2020. "How Strong Is the Evidence that Gut Microbiota Composition Can Be Influenced by Lifestyle Interventions in a Cardio-Protective Way?" *Atherosclerosis* 311: 124–142. https://doi.org/10.1016/j.atherosclerosis.2020.08.028. www.ncbi.nlm.nih.gov/pubmed/32981713.

Ghaffar, T., F. Ubaldi, V. Volpini, F. Valeriani, and V. Romano Spica. 2024. "The Role of Gut Microbiota in Different Types of Physical Activity and Their Intensity: Systematic Review and Meta-Analysis." *Sports (Basel)* 12 (8). https://doi.org/10.3390/sports12080221. www.ncbi.nlm.nih.gov/pubmed/39195597.

Giron, M., M. Thomas, D. Dardevet, C. Chassard, and I. Savary-Auzeloux. 2022. "Gut Microbes and Muscle Function: Can Probiotics Make Our Muscles Stronger?" *J Cachexia Sarcopenia Muscle* 13 (3): 1460–1476. https://doi.org/10.1002/jcsm.12964. www.ncbi.nlm.nih.gov/pubmed/35278043.

Grosicki, G. J., R. A. Fielding, and M. S. Lustgarten. 2018. "Gut Microbiota Contribute to Age-Related Changes in Skeletal Muscle Size, Composition, and Function: Biological Basis for a Gut-Muscle Axis." *Calcif Tissue Int* 102 (4): 433–442. https://doi.org/10.1007/s00223-017-0345-5. www.ncbi.nlm.nih.gov/pubmed/29058056.

Grosicki, G. J., S. P. Langan, J. R. Bagley, A. J. Galpin, D. Garner, J. T. Hampton-Marcell, J. M. Allen, and A. T. Robinson. 2023. "Gut Check: Unveiling the Influence of Acute Exercise on the Gut Microbiota." *Exp Physiol* 108 (12): 1466–1480. https://doi.org/10.1113/EP091446. www.ncbi.nlm.nih.gov/pubmed/37702557.

Hampton-Marcell, J. T., T. W. Eshoo, M. D. Cook, J. A. Gilbert, C. A. Horswill, and R. Poretsky. 2020. "Comparative Analysis of Gut Microbiota Following Changes in Training Volume Among Swimmers."

Int J Sports Med 41 (5): 292–299. https://doi.org/10.1055/a-1079-5450. www.ncbi.nlm.nih.gov/pubmed/31975357.

Huiberts, R. O., R. C. I. Wüst, and S. van der Zwaard. 2024. "Concurrent Strength and Endurance Training: A Systematic Review and Meta-Analysis on the Impact of Sex and Training Status." Sports Med 54 (2): 485–503. https://doi.org/10.1007/s40279-023-01943-9. www.ncbi.nlm.nih.gov/pubmed/37847373.

Iorra, F. Q., P. G. Rodrigues, P. M. Bock, M. P. Guahnon, S. Eller, T. F. de Oliveira, L. Birk, P. S. Schwarz, M. Drehmer, K. V. Bloch, F. V. Cureau, and B. D. Schaan. 2025. "Gut Microbiota Metabolite TMAO and Adolescent Cardiometabolic Health: A Cross-Sectional Analysis." J Endocr Soc 9 (5): bvaf055. https://doi.org/10.1210/jendso/bvaf055. www.ncbi.nlm.nih.gov/pubmed/40242209.

Jones, A. M., and B. S. Kirby. 2025. "Physiological Resilience: What Is It and How Might It Be Trained?" Scand J Med Sci Sports 35 (3): e70032. https://doi.org/10.1111/sms.70032. www.ncbi.nlm.nih.gov/pubmed/40024804.

Kern, T., M. B. Blond, T. H. Hansen, M. Rosenkilde, J. S. Quist, A. S. Gram, C. T. Ekstrøm, T. Hansen, and B. Stallknecht. 2020. "Structured Exercise Alters the Gut Microbiota in Humans with Overweight and Obesity-A Randomized Controlled Trial." Int J Obes (Lond) 44 (1): 125–135. https://doi.org/10.1038/s41366-019-0440-y. www.ncbi.nlm.nih.gov/pubmed/31467422.

Knight, R., A. Vrbanac, B. C. Taylor, A. Aksenov, C. Callewaert, J. Debelius, A. Gonzalez, T. Kosciolek, L. I. McCall, D. McDonald, A. V. Melnik, J. T. Morton, J. Navas, R. A. Quinn, J. G. Sanders, A. D. Swafford, L. R. Thompson, A. Tripathi, Z. Z. Xu, J. R. Zaneveld, Q. Zhu, J. G. Caporaso, and P. C. Dorrestein. 2018. "Best Practices for Analysing Microbiomes." Nat Rev Microbiol 16 (7): 410–422. https://doi.org/10.1038/s41579-018-0029-9. www.ncbi.nlm.nih.gov/pubmed/29795328.

Lefevre, C., and L. B. Bindels. 2022. "Role of the Gut Microbiome in Skeletal Muscle Physiology and Pathophysiology." Curr Osteoporos Rep 20 (6): 422–432. https://doi.org/10.1007/s11914-022-00752-9. www.ncbi.nlm.nih.gov/pubmed/36121571.

Lim, C., E. A. Nunes, B. S. Currier, J. C. McLeod, A. C. Q. Thomas, and S. M. Phillips. 2022. "An Evidence-Based Narrative Review of Mechanisms of Resistance Exercise-Induced Human Skeletal Muscle Hypertrophy." Med Sci Sports Exerc 54 (9): 1546–1559. https://doi.org/10.1249/MSS.0000000000002929. www.ncbi.nlm.nih.gov/pubmed/35389932.

Liu, C., W. H. Cheung, J. Li, S. K. Chow, J. Yu, S. H. Wong, M. Ip, J. J. Y. Sung, and R. M. Y. Wong. 2021. "Understanding the Gut Microbiota and Sarcopenia: A Systematic Review." J Cachexia Sarcopenia Muscle 12 (6): 1393–1407. https://doi.org/10.1002/jcsm.12784. www.ncbi.nlm.nih.gov/pubmed/34523250.

Liu, Y., Y. Wang, Y. Ni, C. K. Y. Cheung, K. S. L. Lam, Z. Xia, D. Ye, J. Guo, M. A. Tse, G. Panagiotou, and A. Xu. 2020. "Gut Microbiome Fermentation Determines the Efficacy of Exercise for Diabetes Prevention." Cell Metab 31 (1): 77–91.e5. https://doi.org/10.1016/j.cmet.2019.11.001. www.ncbi.nlm.nih.gov/pubmed/31786155.

Longoria, C. R., J. J. Guers, and S. C. Campbell. 2022. "The Interplay between Cardiovascular Disease, Exercise, and the Gut Microbiome." Rev Cardiovasc Med 23 (11): 365. https://doi.org/10.31083/j.rcm2311365. www.ncbi.nlm.nih.gov/pubmed/39076202.

Mach, N., and D. Fuster-Botella. 2017. "Endurance Exercise and Gut Microbiota: A Review." J Sport Health Sci 6 (2): 179–197. https://doi.org/10.1016/j.jshs.2016.05.001. www.ncbi.nlm.nih.gov/pubmed/30356594.

Mancin, L., G. D. Wu, and A. Paoli. 2023. "Gut Microbiota-Bile Acid-Skeletal Muscle Axis." Trends Microbiol 31 (3): 254–269. https://doi.org/10.1016/j.tim.2022.10.003. www.ncbi.nlm.nih.gov/pubmed/36319506.

Min, L., A. Ablitip, R. Wang, T. Luciana, M. Wei, and X. Ma. 2024. "Effects of Exercise on Gut Microbiota of Adults: A Systematic Review and Meta-Analysis." Nutrients 16 (7). https://doi.org/10.3390/nu16071070. www.ncbi.nlm.nih.gov/pubmed/38613103.

Moitinho-Silva, L., M. Wegener, S. May, F. Schrinner, A. Akhtar, T. J. Boysen, E. Schaeffer, C. Hansen, T. Schmidt, M. C. Rühlemann, M. Hübenthal, P. Rausch, M. T. Kondakci, W. Maetzler, S. Weidinger, M. Laudes, P. Süß, D. Schulte, R. Junker, F. Sommer, B. Weisser, C. Bang, and A. Franke. 2021. "Short-Term Physical Exercise Impacts on the Human Holobiont Obtained by a Randomised Intervention Study." BMC Microbiol 21 (1): 162. https://doi.org/10.1186/s12866-021-02214-1. www.ncbi.nlm.nih.gov/pubmed/34078289.

Motiani, K. K., M. C. Collado, J. J. Eskelinen, K. A. Virtanen, E. Löyttyniemi, S. Salminen, P. Nuutila, K. K. Kalliokoski, and J. C. Hannukainen. 2020. "Exercise Training Modulates Gut Microbiota Profile and Improves Endotoxemia." Med Sci Sports Exerc 52 (1): 94–104. https://doi.org/10.1249/MSS.0000000000002112. www.ncbi.nlm.nih.gov/pubmed/31425383.

Nikkhah, A., H. S. Ejtahed, F. Ettehad Marvasti, M. Taghavi, A. Pakmehr, F. Hajipour, and B. Larijani. 2023. "The Critical Role of Gut Microbiota Dysbiosis in Skeletal Muscle Wasting: A Systematic Review." J

Appl Microbiol 134 (1). https://doi.org/10.1093/jambio/lxac014. www.ncbi.nlm.nih.gov/pubmed/36626794.

Ortiz-Alvarez, L., H. Xu, and B. Martinez-Tellez. 2020. "Influence of Exercise on the Human Gut Microbiota of Healthy Adults: A Systematic Review." *Clin Transl Gastroenterol* 11 (2): e00126. https://doi.org/10.14309/ctg.0000000000000126. www.ncbi.nlm.nih.gov/pubmed/32463624.

Qiu, Y., J. Yu, Y. Li, F. Yang, H. Yu, M. Xue, F. Zhang, X. Jiang, X. Ji, and Z. Bao. 2021. "Depletion of Gut Microbiota Induces Skeletal Muscle Atrophy by FXR-FGF15/19 Signalling." *Ann Med* 53 (1): 508–522. https://doi.org/10.1080/07853890.2021.1900593. www.ncbi.nlm.nih.gov/pubmed/33783283.

Resende, A. S., G. S. F. Leite, and A. H. Lancha Junior. 2021. "Changes in the Gut Bacteria Composition of Healthy Men with the Same Nutritional Profile Undergoing 10-Week Aerobic Exercise Training: A Randomized Controlled Trial." *Nutrients* 13 (8). https://doi.org/10.3390/nu13082839. www.ncbi.nlm.nih.gov/pubmed/34444999.

Rivera, K., L. Gonzalez, L. Bravo, L. Manjarres, and M. E. Andia. 2024. "The Gut-Heart Axis: Molecular Perspectives and Implications for Myocardial Infarction." *Int J Mol Sci* 25 (22). https://doi.org/10.3390/ijms252212465. www.ncbi.nlm.nih.gov/pubmed/39596530.

Schumann, M., J. F. Feuerbacher, M. Sünkeler, N. Freitag, B. R. Rønnestad, K. Doma, and T. R. Lundberg. 2022. "Compatibility of Concurrent Aerobic and Strength Training for Skeletal Muscle Size and Function: An Updated Systematic Review and Meta-Analysis." *Sports Med* 52 (3): 601–612. https://doi.org/10.1007/s40279-021-01587-7. www.ncbi.nlm.nih.gov/pubmed/34757594.

Silva, J. S. C., C. S. Seguro, and M. M. V. Naves. 2022. "Gut Microbiota and Physical Exercise in Obesity and Diabetes – A Systematic Review." *Nutr Metab Cardiovasc Dis* 32 (4): 863–877. https://doi.org/10.1016/j.numecd.2022.01.023. www.ncbi.nlm.nih.gov/pubmed/35227549.

Suryani, D., M. Subhan Alfaqih, J. W. Gunadi, N. Sylviana, H. Goenawan, I. Megantara, and R. Lesmana. 2022. "Type, Intensity, and Duration of Exercise as Regulator of Gut Microbiome Profile." *Curr Sports Med Rep* 21 (3): 84–91. https://doi.org/10.1249/JSR.0000000000000940. www.ncbi.nlm.nih.gov/pubmed/35245243.

Tabone, M., C. Bressa, J. A. García-Merino, D. Moreno-Pérez, E. C. Van, F. A. Castelli, F. Fenaille, and M. Larrosa. 2021. "The Effect of Acute Moderate-Intensity Exercise on the Serum and Fecal Metabolomes and the Gut Microbiota of Cross-Country Endurance Athletes." *Sci Rep* 11 (1): 3558. https://doi.org/10.1038/s41598-021-82947-1. www.ncbi.nlm.nih.gov/pubmed/33574413.

Taniguchi, H., K. Tanisawa, X. Sun, T. Kubo, Y. Hoshino, M. Hosokawa, H. Takeyama, and M. Higuchi. 2018. "Effects of Short-Term Endurance Exercise on Gut Microbiota in Elderly Men." *Physiol Rep* 6 (23): e13935. https://doi.org/10.14814/phy2.13935. www.ncbi.nlm.nih.gov/pubmed/30536648.

Theodoridis, X., A. Papaemmanouil, N. Papageorgiou, C. Savopoulos, M. Chourdakis, and A. Triantafyllou. 2025. "The Association Between Lifestyle Interventions and Trimethylamine N-Oxide: A Systematic-Narrative Hybrid Literature Review." *Nutrients* 17 (7). https://doi.org/10.3390/nu17071280. www.ncbi.nlm.nih.gov/pubmed/40219037.

Varghese, S., S. Rao, A. Khattak, F. Zamir, and A. Chaari. 2024. "Physical Exercise and the Gut Microbiome: A Bidirectional Relationship Influencing Health and Performance." *Nutrients* 16 (21). https://doi.org/10.3390/nu16213663. www.ncbi.nlm.nih.gov/pubmed/39519496.

Zhao, X., Z. Zhang, B. Hu, W. Huang, C. Yuan, and L. Zou. 2018. "Response of Gut Microbiota to Metabolite Changes Induced by Endurance Exercise." *Front Microbiol* 9: 765. https://doi.org/10.3389/fmicb.2018.00765. www.ncbi.nlm.nih.gov/pubmed/29731746.

CHAPTER 7

Dietary Polyphenols and the Gut Microbiome

Tatiana Diacova and Zhaoping Li

7.1 BI-DIRECTIONAL RELATIONSHIP BETWEEN HOST HEALTH AND THE GUT MICROBIOME

Gut microbiome and the host have a strong bi-directional relationship significantly affecting each other's wellbeing. The major roles gut microbiome plays in host health include nutrient metabolism, xenobiotic/drug metabolism, maintenance of structure/function of the gut barrier and gastrointestinal (GI) tract, and the prevention of translocation of intestinal pathogens (Jandhyala et al., 2015). It can also mediate the association between certain food components and metabolic diseases like type 2 diabetes mellitus (T2DM) (Chen et al., 2021). In addition, it can affect energy balance, metabolism, and hormone secretion, exacerbating obesity and diabetic progression through various microbial metabolites including short-chain fatty acids (SCFAs), bile acids (BAs), and trimethylamine (TMA) N-oxide (TMAO) among others (Chen et al., 2021; Dabke et al., 2019; Metwaly et al., 2022; Liu et al., 2021; Fujisaka et al., 2023). Gut microbiota may also be able to help prevent development of obesity by fermenting indigestible carbohydrates (CHOs) and consequently inhibiting appetite and increasing energy utilization and lipid oxidation by the host (Chen et al., 2021; Dabke et al., 2019; Metwaly et al., 2022; Liu et al., 2021; Fujisaka et al., 2023). At the same time, other gut microbiota can contribute to the development of obesity by increasing host energy absorption, central appetite, and enhancing fat storage, which may lead to chronic inflammation and circadian rhythm regulation (Liu et al., 2021).

Host health, in its turn, can also have an extensive effect on gut microbiota composition and functionality. For instance, the presence of metabolic disorder in the host may disrupt normal metabolic processes of converting food to energy on the cellular level (Pulok et al., 2020). This affects critical cell biochemical reactions, which may increase the risk of cardiovascular disease, T2DM, obesity among others (Pulok et al., 2020). T2DM can then contribute to a decrease in the relative abundance of generally beneficial *Bifidobacteria* and *Akkermansia*, while also increasing *Dallella* (Chen et al., 2021; Dabke et al., 2019; Metwaly et al., 2022; Liu et al., 2021; Fujisaka et al., 2023). Obesity can also affect the gut microbiota. For instance, evidence demonstrates that *Bacteroides thetaiotaomicron* is significantly decreased in individuals with obesity, also negatively correlating with serum glutamate concentrations (Chen et al., 2021; Dabke et al., 2019; Metwaly et al., 2022; Liu et al., 2021; Fujisaka et al., 2023). In addition, the relative abundance of *Akkermansia muciniphila*, *Faecalibacterium prausnitzii*, and *Bacteroides* seems to be decreasing with obesity, while the relative abundance of the phylum Firmicutes increases significantly (Chen et al., 2021; Dabke et al., 2019; Metwaly et al., 2022; Liu et al., 2021; Fujisaka et al., 2023). In addition, the presence of hypertension has been shown to alter microbial diversity, which, in turn, alters production of microbial metabolites

DOI: 10.1201/9781003638292-7

(e.g., TMAO and H2S) that affect vascular tone, inflammation, and nervous system signaling. Perturbations in the gut microbiota may also contribute to increase in blood pressure (Chen et al., 2021; Dabke et al., 2019; Metwaly et al., 2022; Liu et al., 2021; Fujisaka et al., 2023). Atherosclerosis is another cardiovascular condition that has a bi-directional relationship with the gut microbiome, as live oral bacterial DNA has been detected in atherosclerotic plaques (Chen et al., 2021; Dabke et al., 2019; Metwaly et al., 2022; Liu et al., 2021; Fujisaka et al., 2023). The presence of atherosclerotic plaques may, in turn, affect gut microbiota composition and/or functionality. They may increase intestinal permeability, which allow for more lipopolysaccharide (LPS) entering the circulation, triggering foam cell formation along with endothelial dysfunction and thrombosis (Chen et al., 2021; Dabke et al., 2019; Metwaly et al., 2022; Liu et al., 2021; Fujisaka et al., 2023).

7.2 BI-DIRECTIONAL RELATIONSHIP BETWEEN DIET AND THE GUT MICROBIOME

Examples of diets that have shown a significant effect on gut microbiome include the Western diet, Mediterranean diet, as well as vegetarian and vegan diets. Western diet is rich in saturated fats and simple carbohydrates. Individuals following this diet have displayed increased levels of *Bacteroides*, *Lachnospiraceae*, and *Roseburia* and decreased levels of *F. prausnitzii* and *Ruminococcus* (Perler et al., 2023). High animal protein content in this diet leads to production of TMA and its conversion to TMAO by gut microbes. Elevated levels of TMAO contribute to endothelial damage and decreased endothelial cholesterol removal, as well as platelet hyperactivity. This further contributes to the development of atherosclerosis and atherothrombosis (Perler et al., 2023).

Mediterranean and vegetarian/vegan diets, on the contrary, are rich in fruits, vegetables, nuts, and olive oil. All these foods are rich in fiber and (poly)phenolic compounds, which are considered prebiotic food components (Li et al., 2021). Prebiotics are the compounds that microbes in the gut can utilize for energy (metabolize). Microbial metabolites produced as a result have shown the potential to support metabolic health, promote gut microbial diversity, contribute to improving insulin sensitivity, and mitigate inflammatory processes (Barber et al., 2023; Strasser et al., 2021; Ross et al., 2024).

7.3 BI-DIRECTIONAL RELATIONSHIP BETWEEN POLYPHENOLS AND THE GUT MICROBIOME

(Poly)phenolic compounds are secondary plant metabolites, characterized by an aromatic ring and several attached hydroxyl groups. These compounds offer protection to the plant from pathogens, free oxygen radicals, UV rays, and parasites (Gade et al., 2023). (Poly)phenols are divided into two main groups: flavonoids (flavones, flavanones, flavonols, flavan-3-ols, anthocyanidins, and isoflavones) and non-flavonoids (phenolic acids, lignans, and stilbenes).

7.3.1 Effects of the Gut Microbiome on (Poly)phenols

The chemical structure of (poly)phenols determines their bioavailability with simpler structures being more metabolizable and therefore more bioavailable. Examples of simple structures are isoflavones, phenolic acids, quercetin, flavanones, and glycosides, while examples of larger and less metabolizable compounds include proanthocyanidins, catechins, and anthocyanins (Ross et al., 2024; Gade et al., 2023).

(Poly)phenols are present in foods mainly in a conjugated form, as O-glycosides (De-Souza et al., 2015). A small part of (poly)phenolic compounds undergoes some extent of metabolism by human digestive enzymes and acids in the oral cavity, stomach, and small intestine, eventually taking on the form of aglycones via hydroxylation reactions (phase I drug metabolism) (De-Souza et al., 2015; Kamonpatana et al., 2012). Enzymes that participate in this transformation include cytochrome P450 and glucosidase enzymes (De-Souza et al., 2015; Kamonpatana et al., 2012). After undergoing these transformations, the aglycones are able to travel by passive diffusion or via protein carriers, from the gut lumen into the enterocyte cytosol (Kobayashi et al., 2013; Rein et al., 2013). Several hydroxycinnamic acids (e.g., ellagitannins (ETs)) are not metabolized by host enzymes in the small intestine and, as glycosides, travel all the way to the colon to be metabolized to aglycones by the gut microbes (Jaganath et al., 2006). Once aglycones are absorbed into the enterocytes or colonocytes, they travel through the portal vein to the liver, where they are further conjugated to O-glucuronides and O-sulfates (phase II drug metabolism). Enzymes that participate in this are conjugating and detoxifying enzymes including UDP-glucuronosyltransferases, catechol-O-methyltransferases, sulfotransferases, glutathione transferases, quinone reductases) (Stevens et al., 2016; Aura et al., 2008; Cardona et al., 2013). Some of these conjugates are then excreted into the bile and re-enter the small intestine to go through the metabolic cycle again (Stevens et al., 2016; Aura et al., 2008; Cardona et al., 2013). The final phenolic conjugates are then transported to the bloodstream by plasma proteins until they are excreted in urine (Monagas et al., 2010; Crespy et al., 2001; Ouzzine et al., 2003).

Once the gut microbes come in contact with the (poly)phenolic compounds in the large intestine, they alter their chemical structure even further utilizing a plethora of enzymes (e.g., β-glucosidase, β-glucuronidase, and α-rhamnosidase) (Cheng et al., 2023). Gut microbes metabolize (poly) phenols into bioactive metabolites, in most cases increasing their bioactivity and biological effects. These metabolites often have enhanced anti-inflammatory and antioxidant activities compared to the parent compounds (Cheng et al., 2023).

7.3.2 Ellagitannins, Isoflavones, and Metabotypes

ETs and isoflavones are examples of polyphenolic compounds that are extensively metabolized by the gut microbes (Garcia-Villalba et al., 2022; Laudani et al., 2024; Baky et al., 2022; Lv et al., 2024). What is unique about these specific compounds is the overwhelming evidence that humans exhibit differential capacity for production of various ET and isoflavone metabolites and this capacity seems to be mediated by the gut microbiota composition and functionality (Garcia-Villalba et al., 2022; Laudani et al., 2024; Baky et al., 2022; Lv et al., 2024; Iglesias-Aguirre et al., 2023).

7.3.2.1 Ellagitannins

ETs are abundantly found in foods with the main sources being walnuts, pomegranates, and berries (Garcia-Villalba et al., 2022; Banc et al., 2023). They are usually not absorbed by humans in their original form due to their large chemical structure and polarity (Garcia-Villalba et al., 2022; Banc et al., 2023). In the stomach and duodenum, acid- and base-sensitive ETs get broken down into ellagic acid (EA), which is poorly absorbed due to its low solubility and tendency to bind calcium and magnesium (Ascacio-Valdes et al., 2011). EA then travels to the distal parts of the GI tract and is metabolized by the gut microbes into urolithin metabolites (Uros) in the large intestine (Garcia-Villalba et al., 2022; Banc et al., 2023; Ascacio-Valdes et al., 2011). These metabolites then enter the enterohepatic circulation. Metabolism of ETs differs between individuals due to differences in the gut microbiota composition and functionality. This results in 3 Uro metabotypes: metabotype A or UM-A (individuals that produce mostly urolithin A or UroA metabolite), metabotype B or UM-B (individuals that produce UroA, as well as urolithin B or UroB and isourolithin A or IsoUroA), and metabotype 0 or UM-0 (non-producers of Uros) (Cortes-Martin et al., 2018). UM-A individuals usually have better levels of metabolic markers, lower abdominal adiposity, higher fasting insulin, and high-density lipoprotein (HDL) cholesterol levels (Selma et al., 2018). UM-B individuals are usually less metabolically healthy, being characterized by higher blood lipid/lipoprotein levels and more pronounced gut microbial composition and functionality perturbations (Selma et al., 2018). UM-0 individuals usually display higher levels of inflammation and metabolic dysfunction. Interestingly, supplementation with Uro-A in individuals with metabolic syndrome improved markers of metabolic health only in UM-B individuals and not the other two metabotype groups (Selma et al., 2018). This suggests that the gut microbiome may play a crucial role in the extent of health benefits individuals may be able to harvest from consumption of ET-rich foods.

7.3.2.2 Effects of Urolithin Metabolites on Host Health

Evidence shows that *Gordonibacter* and *Ellagibacter* are the two major microbial species known to participate in ET metabolism (Matsumura et al., 2023; Tomas-Barberan et al., 2014, 2017). Certain lactic acid bacteria, such as *Lactobacillus plantarum*, are known to produce tannase enzymes involved in the hydrolysis of ETs as well (Matsumura et al., 2023). Uro metabolites have shown several health benefits for the host including neuroprotection, anti-cancer properties, and promotion of growth of beneficial microbes (e.g., *Gordonibacter*) fostering microbial communities capable of urolithin production (Tomas-Barberan et al., 2017). Uro metabolites may also be able to improve gut barrier and enzyme function. Evidence shows that EA administration increased expression of tight junction proteins (ZO-1 and occludin) and enhanced digestive enzymes (e.g., sucrase, lactase), indirectly supporting healthy microbiota through improved intestinal environment (Banc et al., 2023). Another potential benefit of Uro metabolites is the suppression of perturbation in gut microbial communities in individuals with various disease states. For instance, evidence shows that the detrimental gut microbial shifts in high-fat diet (HFD) models and inflammatory bowel conditions were improved with ET administration. ETs showed the potential to enhance antioxidative enzymes (superoxide dismutase (SOD), glutathione peroxidase (GPx)), reduce inflammatory cytokines (e.g., TNF-α and IL-6), and decrease gut permeability and endotoxemia (Banc et al., 2023). Moreover, Uro metabolites have been detected in plasma and urine of men with prostate cancer after pomegranate extract consumption (Banc et al., 2023). Moreover, both UroA and UroB conjugates were found in normal and malignant mammary tissues in breast cancer models (Banc et al., 2023). Uro metabolites may also be participating in slowing down the aging process by improving mitochondrial gene expression and cellular health markers (Kothe et al., 2023). UroA can help reduce body fat, promote autophagy, and improve mitochondrial function, which has been confirmed by multiple clinical trials (Kothe et al., 2023). In addition, Uro metabolites may have the potential to reinforce the intestinal barrier, increase tight junction protein expression, and reduce intestinal inflammation in models of colitis and inflammatory bowel syndrome (IBS) (Espin et al., 2013).

7.3.2.3 Isoflavones

Isoflavones are less abundant in foods and are generally just found in soybeans. The two prominent examples of isoflavones are genistein and daidzein. Both are broken down by the human digestive enzymes lactase-phlorizin hydrolase and cytosolic beta-glucosidase turning these compounds into isoflavone aglycones (Matsumura et al., 2023). After that, endogenous phase I and II enzymes metabolize these aglycones to glucuronides and sulfates (Matsumura et al., 2023). Unabsorbed isoflavones travel all the way to the colon where they are metabolized by the gut microbes into the major compound – equol (Baky et al., 2022). Equol is highly bioavailable blood–brain barrier permeable, and highly selective for estrogen receptor β, enhancing its therapeutic potential compared to its precursor daidzein (Sekikawa et al., 2022).

Microbes involved in isoflavone metabolism include *Eggerthella* spp., *Enterococcus faecium*, *Adlercreutzia equolifaciens*, and *Slackia equolifaciens* (Baky et al., 2022). Only individuals who have these microbes present in the gut can convert isoflavones to equol. Interestingly, 50–70% of East Asians and only 20–30% of Westerners are able to produce equol after isoflavone consumption (Sekikawa et al., 2022).

7.3.2.4 Effects of Equol Metabolites on Host Health

Some of the effects of equol on host health include relief of menopausal symptoms (reduction in hot flashes), improved bone health (preservation of lumbar spine bone density and reduction of resorption through anti-osteoclast effects), anticancer effects (increase in protective estrogen metabolite ratio and lower breast cancer risk), as well as cardio- and neuroprotection (reduction in LDL-C and inflammation, increase in adiponectin, improvement in glucose metabolism, etc.) (Matsumura et al., 2023). Isoflavone metabolites may also be able to modulate gut microbiota by increasing the relative abundance of generally beneficial bacteria including *Bifidobacterium*, *Akkermansia*, *Eubacterium*, Firmicutes, and *Bacteroides*, therefore also increasing production of SCFAs (e.g., butyrate) (Laudani et al., 2024).

7.3.3 Other (Poly)phenols and Their Metabolite Effects on Host Health

7.3.3.1 Flavan-3-Ols

Major sources of flavan-3-ols are cocoa, tea, apples, grapes, berries, plums, apricots, and nuts (Aron et al., 2008). These compounds undergo both phase I and II metabolism, as well as metabolism by the gut microbes (Matsumura et al., 2023). The resulting metabolites exhibit anti-inflammatory and antioxidant activities (Matsumura et al., 2023). Catechins, for instance, after being metabolized into phenyl-γ-valerolactones by intestinal bacteria, have shown the potential to regulate cellular proteolysis and exert neuroprotective effects (Matsumura et al., 2023).

7.3.3.2 *Condensed Tannins*

Astringent persimmon and red wine are the main sources of condensed tannins (Soares et al., 2020). Condensed tannins are degraded by gut microbes to lower molecular weight fragments (Sallam et al., 2021). These fragments or metabolites have demonstrated the ability to reduce colitis severity and decrease expression of gene coding for pro-inflammatory cytokines and chemokines (Sallam et al., 2021).

7.3.3.3 *Flavonols*

The main flavonol is quercetin, which is abundantly found in most fruits, vegetables, and grains (Xiong et al., 2023). Intestinal bacteria catabolize quercetin glycosides into phenolic acids like 3,4-dihydroxyphenylacetic acid (Xiong et al., 2023). This acid has exhibited the ability to be effective at scavenging free radicals and inducing phase II enzymes (Xiong et al., 2023). Other phenolic acids that form as a result of quercetin microbial metabolism have displayed antioxidant effects as well as the ability to support intestinal homeostasis and prevent colitis and insulin resistance (Xiong et al., 2023).

7.3.3.4 *Phenylpropanoids*

Major sources of phenylpropanoids are coffee (chlorogenic acid) and sesame seeds (sesamin) (Neelam et al., 2020). Gut bacteria metabolize chlorogenic acid into dihydrocaffeic acid and related metabolites, exerting effects on obesity, NAFLD, and neuroinflammation (Gonthier et al., 2003). Sesamin, in turn, is metabolized into its more active forms that increase the relative abundance of generally beneficial bacteria including *Lactobacillus* and *Bifidobacterium* (Gonthier et al., 2003).

7.3.3.5 *Stilbenoids*

Grape, red wine, and peanuts are the main sources of stilbenoids (Jaimes et al., 2019). These polyphenolic compounds are metabolized by the gut microbiome into dihydro-resveratrol (DHR) (Jaimes et al., 2019; Jarosova et al., 2019). DHR is known to alter gut microbiota composition, improve intestinal barrier, and be protective against obesity, metabolic syndrome, and neurodegeneration (Jaimes et al., 2019; Jarosova et al., 2019).

7.3.3.6 *Curcuminoids*

The main source of curcuminoids is turmeric (Jaimes et al., 2019). Curcuminoids are generally poorly absorbed and are biotransformed by gut bacteria into active metabolites like dihydrocurcumin (Scazzocchio et al., 2020). Dihydrocurcumin is known for its anti-inflammatory, neuroprotective as well as gut microbiome modulatory effects (Scazzocchio et al., 2020).

7.3.4 Effects of Polyphenols on the Gut Microbiome

Just as the gut microbiome has significant effects on the dietary polyphenols, polyphenols can also have an effect on the gut microbes. For instance, dietary polyphenols have shown the potential to alter **α**- and **β**-diversity and promote generally beneficial bacteria including *Akkermansia*, *Bifidobacteria*, and *Lactobacilli* (Cheng et al., 2023). Depending on their chemical structure and the dose consumed, (poly)phenolic compounds are also able to exert antimicrobial effects and suppress the growth of generally detrimental bacteria in the gut (e.g., *Helicobacter*, *Enterococcus*, and *Clostridium perfringens*) (Cheng et al., 2023). For instance, many (poly)phenolic compounds can disrupt Gram-positive bacterial cell membranes, increasing their cell permeability and inhibiting growth (Wang et al., 2022). Polyphenols selectively inhibit pathogenic bacteria (*Salmonella*, *Escherichia coli*) while sparing or even supporting generally beneficial ones like lactic acid bacteria (Wang et al., 2022). For instance, tea catechins (EGCG) bind to lipid membranes, disrupt biofilms, reduce mucus production, and neutralize bacterial toxins (Wang et al., 2022). They also have the ability to insert themselves into bacterial membranes via hydrogen bonding and disrupt membrane structure (Wang et al., 2022). In addition, polyphenols inhibit essential bacterial enzymes like DNA gyrase, topoisomerase, and tyrosine kinases (Wang et al., 2022).

7.4 CONCLUDING REMARKS

- There is a clear multidirectional relationship between diet, gut microbiome, and host health.
- Different foods and food components act differently on the gut microbiome, which ultimately affects the whole-body function and overall health.

- Dietary polyphenols are an example of food components that are both extensively affected by the gut microbiome and capable of affecting the gut microbiome in significant ways.
- Gut microbes help metabolize polyphenols, producing more bioactive and bioavailable metabolites that can provide significant health benefits.
- Just like the gut microbes are affecting the dietary polyphenols, these components have an effect on the gut microbes by nourishing the beneficial and suppressing the detrimental ones.
- Not everyone may be able to benefit from consumption of polyphenol-rich foods, as the capacity to produce the beneficial microbial metabolites is mediated by the gut microbiome composition/functionality.

REFERENCES

Aron PM, Kennedy JA. (2008) Flavan-3-ols: nature, occurrence and biological activity. *Mol Nutr Food Res* 52(1):79–104.

Ascacio-Valdés JA, Buenrostro-Figueroa JJ, Aguilera-Carbó A, Prado-Barragán A, Rodríguez-Herrera R, Aguilar CN (2011) Ellagitannins: biosynthesis, biodegradation and biological properties. *J Med Plants Res* 5(19):4696–4703.

Aura AM (2008) Microbial metabolism of dietary phenolic compounds in the colon. *Phytochem Rev* 7:407–429.

Baky MH, Elshahed M, Wessjohann L, Farag MA (2022) Interactions between dietary flavonoids and the gut microbiome: a comprehensive review. *Br J Nutr* 128(4):577–591.

Banc R, Rusu ME, Filip L, Popa DS (2023) The impact of Ellagitannins and their metabolites through gut microbiome on the gut health and brain wellness within the gut-brain axis. *Foods* 12(2):270.

Barber TM, Kabisch S, Pfeiffer AFH, Weickert MO (2023) The effects of the mediterranean diet on health and gut microbiota. *Nutrients* 15(9):2150.

Cardona F, Andrés-Lacueva C, Tulipani S, Tinahones FJ, Queipo-Ortuño MI (2013) Benefits of polyphenols on gut microbiota and implications in human health. *J Nutr Biochem* 24:1415–1422.

Chen Y, Zhou J, Wang L (2021) Role and mechanism of gut microbiota in human disease. *Front Cell Infect Microbiol* 11:625913.

Cheng H, Zhang D, Wu J, Liu J, Zhou Y, Tan Y, Feng W, Peng C (2023) Interactions between gut microbiota and polyphenols: a mechanistic and metabolomic review. *Phytomedicine* 119:154979.

Cortés-Martín A, García-Villalba R, González-Sarrías A, Romo-Vaquero M, Loria-Kohen V, Ramírez-de-Molina A et al (2018) The gut microbiota urolithin metabotypes revisited: the human metabolism of ellagic acid is mainly determined by aging. *Food & Function* 9(8):4100–4106.

Crespy V, Morand C, Besson C, Manach C, Démigné C, Rémésy C (2001) Comparison of the intestinal absorption of quercetin, phloretin and their glucosides in rats. *J Nutr* 131:2109–2114.

Dabke K, Hendrick G, Devkota S (2019) The gut microbiome and metabolic syndrome. *J Clin Invest* 129(10):4050–4057.

De-Souza JE, Casanova LM, Costa SS (2015) Bioavailability of phenolic compounds: a major challenge for drug development? *Rev Fitos* 9:55–67.

Espín JC, Larrosa M, García-Conesa MT, Tomás-Barberán F (2013) Biological significance of urolithins, the gut microbial ellagic Acid-derived metabolites: the evidence so far. *Evid Based Complement Alternat Med* 2013:270418.

Fujisaka S, Watanabe Y, Tobe K (2023) The gut microbiome: a core regulator of metabolism. *J Endocrinol* 256(3):e220111.

Gade A, Kumar MS (2023) Gut microbial metabolites of dietary polyphenols and their potential role in human health and diseases. *J Physiol Biochem* 79(4):695–718.

García-Villalba R, Giménez-Bastida JA, Cortés-Martín A, Ávila-Gálvez MÁ, Tomás-Barberán FA, Selma MV, Espín JC, González-Sarrías A (2022) Urolithins: a comprehensive update on their metabolism, bioactivity, and associated gut microbiota. *Mol Nutr Food Res* 66(21):e2101019.

Gonthier MP, Verny MA, Besson C, Rémésy C, Scalbert A (2003). Chlorogenic acid bioavailability largely depends on its metabolism by the gut microflora in rats. *J Nutr* 133(6):1853–1859.

Iglesias-Aguirre CE, Romo-Vaquero M, Selma MV, Espín JC (2023) Unveiling metabotype clustering in resveratrol, daidzein, and ellagic acid metabolism: prevalence, associated gut microbiomes, and their distinctive microbial networks. *Food Res Int* 173:113470.

Jaganath IB, Mullen W, Edwards CA, Crozier A (2006) The relative contribution of the small and large intestine to the absorption and metabolism of rutin in man. *Free Radic. Res* 40:1035–1046.

Jaimes JD, Jarosova V, Vesely O, Mekadim C, Mrazek J, Marsik P, Killer J, Smejkal K, Kloucek P, Havlik J (2019) Effect of selected stilbenoids on human fecal microbiota. *Molecules* 24(4):744.

Jandhyala SM, Talukdar R, Subramanyam C, Vuyyuru H, Sasikala M, Nageshwar Reddy D (2015) Role of the normal gut microbiota. *World J Gastroenterol* 21(29):8787–803.

Jarosova V, Vesely O, Marsik P, Jaimes JD, Smejkal K, Kloucek P, Havlik J (2019) Metabolism of stilbenoids by human faecal microbiota. *Molecules* 24(6):1155.

Kamonpatana K, Giusti MM, Chitchumroonchokchai C, Morenocruz M, Riedl KM, Kumar P, Failla ML (2012) Susceptibility of anthocyanins to ex vivo degradation in human saliva. *Food Chem* 135:738–747.

Kobayashi S, Shinohara M, Nagai T, Konishi Y (2013) Transport mechanisms for soy isoflavones and microbial metabolites dihydrogenistein and dihydrodaidzein across monolayers and membranes. *Biosci Biotechnol Biochem* 77:2210–2217.

Kothe B, Klein S, Petrosky SN. (2023) Urolithin a as a potential agent for prevention of age-related disease: a scoping review. *Cureus* 15(7):e42550.

Laudani S, Godos J, Romano GL, Gozzo L, Di Domenico FM, Dominguez Azpíroz I, Martínez Diaz R, Giampieri F, Quiles JL, Battino M, Drago F, Galvano F, Grosso G (2024) Isoflavones effects on vascular and endothelial outcomes: how is the gut microbiota involved? *Pharmaceuticals (Basel)* 17(2):236.

Li HY, Zhou DD, Gan RY, Huang SY, Zhao CN, Shang A, Xu XY, Li HB (2021) Effects and mechanisms of probiotics, prebiotics, synbiotics, and postbiotics on metabolic diseases targeting gut microbiota: a narrative review. *Nutrients* 13(9):3211.

Liu BN, Liu XT, Liang ZH, Wang JH (2021) Gut microbiota in obesity. *World J Gastroenterol* 27(25):3837–3850.

Lv J, Jin S, Zhang Y et al (2024) Equol: a metabolite of gut microbiota with potential antitumor effects. *Gut Pathog* 16:35.

Matsumura Y, Kitabatake M, Kayano SI, Ito T (2023) Dietary phenolic compounds: their health benefits and association with the gut microbiota. *Antioxidants (Basel)* 12(4):880.

Metwaly A, Reitmeier S, Haller, D (2022) Microbiome risk profiles as biomarkers for inflammatory and metabolic disorders. *Nat Rev Gastroenterol Hepatol* 19: 383–397.

Monagas M, Urpi-Sarda M, Sánchez-Patán F, Llorach R, Garrido I, Gómez-Cordovés C, Andres-Lacueva C, Bartolomé B (2010) Insights into the metabolism and microbial biotransformation of dietary flavan-3-ols and the bioactivity of their metabolites. *Food Funct* 1:233–253.

Mukherjee PK, Harwansh RK, Bahadur S, Chanda J, Biswas S, Banerjee S (2020) Chapter 31 – Enzyme inhibition assay for metabolic disorders—exploring leads from medicinal plants. Editor(s): Ashish S. Verma, Anchal Singh, Animal Biotechnology (Second Edition), Academic Press, Pages 631–653, ISBN 9780128117101.

Neelam, Khatkar A, Sharma KK (2020). Phenylpropanoids and its derivatives: biological activities and its role in food, pharmaceutical and cosmetic industries. *Crit Rev Food Sci Nutr* 60(16):2655–2675.

Ouzzine M, Barré L, Netter P, Magdalou J, Fournel-Gigleux S (2003) The human UDP-glucuronosyltransferases: structural aspects and drug glucuronidation. *Drug Metab Rev* 35:287–303.

Perler BK, Friedman ES, Wu GD (2023) The role of the gut microbiota in the relationship between diet and human health. *Annu Rev Physiol* 85:449–468.

Rein MJ, Renouf M, Cruz-Hernandez C, Actis-Goretta L, Thakkar SK, da Silva Pinto M (2013) Bioavailability of bioactive food compounds: a challenging journey to bioefficacy. *Br J Clin Pharmacol* 75:588–602.

Ross FC, Patangia D, Grimaud G, Lavelle A, Dempsey EM, Ross RP, Stanton C (2024) The interplay between diet and the gut microbiome: implications for health and disease. *Nat Rev Microbiol* 22(11):671–686.

Sallam IE, Abdelwareth A, Attia H, Aziz RK, Homsi MN, von Bergen M, Farag MA (2021) Effect of gut microbiota biotransformation on dietary tannins and human health implications. *Microorganisms* 9(5):965.

Scazzocchio B, Minghetti L, D'Archivio M (2020) Interaction between gut microbiota and curcumin: a new key of understanding for the health effects of curcumin. *Nutrients* 12(9):2499.

Sekikawa A, Wharton W, Butts B, Veliky CV, Garfein J, Li J, Goon S, Fort A, Li M, Hughes TM (2022) Potential protective mechanisms of S-equol, a metabolite of soy isoflavone by the gut microbiome, on cognitive decline and dementia. *Int J Mol Sci* 23(19):11921.

Selma MV, González-Sarrías A, Salas-Salvadó J, Andrés-Lacueva C, Alasalvar C, Örem A et al. (2018) The gut microbiota metabolism of pomegranate or walnut ellagitannins yields two urolithin-metabotypes that correlate with cardiometabolic risk biomarkers: comparison between normoweight, overweight-obesity and metabolic syndrome. *Clin Nutr* 37(3):897–905.

Soares S, Brandão E, Guerreiro C, Soares S, Mateus N, de Freitas V (2020) Tannins in food: insights into the molecular perception of astringency and bitter taste. *Molecules* 25(11):2590.

Stevens JF, Maier CS (2016) The chemistry of gut microbial metabolism of polyphenols. *Phytochem. Rev* 15:425–444.

Strasser B, Wolters M, Weyh C, Krüger K, Ticinesi A (2021) The effects of lifestyle and diet on gut microbiota composition, inflammation and muscle performance in our aging society. *Nutrients* 13(6):2045.

Tomás-Barberán FA, García-Villalba R, González-Sarrías A, Selma MV et al (2014). Ellagic acid metabolism by human gut microbiota: consistent observation of three urolithin phenotypes in intervention trials, independent of food source, age, and health status. *J Agri Food Chem* 62(28):6535–6538.

Tomás-Barberán FA, González-Sarrías A, García-Villalba R, Núñez-Sánchez MA, Selma MV, García-Conesa MT et al (2017) Urolithins, the rescue of "old" metabolites to understand a "new" concept: metabotypes as a nexus among phenolic metabolism, microbiota dysbiosis, and host health status. *Mol Nutr Food Res* 61(1):1500901.

Wang X, Qi Y, Zheng H (2022) Dietary polyphenol, gut microbiota, and health benefits. *Antioxidants (Basel)* 11(6):1212.

Xiong HH, Lin SY, Chen LL, Ouyang KH, Wang WJ (2023) The interaction between flavonoids and intestinal microbes: a review. *Foods* 12(2):320.

CHAPTER 8

The Impact of Ultra-Processed Foods on the Microbiome and Human Health

Olivia Lutz and Sunil Thomas

8.1 INTRODUCTION

The human body is estimated to host approximately 30 trillion colonizing microorganisms, collectively known as the microbiota. These microbial communities play an essential role in maintaining physiological homeostasis, influencing digestion, immune function, metabolism, and even neurocognitive processes. The composition and function of the microbiota are shaped largely by the diet of the host. Diets rich in diverse, minimally processed foods tend to promote the growth of beneficial microbes, supporting overall health. In contrast, diets that foster a dysbiotic microbial environment—characterized by reduced diversity and an imbalance of microbial species—are associated with a wide range of pathologies (Thomas et al., 2017).

In recent decades, ultra-processed foods (UPFs) have emerged as a dominant dietary component worldwide. Defined within the NOVA food classification system, UPFs are industrial formulations that are energy-dense, extensively altered from their original food sources, and typically high in additives not found in traditional household kitchens. These include hydrogenated oils, flavor enhancers, colorants, artificial sweeteners, protein isolates, and emulsifiers. Common examples include sugar-sweetened beverages, packaged snacks, processed meats, confectionery, and ready-to-eat convenience meals. Their widespread adoption reflects major shifts in global food systems—driven by industrialization, urbanization, and globalization—which have increased the availability, affordability, and desirability of these products (Rondinella et al., 2025).

Growing evidence indicates that UPFs exert profound effects on gut health. Their characteristic of low fiber content, high levels of synthetic additives, and emulsifying agents contribute to decreased microbial diversity, reduced abundance of key beneficial species such as *Akkermansia muciniphila* and *Faecalibacterium prausnitzii*, and expansion of pro-inflammatory taxa. These microbial alterations can impair intestinal barrier integrity, increasing gut permeability—a condition often referred to as "leaky gut." The resulting low-grade, chronic inflammation has been implicated in a spectrum of disorders, including metabolic syndrome, type 2 diabetes, irritable bowel syndrome, cardiovascular disease (CVD), and colorectal cancer. Emerging research further suggests that UPF-induced microbial dysbiosis may disrupt the gut–brain axis, with potential implications for cognitive function, mood regulation, and mental health outcomes (Rondinella et al., 2025).

Given the central role of the microbiome in maintaining host health, understanding the mechanisms through which UPFs influence microbial composition and function is critical. Dietary strategies, including increased intake of fiber-rich

DOI: 10.1201/9781003638292-8

foods, fermented products, and probiotics, have been proposed as potential interventions to counteract the harmful effects of UPFs on gut ecology. This review examines the current evidence on how UPFs shape the gut microbiome and highlights the implications for human health.

8.2 NOVA CLASSIFICATION OF FOOD

The NOVA classification system (*a term, not an acronym*) categorizes foods based on the nature, extent, and purpose of the industrial processing they undergo. In this framework, food processing encompasses the physical, biological, and chemical techniques applied to raw materials after their separation from nature and before they are prepared for consumption. Processing may include simple operations such as cleaning and chopping, or complex industrial techniques such as hydrogenation, extrusion, and chemical modification (Monteiro et al., 2018).

Foods can be consumed in various ways: directly as whole items (e.g., fruits, nuts, milk), as ingredients or components of meals (e.g., grains, vegetables, meat, eggs), or as products used in cooking and food preparation (e.g., oils, butter, sugar). They may also be manufactured to be consumed immediately, with minimal or no preparation, such as packaged snacks, soft drinks, sliced bread, cheese, and a wide array of ready-to-heat frozen meals. Based on these distinctions, NOVA groups all foods and food products into four categories, which together reflect increasing degrees of processing (Monteiro et al., 2018).

8.2.1 Group 1: Unprocessed or Minimally Processed Foods

Group 1 includes unprocessed, or natural, foods—such as edible parts of plants (fruits, seeds, leaves, stems, roots) and animals (muscle tissue, organs, eggs, milk)—as well as fungi, algae, and water. Minimally processed foods are natural foods altered only through techniques that preserve them, extend their shelf life, or make them safe and palatable. These methods include removal of inedible components, drying, grinding, milling, freezing, chilling, pasteurization, boiling, non-alcoholic fermentation, vacuum packaging, or simple packaging.

The essential characteristic of Group 1 foods is that they remain recognizably close to their natural state. These foods typically form the foundation of home-prepared meals or restaurant dishes, often combined with processed culinary ingredients (Group 2) to create soups, salads, stews, baked goods, and other freshly prepared dishes.

8.2.2 Group 2: Processed Culinary Ingredients

Processed culinary ingredients consist of substances derived from Group 1 foods or extracted directly from nature. Examples include vegetable oils, butter, sugar, honey, and salt. These products are produced through processes such as pressing, refining, milling, crushing, or drying. The purpose of these ingredients is not direct consumption. Instead, they serve to season, cook, and prepare dishes made primarily from Group 1 foods. Processed culinary ingredients enable the preparation of homemade or professionally prepared meals, from breads and sauces to stews, desserts, and beverages. In essence, they function as building blocks for traditional culinary practices rather than as stand-alone foods.

8.2.3 Group 3: Processed Foods

Processed foods are created by combining Group 1 foods with Group 2 ingredients—typically salt, oil, sugar, or other culinary additives. Examples include canned vegetables, bottled fruits, cheeses, salted nuts, cured meats, jams, and freshly baked breads. Processing methods range from canning and bottling to fermentation, preservation, and simple cooking. These foods usually contain only two or three ingredients and remain identifiable as modified versions of their original food sources. They are often consumed alone or incorporated into meals. The primary goal of processing in this group is to increase durability and enhance sensory qualities without completely transforming the food's natural structure.

8.2.4 Group 4: Ultra-Processed Foods

UPFs differ fundamentally from processed foods in that they are typically formulations of ingredients, many of which are not recognizable as whole foods. UPFs are made predominantly or entirely from substances extracted or derived from foods, combined with additives designed to improve shelf life, palatability, texture, or appearance. Common UPFs include soft drinks, packaged sweet or savory snacks, confectionery, reconstituted meat products, instant noodles, flavored yogurts, sugary breakfast cereals, and ready-to-heat frozen meals.

UPFs typically contain long and complex ingredient lists made up of substances rarely used in home cooking. These often include basic culinary components such as added sugars, refined oils, fats, and salt, which are used in amounts far exceeding those found in minimally processed foods. Many UPFs also rely on extracted food constituents like casein, lactose, whey, and gluten. These ingredients are separated from their natural food matrices to enhance texture, boost protein content, or modify flavor, but in doing so, they lose the nutritional balance present in whole foods. Additionally, industrial derivatives such as hydrogenated or esterified oils, hydrolyzed vegetable proteins, maltodextrin, soy isolates, invert sugar, and high-fructose corn syrup (FCS) (HFCS) are commonly incorporated to intensify sweetness, prolong shelf life, or create specific mouthfeel characteristics that make these products highly palatable and often addictive.

A defining feature of UPFs is their heavy use of additives, many of which serve technological rather than nutritional purposes. These can include preservatives, stabilizers, and antioxidants designed to prevent spoilage and maintain product consistency over long periods. Sweeteners, artificial flavors, and flavor enhancers are frequently introduced to replicate or exaggerate natural tastes, while colorants and color stabilizers create a visually appealing appearance that may not reflect the food's true quality. Other additives—such as emulsifiers, humectants, anti-foaming agents, glazing agents, and bulking or anti-bulking agents—modify texture, moisture, and structure in ways that make the products more uniform and commercially convenient. Even specialized substances like carbonating and firming agents may be included to further manipulate the sensory experience. Together, these ingredients form highly engineered products that differ significantly from whole or minimally processed foods, raising growing concerns about their long-term effects on metabolic health and dietary behavior.

Many of the industrial processes used to make UPFs—such as extrusion, molding, hydrogenation, hydrolysis, and spray-drying—have no equivalents in domestic or artisanal food preparation. UPFs often require multiple steps and complex processing sequences, which is why they are termed "ultra-processed."

The overarching aim of ultra-processing is to create food products that are highly palatable, convenient, affordable, and profitable, often using low-cost ingredients and intensive marketing strategies. These products are engineered to appeal to consumers' sensory preferences while displacing traditional foods from the diet (Monteiro et al., 2018).

8.3 HISTORY OF ULTRA-PROCESSED FOOD

Throughout the 20th century, the purpose and nature of food processing underwent a fundamental transformation. Early industrial food processing—emerging in the late 19th and early 20th centuries—was primarily focused on improving food safety, shelf life, and occasionally nutritional value. Canning reduced microbial risks, pasteurization made milk safer, and fortification programs helped address nutrient deficiencies. However, as the century progressed, the aims of food processing shifted dramatically. Convenience, palatability, and large-scale industrial efficiency became dominant priorities, paving the way for today's UPF landscape (Huebbe & Rimbach, 2020).

8.3.1 Postwar Economic Growth and the Demand for Convenience

Following the economic recovery after World War I and especially World War II, industrialized high-income countries experienced rapid urbanization, rising household incomes, and major changes in family structure. With more women entering the workforce and urban living reducing access to fresh, home-grown foods, domestic time for cooking declined sharply. As a result, consumers increasingly sought foods that were quick to prepare, required minimal skill, and fit into new, busier lifestyles.

The food industry rapidly responded. By the mid-20th century, companies began developing products that shifted more and more aspects of food preparation from the home kitchen to the factory. This era saw the emergence of ready-to-cook, ready-to-heat, and ultimately ready-to-eat meals—foods designed to require virtually no preparation. These products relied on intensified processing techniques such as extrusion, hydrogenation, fractionation of ingredients, and artificial flavor engineering.

8.3.2 Industrial Reorganization and the Rise of Long Supply Chains

Simultaneously, the structure of the food industry changed. Production of raw agricultural goods became increasingly separated from the processing sector, allowing manufacturers to source ingredients globally. Innovations in packaging, freezing, and transportation extended shelf life and made it possible for food products—or their isolated components—to travel long distances. This expanded supply chain heightened the importance of the "in-between" stages of food processing, where raw materials were transformed into standardized, storable commodities. Modern food systems thus began to rely on an international network of producers, processors, distributors, and retailers, distancing consumers from the origins of what they ate.

8.3.3 Animal Production, Refrigeration, and Shifting Macronutrient Patterns

Major advances in animal agriculture also shaped modern dietary trends. The introduction of scientifically optimized broiler chickens in the 1950s fueled a global boom in poultry production. At the same time, the widespread adoption of household refrigerators and freezers enabled families to purchase and store perishable foods—milk, eggs, cheese, and meat—more easily than ever before. These technological shifts contributed to the rising consumption of animal-based foods and fats throughout much of the 20th century.

By the early 1970s, dietary fat intake in many industrialized countries had reached historic highs, largely due to increased consumption of meat and dairy. Meanwhile, carbohydrate intake declined, reflecting a long-term reduction in staple foods such as potatoes and whole grains. However, growing scientific concerns in the 1960s about saturated fat and cholesterol—particularly their association with CVD—triggered major dietary changes. Both households and the food industry reduced their use of animal fats like butter and lard, replacing them with industrially refined vegetable oils, notably soybean oil (SO) in the United States.

8.3.4 The Surge of Refined Sugars and the New Nutrition Transition

The shift away from animal fats had unintended consequences. As saturated fats decreased, total carbohydrate intake rose—primarily in the form of refined sugars. From the 1960s onward, consumption of sugar-sweetened beverages, confectionery, and processed breakfast cereals increased sharply in high-income countries. Over time, similar trends spread to middle- and low-income nations as global trade liberalization and market deregulation opened domestic markets to transnational food corporations.

During this period, intake of dietary fiber declined, widening the nutritional gap between traditional diets based on whole foods and modern diets dominated by industrially processed products. This shift—often described as the third major nutritional transition—was closely tied to aggressive global marketing strategies, the expansion of convenience foods, and the rise of corporate conglomerates selling not only processed foods but also tobacco and alcoholic beverages.

The global spread of UPFs coincided with steep increases in average body mass index (BMI), waist circumference, and obesity prevalence across many regions of the world. These trends suggest a marked deterioration in dietary quality, driven in part by energy-dense, nutrient-poor products high in sugar, refined starches, fats, and additives (Alomari & Almoraie, 2025).

8.3.5 Displacement of Traditional Diets

As food markets globalized, many countries experienced a rapid displacement of traditional staples by ultra-processed alternatives. This shift destabilized long-standing culinary practices and food cultures. For example, legumes and pulses—historically central to many regional diets for their protein, fiber, and nutrient density—saw notable declines in consumption as instant noodles, packaged snacks, and sugary beverages became widely accessible and heavily marketed.

The erosion of these traditional plant-based foods illustrates a broader pattern: as industrial food processing intensifies, it not only reshapes individual food choices but also transforms entire cultural dietary patterns. The historical rise of UPFs thus represents not merely a technological evolution but a structural, economic, and social reconfiguration of the human diet (Huebbe & Rimbach, 2020).

8.4 MAJOR INGREDIENTS IN ULTRA-PROCESSED FOOD AND ITS IMPACT ON HEALTH

8.4.1 Chemical Bleaching of Wheat Flour: Processes and Potential Health Implications

Flour milled from freshly ground wheat naturally exhibits a pale yellow hue, a coloration attributed to its intrinsic carotenoid pigments. In this fresh state, the flour tends to yield doughs that are sticky, difficult to handle, and less predictable during cooking. As the flour is stored, however, it undergoes a gradual natural aging process driven by oxidative reactions affecting both carotenoids and the sulfhydryl groups of protein systems. Over time, this oxidation bleaches the pigments and alters protein interactions, resulting in a whiter, softer, and more aerated flour that is generally more suitable for producing high-quality bakery products (Mellado-Ortega & Hornero-Méndez, 2017).

To hasten these naturally occurring modifications, the food industry has long relied on chemical treatments designed to improve both the color and the functional properties—such as gluten behavior and pasting characteristics—of wheat flour. Commonly used bleaching agents include benzoyl peroxide, chlorine gas, chlorine dioxide, nitrosyl chloride, and nitrogen oxides (Chittrakorn et al., 2014). Historically, compounds such as chlorine gas, benzoyl peroxide, and potassium bromate were widely adopted to expedite flour maturation, enhancing baking performance and visual appeal. However, growing toxicological evidence has prompted regulatory changes. For instance, potassium bromate has been associated with kidney damage and carcinogenicity in animal models, leading to its prohibition in regions such as the European Union, Canada, and Brazil, though it remains permissible in the United States. Likewise, chlorine gas treatments can generate potentially harmful byproducts—such as chlorinated amino acid and protein derivatives—raising additional safety concerns. As a result, several bleaching agents have been restricted or banned in the United Kingdom and the European Union (Hou et al., 2025).

One historically significant method, known as the agene process, involved bleaching flour with nitrogen trichloride. In use from the early 20th century until approximately 1949–1950, this process produced a toxic byproduct, methionine sulfoximine (MSO). It has been estimated that as much as 80% of flour in the United Kingdom was treated via the agene method during its peak use. MSO is now recognized as a potent inhibitor of two critical biochemical pathways: the synthesis of glutathione (GSH) and glutamine. Reduced glutathione levels impair the body's antioxidant defenses, heightening vulnerability to oxidative stress, while diminished glutamine synthesis can lead to elevated levels of free glutamate and ammonia. Neuronal tissues are particularly susceptible to these metabolic disturbances. As proposed by Shaw and Bains (1998), chronic dietary exposure to MSO may have contributed to long-term neurotoxicity, potentially offering insight into the etiology of neurodegenerative diseases such as Alzheimer's disease (AD), Parkinson's disease (PD), and amyotrophic lateral sclerosis (ALS). Their hypothesis suggests that certain neurological disorders may arise, at least in part, from toxic compounds introduced through processed foods.

Another compound of concern is alloxan (2,4,5,6-tetraoxypyrimidine or 2,4,5,6-pyrimidinetetrone), a possible minor side product formed during the oxidation reactions associated with chemical flour bleaching. Giaccone et al. (2017) identified alloxan in bleached flour samples. Alloxan is known for its toxicological activity on pancreatic β-cells, where it exerts a diabetogenic effect. Structurally analogous to glucose, it acts via two principal mechanisms: (1) Selective inhibition of glucose-stimulated insulin secretion, achieved through targeted inactivation of glucokinase, and (2) Induction of reactive oxygen species (ROS), which can damage proteins, lipids, and nucleic acids through oxidative stress.

The presence of such compounds has prompted increased scrutiny of chemical bleaching practices and renewed interest in alternative methods that maintain flour quality without introducing harmful byproducts.

8.4.2 Sugar

A high intake of added sugars is strongly associated with numerous adverse health outcomes. Excess consumption contributes to weight gain, overweight, and obesity, as added sugars provide energy-dense but nutrient-poor calories that can promote positive energy balance. Over time, this can increase the risk of type 2 diabetes mellitus by exacerbating insulin resistance and impairing glucose metabolism. High added sugar intake is also linked to elevated serum triglycerides, increased total and low-density lipoprotein (LDL) cholesterol, and dyslipidemia, which are key risk factors for CVD. Furthermore, excessive sugar consumption has been associated with higher blood pressure (BP), hypertension, and an increased likelihood of stroke and coronary heart disease. Beyond cardiometabolic effects, diets high in added sugars are implicated in certain cancers and dental caries, highlighting their broad and systemic health impact.

One of the underlying concerns is that foods rich in added sugars are typically "empty calories," providing minimal essential nutrients, dietary fiber, or bioactive compounds. Frequent consumption of such foods can displace more nutrient-dense options, including fruits, vegetables, whole grains, and lean proteins, leading to a paradoxical state in which individuals are simultaneously overfed yet undernourished. This displacement effect not only exacerbates energy imbalance but also undermines the intake of micronutrients necessary for maintaining metabolic and immune health, creating long-term vulnerabilities to chronic disease (Martínez Steele et al., 2016).

Reducing the consumption of UPFs represents a practical and effective strategy for lowering added sugar intake, particularly in countries like the United States where UPFs contribute a substantial proportion of total dietary sugar. UPFs—such as sugar-sweetened beverages, packaged snacks, breakfast cereals, and confectionery—are disproportionately high in added sugars and low in fiber and micronutrients. By shifting dietary patterns toward minimally processed, nutrient-rich foods, individuals can decrease overall sugar consumption while improving dietary quality, supporting weight management, and reducing the risk of metabolic and CVDs. Public health interventions, educational campaigns, and policy measures targeting sugar reduction in processed foods could therefore have a meaningful impact on population health outcomes (Martínez Steele et al., 2016).

8.4.3 Artificial Sweeteners

Artificial sweeteners, or non-nutritive sweeteners (NNS), such as saccharin, sucralose, aspartame, acesulfame-K (Ace-K), cyclamate, and plant-derived stevia glycosides, are widely used in foods and beverages marketed as "diet," "lite," "zero sugar," or "sugar-free." These compounds are hundreds of times sweeter than sucrose on a molar basis while contributing virtually no calories, making them appealing as tools for weight control and diabetes prevention. For many years, they were assumed to be safe and metabolically inert substitutes for sugar, functioning simply as sweetness enhancers without altering gastrointestinal or metabolic processes in any meaningful way.

Over the last decade, however, research from both animal models and human studies has increasingly challenged this assumption. A growing body of evidence shows that artificial sweeteners can trigger metabolic disturbances, particularly impairments in glucose homeostasis, which contradict the very purpose for which they are often consumed. These adverse effects arise through a variety of mechanisms, including alterations to the gut microbiome, changes in hormone signaling, and behavioral influences on appetite and reward pathways. Pioneering studies by Suez and colleagues in 2014, followed by more recent work in 2015, have consistently shown that these sweeteners are far from biologically neutral.

A major breakthrough came from experiments conducted at the Weizmann Institute, which demonstrated that saccharin, sucralose, and aspartame induced glucose intolerance in mice through microbiome-dependent pathways. Mice given artificial sweeteners developed impaired glucose tolerance compared with controls receiving either water or sugar water. The critical finding was that germ-free mice—those without a microbiome—did not experience glucose intolerance after NNS exposure. This established that the gut microbiota is not just associated with the adverse metabolic effects of artificial sweeteners but is essential for causing them.

The causal role of disrupted microbial communities was confirmed through fecal microbiota transplantation. When microbiota from NNS-exposed mice were transferred to germ-free animals, the recipients developed glucose intolerance despite never consuming artificial sweeteners. This elegant experiment provided definitive proof that dysbiosis alone can transmit metabolic dysfunction. Further analyses revealed consistent features of NNS-induced dysbiosis: reduced microbial diversity, shifts toward more *Bacteroides* and certain *Clostridiales*, and decreases in beneficial genera such as *Bifidobacterium* and *Lactobacillus*. Functional alterations accompanied these shifts, including changes in pathways related to carbohydrate metabolism and short-chain fatty acid (SCFA) production.

Several mechanisms appear to drive these microbiome alterations. Contrary to earlier assumptions that artificial sweeteners pass through the gastrointestinal tract unchanged, research now shows that many gut microbes can interact with, metabolize, or respond to these compounds. Some

Bacteroides species can cleave sucralose's glycosidic bonds, producing metabolites whose effects on host physiology remain unclear. Artificial sweeteners may also interfere with bacterial processing of complex carbohydrates by inhibiting polysaccharide utilization loci (PULs), reducing fiber fermentation efficiency, and lowering SCFA production—an outcome that can adversely influence host metabolic health.

Beyond their microbiome effects, artificial sweeteners may disrupt the host's metabolic regulation through direct interactions with sweet-taste receptors (T1R2/T1R3) expressed on enteroendocrine cells throughout the gut. These receptors typically respond to glucose, stimulating the secretion of incretin hormones such as GLP-1 and glucose-dependent insulinotropic polypeptide (GIP) that regulate insulin release and appetite. When artificial sweeteners activate these receptors without accompanying calories or glucose, they may create mismatches in hormonal signaling that contribute to glucose intolerance. Additionally, repeated consumption of NNS may alter brain reward pathways, increasing cravings for sweetness and potentially promoting overall higher caloric intake—an effect that may help explain the paradoxical association between artificial sweetener use and weight gain in some populations.

Importantly, not all individuals respond to artificial sweeteners in the same way. Studies have shown that baseline microbiome composition strongly influences whether someone becomes a "responder," developing glucose intolerance, or a "non-responder," showing minimal metabolic change. Responders tend to harbor microbial communities predisposed to dysbiosis upon exposure to NNS, while others possess more resilient microbiota. This variability underscores the need for personalized nutrition approaches rather than one-size-fits-all dietary recommendations. Even stevia, often marketed as the "natural" alternative, can alter the microbiome—sometimes beneficially, sometimes adversely—depending on dose, formulation, and individual microbial ecology. Together, these findings reveal that artificial sweeteners, despite their calorie-free allure, can significantly alter gut microbiota and metabolic health in ways that demand much more nuanced consideration.

8.4.4 Use of Salt for Taste and Preservation

Elevated BP, or hypertension, is a major modifiable risk factor for CVD, the leading cause of morbidity and mortality worldwide. Effective BP management is crucial not only for individuals with diagnosed hypertension but also for those with high-normal BP, as even modest elevations can increase the risk of cardiovascular events. Behavioral factors—including tobacco use, physical activity, and diet—play a significant role in regulating BP. Among these, dietary patterns have emerged as a critical determinant, with growing evidence highlighting the impact of UPFs on cardiovascular health.

UPFs are industrially produced products that are typically energy-dense, high in salt and sugar, and low in fiber, micronutrients, and other bioactive compounds. They often contain saturated and trans fats, refined carbohydrates, artificial additives, and flavor enhancers, with little, if any, whole-food content (Shim et al., 2022). Their nutrient-poor yet highly palatable composition encourages overconsumption, contributing to metabolic and cardiovascular disturbances. The high sodium content of many UPFs, in particular, has been strongly linked to increased BP and hypertension risk.

Multiple epidemiological studies support this association. Oladale et al. (2024) demonstrated that individuals with high UPF consumption have a significantly elevated risk of developing hypertension. Similar findings were reported in a Brazilian cohort by Scaranni et al. (2021) and replicated in a Korean population (Shim et al., 2022), highlighting the consistency of these associations across diverse dietary and cultural contexts. These studies suggest that the rising prevalence of UPFs in global diets may be a key driver of increasing hypertension rates.

Several physiological pathways connect UPF consumption to elevated BP. Excess dietary sodium disrupts renal sodium homeostasis and extrarenal sodium handling, leading to water retention and plasma volume expansion. Additionally, UPFs may exert direct effects on vascular walls, promoting endothelial stiffness and increased peripheral resistance. Systemic and local neuro-hormonal pathways—including the renin–angiotensin–aldosterone system and sympathetic nervous system—further contribute to BP elevation, particularly in individuals with salt-sensitive phenotypes. Chronic consumption of UPFs can also trigger metabolic, hemodynamic, and inflammatory changes that exacerbate hypertension risk (Juul et al., 2021).

Dietary sodium-to-potassium balance is another critical factor influencing cardiovascular risk.

Epidemiological evidence indicates that a high sodium-to-potassium ratio (≥1.0) is associated with greater CVD mortality, whereas higher potassium intake is protective. In the United States, commercially processed foods—many of which are UPFs—constitute the primary source of sodium, while minimally processed foods such as fruits, vegetables, and dairy provide potassium (Juul et al., 2021). Diets dominated by UPFs therefore increase sodium intake while reducing potassium consumption, shifting the sodium-to-potassium ratio in a direction that favors hypertension and CVD.

Beyond sodium, the low fiber and micronutrient content of UPFs may indirectly contribute to BP dysregulation. Dietary fiber supports gut health, modulates inflammatory pathways, and improves insulin sensitivity, all of which influence vascular function and BP. Conversely, the refined carbohydrates, added sugars, and industrial fats in UPFs can exacerbate insulin resistance, endothelial dysfunction, and systemic inflammation, creating a metabolic environment conducive to hypertension. Thus, the impact of UPFs on BP is multifactorial, encompassing both direct sodium-mediated effects and broader metabolic consequences.

Salt is commonly added to UPFs not only to intensify flavor but also to inhibit the growth of microorganisms, thereby extending shelf life (Rysová & Šmídová, 2021). Beyond its functional roles, salt can also contribute to habitual overconsumption. Research suggests that high salt intake may have addictive properties, influencing neural reward pathways and reinforcing preferences for salty foods (Morris et al., 2008). As a result, the use of salt in UPFs can simultaneously enhance product appeal and promote repeated consumption.

Overall, high consumption of UPFs represents a significant and modifiable dietary risk factor for elevated BP and subsequent CVD. The combination of high sodium, low potassium, poor nutrient density, and inflammatory potential makes UPFs particularly detrimental to cardiovascular health. Reducing reliance on these foods and prioritizing minimally processed, potassium- and fiber-rich whole foods may help lower BP, improve sodium-to-potassium balance, and mitigate long-term cardiovascular risk.

8.4.5 Emulsifiers: Disrupting the Mucus Barrier and Promoting Inflammation

Emulsifiers are amphiphilic compounds designed to stabilize mixtures of oil and water by lowering surface tension at the interface between hydrophobic and hydrophilic phases. Their ability to bind simultaneously to both environments makes them essential for creating smooth, uniform textures in processed foods. Because they prevent ingredient separation, enhance mouthfeel, and extend shelf life, emulsifiers have become almost ubiquitous in modern industrial food production. They appear in an enormous range of products—baked goods, margarine, ice cream, salad dressings, processed dairy alternatives, sauces, spreads, and plant-based meat substitutes—making them one of the most frequently consumed classes of food additives in industrialized diets.

The emulsifiers most commonly found in processed foods include mono- and diglycerides, which are synthesized by combining glycerol with fatty acids and represent the single most widely used class of these additives. Polysorbates such as polysorbate-80 (P80) and polysorbate-20 (P20)—polyoxyethylene sorbitan esters—are used extensively to solubilize fats and ensure consistent texture. Additional emulsifying and stabilizing agents include carboxymethylcellulose (CMC), a chemically modified cellulose derivative; soy lecithin, a phospholipid-rich extract from soybeans; carrageenan, a sulfated polysaccharide obtained from red seaweed; and a variety of plant-derived gums such as guar gum and xanthan gum. Although these compounds differ structurally, many share the common feature of possessing both hydrophobic and hydrophilic regions, a property that underlies their functional effects in food—and, increasingly recognized, their biological effects in the gut.

Over the past decade, mechanistic and experimental research has revealed that dietary emulsifiers are not biologically inert. Instead, they can compromise intestinal barrier function by directly interacting with the mucus layer that protects the epithelial surface. The amphiphilic nature of emulsifiers allows them to insert into the mucin network, which is normally stabilized by a complex interplay of hydrophobic interactions, hydrogen bonds, and electrostatic forces. Mucin glycoproteins possess both protein-rich hydrophobic regions and highly glycosylated hydrophilic domains, and their ability to self-assemble into a cohesive gel is critical for maintaining a functional barrier. By disrupting these stabilizing interactions, emulsifiers reduce mucus viscosity and thickness, weakening its ability to prevent bacterial contact with epithelial cells.

Evidence from experimental studies provides compelling support for this mechanism. In vitro models show that physiologically relevant concentrations of CMC and P80 impair the structural integrity of mucus, increasing its permeability and allowing greater bacterial translocation. In vivo investigations confirm these findings: mice fed emulsifier-enriched diets develop thinner mucus layers and exhibit markedly reduced separation between gut bacteria and the intestinal epithelium. Bacteria also penetrate more deeply into crypts, an abnormal pattern of microbial encroachment that signals the early breakdown of mucosal defense systems.

As the mucus barrier becomes compromised, bacteria gain closer access to epithelial cells, increasing stimulation of pattern recognition receptors such as Toll-like receptors (TLRs) and NOD-like receptors (NLRs). These receptors detect bacterial molecular patterns including lipopolysaccharide (LPS), peptidoglycan, and flagellin. Chronic activation of these innate immune sensors initiates low-grade inflammation and amplifies production of pro-inflammatory cytokines such as TNF-α, IL-1β, IL-6, and IL-17. This low-level but persistent inflammatory state resembles metabolic endotoxemia, a phenomenon increasingly linked to obesity, insulin resistance, and other elements of metabolic syndrome.

Pioneering work from Chassaing et al. (2015) provided some of the clearest evidence that emulsifiers can induce both inflammatory and metabolic disease. In controlled experiments, mice consuming diets containing human-relevant concentrations of CMC or P80 developed a suite of concerning phenotypes: chronic intestinal inflammation, increased immune cell infiltration, elevated fasting glucose, impaired glucose tolerance, weight gain, fat accumulation, and heightened susceptibility to colitis. These effects closely mirror metabolic syndrome and inflammatory bowel conditions in humans, suggesting that emulsifiers may contribute to disease risk in populations consuming large quantities of processed foods.

A crucial element of these findings is that emulsifier-induced pathology was entirely dependent on the presence of an intact microbiome. Germ-free mice exposed to the same emulsifiers displayed none of the inflammatory or metabolic abnormalities observed in conventional mice. This indicates that emulsifiers exert their harmful effects not through direct toxicity to the host, but by reshaping microbial communities in ways that destabilize the gut environment. These results also highlight a major limitation of traditional toxicology testing, which rarely incorporates microbiome-dependent modes of action and therefore may overlook health effects that emerge only in the context of host–microbe interactions.

Microbiome analyses reveal that emulsifier exposure induces marked shifts in community structure. Beneficial taxa such as Bacteroidales and the anti-inflammatory species *F. prausnitzii* decrease significantly, while Proteobacteria—including various *Escherichia* species—expand disproportionately. These dysbiotic microbial communities express more pro-inflammatory genes, produce increased quantities of flagellin, and exhibit greater mucolytic activity, all of which exacerbate mucus degradation and promote closer bacterial–epithelial interactions. This altered ecosystem appears primed to sustain a state of chronic, low-grade inflammation.

Remarkably, emulsifier-induced dysbiosis is sufficient to transmit disease phenotypes even in the absence of direct emulsifier consumption. When fecal microbiota from emulsifier-exposed mice were transplanted into germ-free recipients, the recipients developed glucose intolerance, increased adiposity, and signs of inflammation despite never ingesting emulsifiers. These experiments provide definitive evidence that emulsifier-driven microbiome alterations are causal drivers—not merely correlates—of metabolic and inflammatory disturbances.

Beyond their effects on mucus integrity and immune activation, emulsifiers may influence metabolic processes through additional mechanisms. Some evidence suggests that they can alter lipid digestion and absorption, potentially increasing postprandial lipemia and promoting the formation of atherogenic lipoprotein particles. Emulsifiers may also disrupt bile acid metabolism, which is critical for shaping the gut microbiome and regulates host metabolic pathways through receptors such as FXR and TGR5. Altered bile acid signaling could therefore contribute to changes in glucose homeostasis, energy expenditure, and inflammatory tone. Although these secondary pathways require further investigation, they underscore the likelihood that the metabolic impact of emulsifiers extends far beyond the gut lumen.

8.4.6 Xanthan Gum

Xanthan gum, a microbial exopolysaccharide produced via fermentation by *Xanthomonas campestris*, has become one of the most prevalent additives in the modern food supply (Ostrowski et al., 2022). Its exceptional functional properties—such as providing thickening, stabilizing, and emulsifying capabilities across a wide range of temperatures and pH levels—have made it highly valuable in the food industry. Today, xanthan gum is found in an extensive array of processed products, including salad dressings, sauces, ice creams, baked goods, gluten-free formulations, and sugar-free syrups. Its ubiquity means that daily exposure is now routine for most consumers, often occurring without conscious awareness.

Because xanthan gum is a complex, high–molecular weight polysaccharide, it might initially seem to contribute positively to gut health by acting as a source of fermentable dietary fiber. Indeed, certain gut microbes—especially specialized *Bacteroides* species—harbor PULs capable of breaking down xanthan gum's highly branched molecular structure. These bacteria metabolize its carbohydrate components into SCFAs such as acetate and propionate, which provide metabolic fuel for host tissues and confer important immunological and metabolic benefits. Thus, at first glance, xanthan gum may appear to function similarly to traditional plant-derived fibers.

However, concerns arise when examining the broader ecological consequences of substituting industrial polysaccharides for natural dietary fibers. The gut microbiome is organized around distinct ecological niches, with each bacterial species equipped with a specialized enzymatic toolkit. Keystone fiber-degrading species—including *Ruminococcus bromii*, *F. prausnitzii*, *Eubacterium rectale*, and members of the *Roseburia* genus—play irreplaceable roles in breaking down cellulose, hemicellulose, pectin, resistant starch, and other structural polysaccharides from whole plant foods. These microbes form the backbone of fiber fermentation in the human colon and produce butyrate, the SCFA most critical for colonocyte energy supply and epithelial health.

When diets shift away from diverse plant-derived polysaccharides toward simplified industrial additives like xanthan gum, microbial competition can change in ways that disadvantage these keystone species. Organisms that efficiently degrade xanthan gum may gain a growth advantage over traditional fiber-degrading microbes. Over time, this can lead to measurable reductions in populations of bacteria specialized for processing complex plant fibers. If this trend persists across long-term dietary patterns—or across generations—microbial communities may gradually lose metabolic pathways needed to break down the wide array of polysaccharides found in whole plant foods, reducing the gut ecosystem's overall resilience and functional capacity.

These concerns are especially relevant in industrialized societies where habitual fiber intake already falls far below recommended levels. If xanthan gum and other industrial polysaccharides displace natural fibers in the diet, the microbiome may become progressively less capable of fermenting the diverse fibers that support metabolic health. This could create a self-perpetuating cycle: a fiber-poor diet leads to the loss of fiber-degrading microbes, which in turn diminishes the body's ability to benefit from fiber, making plant-rich diets more challenging to reintroduce effectively. This ecological drift in the microbiome represents an underappreciated consequence of modern food processing.

Sugar-free syrups provide a clear example of this issue. Marketed as healthier alternatives due to the absence of sugar and the promise of negligible caloric content, these products often contain a mixture of artificial sweeteners, xanthan gum or similar polysaccharide thickeners, preservatives, and synthetic flavoring agents. While the marketing highlights sugar reduction, it rarely acknowledges that these additives—many of which have documented effects on gut microbial composition—can collectively disrupt the gut ecosystem. The simultaneous presence of artificial sweeteners (which can impair glucose tolerance through microbiome alterations), xanthan gum (which may shift ecological niches away from natural fiber degraders), and other synthetic compounds creates complex exposure scenarios whose cumulative or interactive effects remain poorly understood.

Ultimately, understanding the ecological implications of replacing natural dietary fibers with industrial polysaccharides like xanthan gum requires recognizing the microbiome as a dynamic ecosystem shaped by selective pressures. Although xanthan gum is fermentable by some beneficial microbes, its widespread use in processed foods may inadvertently reshape microbial communities in ways that reduce metabolic flexibility and fiber-processing capacity. As diets become increasingly dominated by engineered ingredients, the long-term health implications for microbial ecology—and therefore host physiology—deserve closer scientific and public attention.

8.4.7 Fat and Oil

Potato chips are among the most widely consumed UPFs worldwide. Their defining sensory characteristics include a high salt content and substantial amounts of added oil, both of which contribute to their flavor, texture, and overall palatability. Typically, potato chips contain between 35 and 45% oil by weight (Latif et al., 2020). This high fat content, combined with refined starch and added sodium, plays a significant role in their energy density and potential impact on dietary health.

The rising consumption of UPFs has been identified as a major contributor to the global obesity epidemic. These products are typically energy-dense, high in added sugars, unhealthy fats, and sodium, and designed to promote overconsumption through enhanced palatability and convenience. A growing body of evidence indicates that the higher intake of UPFs is associated not only with increased risk of obesity but also with a greater prevalence of metabolic syndrome and related cardiometabolic disorders. Studies have shown that frequent consumption of UPFs can lead to elevations in total cholesterol and LDL cholesterol, further compounding long-term health risks (Poti et al., 2017; Nouri et al., 2023). These findings highlight the significant public health implications of widespread UPF consumption.

8.4.8 Synthetic Food Color

Synthetic food colorants are among the most unnecessary yet widely used additives in the modern food supply. Their purpose is purely aesthetic: to make processed foods appear more vibrant, uniform, and visually enticing. Despite offering no nutritional benefit, these dyes are ubiquitous in UPFs, especially those targeted toward children. Candies, fruit-flavored drinks, breakfast cereals, baked goods, dessert mixes, and snack products frequently rely on synthetic colorants to create bright, appealing hues that enhance marketability.

The most commonly used artificial dyes include tartrazine (Yellow 5), sunset yellow (Yellow 6), allura red AC (Red 40), brilliant blue FCF (Blue 1), and indigotine (Blue 2). Many of these compounds belong to the azo dye family, distinguished by the presence of a nitrogen–nitrogen double bond (N=N) linking aromatic rings. While this structural arrangement gives the dyes their stability and intense coloration, it also determines how they are processed within the human gastrointestinal tract—particularly by gut microbes.

A key concern centers on the interaction between azo dyes and bacterial azoreductase enzymes. Numerous gut bacteria possess these enzymes, which are capable of reducing and cleaving the N=N bond in azo dyes. This metabolic reaction transforms the original dye molecules into smaller aromatic amines—compounds with biological properties that can differ dramatically from the parent dye. While synthetic colorants are typically evaluated for safety in their unmodified form, these microbial metabolites have often undergone far less rigorous toxicological testing.

The aromatic amines generated from dye metabolism are of special interest because some are structurally related to known mutagenic or carcinogenic compounds. Although definitive evidence linking food dye–derived aromatic amines to cancer remains limited and debated, their potential bioactivity underscores a gap in traditional safety assessments. Most regulatory evaluations do not fully account for the biochemical transformations that occur in the gut, despite increasing recognition that microbial metabolism can profoundly alter compound toxicity and biological effects.

In addition to concerns about metabolite formation, accumulating research indicates that synthetic colorants can disrupt gut microbiome composition. Experimental studies in rodents and ex vivo human microbiota models show that common food dyes reduce populations of beneficial Firmicutes and Bacteroidetes while encouraging the growth of Proteobacteria, a phylum often associated with dysbiosis and intestinal inflammation. Dye exposure has been linked to elevated levels of inflammatory markers such as fecal calprotectin and lipocalin-2, indicating that these additives may exacerbate or promote gut inflammatory states.

The mechanisms underlying dye-induced dysbiosis appear multifactorial. Some bacterial species may be directly harmed by dye compounds or their aromatic amine metabolites, experiencing oxidative stress or inhibited growth. Conversely, bacteria equipped with azoreductase enzymes may gain competitive advantages from their ability to metabolize these xenobiotics, thereby altering ecological balance. The metabolic burden associated with processing synthetic dyes may also divert bacterial energy away from beneficial functions such as fiber fermentation, further influencing community structure and function.

Synthetic colorants have also been shown to stimulate pro-inflammatory signaling in host tissues. In rodent models, chronic exposure to commonly used dyes increases intestinal expression of TNF-α, IL-1β, IL-6, and interferon-γ—cytokines strongly implicated in the initiation and progression of inflammatory bowel disease. Although more research is needed to determine whether typical dietary exposure contributes to inflammatory bowel disease (IBD) or other chronic conditions in humans, the parallels between experimental findings and known inflammatory pathways warrant careful consideration.

Importantly, the levels of food dyes used in many studies reflect real-world exposure, particularly among children. Analyses of commercial products show that a single serving of certain brightly colored cereals, candies, or fruit beverages can contain 30–40 mg of synthetic dyes. Children who consume multiple servings of such foods daily may reach intake levels comparable to those associated with microbiome and inflammatory changes in experimental models. This raises questions about cumulative, long-term effects in populations with high processed–food consumption.

Regulatory responses differ sharply across regions. The European Union has adopted a more precautionary stance, requiring warning labels for products containing specific azo dyes and imposing stricter limits on their use. In contrast, U.S. regulations remain more permissive, reflecting divergent interpretations of available evidence and differing philosophical approaches to risk assessment. As research continues to illuminate the complex interplay between synthetic colorants, microbial metabolism, and host health, these regulatory differences highlight the ongoing debate over how best to protect consumers in an evolving scientific landscape.

8.5 MECHANISMS OF MICROBIOME DISRUPTION BY ULTRA-PROCESSED FOODS

UPFs now constitute 50–60% of total energy intake in countries including the United States, Canada, and the United Kingdom, with even higher proportions among children, adolescents, and socioeconomically disadvantaged populations (Lane et al., 2024). Common examples include packaged breads and baked goods made with refined white flour, breakfast cereals, sweetened beverages (both sugar-sweetened and artificially sweetened with compounds like stevia, aspartame, or sucralose), reconstituted meat products, instant soups and noodles, pre-prepared meals, sugar-free syrups stabilized with xanthan gum, diet sodas, and mass-produced snack foods containing synthetic colorants.

UPFs are typically low in natural dietary fiber, a key nutrient that supports digestive health, stabilizes blood sugar, and nourishes beneficial gut microbes. Because the original plant or animal ingredients are heavily altered, much of the fiber is removed or destroyed during processing. In place of whole ingredients, UPFs often rely on refined carbohydrates, starches, and artificial thickeners that provide energy but little nutritional value. This lack of fiber contributes to rapid spikes in blood glucose, reduced satiety, and a higher likelihood of overeating—factors closely tied to weight gain and metabolic dysfunction.

Alongside being fiber-poor, UPFs often contain high amounts of added sugars or sugar substitutes, as well as emulsifiers, artificial colors, salt, preservatives, and other additives designed to enhance taste, texture, appearance, or shelf life. Although these compounds can make products appealing and convenient, many have been associated with adverse health outcomes. Excess added sugars promote inflammation, insulin resistance, and fatty liver disease, while certain emulsifiers and artificial sweeteners may disrupt gut microbiota and impair metabolic health. Food dyes and preservatives have also raised concerns regarding behavioral effects in children and long-term disease risk. Together, these components make heavy consumption of UPFs a significant contributor to modern health problems, including obesity, hypertension, CVD, type 2 diabetes, and gastrointestinal disorders.

8.5.1 Fiber Depletion: Starving the Beneficial Microbiome

Dietary fiber consists of a diverse group of plant-derived polysaccharides that resist digestion by human enzymes but undergo fermentation by gut microbes. These fibers serve as the primary energy source for many beneficial bacteria and are critical for maintaining microbial diversity and gut health. Yet average fiber intake in the United States is only about 15 g/day, far below the recommended 25–35 g, and a small fraction of the 80–120 g consumed daily by contemporary hunter-gatherers and rural populations still eating traditional plant-based diets.

UPFs contribute substantially to this fiber deficit. Refining grains removes 70–80% of their natural fiber content: a slice of commercial white bread contains less than 1 g of fiber, compared with 2–3 g in whole wheat bread and 3–4 g in traditional stone-ground whole-grain bread. Because grain-based products make up a large share of the modern American diet, these losses carry significant nutritional consequences.

Fiber removal also occurs during the processing of fruits and vegetables. Juice extraction discards most fibrous pulp—apple juice contains virtually no fiber, whereas a whole apple provides about 4 g. Instant mashed potatoes lack the resistant starch and fiber found in whole potatoes with skins (Li et al., 2025). Even mechanical processing—chopping, grinding, homogenizing—can reduce the physiological benefits of fiber by disrupting cell walls and reducing particle size, making fiber less effective in modulating digestion and metabolism.

The metabolic consequences of widespread fiber depletion are profound. When dietary fiber is scarce, colonic microbes must shift to alternative substrates, including mucus glycoproteins, amino acids, and other host-derived compounds. This transition sets off several negative biological cascades.

8.5.1.1 Mucus Layer Erosion

The intestinal mucus layer consists of a dense inner region that excludes bacteria and a looser outer layer that supports microbial life. Under normal conditions, mucin-degrading species such as *A. muciniphila* and *Bacteroides* fragilis participate in a balanced cycle of mucus breakdown and renewal. In low-fiber environments, however, these bacteria increase mucin consumption to make up for lost dietary substrates. When degradation outpaces synthesis, the mucus layer thins, allowing bacteria to encroach upon epithelial surfaces. This proximity activates TLRs and NLRs, triggering inflammatory pathways and disrupting the spatial organization that normally maintains immune homeostasis.

8.5.1.2 Increased Protein Fermentation

Low-fiber diets force microbes to rely more heavily on fermentation of amino acids. Metabolism of aromatic amino acids and branched-chain amino acids yields metabolites such as phenols, indoles, ammonia, hydrogen sulfide, and branched-chain fatty acids. While some compounds—like indole-3-propionic acid (IPA)—are beneficial, excessive protein fermentation is associated with intestinal inflammation, impaired insulin sensitivity, and systemic metabolic dysfunction.

8.5.1.3 Reduced Production of Short-Chain Fatty Acids (SCFAs)

SCFAs—acetate, propionate, and especially butyrate—are the principal metabolic products of fiber fermentation and play critical roles in gut and systemic physiology. Butyrate supplies 60–70% of the energy required by colonocytes, making it essential for maintaining epithelial integrity. When fiber intake declines, butyrate levels fall, compromising colonocyte metabolism and weakening the gut barrier.

Beyond serving as a fuel, butyrate regulates gene expression by inhibiting histone deacetylases (HDACs) and activates G protein-coupled receptor (GPCRs) such as GPR43 and GPR41 on intestinal and immune cells. Through these mechanisms, SCFAs modulate inflammation, support tight-junction integrity, influence gut motility, regulate appetite hormones (GLP-1, peptideYY (PYY)), and help maintain overall metabolic balance. Low-fiber diets therefore have far-reaching consequences that extend well beyond the gastrointestinal tract.

Microbiome studies reinforce these findings. High-fiber diets promote a diverse microbial community enriched with species such as *Prevotella*, *Roseburia*, *E. rectale*, and *F. prausnitzii* (Sokol et al., 2008)—bacteria equipped with extensive carbohydrate-active enzymes (CAZymes) capable of breaking down complex plant polysaccharides and producing butyrate (Atzeni et al., 2022). In contrast, low-fiber, UPF-rich diets reduce microbial diversity, encourage expansion of pro-inflammatory Proteobacteria (e.g., *Escherichia*, *Shigella*, *Desulfovibrio*), and diminish the gut's capacity to generate beneficial metabolites. These shifts are associated with greater intestinal permeability, heightened systemic inflammation, insulin resistance, and increased risk of inflammatory bowel disease.

8.6 MICROBIOME ALTERATIONS LINKED TO INGREDIENTS IN ULTRA-PROCESSED FOODS

8.6.1 Microbiome Changes Associated with Dietary Sugar

Dietary sugars—particularly fructose—have emerged as major dietary drivers of microbiome disruption and metabolic disease. Fructose is widely consumed through processed foods, sweetened beverages, and HFCS, and its excessive intake has been closely linked to CVDs and cardiac arrhythmias. Traditionally, fructose metabolism was thought to occur primarily in the liver, but recent evidence shows that the small intestine is a major site of initial fructose processing. When consumption exceeds intestinal metabolic capacity, unabsorbed fructose reaches the colon, where it interacts with and is metabolized by the gut microbiota. This excess fructose induces microbial dysbiosis, increases intestinal permeability, and triggers inflammatory pathways. Microbial products such as LPS, trimethylamine N-oxide (TMAO), and SCFAs further modulate systemic inflammation and cardiovascular function. These findings support a model in which high-fructose diets disrupt the heart–gut axis, creating an inflammatory milieu that promotes arrhythmogenesis (Cheng et al., 2021). Understanding how sugar-induced dysbiosis contributes to cardiac inflammation may reveal mechanistic pathways underlying cardiac arrhythmia development.

HFCS has been of particular concern due to its widespread use in soft drinks and packaged foods. Excessive HFCS consumption is strongly associated with obesity and metabolic syndrome, but emerging research indicates that it can also directly affect the microbiota in ways that promote inflammation. Chen et al. (2024) examined the effects of 30% FCS in mice over a 16-week period and found pronounced fat accumulation, hepatic steatosis, and inflammatory injury in both the intestine and liver. FCS markedly increased the abundance of Muribaculaceae in vivo and in vitro, with this genus positively correlating with markers of metabolic dysfunction. Functional analysis revealed that FCS enhanced microbial pathways such as the pentose phosphate pathway and arachidonic acid metabolism. Metabolomic profiling confirmed elevated levels of prostaglandins—pro-inflammatory metabolites derived from arachidonic acid. These findings demonstrate that HFCS can drive the microbiota to synthesize inflammatory mediators, providing a novel mechanistic link between fructose intake and metabolic inflammation.

HFCS consumption also appears to contribute to carcinogenesis in the colon. Goncalves et al. (2019) investigated the effects of daily HFCS administration in adenomatous polyposis coli (APC) mutant mice, a model predisposed to colorectal cancer. Remarkably, HFCS increased tumor size and grade even in the absence of obesity or metabolic syndrome, indicating a direct tumor-promoting effect. HFCS elevated fructose in the intestinal lumen and glucose in the blood, and tumors readily transported both sugars. Within the tumor microenvironment, fructose was converted into fructose-1-phosphate, stimulating glycolysis and fatty acid synthesis—metabolic pathways that support rapid tumor growth. These data suggest that even moderate combined glucose and fructose intake can accelerate intestinal tumorigenesis.

Beyond cancer risk, chronic fructose consumption has long been associated with obesity and other metabolic disorders. Beisner et al. (2020) conducted a controlled dietary intervention to examine how different fructose sources influence the human gut microbiome. Participants sequentially consumed four diets: a low-fructose diet (<10 g/day), a fruit-rich diet (100 g/day fructose), another low-fructose phase, and finally a high-fructose syrup (HFS) diet (100 g/day fructose). Microbiota profiling revealed that fructose source significantly shaped microbial communities. The fruit-rich diet—high in both fructose and dietary fiber—shifted the microbiota toward increased Firmicutes, including beneficial butyrate-producing taxa such as *Faecalibacterium*, *Anaerostipes*, and *Erysipelatoclostridium*, while reducing Bacteroidetes and genera such as *Parabacteroides*. In contrast, the HFS diet produced an opposite profile, decreasing Firmicutes and increasing Bacteroidetes, with notable reductions in beneficial taxa such as *Ruminococcus*, *Faecalibacterium*, and *Erysipelatoclostridium*. These microbial shifts correlated with host lipid markers: Bacteroidetes abundance positively correlated with plasma cholesterol and LDL levels, whereas Firmicutes abundance negatively correlated. This suggests that fructose from whole fruit may support microbial communities that promote digestive and metabolic health, whereas fructose from syrup may promote dysbiosis and adverse metabolic profiles.

More detailed genus-level analysis uncovered additional diet-specific microbial signatures. Ten genera—including *Parabacteroides*, *Alistipes*, *Odoribacter*, *Oscillibacter*, *Faecalibacterium*, *Barnesiella*, *Erysipelatoclostridium*, *Ruminococcus*, *Anaerostipes*, and *Veillonella*—were significantly altered across diet phases. Fruit consumption increased beneficial genera such as *Anaerostipes*, *Faecalibacterium*, and *Erysipelatoclostridium*, while decreasing potentially harmful or inflammation-associated genera such as *Alistipes*, *Oscillibacter*, and *Odoribacter*. Conversely, the HFS diet reduced key beneficial taxa including *Ruminococcus* and increased genera such as *Barnesiella* and *Veillonella*. Although lean and obese subjects exhibited similar directional shifts, only the reduction in *Ruminococcus* after HFS intake reached significance in lean individuals. Overall, these findings indicate that not all forms of fructose exert equivalent effects on the microbiome: fructose delivered with dietary fiber (as in fruit) supports beneficial microbial communities, whereas refined fructose syrups promote dysbiosis linked to metabolic dysfunction.

8.6.2 Microbiome Alterations Associated with Artificial Sweeteners

8.6.2.1 Microbiome Effects of Aspartame

Non-caloric artificial sweeteners (NAS) are among the most frequently consumed food additives worldwide, used by individuals across all body-weight categories. Although originally promoted as metabolically inert sugar substitutes, accumulating evidence shows that NAS can profoundly influence host physiology by altering the structure and function of the gut microbiome. Seminal work by Suez et al. (2014) demonstrated that consumption of common NAS formulations induces glucose intolerance by driving dysbiosis and shifting microbial metabolic activity. These findings revealed that NAS are not biologically passive compounds; rather, they interact with the gut microbiota in ways that may contribute to cardiometabolic disease risk.

Animal studies and limited human trials suggest that NAS—particularly aspartame—can produce oxidative and inflammatory effects. Aspartame and its metabolites, even at doses within recommended safety limits, may disrupt the oxidant/antioxidant balance and induce oxidative stress. These disturbances can compromise cell membrane integrity and impair cellular function across diverse tissues, ultimately contributing to systemic inflammation (Choudhary & Pretorius, 2017). Although the precise molecular mechanisms remain under investigation, redox imbalance, alterations in SCFA metabolism, and changes in bacterial signaling molecules are believed to play important roles.

Maternal consumption studies provide additional insight into NAS-induced microbiome disruption. In pregnant Sprague Dawley rats fed a high-fat/sucrose (HFSD) diet with or without aspartame supplementation (5–7 mg/kg body weight for 18 weeks), offspring from aspartame-exposed dams exhibited increased body fat at weaning and impaired glucose tolerance compared with offspring from HFSD-only dams. These physiological differences correlated with significant alterations in maternal and offspring microbiota. Dams receiving aspartame displayed higher levels of *A. muciniphila* and Enterobacteriaceae, whereas the aspartame-supplemented group showed lower levels of Enterococcaceae, *Enterococcus*, and *Parasutterella*, and elevated levels of *Clostridium* cluster IV in the cecum (Conz et al., 2023). Fecal microbiota transplantation from the offspring into germ-free mice reproduced many of the metabolic disturbances—direct evidence that the NAS-altered microbiota itself mediates adiposity and glucose intolerance. Both male and female offspring also showed increased Porphyromonadaceae, linking early-life NAS exposure to long-term microbial changes.

Human data indicate that NAS can also affect microbial communities outside the gut. Aspartame consumption has been shown to reduce the abundance of oral bacterial taxa such as *Porphyromonas* and *Prevotella nanceiensis*, indicating that artificial sweeteners may have multi-site microbial effects (Conz et al., 2023). Since the oral cavity serves as an entry point for microbial colonization of the gastrointestinal tract, such alterations could influence downstream microbial assembly and host immunity.

Controlled mouse studies further highlight the microbiome-disruptive potential of aspartame. Animals consuming aspartame exhibited higher relative abundances of Providencia

(Proteobacteria) and *Enorma* (Actinobacteria), and lower levels of the beneficial butyrate-producing genus *Butyrivibrio* (Firmicutes). Similar to animals given non-aspartame artificial sweeteners (NANS), the aspartame group displayed elevated abundances of *Salmonella*, *Klebsiella*, and *Escherichia/Shigella*, taxa frequently associated with inflammation and gastrointestinal pathology. In contrast, beneficial or commensal genera such as *Parvimonas*, *Arcobacter*, and *Streptococcus* were reduced compared with controls.

Aspartame exposure produced additional shifts in both core and non-core microbial genera. Notably, the relative abundance of *Lactobacillus*, a critical genus for gut barrier function and immune regulation, was significantly reduced. The same pattern was observed for *Fusobacterium*. Among non-core bacteria, an unidentified genus from the family Neisseriaceae increased more than 11-fold, along with the genera *Hydrogenophaga* (Proteobacteria) and *Leifsonia* (Actinobacteria). Conversely, *Roseomonas*, *Lysinibacillus*, and *Aeromonas* declined. These substantial shifts highlight the wide taxonomic range of microbes affected by aspartame.

Hosseini et al. (2023) extended this research by comparing the effects of non-sugar sweeteners (NSS)—both aspartame (ASP) and non-aspartame sweeteners (NANS)—on microbial communities in both stool and the duodenum, a region rarely examined in dietary studies. Interestingly, duodenal levels of *Escherichia* and *Klebsiella*, known disruptors of upper-gut microbial balance, were lower in both ASP and NANS groups compared with controls. Despite this, aspartame still induced many of the microbial alterations described above, demonstrating site-specific effects along the intestinal tract. Core microbial genera such as *Lactobacillus* again declined, while less common or opportunistic taxa—including the Neisseriaceae-related genus, *Hydrogenophaga*, and *Leifsonia*—expanded substantially. These findings underscore that NAS exposure produces complex, region-specific, and dose-dependent microbiome shifts that may contribute to metabolic and inflammatory outcomes.

8.6.2.2 Microbiome Effects of Acesulfame-K

Ace-K is a widely used low-calorie artificial sweetener incorporated into many processed foods and beverages. Despite its extensive use, the available toxicity data remain limited and insufficient for drawing firm conclusions about its long-term safety. Nevertheless, early investigations have identified several concerning biological effects. Ace-K has demonstrated genotoxic properties in experimental settings and has been shown to inhibit glucose fermentation by intestinal bacteria, suggesting it may interfere with normal microbial metabolic activity. Structurally, Ace-K belongs to the sulfonamide class—alongside sodium saccharin and sodium cyclamate—a group of compounds known for their antimicrobial characteristics. These features collectively raise questions about the potential for Ace-K to disrupt the gut microbial ecosystem (Bian et al., 2017).

Research in animal models provides further insight into how Ace-K may influence host physiology, particularly in a sex-dependent manner. Studies by Bian et al. (2017) revealed that Ace-K exposure leads to significant gender-specific alterations in body weight and gut microbiota composition. Male mice receiving Ace-K gained substantially more weight than untreated controls. This weight gain coincided with notable increases in the genus *Bacteroides* and measurable shifts in *Anaerostipes* and *Sutterella*. In contrast, female mice exhibited a markedly different response: after four weeks of Ace-K consumption, the relative abundance of several beneficial or commensal genera—*Lactobacillus*, *Clostridium*, an unclassified *Ruminococcaceae* genus, and an unclassified *Oxalobacteraceae* genus—declined sharply. Conversely, the abundance of *Mucispirillum*, a genus often associated with inflammation or mucosal disruption, increased. These findings suggest that Ace-K can perturb the gut microbiome in fundamentally different ways depending on biological sex.

Additional studies have reinforced these observations. In 8-week-old CD-1 mice administered Ace-K by gavage for four weeks at 37.5 mg/kg/day, researchers used 16S rRNA sequencing and metabolomic profiling to assess microbial and metabolic changes. The results mirrored earlier findings: male mice again displayed substantial increases in *Bacteroides*, as well as shifts in *Anaerostipes* and *Sutterella*. Female mice showed broad reductions across multiple genera, including *Lactobacillus* and *Clostridium*, along with increased *Mucispirillum*. Importantly, Ace-K-induced gender-specific body weight changes, favoring weight gain in males but not in females. These microbial alterations were paired with shifts in functional genes related to energy metabolism and detectable differences in fecal metabolites, underscoring Ace-K's capacity to influence not only microbial composition but also metabolic outputs in the gut (Conz et al., 2023).

Human studies, though more limited, have begun to examine similar patterns. Sylvetsky et al. (2024) evaluated the effects of consuming sucralose- and Ace-K-containing diet soda three times daily for one or eight weeks in healthy young adults. After eight weeks, participants exhibited increased relative abundance of Proteobacteria—particularly members of the Enterobacteriaceae family, which are often associated with dysbiosis or inflammation. Increases in two Proteobacteria taxa were already detectable after just one week of diet soda consumption compared with sparkling water controls. Furthermore, three taxa within the *Bacteroides* genus were found to increase after one week of intake. Although these findings do not establish causation, they highlight the possibility that routine consumption of Ace-K-containing products may subtly but measurably alter gut microbiota composition in humans.

Together, these studies suggest that Ace-K, long considered metabolically inert, may have meaningful biological effects on both microbial ecology and host metabolic pathways. Continued research in both animals and humans is essential to clarify the long-term implications of chronic Ace-K consumption.

8.6.2.3 Impact of Sucralose on the Microbiome

Sucralose, one of the most widely consumed NNS, has been increasingly scrutinized for its potential effects on the gut microbiome and host physiology. Emerging evidence suggests that sucralose is not biologically inert; instead, it can substantially alter microbial communities and impair immune function. Morder et al. (2025) demonstrated that sucralose consumption disrupts the gut microbiota in ways that restrict T-cell metabolism and diminish immune activity. In both preclinical cancer models and patients receiving anti-PD-1 immune checkpoint inhibitors, sucralose intake was associated with reduced T-cell function and poor therapeutic response. A key mechanism involved a notable decrease in microbiota-accessible arginine, an amino acid essential for cytotoxic T-cell activity. Remarkably, restoring arginine availability—either through amino acid supplementation or fecal microbiota transfer from anti-PD-1–responsive mice—fully rescued immune function and treatment efficacy. These findings reveal that sucralose induces a destabilized gut microbial environment that ultimately compromises the host's ability to mount an effective antitumor immune response.

At the microbial taxonomic level, sucralose consumption produced consistent and significant shifts. Morder et al. (2025) reported increased abundance of the Firmicutes and Proteobacteria phyla, accompanied by a relative outgrowth of several Gram-positive bacterial groups, particularly Clostridiaceae and Lachnospiraceae. This microbial imbalance, or dysbiosis, appears to be closely linked to the observed immune dysfunction. The authors proposed that these phenotypic and functional changes within the microbiota contribute directly to resistance against immune checkpoint inhibitor therapy. To better understand the functional consequences of these microbial alterations, the researchers performed both metagenomic and metabolomic analyses. Pathway-level investigations revealed widespread disruptions in amino acid metabolism, especially pathways associated with arginine degradation. Enzymes involved in arginine catabolism increased significantly in sucralose-exposed animals. Stool metabolomics confirmed reduced levels of arginine and its related metabolites, including citrulline, in sucralose-treated mice. Importantly, arginine depletion extended beyond the gut lumen, with significant reductions in serum and tumor interstitial fluid. Sucralose exposure also downregulated the amino acid transporter Slc7a3, further limiting arginine uptake and exacerbating T-cell dysfunction. Notably, citrulline supplementation restored anti-PD-1 response even in the continued presence of sucralose, highlighting the central role of arginine availability in immune regulation.

Additional animal studies further support sucralose's capacity to influence the gut microbiome. Zheng et al. (2022) reported that even low doses of sucralose significantly altered microbial communities in different intestinal regions of mice. Increases in genera such as *Tenacibaculum*, *Ruegeria*, Staphylococcus, and *Allobaculum* were observed in the jejunum, ileum, and colon, while declines in *Lachnoclostridium* and members of the Lachnospiraceae family occurred in the cecum. These findings highlight the sensitivity of the gut microbiota to sucralose and suggest that even modest consumption can produce measurable ecological shifts.

Human studies, though more limited, similarly indicate that sucralose may influence microbial composition and metabolic health. In an open-label clinical trial, Mendez-Garcia et al. (2022) evaluated the effects of daily sucralose consumption in healthy young adults over a ten-week period. Participants who consumed 48 mg of sucralose per day experienced significant alterations in the abundance of certain Firmicutes species, including a threefold increase in *Blautia coccoides* and a reduction to one-third of baseline levels of *Lactobacillus acidophilus*. Notably, these microbial changes were accompanied by metabolic changes: sucralose consumers displayed higher serum insulin levels and an increased area under the glucose curve during oral glucose tolerance testing. These findings suggest that long-term sucralose intake can induce gut dysbiosis that correlates with impaired glucose regulation.

Collectively, current research indicates that sucralose consumption can reshape the gut microbiome, alter amino acid metabolism, disrupt immune function, and potentially contribute to metabolic dysregulation. While more human studies are needed to clarify the magnitude and clinical relevance of these effects, existing evidence challenges the long-held assumption that sucralose is metabolically inert and highlights the importance of reevaluating its widespread use.

8.7 HOST MICROBIOME CHANGES ASSOCIATED WITH HIGH DIETARY SALT INTAKE

High dietary salt intake has emerged as a powerful modifier of the host gut microbiome, influencing both microbial community structure and microbial metabolic function in humans and animal models. Across studies, excessive sodium consumption consistently reshapes gut ecosystems, disrupts microbial homeostasis, and triggers host immune and metabolic responses.

One of the most well-characterized effects of high-salt diets (HSD) is the rapid depletion of *Lactobacillus* species. In both mice and humans, sodium-rich diets dramatically reduce *Lactobacillus* abundance, with *Lactobacillus murinus*—a mouse-specific species—being particularly sensitive. This depletion is reversible; when mice previously exposed to 14 days of high salt were returned to a normal diet, *L. murinus* abundance recovered. Functional studies further highlight the significance of *Lactobacillus* in host health: supplementation with *L. murinus* or *Lactobacillus reuteri* in salt-sensitive mice lowered BP and reduced TH17 cell activity, demonstrating that commensal bacteria can mitigate salt-induced hypertension. In a small human cohort, 14 days of high sodium intake (5,500 mg/day) led to a nearly 90% loss of *Lactobacillus* species accompanied by elevated circulating TH17 cells, suggesting that these bacteria are highly sodium-sensitive and that their loss may contribute to inflammation and BP dysregulation (Smiljanec & Lennon, 2019).

Lactobacillus species play essential roles in host immunity and gut ecosystem stability, including inhibiting pathogen growth, supporting anti-inflammatory pathways, and shaping overall microbial community structure. Populations consuming Western-style diets—typically high in sodium—show lower *Lactobacillus* levels than individuals in agricultural, nonindustrialized settings. This pattern suggests that modern dietary patterns may contribute to microbiota-associated chronic diseases, though more research is needed to clarify causal relationships.

Beyond *Lactobacillus*, high salt intake also affects other major microbial groups. Several genera within the order *Clostridiales* decrease significantly under high-salt conditions, while others increase. For example, *Christensenellaceae*, *Erwinia*, and Corynebacteriaceae increase after eight weeks of high-salt feeding in mice. At the same time, families such as Lachnospiraceae and genera including *Ruminococcaceae* and *Oscillospira* rise with prolonged high-salt exposure. These shifts correspond with worsened colitis in murine models, indicating that sodium may exacerbate inflammatory bowel conditions by promoting pro-inflammatory or mucolytic taxa. In contrast, mice on standard-salt diets maintain higher *Lactobacillus* levels and lower abundances of Lachnospiraceae and *Ruminococcaceae*. High salt intake also consistently correlates with reduced overall microbial diversity—a hallmark of dysbiosis. Importantly, microbial taxa differ in their intrinsic salt tolerance; several salt-tolerance genes (SMG3, SMG5, SMG9, SMG25) increase in expression under high-sodium conditions, reflecting microbial adaptation to osmotic stress (Smiljanec & Lennon, 2019).

Salt also influences microbial metabolism, particularly SCFA production. In HSD, intestinal levels of the SCFA butyrate decline, even though butyrate-producing *Roseburia* increase in abundance—suggesting impaired SCFA synthesis or altered substrate availability. Depletion of lactate-producing *Lactobacillus* may contribute to this reduction because lactate often serves as a substrate for butyrate-producing bacteria via cross-feeding. Conversely, levels of acetate and propionate increase in feces and plasma under high-salt conditions in rodents. These metabolites activate the SCFA receptor Olfr78, which promotes renin secretion and elevates BP. Thus, SCFAs may exert divergent physiological effects under high-salt conditions: acetate and propionate potentially increasing BP, while butyrate may confer protective benefits (Smiljanec & Lennon, 2019).

High salt–induced taxonomic changes extend beyond *Lactobacillus* and Clostridia. Mice fed HSD display increased Lachnospiraceae and *Ruminococcaceae*, and an elevated Firmicutes-to-Bacteroidetes (F/B) ratio, a widely used indicator of gut microbial imbalance. *Ruminococcus* taxa are known mucin degraders and have been implicated in Crohn's disease, suggesting that sodium-driven expansion of mucolytic organisms may compromise the gut barrier and promote inflammation. Alterations in the F/B ratio, whether an increase or a decrease, often reflect dysbiosis and have been linked to multiple metabolic and inflammatory disorders (Wang et al., 2024).

Studies in rats further confirm that high salt intake significantly alters the gut microbiome, often before any physiological symptoms appear. Increased abundances of *Alloprevotella*, *Prevotella* 9, *Allobaculum*, and *Turicibacter* were observed, whereas *Prevotella* NK3B31 and *Helicobacter* declined. After eight weeks of high salt feeding, reductions were noted in *Oscillibacter*, *Pseudoflavonifractor*, *Clostridium* XIVa, *Johnsonella*, and *Rothia*, while *Parasutterella* increased. These findings reinforce that high salt intake produces broad and measurable shifts in microbial community composition independent of early clinical symptoms (Wang et al., 2024).

More mechanistic insights come from Hamad et al. (2022), who evaluated intestinal microbial communities across diets containing varying sodium levels. At the phylum level, the dominant groups were Firmicutes (47.5%), Bacteroidetes (37%), Verrucomicrobiota (13%), Proteobacteria (9.3%), and Actinobacteriota (4.85%). Notably, both Proteobacteria and Verrucomicrobiota increased significantly under 10% NaCl diets. Although many studies report an increased F/B ratio with high salt, Hamad et al. observed the opposite trend: both 4 and 10% salt reduced Firmicutes and enriched Bacteroidetes. These discrepancies highlight the context-dependent nature of sodium's effects—differences in host species, salt concentration, and diet composition may all influence outcomes.

At the family level, profound shifts occurred under high-salt conditions. Beneficial groups such as Bifidobacteriaceae, Peptostreptococcaceae, and Lactobacillaceae were depleted in a dose-dependent fashion from low-salt to HSD. Meanwhile, families associated with inflammation or metabolic dysfunction—Akkermansiaceae, Rikenellaceae, Staphylococcaceae, and Prevotellaceae—were enriched, especially under 10% NaCl conditions. Prevotellaceae enrichment is noteworthy, as this group has been linked to chronic inflammatory diseases including rheumatoid arthritis.

Genus-level patterns reveal similar sodium-sensitive trends. Lactic acid–producing taxa such as *Bifidobacterium*, *Lactobacillus*, *Blautia*, and *Faecalibaculum* declined steadily with increasing salt concentration, confirming that these beneficial microbes are salt-sensitive. In contrast, genera such as *Akkermansia*, *Tuzzerella*, and *Alistipes* were markedly enriched at 10% NaCl, consistent with their known associations with inflammation and metabolic disorders. Together, these findings indicate that high salt intake reshapes the gut microbiome in a dose-dependent manner, characterized by loss of probiotic bacteria and enrichment of potentially pathogenic or inflammation-associated taxa.

8.8 IMPACT OF EMULSIFIERS ON THE GUT MICROBIOME

Food additives are widely incorporated into modern industrial food production to enhance texture, stability, palatability, and shelf-life. Among these, emulsifiers—substances that stabilize mixtures of fat and water—are some of the most pervasive ingredients in UPFs. They are routinely added to products such as baked goods, confectioneries, dairy and non-dairy desserts, sauces, edible oils, syrups, ultra-processed fruits and vegetables, and cereals. Globally, the most commonly used emulsifiers include lecithins (E322), monoglycerides and diglycerides (MDG) of fatty acids (E471), guar gum (E412), xanthan gum (E415), carrageenans (E407), and celluloses (E460–469), with prevalence ranging from approximately 2 to 14% of products in the European food supply. Their ubiquity has raised concerns, as growing evidence suggests that certain emulsifiers can profoundly alter intestinal microbial ecology and host metabolic health (Salame et al., 2024).

Recent experimental studies have demonstrated that emulsifiers have the capacity to directly modulate the structure, function, and spatial organization of the gut microbiota. In vitro, animal, and short-term human intervention studies show that consumption of emulsifiers can lead to dysbiosis, characterized by shifts in microbial community composition, increases in pro-inflammatory taxa, and disruption of the protective mucus barrier. These changes promote chronic low-grade inflammation, a known driver of metabolic disorders. Salame et al. (2024), using a large population-based cohort of French adults, identified significant associations between higher emulsifier intake and increased risk of type 2 diabetes (T2D). Seven individual emulsifiers—including carrageenans (E407), tripotassium phosphate (E340), acetylated tartaric acid esters of mono- and diglycerides (E472e), sodium citrate (E331), guar gum (E412), gum arabic (E414), and xanthan gum (E415)—as well as total carrageenan exposure (E407–407a) were all positively associated with T2D risk. These findings suggest that emulsifier intake may contribute to metabolic disease development at the population level.

Controlled animal studies provide mechanistic insight into these epidemiological observations. In a mouse model, sucrose fatty acid esters and CMC were found to induce hyperglycemia and hyperinsulinemia, while lecithin, sucrose fatty acid esters, and CMC disrupted glucose homeostasis in an in vitro insulin-resistance model. MDG impaired circulating lipid and glucose metabolism. Importantly, all tested emulsifiers altered gut microbial diversity and induced dysbiosis. While lecithin, sucrose fatty acid esters, and CMC did not significantly change mucus–bacterial interactions, MDG promoted bacterial encroachment into the normally sterile inner mucus layer and increased systemic inflammation through elevated circulating LPS. Collectively, these results suggest that several common dietary emulsifiers can adversely influence metabolic health by altering the gut microbiota and stimulating inflammatory pathways (Panyod et al., 2024).

The microbial consequences of emulsifier exposure vary by compound. In control animals, the gut microbiota was enriched in *Olsenella*, a genus associated with leanness. Lecithin exposure, however, was associated with increases in *Faecalibaculum*, *Enterorhabdus*, and *Muribaculum*, while sucrose fatty acid esters correlated with [*Eubacterium*] *xylanophilum* group, *Clostridium sensu stricto* 1, and *Akkermansia*, and CMC exposure correlated with *Alloprevotella*, *Acetatifactor*, Muribaculaceae, Clostridia vadinBB60 group, *Blautia*, and UCG-010. Across treatments, emulsifier consumption significantly altered both α-diversity and β-diversity, confirming broad disruptions to microbial ecology, each emulsifier producing a distinct microbiome signature linked to insulin-resistance biomarkers.

More detailed compositional analyses show that lecithin increased a range of disease-associated bacteria, including *Streptococcus*, [*Eubacterium*] *coprostanoligenes* group, *Enterobacter*, *Lachnoclostridium*, *Desulfovibrio*, and additional genera such as *Bifidobacterium*, *Lactobacillus*, and *Candidatus arthromitus*. Simultaneously, lecithin reduced potentially beneficial microbes such as *Oscillibacter*, *Parasutterella*, *Dubosiella*, *Turicibacter*, and members of Prevotellaceae, Coriobacteriaceae, and Tyzzerella. Sucrose fatty acid esters enriched disease-linked taxa including *C. sensu stricto* 1, Lachnospiraceae UCG-006, and [*E.*] *xylanophilum* group, while depleting beneficial microbes such as Muribaculaceae, *Oscillibacter*, *Faecalibaculum*, *Parasutterella*, and *Olsenella*. CMC exposure elevated disease-associated bacteria such as *Blautia*, *Staphylococcus*, and [*E.*] *coprostanoligenes* group, and reduced many beneficial microbes including *Muribaculum*, *Faecalibaculum*, *Parasutterella*, *Dubosiella*, Tyzzerella, and [*Eubacterium*] *siraeum* group. These collective patterns point toward a consistent trend in which emulsifiers enrich inflammatory or dysbiosis-associated taxa while depleting beneficial commensals.

The impact of MDG was similarly unfavorable. Eleven genera were significantly depleted and five enriched following MDG exposure. Reduced genera included beneficial taxa such as Muribaculaceae, *Parabacteroides*, Lachnospiraceae NK4A136 group, *Akkermansia*, *Collinsella*, and Coriobacteriaceae UCG-002, as well as *Alistipes*, *Alloprevotella*, ASF356, and others. Enriched genera included potentially pathogenic or inflammatory microbes such as *Enterorhabdus*, *Jeotgalicoccus*, and *Atopostipes*, as well as *Lactococcus* and various uncultured taxa. These findings reinforce concerns that MDG consumption may destabilize gut microbial communities and promote dysbiosis (Panyod et al., 2024).

Many of these studies rely on 16S rRNA gene sequencing, which further elucidates how emulsifiers alter microbial communities in controlled in vitro systems. Regardless of emulsifier exposure, the incubation environment itself induced major shifts in community structure: increases in *Escherichia/Shigella* (from ~0.02 to ~16%), increases in *Bacteroides*, and steep reductions in carbohydrate-fermenting genera such as *Faecalibacterium* and *Prevotella*. These shifts likely reflect the nutrient composition of the experimental media—high in protein and low in carbohydrates—favoring protein-fermenting bacteria like *Escherichia/Shigella* and generalists like *Bacteroides*, while disadvantaging fiber-specialists such as *Prevotella* and *Faecalibacterium* (Panyod et al., 2024).

Finally, work by Miclotte et al. (2020) analyzing the effects of five dietary emulsifiers on human fecal microbiota over 48 hours demonstrated substantial emulsifier- and donor-dependent variability. Among the compounds tested, rhamnolipids and sophorolipids caused the most pronounced microbiota disruptions, followed by soy lecithin, while CMC and P80 induced the smallest changes. Rhamnolipids produced the strongest reductions in diversity and drove increases in Enterobacteriaceae, *Fusobacterium*, and *Escherichia/Shigella*, while suppressing Bacteroidetes, *Barnesiella*, and *Bacteroides*. Sophorolipids similarly increased *Escherichia/Shigella*, *Acidaminococcus*, and *Phascolarctobacterium*, while decreasing multiple Bacteroidetes taxa. Soy lecithin induced more moderate shifts, increasing *Acidaminococcus*, Porphyromonadaceae (unclassified), and *Sutterella*, while decreasing *Flavonifractor* and *Pseudoflavonifractor*. These findings highlight the capacity of different emulsifiers to disrupt human gut microbial communities to varying degrees, reinforcing concerns about their widespread use.

8.9 XANTHAN GUM MODULATES THE HOST GUT MICROBIOME

Xanthan gum is a highly viscous, soluble dietary fiber that forms a thick, non-diffusible aqueous matrix in the gastrointestinal tract. By increasing the viscosity of luminal contents, it slows the diffusion of nutrients toward the intestinal mucosa and effectively prolongs gastrointestinal transit time. This increased mucosal thickness can delay nutrient absorption and modify postprandial metabolic responses. Early physiological studies demonstrated that xanthan gum reduces the rate of nutrient uptake by increasing luminal viscosity (Fuse et al., 1989), and more recent research suggests that its consumption is associated with improved glucose homeostasis and decreased hyperlipidemia (Nagasawa et al., 2022).

In vivo administration of xanthan gum has been shown to shift microbial community structure across multiple taxonomic levels. Nagasawa et al. (2022) reported that animals fed xanthan gum exhibited increased abundances of several bacterial orders and families, including Christensenellales, Erysipelotrichales, *Christensenellaceae*, Erysipelotrichaceae, and the (E.) *coprostanoligenes* group. At the genus level, taxa such as UBA1819, *Christensenellaceae* R-7 group, and the coprostanoligenes group were enriched relative to controls. In contrast, the species *Alistipes indistinctus* was significantly reduced in the xanthan gum group, while Bacterium YE57 showed a trend toward increased abundance.

These community shifts were functionally relevant: the relative abundance of Erysipelotrichales and *Christensenellaceae* positively correlated with GLP-1 and GLP-1r expression in the ileum, suggesting that xanthan gum–induced microbiome remodeling may influence incretin signaling. This mechanistic link supports the observation that xanthan gum–based thickeners can improve glucose and lipid metabolism.

Further evidence of xanthan gum's microbiome-mediated metabolic effects comes from the work of Xu et al. (2022). In both type 2 diabetic (T2D) mice and in vitro fecal fermentation systems, xanthan gum significantly altered colonic microbial composition by reducing the Firmicutes/Bacteroidetes ratio—typically elevated in metabolic disease—and increasing the abundance of Bacteroidales and *Prevotella* species. These changes were accompanied by an 83% increase in butyric acid production during fermentation, indicating that xanthan gum serves as a fermentable substrate that boosts SCFA generation.

Importantly, degradation of xanthan gum stimulated hepatic expression of the SCFA receptors GPR41 and GPR43, which play key roles in energy regulation, insulin sensitivity, and inflammatory modulation. Together, these changes suggest that xanthan gum can ameliorate glucose metabolism in T2D mice not only by modifying microbial ecology but also by activating SCFA-dependent metabolic pathways.

Although xanthan gum is generally considered safe and beneficial at physiological doses, some evidence suggests that excessive intake or host susceptibility may lead to adverse outcomes. Certain microbial taxa that proliferate in response to xanthan gum—such as *Ruminococcus gnavus* and members of the Enterobacteriaceae family—are known opportunistic bacteria associated with mucosal inflammation.

A study in Wistar rats (Spiller et al., 2025) reported that high-dose xanthan gum induced increases in pro-inflammatory cytokines IL-1β and TNF-α, along with unfavorable modulation of epithelial tight-junction proteins, including increased expression of Claudin-2, which is typically associated with intestinal permeability. These findings raise the possibility that, under high-exposure conditions or in individuals with underlying dysbiosis, xanthan gum may compromise epithelial barrier integrity and promote an inflammatory milieu.

8.10 DIETARY OILS MODULATES THE GUT MICROBIOME

Dietary oils exert profound effects on human health, and thermal processing—such as deep-frying or high-temperature cooking—can substantially alter their chemical composition and biological activity. Palm oil is one of the most widely used oils in the food-processing industry; however, its health impacts remain controversial. Ruan et al. (2021) compared the effects of thermally oxidized palm oil and canola oil on the gut microbiota. To generate high-fat diets (HFDs), palm oil or canola oil was heated at 180°C for 10 hours. Rats were then fed these diets for three months, after which hematological parameters, gut microbial composition, and intestinal gene-expression profiles were assessed. Heated canola oil consumption increased plasma total cholesterol and LDL-cholesterol levels relative to unheated canola oil, whereas heated palm oil did not elicit these changes. Notably, intake of heated palm oil significantly elevated the relative abundance of *Lactobacillus* and *Roseburia* compared with non-heated palm oil or either canola-oil group. In addition, expression of IL-22 in the intestine was increased in rats consuming heated palm oil, while expression of ZO-1 and GPR41 was reduced. Collectively, these findings suggest that thermal processing may enhance palm oil's ability to promote beneficial *Lactobacillus* proliferation, while diminishing the cholesterol-modulating effects typically associated with canola oil (Ruan et al., 2021).

Over the past several decades, global consumption of SO has risen sharply. Diet is a major determinant of gut microbiome composition, particularly in the context of high-fat intake. Accumulating evidence links diet-induced dysbiosis to numerous disease states, including CVD and atherosclerosis, in both humans and animal models. To evaluate the consequences of high SO intake, C57BL/6 mice were supplemented orally with a SO emulsion (SOE) for one month, followed by the assessment of atherosclerosis-related biomarkers and gut microbiota profiling via 16S rRNA sequencing of fecal DNA. SOE supplementation resulted in significant compositional shifts in 64 microbial taxa, including increases in Bacteroidetes, *Mucispirillum*, *Prevotella*, and *Ruminococcus*, along with decreased Firmicutes—patterns previously linked with atherosclerosis risk. Of these altered taxa, 40 showed significant correlations with at least one atherosclerosis-associated biomarker (FDR < 0.05), and 13 correlated positively with the average of all biomarkers. Microbial functional-pathway analysis revealed enrichment in amino-acid metabolic pathways implicated in CVD. These results demonstrate that SOE supplementation induces dysbiosis associated with atherosclerotic processes, suggesting that microbiome alterations may serve as mediators or biomarkers of cardiovascular risk (Korach-Rechtman et al., 2020).

Neuroinflammation is a central pathological mechanism driving neurodegenerative diseases, and growing evidence indicates that dietary fat intake and gut health are closely intertwined with brain inflammatory responses. To explore this relationship, 8-week-old C57BL/6J mice were subjected to a 20-week intervention involving diets containing either lard or SO at two fat-energy levels (15 and 35%). At 35% fat energy, both oils induced neuroinflammation, but the effect was substantially more severe in mice fed SO. In these animals, neuronal structural integrity was compromised, inflammatory cytokines were upregulated, antioxidant defenses in the brain were reduced, and the TLR4/MyD88/NF-κB p65 inflammatory pathway was strongly activated. This cascade disrupted the brain–gut barrier, leading to reductions in *Akkermansia* and unclassified Lachnospiraceae, as well as an expansion of *Dubosiella*, ultimately resulting in aggravated neuroinflammatory damage. These findings indicate that SO elicits more severe neuroinflammation than lard under high-fat dietary conditions (Liu et al., 2024).

HFDs are well known to modulate gut microbiota and contribute to obesity, systemic inflammation, and hepatic steatosis. Although fish oil and SO are often incorporated into healthy dietary patterns, the effects of these fats in the absence of sucrose on gut dysbiosis and its association with liver steatosis are less clear. To address this gap, C57BL/6 mice were fed sucrose-free SO-based (SF-Soy-HFD) or fish-oil-based (SF-Fish-HFD) HFDs for 24 weeks. Despite similar effects on body and liver weights, 16S rRNA sequencing revealed distinct patterns of dysbiosis between the two diet groups. The SF-Soy-HFD increased the abundance of Bacteroidetes, Firmicutes, and Deferribacteres, while reducing Verrucomicrobia. Compared with SF-Fish-HFD controls, the SF-Soy-HFD group exhibited a higher Clostridia/Bacteroidia ratio and a markedly lower Verrucomicrobiaceae/S24_7 ratio. The SF-Soy-HFD also enriched taxa such as S24_7, *Clostridiales*, *Allobaculum*, Coriobacteriaceae, *Adlercreutzia*, *Christensenellaceae*, *Lactococcus*, and *Oscillospira*, while reducing *Akkermansia*, a key species involved in maintaining gut barrier function. Microbiome functional predictions linked these community shifts to host pathways involved in fatty-liver progression and inflammation. Mice consuming the SF-Soy-HFD developed liver steatosis and showed elevated expression of genes involved in de novo lipogenesis and cholesterol synthesis. Fat export via Mttp was reduced, and hepatic inflammatory markers (TNFa and IL1b) were significantly upregulated. Overall, SF-Soy-HFD feeding induced gut dysbiosis that was associated with steatosis, hepatic inflammation, and impaired glucose regulation (Jacob et al., 2024).

8.11 CONCLUSION

UPFs, with their high levels of refined sugars, bleached flour, unhealthy fats, additives, and low nutrient density, disrupt the delicate symbiosis that normally exists between humans and their gut microbiota. These foods induce obesity, promote microbial imbalances, weaken intestinal integrity, and impair metabolic and immune functions that depend on a diverse and stable microbial community. In contrast, diets rich in whole, minimally processed foods nourish beneficial microbes and help sustain mutualistic relationships essential for health. Thus, reducing UPF intake is central to preserving the intricate host–microbe symbiosis that underpins long-term well-being.

ACKNOWLEDGMENTS

The author (ST) acknowledges Sharpe-Strumia Research Foundation, W.W. Smith Charitable Trust and Abraham Thomas Foundation for providing the resources for this work.

REFERENCES

Alomari WD, Almoraie NM. Ultra-processed food intake and its association with obesity risk factors, Mediterranean diet, and nutrient intake of adults. *Front Nutr*. 2025; 12:1577431.

Atzeni A, Martínez MÁ, Babio N, Konstanti P, Tinahones FJ, Vioque J, ..., & Salas-Salvadó J. Association between ultra-processed food consumption and gut microbiota in senior subjects with overweight/obesity and metabolic syndrome. *Front. Nutr.* 2022;9:976547.

Beisner J, Gonzalez-Granda A, Basrai M, Damms-Machado A, Bischoff SC. Fructose-induced intestinal microbiota shift following two types of short-term high-fructose dietary phases. *Nutrients*. 2020 Nov 10;12(11):3444. doi: 10.3390/nu12113444.

Bian X, Chi L, Gao B, Tu P, Ru H, Lu K. The artificial sweetener acesulfame potassium affects the gut microbiome and body weight gain in CD-1 mice. *PLoS One*. 2017; 12(6):e0178426.

Chassaing B, Koren O, Goodrich JK, Poole AC, Srinivasan S, Ley RE, Gewirtz AT. Dietary emulsifiers impact the mouse gut microbiota promoting colitis and metabolic syndrome. *Nature*. 2015 Mar 5;519(7541):92–96. doi: 10.1038/nature14232.

Chen Q, Luo Y, Shen Y, Li X, Yang H, Li J, Wang J, Xiao Y. Fructose corn syrup induces inflammatory injury and obesity by altering gut microbiota and gut microbiota-related arachidonic acid metabolism. *J Nutr Biochem*. 2024; 124:109527.

Cheng WL, Li SJ, Lee TI, Lee TW, Chung CC, Kao YH, Chen YJ. Sugar fructose triggers gut dysbiosis and metabolic inflammation with cardiac arrhythmogenesis. *Biomedicines*. 2021 Jun 25; 9(7):728.

Chittrakorn S, Earls D, MacRitchie F. Ozonation as an alternative to chlorination for soft wheat flours. *J Cereal Sci*. 2014; 60: 217–221.

Choudhary AK, Pretorius E. Revisiting the safety of aspartame. *Nutr Rev*. 2017 Sep 1; 75(9):718–730.

Conz A, Salmona M, Diomede L. Effect of Non-nutritive sweeteners on the gut microbiota. *Nutrients*. 2023;15(8):1869.

Fuse K, Bamba T, Hosoda S. Effects of pectin on fatty acid and glucose absorption and on thickness of unstirred water layer in rat and human intestine. *Dig Dis Sci.* 1989; 34(7):1109–1116.

Giaccone V, Cammilleri G, Di Stefano V, Pitonzo R, Vella A, Pulvirenti A, Lo Dico GM, Ferrantelli V, Macaluso A. First report on the presence of Alloxan in bleached flour by LC-MS/MS method. *J Cereal Sci.* 2017; 77: 120–125.

Goncalves MD, Lu C, Tutnauer J, Hartman TE, Hwang SK, Murphy CJ, Pauli C, Morris R, Taylor S, Bosch K, Yang S, Wang Y, Van Riper J, Lekaye HC, Roper J, Kim Y, Chen Q, Gross SS, Rhee KY, Cantley LC, Yun J. High-fructose corn syrup enhances intestinal tumor growth in mice. *Science.* 2019; 363(6433):1345–1349.

Hamad I, Cardilli A, Côrte-Real BF, Dyczko A, Vangronsveld J, Kleinewietfeld M. High-salt diet induces depletion of lactic acid-producing bacteria in murine gut. *Nutrients.* 2022; 14(6):1171.

Hosseini A, Barlow GM, Leite G, Rashid M, Parodi G, Wang J, Morales W, Weitsman S, Rezaie A, Pimentel M, Mathur R. Consuming artificial sweeteners may alter the structure and function of duodenal microbial communities. *iScience.* 2023; 26(12):108530.

Hou L, Li S, Ou Y, Zhu L. Flour bleaching: over a century of health risks and controversies. *Food, Nutrition and Health* 2025; 2:17.

Huebbe P, Rimbach G. Historical reflection of food processing and the role of legumes as part of a healthy balanced diet. *Foods.* 2020; 9(8):1056.

Jacob T, Sindhu S, Hasan A, Malik MZ, Arefanian H, Al-Rashed F, Nizam R, Kochumon S, Thomas R, Bahman F, Shenouda S, Wilson A, Akther N, Al-Roub A, Abukhalaf N, Albeloushi S, Abu-Farha M, Al Madhoun A, Alzaid F, Thanaraj TA, Koistinen HA, Tuomilehto J, Al-Mulla F, Ahmad R. Soybean oil-based HFD induces gut dysbiosis that leads to steatosis, hepatic inflammation and insulin resistance in mice. *Front Microbiol.* 2024; 15:1407258.

Juul F, Vaidean G, Lin Y, Deierlein AL, Parekh N. Ultra-processed foods and incident cardiovascular disease in the framingham offspring study. *Journal of the American College of Cardiology.* 2021 Mar 30;77(12):1520–1531.

Korach-Rechtman H, Rom O, Mazouz L, Freilich S, Jeries H, Hayek T, Aviram M, Kashi Y. Soybean oil modulates the gut microbiota associated with atherogenic biomarkers. *Microorganisms.* 2020; 8(4):486.

Lane MM, Gamage E, Du S, Ashtree DN, McGuinness AJ, Gauci S, ..., & Segasby T, Marx W. Ultra-processed food exposure and adverse health outcomes: Umbrella review of epidemiological meta-analyses. *BMJ.* 2024 Feb 28;384:e077310. doi: 10.1136/bmj-2023-077310.

Latif NAM, Ropi AAM, Mohamad AMD, Shaharuddin S. Fat reduction and characteristic enhancement of edible composite coating (Pectin-Maltodextrin) on fried potato chips. *Materials Today: Proceedings* 2020; 31: A79–A84.

Li J, Lang W, Han S, Wu X, Hao F, Zhou Y, Du R, ..., & Song C. Insights into the mechanisms and functional effects of insoluble dietary fiber modification: a review. *Foods.* 2025 Dec 23;15(1):38. doi: 10.3390/foods15010038.

Liu X, Tao R, Guo F, Zhang L, Qu J, Li M, Wu X, Wang X, Zhu Y, Wen L, Wang J. Soybean oil induces neuroinflammatory response through brain-gut axis under high-fat diet. *J Tradit Complement Med.* 2024; 14(5):522–533.

Martínez Steele E, Baraldi LG, Louzada ML, Moubarac JC, Mozaffarian D, Monteiro CA. Ultra-processed foods and added sugars in the US diet: evidence from a nationally representative cross-sectional study. *BMJ Open.* 2016; 6(3):e009892.

Mellado-Ortega E, Hornero-Méndez D. Lutein esterification in wheat flour increases the carotenoid retention and is induced by storage temperatures. *Foods.* 2017;6 (12):111.

Méndez-García LA, Bueno-Hernández N, Cid-Soto MA, De León KL, Mendoza-Martínez VM, Espinosa-Flores AJ, Carrero-Aguirre M, Esquivel-Velázquez M, León-Hernández M, Viurcos-Sanabria R, Ruíz-Barranco A, Cota-Arce JM, Álvarez-Lee A, De León-Nava MA, Meléndez G, Escobedo G. Ten-week sucralose consumption induces gut dysbiosis and altered glucose and insulin levels in healthy young adults. *Microorganisms.* 2022;10(2):434.

Miclotte L, De Paepe K, Rymenans L, Callewaert C, Raes J, Rajkovic A, Van Camp J, Van de Wiele T. Dietary emulsifiers alter composition and activity of the human gut microbiota in vitro, irrespective of chemical or natural emulsifier origin. *Front. Microbiol.* 2020; 11:577474.

Monteiro CA, Cannon G, Moubarac JC, Levy RB, Louzada MLC, Jaime PC. The UN decade of nutrition, the NOVA food classification and the trouble with ultra-processing. *Public Health Nutr.* 2018; 21(1):5–17.

Morder KM, Nguyen M, Wilfahrt DN, Dahmani ZL, Burr ABP, Xie B, Morikone M, Nieves-Rosado H, Gunn WG, Hurd DE, Wang H, Mullett SJ, Bossong K, Gelhaus SL, Rajasundaram D, Kane LP, Delgoffe GM, Das J, Davar D, Overacre-Delgoffe AE. Sucralose consumption ablates cancer immunotherapy response through microbiome disruption. *Cancer Discov.* 2025; 15(11):2278–2297.

Morris MJ, Na ES, Johnson AK. Salt craving: the psychobiology of pathogenic sodium intake. *Physiol Behav.* 2008; 94(5):709–721.

Nagasawa Y, Katagiri S, Nakagawa K, Hirota T, Yoshimi K, et al. Xanthan gum-based fluid thickener decreases postprandial blood glucose associated with increase of Glp1 and Glp1r expression in ileum and alteration of gut microbiome. J Funct Foods. 2022; 99:105321.

Nouri M, Eskandarzadeh S, Makhtoomi M, et al. Association between ultra-processed foods intake with lipid profile: a cross-sectional study. Sci Rep. 2023; 13: 7258.

Oladele CR, Khandpur N, Johnson S, Yuan Y, Wambugu V, Plante TB, Lovasi GS, Judd S. Ultra-processed food consumption and hypertension risk in the REGARDS Cohort Study. Hypertension. 2024; 81(12):2520–2528.

Ostrowski MP, La Rosa SL, Kunath BJ, Robertson A, Pereira G, Hagen LH, ..., & Martens EC. Mechanistic insights into consumption of the food additive xanthan gum by the human gut microbiota. Nat Microbiol. 2022 Apr;7(4):556–569. doi: 10.1038/s41564-022-01093-0.

Panyod, S., Wu, WK., Chang, CT. et al. Common dietary emulsifiers promote metabolic disorders and intestinal microbiota dysbiosis in mice. Commun Biol. 2024; 7: 749.

Poti JM, Braga B, Qin B. Ultra-processed food intake and obesity: what really matters for health-processing or nutrient content? Curr Obes Rep. 2017; 6(4):420–431.

Rondinella D, Raoul PC, Valeriani E, Venturini I, Cintoni M, Severino A, Galli FS, Mora V, Mele MC, Cammarota G, Gasbarrini A, Rinninella E, Ianiro G. The detrimental impact of ultra-processed foods on the human gut microbiome and gut barrier. Nutrients. 2025; 17(5):859.

Ruan M, Bu Y, Wu F, Zhang S, Chen R, Li N, Liu Z, Wang H. Chronic consumption of thermally processed palm oil or canola oil modified gut microflora of rats. Food Sci Human Wellness. 2021; 10: 94–102.

Rysová J, Šmídová Z. Effect of salt content reduction on food processing technology. Foods. 2021; 10(9):2237.

Salame C, Javaux G, Sellem L, Viennois E, de Edelenyi FS, Agaësse C, De Sa A, Huybrechts I, Pierre F, Coumoul X, Julia C, Kesse-Guyot E, Allès B, Fezeu LK, Hercberg S, Deschasaux-Tanguy M, Cosson E, Tatulashvili S, Chassaing B, Srour B, Touvier M. Food additive emulsifiers and the risk of type 2 diabetes: analysis of data from the NutriNet-Santé prospective cohort study. Lancet Diabetes Endocrinol. 2024 May; 12(5):339–349.

Scaranni PODS, Cardoso LO, Chor D, Melo ECP, Matos SMA, Giatti L, Barreto SM, da Fonseca MJM. Ultra-processed foods, changes in blood pressure and incidence of hypertension: the Brazilian Longitudinal Study of Adult Health (ELSA-Brasil). Public Health Nutr. 2021 Aug; 24(11):3352–3360.

Shaw CA, Bains JS. Did consumption of flour bleached by the agene process contribute to the incidence of neurological disease? Med Hypotheses. 1998 Dec; 51(6):477–81.

Shim SY, Kim HC, Shim JS. Consumption of ultra-processed food and blood pressure in Korean adults. Korean Circ J. 2022; 52(1):60–70.

Smiljanec K, Lennon SL. Sodium, hypertension, and the gut: does the gut microbiota go salty? Am J Physiol Heart Circ Physiol. 2019; 317(6):H1173–H1182.

Sokol H, Pigneur B, Watterlot L, Lakhdari O, Bermúdez-Humarán LG, Gratadoux JJ, ..., & Langella P. Faecalibacterium prausnitzii is an anti-inflammatory commensal bacterium identified by gut microbiota analysis of Crohn disease patients. Proc Natl Acad Sci U S A. 2008 Oct 28;105(43):16731–16736. doi: 10.1073/pnas.0804812105.

Spiller AL, Costa BGd, Yoshihara RNY, Nogueira EJZ, Castelhano NS, Santos A, Brusco De Freitas M, Magro DO, Yukie Sassaki L. Ultra-processed foods, gut microbiota, and inflammatory bowel disease: a critical review of emerging evidence. Nutrients. 2025; 17(16):2677.

Suez, J., Korem, T., Zeevi, D. et al. Artificial sweeteners induce glucose intolerance by altering the gut microbiota. Nature 2014; 514: 181–186.

Suez J, Korem T, Zilberman-Schapira G, Segal E, Elinav E. Non-caloric artificial sweeteners and the microbiome: findings and challenges. Gut Microbes. 2015; 6(2):149–55.

Sylvetsky AC, Clement RA, Stearrett N, Issa NT, Dore FJ, Mazumder R, King CH, Hubal MJ, Walter PJ, Cai H, Sen S, Rother KI, Crandall KA. Consumption of sucralose- and acesulfame-potassium-containing diet soda alters the relative abundance of microbial taxa at the species level: findings of two pilot studies. Appl Physiol Nutr Metab. 2024; 49(1):125–134.

Thomas S, Izard J, Walsh E, Batich K, Chongsathidkiet P, Clarke G, Sela DA, Muller AJ, Mullin JM, Albert K, Gilligan JP, DiGuilio K, Dilbarova R, Alexander W, Prendergast GC. The host microbiome regulates and maintains human health: a primer and perspective for non-microbiologists. Cancer Res. 2017; 77(8):1783–1812.

Wang X, Lang F, Liu D. High-salt diet and intestinal microbiota: influence on cardiovascular disease and inflammatory bowel disease. Biology. 2024; 13(9):674.

Xu J, Sun W, Li H, Z Gao Z, et al. Xanthan gum oligosaccharides ameliorate glucose metabolism and related gut microbiota dysbiosis in type 2 diabetic mice. Food Bioscience 2022; 50:102002.

Zheng Z, Xiao Y, Ma L, Lyu W, Peng H, Wang X, Ren Y, Li J. Low dose of sucralose alter gut microbiome in mice. Front Nutr. 2022; 9:848392.

CHAPTER 9

Peinosis

THE SHORTENING OF THE COLON WHEN ON A HIGH-FAT–HIGH-PROTEIN DIET

Sunil Thomas

9.1 INTRODUCTION

The global prevalence of obesity is higher than at any other point in human history. Rising disposable income, the low cost of calorie-dense foods, and the unprecedented variety and availability of processed and convenience foods have collectively contributed to widespread weight gain across populations. This nutritional environment—characterized by excess energy intake and often poor nutrient quality—has been a major driver of obesity and its associated lifestyle-related diseases (Thomas et al. 2023).

Beyond its well-recognized links to cardiovascular disease, type 2 diabetes, and metabolic syndrome, obesity is increasingly implicated in chronic inflammatory disorders, including inflammatory bowel disease (IBD). Diets rich in fats, processed sugars, and animal proteins can reshape the gut microbiome, disrupt intestinal barrier integrity, and alter systemic immune responses, thereby creating conditions that may worsen or precipitate IBD (Thomas et al. 2017).

Ulcerative colitis (UC) is a chronic, idiopathic inflammatory disease of the large intestine whose onset and severity have been associated with high-fat–high-protein (HFHP) diets, gut microbial dysbiosis, and metabolomic alterations driven by nutrition and/or circadian disruption related to poor sleep patterns. Identifying diet-responsive factors that impair colonic health may yield new strategies for UC prevention and for improving the effectiveness of emerging UC immunotherapies (Thomas et al. 2023).

In this preclinical investigation, we observed that mice maintained on either a standard diet or a high-fiber diet exhibited improved colonic health metrics relative to mice fed a HFHP diet. Consistent with clinical observations, the HFHP diet induced obesity and significantly shortened colon length. This phenotype also corresponded to a notable reduction in residual nutrient energy in fecal pellets, suggesting the emergence of a distinct diet-associated physiological state. We proposed the term *peinosis* to describe this condition—derived from the Greek *peina* (hunger) and *-osis* (condition)—representing a paradoxical "hunger-like" state in which nutrient availability to the host becomes impaired despite caloric excess (Thomas et al. 2023).

Strikingly, animals on the HFHP diet also displayed measurable muscle weakness, a deficit that could not be fully explained by increased body weight alone, indicating potential diet-induced metabolic or neuromuscular dysfunction. In contrast, mice receiving a high-fiber diet demonstrated the most favorable outcomes, including the longest colon lengths and the absence of muscle weakness, highlighting the

DOI: 10.1201/9781003638292-9

protective role of dietary fiber against diet-driven colonic and systemic impairments.

These findings underscore the importance of diet composition in shaping colonic physiology, whole-body metabolism, and potentially UC susceptibility, offering a foundation for future mechanistic and therapeutic studies.

9.2 DIET INFLUENCES COLON LENGTH

In a short-term experimental study, in animal models, Thomas et al. (2023) monitored the body weight of mice over a 30-day period while feeding them different dietary regimens. The animals that received an HFHP diet showed a clear increase in body weight when compared with mice maintained on a standard diet or a fiber diet. Along with tracking weight, they also examined changes in gut structure by measuring the length of the colon at the end of the study.

The results revealed striking differences between diet groups. Mice fed with food containing antibiotics developed the longest colon among all groups, suggesting that reduced microbial activity may influence intestinal growth. In contrast, mice consuming the HFHP diet exhibited a pronounced shortening of the colon compared with those on the standard diet. When colon length was normalized to body weight, the same pattern persisted: despite gaining more weight, the HFHP group consistently showed significantly shorter colons.

From these findings, they concluded that an HFHP diet is associated with measurable reductions in colon length, pointing to a distinctive shift in gut physiology under this dietary condition. These structural changes may have broader implications for digestion, microbiome composition, and overall gastrointestinal (GI) health, highlighting the importance of diet composition in shaping both metabolic and anatomical outcomes.

Protein expression analysis revealed that mice fed a fiber-rich diet exhibited robust expression of Claudin-5 in the colon, a critical tight junction protein essential for maintaining intestinal barrier integrity. In contrast, Claudin-5 levels were markedly reduced in mice consuming an HFHP diet, indicating compromised gut barrier function. Similarly, BMI-1, a transcription factor and master regulator of GI stem cells that plays a central role in maintaining colon structure and regenerative capacity, was highly expressed in the colons of fiber-fed mice. Mice on the HFHP diet, however, showed minimal BMI-1 expression, suggesting impaired stem cell function and structural integrity of the colon (Thomas et al. 2023).

Collectively, these findings demonstrate that dietary composition directly influences key molecular regulators of gut health. A fiber-rich diet promotes the expression of proteins essential for maintaining tight junction integrity and supporting stem cell-mediated tissue homeostasis, whereas an HFHP diet suppresses these critical pathways. This suggests that long-term consumption of HFHP diets may compromise colon structure and barrier function, potentially predisposing the gut to inflammation, dysfunction, and reduced regenerative capacity. In contrast, fiber-rich diets appear protective, supporting both intestinal integrity and the physiological resilience of the colon.

9.3 DIET INFLUENCES THE STATUS OF ENTERIC NEURONS

The enteric nervous system (ENS) is a complex and highly autonomous network of neurons that lines the GI tract. Often referred to as the "second brain," the ENS governs essential digestive activities—including motility, secretion, and nutrient processing—largely independent of the central nervous system (CNS). Because disruptions in ENS function are associated with a range of digestive disorders, understanding how external factors such as diet shape its structure and activity is essential. While diet is well known to affect gut microbiota and intestinal physiology, whether diet directly influences enteric neurons has not been widely explored.

To address this gap, Thomas et al. (2023) evaluated the number and distribution of ENS-associated cells in mice fed different dietary regimens. Using Neuronal Nuclear antigen (NeuN) and glial fibrillary acidic protein (GFAP) immunostaining as indicators of neuronal and glial health, the researchers analyzed gut tissue across all diet groups. NeuN, a widely used marker of mature neurons, displayed strong expression in the muscularis mucosa in most conditions. However, mice fed an HFHP diet showed a striking reduction in NeuN staining, pointing to either a loss of neurons or a shift in neuronal phenotype. Quantitative measurements confirmed this decline, revealing significantly lower NeuN levels in this group compared with mice on standard or antibiotic-supplemented diets.

Conversely, GFAP expression—representing glial activation—was elevated in the mucosal layer of mice consuming the HFHP diet. This increase suggests a potential compensatory glial response or altered neuronal–glial communication under this dietary stress. Taken together, these findings indicate that diet composition can meaningfully influence the physiological state of enteric neurons. In particular, an HFHP diet appears to drive neuronal alterations accompanied by increased glial activation, ultimately reshaping the functional environment of the ENS and potentially contributing to diet-associated GI changes.

9.4 IMPACT OF A HIGH-FAT–HIGH-PROTEIN DIET ON FECAL OUTPUT AND NUTRIENT CONTENT

Mice consuming an HFHP diet produced noticeably fewer fecal pellets compared to mice on other dietary regimens, particularly during months 1 and 7 of the study. Not only was the number of pellets reduced, but the weight of each pellet was also significantly lower than that of mice fed standard, high-fiber, or high-carbohydrate diets. Even when normalized to body size, the fecal pellets of HFHP-fed mice remained smaller, indicating that this diet substantially affects intestinal transit and fecal bulk independently of overall body weight. These findings suggest that an HFHP diet may lead to decreased fecal output, potentially reflecting altered digestion, absorption, or gut motility.

To further understand the functional consequences of these changes, we analyzed the macronutrient content—protein, carbohydrate, and lipid—remaining in the fecal pellets. Remarkably, fecal pellets from HFHP-fed mice contained the lowest levels of these nutrients, suggesting that the majority of ingested macronutrients were absorbed or metabolized before excretion. In contrast, fecal pellets from mice on a high-fiber diet retained the highest nutrient content, indicating that fiber-rich diets promote greater bulk and nutrient retention within the feces.

These observations highlight how diet composition influences not only the quantity but also the quality of fecal matter, reflecting underlying differences in digestion, nutrient absorption, and intestinal physiology. The reduced fecal bulk and nutrient content in HFHP-fed mice may contribute to altered colonic length due to the "hunger-like condition" (peinosis) characterized by low-energy fecal output. Conversely, fiber-rich diets appear to support healthy gut function, providing both structural benefits to the colon and improved regulation of nutrient passage through the GI tract.

Overall, the findings demonstrate that an HFHP diet markedly diminishes fecal output and reduces nutrient content, whereas fiber-rich diets maintain higher fecal mass and nutrient retention. These results demonstrate the critical role of dietary composition in modulating gut physiology, digestion, and nutrient utilization, with potential implications for metabolic health and GI function (Thomas et al. 2023).

9.4.1 Microbiome Changes in Response to a High-Fat–High-Protein Diet

Diet is a major determinant of gut microbiome composition, influencing not only microbial diversity but also the relative abundance of specific bacterial classes and genera. In our study, we examined the effects of various diets—including HFHP, fiber-rich, carbohydrate-rich, standard, and antibiotic-supplemented diets—on the gut microbiota of mice. The results revealed striking shifts in both bacterial classes and genera depending on the dietary regimen (Thomas et al. 2023).

At the class level, distinct patterns emerged across diets. Verrucomicrobiae were most abundant in mice receiving antibiotics, suggesting a potential resilience or opportunistic growth in the absence of competitive microbial communities. Actinobacteria, in contrast, were significantly reduced in both antibiotic-treated and HFHP-fed mice but reached their highest abundance in the fiber diet, highlighting the sensitivity of this class to dietary composition. Bacteroidia showed a similar trend, increasing with antibiotic treatment but reaching minimal levels under the HFHP diet, whereas Bacilli were most abundant in the HFHP group and completely absent in antibiotic-treated mice. Clostridia thrived in the antibiotic-treated mice but were lowest in the carbohydrate-rich diet, while Cyanobacteria were entirely absent in both HFHP and antibiotic-treated groups. Gammaproteobacteria remained at low levels in HFHP and antibiotic-fed mice, indicating a suppressed growth under these conditions.

At the genus level, additional diet-dependent shifts were observed. *Dubosiella* reached its highest abundance in the standard diet but was minimally present in the fiber diet and completely absent in both carbohydrate and HFHP diets. Muribaculaceae levels were lowest in HFHP-fed mice, suggesting that a HFHP environment may suppress this genus. Conversely, HFHP feeding was associated with increased levels of *Faecalibaculum* and *Lactococcus*, highlighting selective enrichment of certain taxa under protein- and fat-rich conditions. *Bifidobacterium*, a genus often linked to gut health, was highest in the fiber diet and minimal in HFHP-fed mice. *Ileibacterium* was abundant in carbohydrate- and fiber-rich diets but nearly absent in HFHP-fed animals.

Overall, these findings demonstrate that an HFHP diet markedly reshapes the gut microbiome, favoring certain bacteria such as Bacilli, *Faecalibaculum*, and *Lactococcus* while suppressing beneficial taxa like *Bifidobacterium*, Muribaculaceae, and *Ileibacterium*. Such microbial shifts may contribute to the physiological and metabolic changes observed in HFHP-fed mice, including altered gut structure, inflammation, and digestive function. These results highlight the profound impact of diet composition on microbial ecology and underscore the importance of nutritional strategies in maintaining a healthy gut microbiome (Thomas et al. 2023).

9.5 LONG-TERM EFFECTS OF DIET ON GUT AND MUSCLE/NERVE PHYSIOLOGY

The long-term impact of different diets on gut and neuromuscular physiology remains poorly understood. To address this, we conducted a seven-month study monitoring mice fed various diets, including HFHP, high-fiber, high-carbohydrate, standard, and antibiotic-supplemented diets. Body weight trajectories revealed significant differences among the groups. Mice on the HFHP diet gained the most weight, showing significant increases compared with the standard diet during months 1, 2, and 6. By month 6, HFHP-fed mice were nearly twice as heavy as those on the high-fiber diet. In contrast, mice on high-fiber or high-carbohydrate diets showed minimal weight gain, indicating the protective effect of these diets against excessive weight accumulation.

Gut physiology was also profoundly affected by diet. Mice on the HFHP diet produced fewer and lighter fecal pellets throughout the study, particularly during months 1 and 7. Even when normalized to body size, the fecal pellets of HFHP-fed mice were significantly smaller than those of mice on other diets. These observations suggest that an HFHP diet reduces intestinal bulk and alters colonic function. To further explore the implications, we assessed colon length and found that HFHP-fed mice had shorter colons compared to other diet groups, pointing to diet-induced structural changes in the gut.

Neuromuscular function was assessed using rotarod balance and wire-mesh hanging tests. Mice consuming an HFHP diet performed poorly in both tests, with significant deficits observed by days 50 and 100, indicating impaired coordination and muscle strength. Antibiotic-fed mice similarly exhibited poor wire-hanging performance, while high fiber–fed mice tended to perform better than other groups. These data suggest that HFHP feeding may compromise neuromuscular health, possibly due to age-associated nerve or muscle deficiencies that are not explained solely by increased body weight.

To examine the potential reversibility of HFHP-induced effects, a subset of mice was switched from an HFHP diet to a fiber diet after 60 days. Following the transition, mouse weight decreased significantly within 10 days and stabilized for the remainder of the 40-day observation period. Fecal pellet weight increased steadily, approaching levels seen in fiber-fed mice. Colon length also improved, suggesting structural recovery. At the molecular level, HFHP feeding reduced expression of tight junction proteins Claudin-5, critical for intestinal barrier integrity. Transitioning to a fiber diet restored these proteins to levels comparable to standard and fiber diets, as confirmed by densitometric analysis, indicating the recovery of intestinal barrier function and protective signaling.

Overall, our study demonstrates that an HFHP diet has deleterious effects on body weight, gut physiology, fecal output, colon structure, and neuromuscular function. In contrast, fiber-rich diets support healthier gut and neuromuscular outcomes, underscoring the importance of diet composition in maintaining overall physiological health and optimizing responses to therapies such as UC immunotherapy (Thomas et al. 2023).

9.6 IMPACT OF THE CAFETERIA DIET ON MICROBIOTA, ENS FUNCTION, AND GASTROINTESTINAL PHYSIOLOGY

Obesity represents one of the most pressing global health challenges, and the widespread consumption of highly processed, energy-dense "junk" foods is a major contributing factor. These foods—characterized by their high palatability, rich fat, and sugar content, and appealing sensory qualities—promote overeating and rapid weight gain. To study the biological consequences of such diets, researchers often rely on animal models. Among these, the cafeteria (CAF) diet has gained significant attention for its ability to closely replicate human dietary habits.

Unlike conventional high-fat or high-sugar diets used in laboratory settings, the CAF diet incorporates the same attractive yet nutritionally poor foods commonly consumed by people, such as hot dogs, cookies, pastries, chips, and muffins. Importantly, it accounts not only for macronutrient composition but also for the variety, novelty, and sensory properties—smell, taste, and texture—that drive human food choice and overconsumption. This diverse assortment of highly palatable items mirrors the modern food environment, where constant dietary choices encourage snacking and hedonic eating.

Because the CAF diet captures both the physiological and behavioral aspects of human food intake, it serves as a superior model for studying obesity and its related complications. Animals on CAF diets display eating patterns, metabolic disturbances, and organ-level changes that closely reflect those seen in humans, making this model particularly valuable for understanding how dietary habits contribute to obesity, gut dysfunction, and chronic disease (Lalanza and Snoeren 2021, Ramírez-Maldonado et al. 2025).

Despite its widespread use, the specific effects of CAF feeding on gut microbial composition during progressive obesity—and the subsequent consequences for the ENS and GI motility—remain incompletely understood (Ramírez-Maldonado et al. 2025).

Ramírez-Maldonado et al. (2025) studied the impact of CAF diet on rodents. CAF-fed mice exhibited a steady increase in body weight, confirming the obesogenic nature of the diet. Strikingly, colon weight decreased as early as week 2, and this reduction persisted through week 8, accompanied by visible colon shrinkage (peinosis). Although the colon weight-to-length ratio remained largely unchanged, CAF feeding had a marked negative impact on cecum weight, which declined progressively from week 2 onward. Inflammatory profiling revealed that the CAF diet induced a distinct cytokine expression signature: IL-6 rose sharply by week 2, whereas TNF-α and IL-1β became significantly elevated by week 8, indicating the development of sustained low-grade inflammation.

To evaluate how these changes influence GI neurobiology, ENS structure and function were assessed at week 8. Quantification of HuC/D neurons revealed increased neuronal density but reduced neuronal body size in CAF-fed mice, suggesting altered neurogenesis or impaired neural maturation. Electrophysiological recordings further demonstrated decreased neuronal excitability, indicating functional impairment of myenteric neurons. Consistent with these findings, ex vivo contractility assays showed that both the amplitude and frequency of spontaneous rhythmic contractions were disrupted in the ileum and colon of CAF-fed mice.

Consumption of CAF diet led to profound disruptions in gut microbial balance, demonstrating a clear pattern of diet-induced dysbiosis. To more precisely characterize these alterations, microbial communities were examined at both the phylum and genus levels across multiple time points. Overall, taxonomic profiling revealed that the gut microbiota of both control (CTRL) and CAF-fed mice were primarily dominated by the Bacteroidetes and Firmicutes phyla, followed by smaller contributions from Campilobacterota and Proteobacteria. Although the Firmicutes/Bacteroidetes (F/B) ratio remained stable between groups at week 2, CAF feeding induced a striking and progressive increase in Proteobacteria at weeks 2 and 8. Simultaneously, a noticeable decline in Campilobacterota was observed by week 8, reflecting a shift toward a dysbiotic state characterized by the expansion of inflammation-associated taxa.

At the genus level, CAF feeding produced substantial changes in microbial composition as early as week 2. Several genera widely considered hallmarks of a healthy gut ecosystem—including *Prevotellaceae* UCG-001, *Lactobacillus*, and *Akkermansia*—were markedly reduced at week 2 and/or week 8. These taxa are known for roles in mucin regulation, short-chain fatty acid production, and overall gut barrier integrity, highlighting the negative functional implications of their depletion. In contrast, genera such as *Bacteroides* showed a gradual, diet-induced increase over time, whereas *Ruminococcus* displayed an early peak at week 2 without further change by week 8. Together, these patterns indicate that a CAF diet not only alters the microbial structure but also favors the expansion of bacteria more commonly associated with metabolic disease and intestinal inflammation.

To further pinpoint the microbial taxa driving differences between CTRL and CAF-fed mice, LEfSe analysis was conducted at weeks 2 and 8—representing early exposure and the period following obesity onset, respectively. At week 2, 17 phylotype biomarkers were enriched in the CTRL group, while 26 were characteristic of CAF-fed mice. By week 8, the imbalance intensified to 13 CTRL-associated biomarkers versus 38 CAF-associated biomarkers, demonstrating progressive divergence in microbial structure. Early CAF-related biomarkers included multiple members of the Proteobacteria phylum and Clostridia class. Several genera enriched at week 2 in CAF-fed mice included the *Lachnospiraceae* NK4A136 group, *Parabacteroides*, *Christensenellaceae*, *Eubacterium* groups, *Butyricimonas*, and *Gordonibacter*. In contrast, genera significantly depleted included *Prevotellaceae* UCG_001, *Muribaculum*, *Blautia*, *Dubosiella*, *Akkermansia*, and *Rikenella*, reflecting a broad loss of beneficial commensals.

By week 8, the microbiota of CAF-fed mice exhibited a dysbiotic pattern distinct from that seen at week 2. Notably, the Bacilli class showed a significant decline, while the Actinobacteriota phylum—including the Coriobacteriia class—increased substantially. At the genus level, biomarkers associated with CAF-induced obesity included *Bacteroides*, *Eubacterium coprostanoligenes* group, *Parabacteroides*, *Christensenellaceae* R7 group, *Ureoplasma*, *Anaerovorax*, *Odoribacter*, *Negativacillus*, *Butyricimonas*, and *Tuzzerella*. Meanwhile, several beneficial or metabolically important genera decreased, such as *Lactobacillus*, *Prevotellaceae* UCG_001, *Paraprevotella*, Lachnospiraceae UCG_001, *Candidatus Stoquefichus*, and *Acetatifactor muris*. These changes reflect a gut microbial ecosystem increasingly dominated by taxa associated with metabolic dysfunction, inflammation, and impaired gut barrier function (Ramírez-Maldonado et al. 2025).

Collectively, the study provides the first comprehensive demonstration that the CAF diet not only reshapes the gut microbiota over time but also triggers low-grade inflammatory responses that disrupt ENS physiology and GI function. These findings highlight the profound and multifactorial impact of diet composition on gut health and underscore the value of the CAF model for investigating diet-induced disorders of metabolism, immunity, and neurogastroenterology.

9.7 MECHANISM OF PEINOSIS

Peinosis refers to a diet-induced pathological state in which intestinal homeostasis progressively deteriorates due to chronic exposure to harmful nutritional patterns. In the context of HFHP diet, peinosis emerges from the combined effects of microbial dysbiosis, impaired epithelial regeneration, heightened inflammation, and altered cell-survival signaling. These interconnected processes gradually reshape the intestinal microenvironment, setting the stage for long-term GI disease.

A sustained HFHP diet profoundly disrupts the gut microbiome by reducing microbial diversity and enriching pro-inflammatory taxa. This dysbiosis triggers elevated production of colonic inflammatory cytokines, which in turn weaken epithelial barrier integrity. At the same time, stem cell–mediated epithelial renewal is suppressed, depriving the intestine of its natural repair capacity. The HFHP diet also accelerates epithelial apoptosis while simultaneously upregulating survivin, an anti-apoptotic protein associated with tumorigenesis. This paradoxical combination—excessive cell death alongside aberrant survivin expression—creates instability within the mucosal lining and fosters a microenvironment conducive to the initiation of IBD and the early stages of colorectal cancer development.

In contrast, transitioning from an HFHP diet to a fiber-rich diet activates the reversal phase of peinosis. Dietary fiber enriches beneficial microbiota, restores fermentation-derived metabolites such as short-chain fatty acids, and promotes normalization of the metabolome. These changes stimulate intestinal stem cell proliferation, enhance epithelial repair, and reduce apoptosis. Inflammatory cytokine levels fall, barrier function improves, and survivin expression declines toward physiological levels. Remarkably, this restorative cascade stabilizes the gut microbiome and reverses measurable tissue damage within roughly 30 days, demonstrating the intestine's exceptional regenerative capacity.

Overall, the mechanism of peinosis highlights the gut as a highly diet-responsive organ system. It underscores how harmful diets can drive a pathological state through intertwined microbial, inflammatory, and epithelial shifts—and how dietary fiber acts as a potent modulator capable of re-establishing intestinal health. These findings emphasize the preventive power of fiber-rich diets in reducing the risk of diet-induced intestinal diseases, including IBD and colorectal cancer (Thomas 2025).

9.8 CONCLUSION

An HFHP and CAF diet profoundly disrupts gut physiology, neuromuscular function, and intestinal barrier integrity. It leads to excessive weight gain, smaller fecal output, shorter colons, and reduced tight junction protein expression. Switching to a fiber-rich diet can reverse many of these adverse effects, restoring gut structure and function. Overall, diet composition is a key determinant of health, highlighting the risks of HFHP and CAF diets and the benefits of fiber for gut and systemic physiology.

ACKNOWLEDGMENTS

The author acknowledges Wawa Foundation, Sharpe-Strumia Research Foundation and W. W. Smith Charitable Trust for providing the resources for this work.

REFERENCES

Lalanza JF, Snoeren EMS. The cafeteria diet: A standardized protocol and its effects on behavior. *Neurosci Biobehav Rev*. 2021; 122:92–119.

Ramírez-Maldonado LM, Guerrero-Castro J, Rodríguez-Mejía JL, Cárdenas-Conejo Y, Bonales-Alatorre EO, Valencia-Cruz G, Anguiano-García PT, Vega-Juárez II, Dagnino-Acosta A, Ruvalcaba-Galindo J, Valdez-Morales EE, Ochoa-Cortes F, Barajas-Espinosa A, Guerrero-Alba R, Liñán-Rico A. Obesogenic cafeteria diet induces dynamic changes in gut microbiota, reduces myenteric neuron excitability, and impairs gut contraction in mice. *Am J Physiol Gastrointest Liver Physiol*. 2025; 328(1):G32–G48.

Thomas S. Molecular mechanisms driving peinosis of the colon in obesity. *Research Square* 2025. https://doi.org/10.21203/rs.3.rs-7401315/v1

Thomas S, Dilbarov N, Kelly J, Mercogliano G, Prendergast GC. Diet effects on colonic health influence the efficacy of Bin1 mAb immunotherapy for ulcerative colitis. *Sci Rep*. 2023; 13(1):11802.

Thomas S, Izard J, Walsh E, Batich K, Chongsathidkiet P, Clarke G, Sela DA, Muller AJ, Mullin JM, Albert K, Gilligan JP, DiGuilio K, Dilbarova R, Alexander W, Prendergast GC. The host microbiome regulates and maintains human health: A primer and perspective for non-microbiologists. *Cancer Res*. 2017; 77(8):1783–1812.

INDEX

For Product Safety Concerns and Information please contact our EU
representative GPSR@taylorandfrancis.com
Taylor & Francis Verlag GmbH, Kaufingerstraße 24, 80331 München, Germany

www.ingramcontent.com/pod-product-compliance
Lightning Source LLC
LaVergne TN
LVHW062240200926
848484LV00006B/1576

9781041069874